MELANOMA

CURRENT CLINICAL ONCOLOGY

Maurie Markman, MD, SERIES EDITOR

Melanoma: *Biologically Targeted Therapeutics,* edited by *ERNEST C. BORDEN,* 2002

Breast Cancer: *A Guide to Detection and Multidisciplinary Therapy,* edited by *MICHAEL H. TOROSIAN*, 2002

Colorectal Cancer: *Multimodality Management,* edited by *LEONARD B. SALTZ,* 2002

Chronic Leukemias and Lymphomas: *Clinical Management,* edited by *GARY J. SCHILLER,* 2003

Cancer of the Lung: *From Molecular Biology to Treatment Guidelines,* edited by *ALAN B. WEITBERG,* 2002

Renal Cell Carcinoma: *Molecular Biology, Immunology, and Clinical Management,* edited by *RONALD M. BUKOWSKI AND ANDREW NOVICK,* 2000

Current Controversies in Bone Marrow Transplantation, edited by *BRIAN J. BOLWELL,* 2000

Regional Chemotherapy: *Clinical Research and Practice,* edited by *MAURIE MARKMAN,* 2000

Intraoperative Irradiation: *Techniques and Results,* edited by *L. L. GUNDERSON, C. G. WILLETT, L. B. HARRISON, AND F. A. CALVO,* 1999

MELANOMA

BIOLOGICALLY TARGETED THERAPEUTICS

Edited by

ERNEST C. BORDEN, MD

Center for Cancer Drug Discovery and Development
Taussig Cancer Center
The Cleveland Clinic Foundation
Cleveland, OH

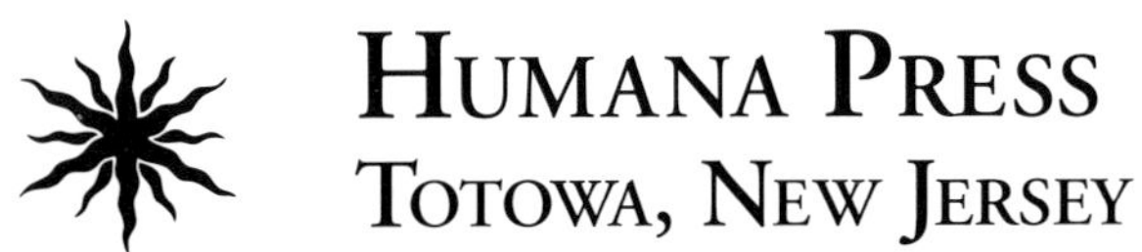
HUMANA PRESS
TOTOWA, NEW JERSEY

999 Riverview Drive, Suite 208
Totowa, New Jersey 07512

www.humanapress.com

This publication is printed on acid-free paper. ∞

ANSI Z39.48-1984 (American National Standards Institute) Permanence of Paper for Printed Library Materials.

Cover design by Patricia F. Cleary.

Cover illustration: Tumor infiltrating lymphocytes surround individual tumor cells as well as small groups of cells (intermediate magnification). *See* discussion and Fig. 11 on pp. 50–51 in Chapter 2 and Color Plate 15, following p. 176.

For additional copies, pricing for bulk purchases, and/or information about other Humana titles, contact Humana at the above address or at any of the following numbers: Tel: 973-256-1699; Fax: 973-256-8341; E-mail: humana@humanapr.com or visit our website at http://humanapress.com

Printed in the United States of America. 10 9 8 7 6 5 4 3 2 1

Library of Congress Cataloging-in-Publication Data

Melanoma : biologically targeted therapeutics / edited by Ernest C. Borden
p. ; cm. -- (Current clinical oncology)
Includes bibliographical references and index.
ISBN 0-89603-876-9 (alk. paper)
1. Melanoma--Immunotherapy. 2. Biological products--Therapeutic use. 3. Proteins--Therapeutic use. I. Borden, Ernest. II. Current clinical oncology (Totowa, N.J.)
[DNLM: 1. Melanoma--therapy. 2. Biological Therapy. 3. Gene Therapy. QZ 200 M51785 2002]
RC280.M37 M446 2002
616.99'47706--dc21

2001039468

INTRODUCTION

Strategies of treatment involving therapeutic proteins, immune cells, or cellular protein targets are those of greatest potential for further reducing mortality from melanoma. Therapeutic proteins or cells may inhibit melanoma cell growth either by augmentation of immune cell function or by inhibition of angiogenesis. Cytokines and melanoma antigens may be used either in vivo as a vaccine to stimulate immune cell function or ex vivo to stimulate or proliferate cells for infusion. Alternatively, alteration in melanoma cell growth can occur through inhibition of protein signal transduction pathways within melanoma cells or in the endothelial cells constituting the necessary angiogenic support for tumor growth. The great promise of these therapies and their cellular targets constitutes the basis for *Melanoma: Biologically Targeted Therapeutics.*

THE CLINICAL PROBLEM

More than four million people will be diagnosed with melanoma in the first decade of the 21st century. Half of those who will die will be individuals who would otherwise have had a life expectancy of another 25 years or more. These individuals will die of systemic metastases, which are present at the time of primary surgery. Despite use of sunscreens, incidence continues to increase in developed countries worldwide. To reduce mortality, there must continue to be a focus on prevention and earlier detection through public education. Early interventions are always preferable to treatment of disseminated metastatic disease. Too frequently, patients at highest risk—those with a prior melanoma and/or a family history—are not counseled by their healthcare providers regarding sun exposure and skin protection. Cure is directly related to the microscopic thickness of the primary lesion. Thus, for early detection and excision of thin lesions, public and professional education should continue to be emphasized. The many excellent public and professional education materials, illustrated with clear color photographs, available through the American Cancer Society, the U.S. National Cancer Institute, other national health agencies, and dermatologic organizations should be more widely used.

Once melanoma is detected, precise staging and appropriate surgery are essential (Chapters 2 and 3). Surgery remains essentially the only curative treatment at this time. The surgical research community has contributed very substantially over the past two decades to reducing both morbidity and mortality, once melanoma is diagnosed *(1–3)*. Initial diagnosis remains excisional biopsy. Adequate (1–2 cm) free margins must be established by re-excision. Effectiveness of limited, potentially curative excision has been established over the past two decades by large international multi-institutional studies *(4–5)*. This has reduced morbidity associated with the wider, deeper excisions of 25 or more years previous. Unless the primary is <1–1.5 mm in thickness when measured by the surgical pathologist, re-excision should include sentinel node biopsy.

Prognostic factors are increasingly able to discriminate those patients at highest risk for recurrent disease (Chapters 2 and 3). Lesion microscopic thickness remains the strongest predictor of outcome (Chapter 2). However, pathologic loss of epidermal continuity (ulceration) and nodal involvement are other critical elements in identifying those patients at highest risk of recurrence. Precise staging by sentinel node biopsy can determine which patients may have residual nodal disease demanding regional node dissection and systemic adjuvant therapies and which patients will not. Nodal involvement is being defined with greater accuracy by sentinel node lymphoscintigraphy *(6)*, which is a surgical innovation of substantial value in primary staging. Since regional nodes are key prognostic factors for survival, the pathologic assessment of the first lymph node draining the site of primary melanoma (sentinel lymph node) is proving to be an important prognostic factor for the prediction of the presence of melanoma in the lymphatic basin. Lymphoscintigraphy, with vital dye blue injection and radiolymphoscintigraphy, showed that a negative sentinel lymph node biopsy virtually eliminates the presence of lymphatic metastases when multiple histologic sections of the sentinel node are examined *(6,7)*.

BIOLOGICAL AND TARGETED THERAPIES

Interest in stimulating host immune response for therapy of melanoma dates back to observations with the nonspecific immunostimulant, Bacillus Calmette-Guerin (BCG). When injected intralesionally into cutaneous metastatic melanoma nodules, tumor regression resulted in injected nodules, and sometimes in uninjected metastases *(8)*. This clinical approach was well-grounded in animal studies, which had demonstrated antitumor effects and augmentation of T cell and particularly macrophage function *(9)*. Other studies began to identify immunologic factors involved in response to murine melanomas *(10)*. Subsequent clinical studies identified only rare effects of BCG on visceral metastases and no effects on preventing recurrence after primary resection in melanoma patients *(11)*. Large clinical studies in other tumors, except local bladder carcinomas, also failed to show clinical effectiveness *(12–13)*. When coupled with difficulties in defining the most potent strains and key chemically defined constituents, interest in BCG as immunotherapy for melanoma waned. However, when coupled with knowledge that melanoma metastases could occasionally spontaneously regress for sometimes months or years, suggesting a host response to tumor *(14)*, these initial studies provided a basis that continues to result in the definition of immunologic response to melanoma.

Essentially concomitant with studies of BCG, a T cell response to melanoma was demonstrated *(15)*. Melanoma-associated antigens began to be defined and led to melanoma being among the first tumors to which monoclonal antibodies were produced *(16–17)*. Studies with interferons (IFNs) and interleukin (IL)-2 demonstrated regressions of metastatic disease *(18–19)*. This substantial progress over the past 20 years has led to a focus on biological and targeted therapies for melanoma, which are the topics of the chapters which follow.

The focus of *Melanoma: Biologically Targeted Therapeutics* is to provide the rationale and background for translating the many promising biological and targeted therapies into new clinical trials and effective therapies. To furnish a framework for the clinical biology of the disease, the first three chapters cover primary identification and management, pathology, and clinical staging. Because outcome from the primary melanoma is, in part, determined by immune and vascular systems of the host, two chapters provide the context from which to better understand specific interventions. This is followed by individual chapters on cytokines, cellular therapies, monoclonal antibodies, targeted inhibitors, and angiogenesis.

IFNs remain the most active adjuvant therapy for melanoma for patients staged as at highest risk for recurrence (Chapters 3 and 9). Additional clinical studies will be required to clarify the role and optimal timing of intervention with IFN in the adjuvant setting. However, one of the most exciting potential areas for adjuvant therapy is the use of vaccines aimed at stimulating T-cell response (Chapters 4–6). Vaccines may also eventually be of benefit for patients with identified sporadic or familial gene mutations. IFN-α2 may additively or synergistically, through for example increase in dendritic cell function, potentiate melanoma antigen recognition or the effect of melanoma vaccine. IL-2, either alone or in combination with other autokines or adoptive cellular therapies, may provide potential to harness the antitumor effectiveness and specificity of T cells (Chapters 4, 5, 7, and 8). Clinical studies of therapies targeted at abnormal melanoma cell proliferative signaling and angiogenesis inhibitors are just beginning (Chapters 11, 12, and 13). The first part of the 21st century should see the beginnings of an understanding of how to effectively utilize IFNs, vaccines, and targeted therapies for melanoma, brought together to increase cure and almost eliminate recurrence. Improvements in outcome for patients with metastatic disease, and probably primary disease, will come through a combination of biological and chemotherapies, an era that has just begun (Chapter 10).

FUTURE

This field is rapidly moving and evolving. New cytokines are being discovered that influence dendritic natural killer (NK) and T-cell function (Chapter 4). These include IL-12, IL-15, IL-18, IL-22, and IL-23 *(20–25)*. Clinical activity of adoptive cellular therapies has been suggested by recent studies in renal carcinoma *(26–27)*. Many groups are beginning to plan and initiate dendritic cell trials

Table 1
Reduction in Melanoma Mortality and Morbidity

- Prevention
- Early detection
- Refine prognostic factors
- New systemic therapies
- Cure

in melanoma *(28–32)*. Cellular allogeneic stem cell transplants after immunosuppression and minimal recipient marrow eradication attempt to harness the graft vs tumor reaction to therapeutic advantage; although to date, this has proven less effective in melanoma than in renal carcinoma, further trials are sure to follow. An allogeneic cellular extract vaccine has been demonstrated in a randomized trial to reduce risk of recurrence from primary disease *(33)*. Angiogenesis may be affected by high constitutive levels of the transcription factor, nuclear factor (NF)κB, and high levels of IL-8 in melanoma *(34)*; both would be potential new targets for anti-angiogenesis therapies. Many of these advances have occurred even since these chapters were written.

Attention to prevention in high risk individuals, more precise staging of primary disease, and the use of biological, cellular and targeted therapies will further reduce mortality from primary melanomas in the first quarter of the 21st century (Table 1). It is the hope of the authors that the approaches and strategies discussed herein will result in an overall reduction in melanoma mortality to less than 5% by the year 2030.

REFERENCES

1. Reintgen D, Balch CM, Kirkwood J, Ross M. Recent advances in the care of the patient with malignant melanoma. *Ann Surg* 1997; 225: 1–14.
2. Mansfield PF, Lee JE, Balch CM. Cutaneous melanoma: current practice and surgical controversies. *Curr Probl Surg* 1994; 31: 253–374.
3. Borden EC, Smith TJ. Melanoma: Adjuvant therapy with interferons. American Society of Clinical Oncology Educational Book, Spring 1999; 120–125.
4. Veronesi U, Cascinelli N. Narrow excision (1-cm margin). A safe procedure for thin cutaneous melanoma. *Arch Surg* 1991; 126: 438–441.
5. Balch CM, Urist MM, Karakousis CP, et al. Efficacy of 2-cm surgical margins for intermediate-thickness melanomas (1 to 4 mm): results of a multi-institutional randomized surgical trial. *Ann Surg* 1993; 218: 262–269.
6. Ross MI, Reintgen D, Balch CM. Selective lymphadenectomy: emerging role for lymphatic mapping and sentinel node biopsy in the management of early stage melanoma. *Semin Surg Oncol* 1993; 9: 219–223.
7. McMasters KM, Reintgen DS, Ross MI, et al. Sentinel lymph node biopsy for melanoma: controversy despite widespread agreement. *J Clin Oncol* 2001; 19: 2851–2855.

8. Morton DL, Eilber FR, Malmgren RA, Wood WC. Immunological factors which influence response to immunotherapy in malignant melanoma. *Surgery* 1970; 68: 158–164.
9. Hersh EM, Gutterman JU, Mavligit GM. BCG as adjuvant immunotherapy for neoplasia. *Ann Rev Med* 1977; 28: 489–515.
10. Kripke ML. Antigenicity of murine skin tumors induced by ultraviolet light. *J Natl Cancer Inst* 1974; 53: 1333–1336.
11. Veronesi U, Adamus J, Aubert C, et al. A randomized trial of adjuvant chemotherapy and immunotherapy in cutaneous melanoma. *N Eng J Med* 1982; 307: 913–916.
12. Morton DL. Active immunotherapy against cancer: present status. *Semin Oncol* 1986; 13: 180–185.
13. Borden EC, Hawkins MJ. Biologic response modifiers as adjuncts to other therapeutic modalities. *Semin Oncol* 1986; 13: 144–152.
14. Cole WH. Efforts to explain spontaneous regression of cancer. *J Surg Oncol* 1981; 17: 201–209.
15. Golub SH, Morton DL. Sensitisation of lymphocytes in vitro against human melanoma-associated antigens. *Nature* 1974; 251: 161–163.
16. Shiku H, Takahashi T, Oettgen HF. Cell surface antigens of human malignant melanoma. II. Serological typing with immune adherence assays and definition of two new surface antigens. *J Exp Med* 1976; 144: 873–881.
17. Dippold WG, Lloyd KO, Li LT, Ikeda H, Oettgen HF, Old LJ. Cell surface antigens of human malignant melanoma: definition of six antigenic systems with mouse monoclonal antibodies. *Proc Natl Acad Sci USA* 1980; 77; 6114–6118.
18. Krown SE, Burk MW, Kirkwood JM, Kerr D, Morton DL, Oettgen HF. Human leukocyte (alpha) interferon in metastatic malignant melanoma: the American Cancer Society phase II trial. *Cancer Treat Rep* 1984; 68: 723–726.
19. Rosenberg SA, Mule JJ, Spiess PJ, Reichert CM, Schwarz SL. Regression of established pulmonary metastases and subcutaneous tumor mediated by the systemic administration of high-dose recombinant interleukin 2. *J Exp Med* 1985; 161: 1169–1188.
20. Tanaka F, Hashimoto W, Okamura H, Robbins PD, Lotze MT, Tahara H. Rapid generation of potent and tumor-specific cytotoxic T lymphocytes by interleukin 18 using dendritic cells and natural killer cells. *Cancer Res* 2000; 60: 4838–4844.
21. Vidal-Vanaclocha F, Fantuzzi G, Mendoza L, et al. IL-18 regulates IL-beta-dependent hepatic melanoma metastasis via vascular cell adhesion molecule-1. *Proc Natl Acad Sci USA* 2000; 97: 734–739.
22. Xie MH, Aggarwal S, Ho WH, et al. Interleukin (IL)-22, a novel human cytokine that signals through the interferon receptor-related proteins CRF2-4 and IL-22R. *J Biol Chem* 2000; 275: 31,335–31,339.
23. Kotenko SV, Izotova LS, Mirochnitchenko OV, et al. Identification of the functional IL-TIF (IL-22) receptor complex: the IL-10R chain (IL-10R{beta}) is a shared component of both IL-10 and IL-TIF (IL-22) receptor complexes. *J Biol Chem* 2000; 276:2725–2732.
24. Oppmann B, Lesley R, Blom B, et al. Novel p19 protein engages IL-12p40 to form a cytokine, IL-23, with biological activities similar as well as distinct from IL-12. *Immunity* 2000; 13: 715–725.
25. Cooper MA, Fehniger TA, Turner SC, et al. Human natural killer cells: a unique innate immunoregulatory role for the CD56 (bright) subset. *Blood* 2001; 97: 3146–3151.
26. Childs RW, Clave E, Tisdale J, Plante M, Hensel N, Barrett J. Successful treatment of metastatic renal cell carcinoma with a nonmyeloablative allogeneic peripheral-blood progenitor-cell transplant: evidence for a graft-versus-tumor effect. *J Clin Oncol* 1999; 17: 2044–2049.
27. Kugler A, Stuhler G, Walden P, et al. Regression of human metastatic renal cell carcinoma after vaccination with tumor cell-dendritic cell hybrids. *Nat Med* 2000; 6: 332–336.

28. Schuler-Thurner B, Dieckmann D, Keikavoussi P, et al. Mage-3 and influenza-matrix peptide-specific cytotoxic T cells are inducible in terminal stage HLA-A2.1+ melanoma patients by mature monocyte-derived dendritic cells. *J Immunol* 2000; 165: 3492–3496.
29. Mackensen A, Herbst B, Chen JL, et al. Phase I study in melanoma patients of a vaccine with peptide-pulsed dendritic cells generated in vitro from CD34 (+) hematopoietic progenitor cells. *Int J Cancer* 2000; 86: 385–392.
30. Thurner B, Haendle I, Roder C, et al. Vaccination with mage-3A1 peptide-pulsed mature, monocyte-derived dendritic cells expands specific cytotoxic T cells and induces regression of some metastases in advanced stage IV melanoma. *J Exp Med* 1999; 190: 1669–1678.
31. Lotze MT, Hellerstedt B, Stolinski L, et al. The role of interleukin-2, interleukin-12, and dendritic cells in cancer therapy. *Cancer J Sci Am* 1997; 3: S109–114.
32. Baggers J, Ratzinger G, Young JW. Dendritic cells as immunologic adjuvants for the treatment of cancer. *J Clin Oncol* 2000; 18: 3879–3882.
33. Sosman JA, Unger JM, Liu P, et al. Significant impact of HLA Class I alleles on outcome in T3NO melanoma patients treated with melacine (MEL), an allogeneic melanoma cell lysate vaccine: prospective analysis of Southwest Onoclogy Group (SWOG)–9035. Proc Am Soc Clin Oncol 2001;20:351a.
34. Huang S, DeGuzman A, Bucana CD, Fidler IJ. Nuclear Factor-kB activity correlates with growth, angiogenesis, and metastasis of human melanoma cells in nude mice. *Clin Cancer Res* 2000; 6: 2573–2581.

Contents

Contributors

BELA ANAND-APTE, MBBS, PhD, *Cole Eye Institute, Department of Ophthalmic Research, The Cleveland Clinic Foundation, Cleveland, OH*

MICHAEL B. ATKINS, MD, *Director of Cutaneous Oncology and Biologic Therapy Programs, Division of Hematology/Oncology, Beth Israel Deaconess Medical Center; Associate Professor of Medicine, Harvard Medical School, Boston, MA*

PHILIP L. BAILIN, MD, FACP, *Department of Dermatology, The Cleveland Clinic Foundation, Cleveland, OH*

ERNEST C. BORDEN, MD, *Director, Center for Cancer Drug Discovery and Development, Taussig Cancer Center, The Cleveland Clinic Foundation, Cleveland, OH*

RONALD M. BUKOWSKI, MD, *Experimental Therapeutics Program, Taussig Cancer Center, The Cleveland Clinic, Cleveland, OH*

PAUL B. CHAPMAN, MD, *Clinical Immunology Service, Department of Medicine, Memorial Sloan-Kettering Cancer Center and Cornell University Joan and Sanford I. Weill Medical College, New York, NY*

PETER A. COHEN, MD, *Center for Surgery Research, The Cleveland Clinic Foundation, Cleveland, OH*

HAMED DAW, MD, *Moll Cancer Center, The Cleveland Clinic Foundation, Cleveland, OH*

JAMES H. FINKE, PhD, *Department of Immunology, The Cleveland Clinic Foundation, Cleveland, OH*

LAWRENCE E. FLAHERTY, MD, *Barbara Ann Karmanos Cancer Institute, Division of Hematology and Oncology, Wayne State University School of Medicine, Detroit, MI*

PAUL L. FOX, PhD, *Lerner Research Institute, Department of Cell Biology, The Cleveland Clinic Foundation, Cleveland, OH*

RUTH HALABAN, PhD, *Department of Dermatology, Yale University School of Medicine, New Haven, CT*

STANLEY P. L. LEONG, MD, *Professor of Surgery, University of California, San Francisco, School of Medicine; Member, UCSF Comprehensive Cancer Center, San Francisco, CA*

JON S. MEINE, MD, *Surgical Dermatology, The Cleveland Clinic Foundation, Cleveland, OH*

JAMES W. MIER, MD, *Director of Cancer Immunotherapy Laboratory, Division of Hematology/Oncology, Beth Israel Deaconess Medical Center; Associate Professor of Medicine, Harvard Medical School, Boston, MA*

Thomas Olencki, do, *Taussig Cancer Center, The Cleveland Clinic Foundation, Cleveland, OH*

Vann P. Parker, PhD, *Clinical Development, Ribozyme Pharmaceuticals, Inc., Boulder, CO*

Philip Agop Philip, MD, PhD, MRCP, *Barbara Ann Karmanos Cancer Institute, Division of Hematology and Oncology, Wayne State University, Detroit, MI*

Christine Poblete-Lopez, MD, *Surgical Dermatology, The Cleveland Clinic Foundation, Cleveland, OH*

Suyu Shu, PhD, *Director, Center for Surgical Research, Division of Surgery, The Cleveland Clinic Foundation, Cleveland, OH*

Charles Tannenbaum, PhD, *Lerner Research Institute, Department of Immunology, The Cleveland Clinic, Cleveland, OH*

Ralph J. Tuthill, MD, *Anatomic Pathology, The Cleveland Clinic Foundation, Cleveland, OH*

Maria C. von Willebrand, MD, PhD, *Department of Dermatology, Yale University School of Medicine, New Haven, CT*

Jedd D. Wolchok, MD, PhD, *Clinical Immunology Service, Department of Medicine, Memorial Sloan-Kettering Cancer Center and Cornell University Joan and Sanford I. Weill Medical College, New York, NY*

Color Plates

Color Plates follow p. 176.

Color Plate 15. Tumor infiltrating lymphocytes (*Fig. 11, Chapter 2*; *see* full caption and discussion on pp. 50–51).

Color Plate 16. Immune-reactive stroma (incomplete regression) (*Fig. 12, Chapter 2*; *see* discussion on p. 53).

Color Plate 17. Micrometastasis in a sentinel lymph node. H&E stain shows a small group of atypical cells of uncertain nature **(A)**. Immunostaining with antibodies to Melan-A (Mart-1) supports the interpretation of micrometastasis of malignant melanoma **(B)**. (*Figs. 13 A,B, Chapter 2*; *see* discussion p. 60–63.)

Color Plate 18. Putative mechanism by which tumor cells can induce immune dysfunction in T cells and dendritic cells. Tumor cells can produce a variety of immunosuppressive products that include IL-10, gangliosides, TGFβ, and PGs. These products can affect T cell signaling and can suppress activation of transcription factors such as NFκB. Blocking NFκB may also reduce expression of certain anti-apoptotic genes that would render T cells more sensitive to apoptosis. IL-10 can also inhibit the Ag-presenting function of DCs. Moreover, some tumors express Fas ligand (Fas-L) that can induce apoptosis in T cells that express Fas receptor. At the same time, some tumor cells that express Fas receptor may themselves be resistant to apoptosis induced by Fas-L expression on the activated T cells. Such resistance, in some cases, appears related to the tumor cells' reduced expression of molecules such as caspase that are essential for activation of apoptotic pathways. (*Fig. 5, Chapter 4*; *see* discussion on p. 122.)

I Perspective on the Clinical Disease

1 Management of Primary Malignant Melanoma

Philip L. Bailin, MD, FACP,
Jon S. Meine, MD,
and Christine Poblete-Lopez, MD

Contents

1. INTRODUCTION

Cutaneous malignant melanoma is widely recognized to be multifactorial in its etiology and development *(1)*. There appears to be an increasingly recognized and documented set of causative environmental factors that may be superimposed upon underlying personal genetic substrate factors. Such combinations lead to a predisposition for developing malignant melanoma.

2. RISK FACTORS AND PRECURSOR LESIONS

Phenotypic traits associated with malignant melanoma are numerous *(2)*. Among those commonly recognized are: fair complexion *(3)*, blue eyes *(4)*, blond or red hair *(5–7)*, inability to tan *(8)*, tendency to freckle *(9)*, and tendency to develop sunburns *(10,11)*.

From: *Current Clinical Oncology, Melanoma: Biologically Targeted Therapeutics*
Edited by: E. C. Borden © Humana Press Inc., Totowa, NJ

The most frequently implicated environmental factor thought to be acting upon these phenotypic targets is UV radiation *(12)*. The incidence of malignant melanoma varies with latitude, gradually increasing with proximity to the equator (after adjustment for skin color) *(13)*. Since the protective effect of the ozone layer decreases across latitude only for the UVB portion of the ultraviolet spectrum, while that for UVA and UVC is relatively constant, UVB is judged to be the critical etiologic factor. Such a view is supported by population migration studies *(14,15)* and by studies focusing on lifestyle changes related to increased outdoor recreation and styles of apparel providing less skin coverage *(16–20)*.

The dosing of UVB is likewise recognized to play a critical etiologic role. While chronic exposure and the total cumulative dosage of UVB received is known to be of utmost importance in carcinogenesis relating to nonmelanoma skin cancers, it is believed that intermittent heavy exposure and, particularly, such levels of exposure resulting in blistering sunburns is most relevant to development of malignant melanoma *(21)*. Individuals with the disease xeroderma pigmentosum are unable to repair UV-induced DNA damage. They have, as a result, an extremely high risk for melanoma and an earlier average age at diagnosis *(22)*.

While UVB is the apparent culprit in natural sunlight, there is evidence that UVA from artificial sources may play an etiologic role. Tanning lights emit high doses of UVA, but studies of such lights used for cosmetic purposes related to increased melanoma incidence are equivocal *(23)*. However, the medical use of UVA plus psoralen compounds (PUVA) is known to increase melanoma risk *(24)*. Immunosuppression is agreed to be a predisposing factor for increased risk of developing malignant melanoma. Suppression secondary to diseases *(25)* or organ transplantation *(26)* have both been implicated.

Most individuals develop malignant melanoma sporadically and have no family history of the disease. However, approximately 3–5% do have such a documented family history *(27)*. Most familial melanoma patients are able to be grouped into a syndrome which has been assigned a variety of names: B-K mole syndrome *(28)*, familial atypical multiple mole melanoma (FAMMM) syndrome *(29)*, dysplastic nevus syndrome *(30)*, large atypical nevus syndrome *(31)*, Clark's nevus syndrome *(32)*, familial atypical mole and melanoma syndrome *(33)*, and classic atypical mole syndrome (CAMS) *(34)*. This syndrome *(35)* (now referred to as atypical mole syndrome) is characterized by the presence of large numbers (>50) of heterogeneous nevi, which occur preferentially on the trunk, buttocks, breasts, and scalp. Clinically, these nevi are atypical, showing one or more of the features (asymmetry, border irregularity, color variegation, and diameter >6 mm) associated with malignant melanoma lesions. Histologically, they show a number of features defined by the National Institutes of Health (NIH) Consensus Conference on Diagnosis and Treatment of Early Melanoma *(36)*:

1. Architectural disorder with asymmetry.
2. Subepidermal fibroplasia (concentric eosinophilic and/or lamellar).
3. Lentiginous melanocytic hyperplasia with spindle and/or epithelioid cell nests bridging adjacent rete ridges.
4. Melanocytic atypia.
5. Dermal lymphocytic infiltration.
6. Intraepidermal melanocytes extending singly or in nests beyond the dermal component ("shoulder" phenomenon).

The relative risk of such individuals for developing a malignant melanoma varies greatly (from approximately twice the average person's risk to 1000 times average) depending mainly on the presence of a family member with melanoma and the number (1, 2, or >2) of such affected family members. Interestingly, a personal history of a preceding malignant melanoma does not confer as high a relative risk as does the positive history of a family member.

The genetics of atypical mole syndrome are not totally understood. It appears to have an autosomal dominant mode of inheritance with incomplete penetrance *(37–39)*. The affected gene was thought to be on chromosome 1 (1p36) *(40,41)*. Other investigators have postulated the genetic locus to be 9p *(42)*, 6 *(43)*, 7 *(44)*, and 10 *(45)*. In truth, it may be polygenic in nature or demonstrate heterogeneity *(46)*.

Melanocytic nevi need not be atypical to confer an increased risk for development of malignant melanoma. Outside the spectrum of familial atypical moles and/or melanoma, it is recognized that the presence of large numbers of benign moles confers increased risk *(47)*. Likewise, the presence of large nonatypical nevi apparently increases risk *(48)*.

Other external factors and personal conditions have occasionally been reported or purported to increase the risk of developing melanoma. These associations are less rigorously proven than those discussed previously. Among such potential causes of increased risk are:

1. Childhood sunburns versus adult sunburn *(49)*.
2. Chronic exposure to fluorescent lighting *(50)*.
3. Use of sunscreen products *(51)*.
4. Excess selenium intake via drinking water *(52)*.
5. Excess alcohol intake *(53,54)*.
6. Long-term use of oral contraceptives *(55–57)*.
7. Exposure to polychlorinated biphenyl compounds *(58)*.

The role of pregnancy as a risk factor for development of malignant melanoma is confusing. There is no dependable evidence to show that relative risk is increased. However, there is good evidence that melanomas appearing during pregnancy may be relatively more advanced and occur in statistically less favorable anatomic sites *(59)*.

3. CLINICAL DETECTION OF MELANOMA

The fact that cutaneous melanoma arises on a readily accessible site offers the physician and the patient a unique and challenging opportunity to diagnose and excise melanoma at an early and curable stage. Since primary tumor thickness remains the single most important prognostic indicator in this malignancy *(60)*, early diagnosis and prompt excision is critical. Despite the recognition of this importance, however, there are still several reasons why this objective is not fulfilled. Patients with suspicious lesions may delay medical assessment due to lack of knowledge, fear, or denial *(2)*. In addition, the physician's diagnostic accuracy of melanoma is not perfect, with the sensitivity of diagnosis on the order of 47 to 97% *(61)*.

The clinical diagnosis of melanoma relies on assessing a constellation of gross morphologic features, in essence, related to the overall degree of symmetry and order of a lesion. The ABCD's of melanoma (asymmetry, border irregularity, color variegation, and diameter greater than 6 mm), as well as surface topography are readily recognizable features utilized in assessing melanocytic lesions. Malignant melanomas have an initial pattern of growth, the radial growth phase, common to all types of melanoma, except nodular melanoma. In general, asymmetry, irregular borders with notching, variation and complexity of color pattern, a diameter >10 mm at time of diagnosis, and obliteration or loss of skin cleavage lines when observed with tangential or side lighting are present at this stage. Pattern of coloration is perhaps the single most important attribute for the detection of melanoma *(62)*. Varying shades of brown, as well as striking aspects of black, blue, gray, white, pink, and red coloration may be found in melanoma. In fact, the presence of red, white, and blue-black hues is particularly suggestive of the diagnosis. Changes of regression, usually corresponding to foci of white, gray, and pink may occur. Loss of pigmentation may involve the lesion and take the form of a halo or occur in distant locations, resulting in a vitiligo-like process known as melanoma-associated leukoderma. Focal black areas, especially if newly developed, are suspicious for melanoma. The most suspicious sign suggesting melanoma is a persistently changing pigmented lesion. The most frequent signs suggesting early melanoma are changes in size and color *(60)*. These should prompt immediate attention. Other findings such as elevation, itching, tenderness, and bleeding generally signify more advanced primary melanoma and, typically, occur over the course of weeks or months.

3.1. Initial Evaluation

The initial evaluation of a patient with a suspected melanoma should include a personal history, a thorough family history, and an appropriate physical examination. The skin examination should encompass the entire skin surface, including the scalp and genitalia. Palpation of regional lymph nodes should be included.

Utilizing a magnifying lens, as well as a Woods lamp, may facilitate the examination. The focus of this evaluation is to identify risk factors, atypical moles, any primary melanoma, and signs and symptoms of metastasis.

3.2. Noninvasive Clinical Techniques

The development of some noninvasive clinical techniques in the assessment of pigmented skin lesions has led to improved clinical diagnostic accuracy of melanoma. These include, to date, epiluminescence microscopy (ELM) or dermoscopy and computerized image analysis.

ELM is a noninvasive in vivo examination technique that permits the visualization of subsurface skin structures. This involves the application of a thin layer of immersion oil to the skin surface, and compression with a handheld device (dermatoscope) or lens is used to examine the pigmented skin lesion. Morphologic structures are observed using this technique that are otherwise not visible to the unaided eye. A new set of clinical terminology, histologic correlation, and diagnostic significance has been subsequently developed based on this ELM morphology for application in the assessment of pigmented lesions (*see* Table 1) *(62)*. The pigment network is one of the most recognizable and important structures to identify to facilitate accurate diagnosis when examining a pigmented skin lesion with ELM. Close examination of the pattern of pigment network allows differentiation of a benign from a malignant pigmented lesion. A benign pattern has regular delicate lines that gradually thin at the margin, and a malignant pattern has irregular, variable, and a widened pigment network that ends abruptly at the periphery *(62)*. ELM features most highly associated with melanoma include a whitish veil, blue-gray areas, radial streaming, and pseudopods. These features are seen considerably more frequently with well-developed melanomas and may be absent in early lesions *(63)*. In the hands of experienced users, ELM has been demonstrated to improve the accuracy of diagnosis of pigmented lesions *(63)*. It must be emphasized that this technique is not absolute and that the presence or absence of dermoscopic features has not been reliably shown to be 100% sensitive or specific for the diagnosis of melanoma. Hence, ELM should merely be used as an aid to the clinical diagnosis of melanoma.

Computerized digital imaging analysis is another noninvasive in vivo technique currently being investigated for the assessment, diagnosis, and monitoring of pigmented skin lesions. This involves acquiring, electronically reproducing, and storing clinical images as numbers or pixels (picture elements). In combination with ELM, digital ELM (DELM) allows for an enhanced discrimination of melanoma from other pigmented skin lesions. This uses computer image analysis programs, which provide objective measurements of changes in pigmented lesions over time, storage and rapid retrieval at extremely low operating cost, transmission of images to experts for further discussion, and extraction of morphologic features for numeric analysis *(62)*. The combination of these techniques

Table 1
Epiluminescence Features of Pigmented Lesions

Surface ELM criteria	*Histologic features*	*Diagnostic significance*
Pigment network	Pigmented rete ridges.	Melanocytic lesion.
Regular	Regular distributed rete.	Benign melanocytic lesion.
Irregular	Irregular distributed rete.	Dysplastic nevi or melanoma.
Broadened pigment network	Broad rete ridges with increased number of atypical melanocytes.	Early melanoma.
Black dots	Collections and clumps of pigmented cells in the cornified layer.	Melanoma.
Pseudopods	Junctional nests at the periphery.	Melanoma.
Radial streaming	Junctional nests arranged radially.	Melanoma, pigmented spindle cell nevus.
Brown globules	Pigmented nests in the papillary dermis and dermal–epidermal junction.	Dermal nevus (if regular). Melanoma (if irregular).
Maple leaf-like areas	Pigmented aggregates of basaloid cells.	Basal cell carcinoma
Comedo-like openings	Horn pseudocysts.	Seborrheic keratosis. Papillary dermal nevus.
Blue-gray veil	Melanoma with areas of regression.	Fibrosis, widened papillary dermis, melanophages.
Depigmentation	Areas lacking melanin in the epidermis and dermis.	Regular and central—benign.
	May be fibroplasia or regression of melanoma.	Irregular and peripheral—malignant.

Adapted from Langley RGB, Sober AJ. New techniques in the early diagnosis of melanoma. In *International Symposium on Melanogenesis and Malignant Melanoma*, Fukoka, December 5–6, 1995. Amsterdam, Elsevier/North Holland, Excerpta Medica International Congress Series 1096.

could have a useful role in assisting the diagnosis of pigmented skin lesions for a nonexpert clinician.

Recent advances in optical imaging technology include the use of a confocal scanning laser microscope in the study of pigmented lesions. The first clinical study used Nd:YAG (1064 nm) laser, which allowed in vivo visualization of cellular level structures within the epidermis and papillary dermis, including circulating erythrocytes and leukocytes in the superficial plexus *(62)*. The output is displayed on a video monitor and recorded on a videotape. It provides high resolution instantaneous and nondestructive reflectance images of the epidermis and papillary dermis *(64)*. Melanin provides strong cytoplasmic contrast *(64)*, making confocal scanning laser microscopy of particular interest in the study of pigmented lesions.

4. CLINICAL CLASSIFICATION

4.1. Four Major Subtypes

(*See* Table 2) *(62)*.

4.1.1. Lentigo Maligna Melanoma (Fig. 1; *see* Color Plate 1, ff. p. 176)

Lentigo maligna melanoma (LMM), which is the least common type of melanoma (usually 4 to 15% of all melanoma patients) *(60)*, arises from lentigo maligna, a type of melanoma in situ (also known as Hutchinson's freckle). It is almost exclusively seen on sun-exposed skin of the head and neck, with the nose and cheeks being the most common sites. A few may be found on the dorsal aspect of the hands, the lower legs, or rarely at other sites *(60)*. LMM occurs in the older age group, with a median age of diagnosis of approximately 65 yr of age. Many years (5 to 15 yr) may elapse before the tumor progresses from their precursor form, lentigo maligna (radial growth phase), to fully evolved LMM (vertical growth phase or invasion). At this point, LMM can be fatal *(65)*. After lentigo maligna reaches the vertical growth phase, however, the prognosis is the same as that associated with other types of malignant melanoma, for all of which the thickness must be taken into consideration *(66)*.

Typically, the lesion is quite large (3 to 6 cm or larger) and flat, although its nodular portion may vary from only a few millimeters to 1 to 2 cm in width. Palpability usually indicates dermal invasion, although clinical examination may be unreliable in early invasive LMM (<1 mm) *(67)*. The colors in the flat areas may include tan, brown, black, and at times, opalescent blue-gray and white. Brown areas may exhibit dark flecks in a black reticular pattern. Lesions may rarely be amelanotic *(68)*, or show signs of regression, present as blue-gray or white areas. They can have extremely convoluted borders with prominent notching and indentation. The appearance of papules, nodules, or one or more or areas of induration within the macular lesion may herald the vertical growth phase. The percentage of lentigo maligna that progresses to LMM is unknown, but estimates of the lifetime risk of developing LMM from lentigo maligna has been calculated as 4.7% at 45 yr and 2.2% at 65 yr of age *(69)*.

Table 2
Comparisons of Clinical Features of Cutaneous Melanoma

Type of melanoma	*Frequency*	*Duration before diagnosis (yr)*	*Mean age at diagnosis (yr)*	*Site*	*Clinical features*
Types with radial growth phases					
Superficial spreading melanoma	70%	1–7	Mid-40s	Any site; lower legs in females, back in both sexes.	Raised border on palpation or inspection; pinks, whites, grays, and blues in brown lesion.
Acral lentiginous melanoma (including subungual melanoma)	10%	1–10	60s	Sole, palms, mucous membranes, subungual.	Flat irregular border; predominantly dark brown to black with highly irregular border with areas of regression; brown-tan macular lesion with variation in pigment pattern; may be amelanotic.
Lentigo maligna melanoma	5%	5–50	70s	Nose, cheeks, temples.	
Type with no radial growth phase					
Nodular melanoma	15%	Months	Mid to late 40s	Any site.	Nodule arises in apparently normal skin or in a nevus; brown to brown-black; may have bluish hues; may be amelanotic.

Modified from Petersdorf RG, et al. (eds.): *Harrison's Principles of Internal Medicine, 10th ed.*, McGraw-Hill, New York, 1983, p 836.

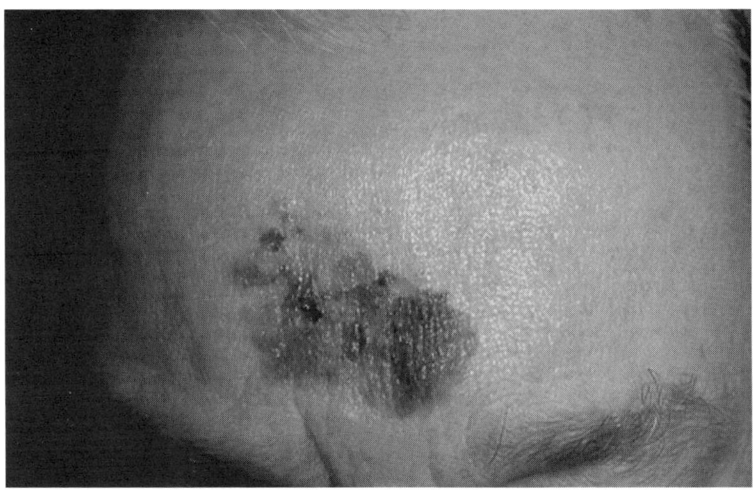

Fig. 1. Lentigo maligna melanoma.

4.1.2. Superficial Spreading Melanoma (*see* Fig. 2; Color Plate 2, ff. p. 176)

Superficial spreading melanoma (SSM) is the most common type of cutaneous melanoma (representing approximately 70% of all melanomas) *(60)*, occurring in the light-skinned population. SSM frequently arises in a preexisting melanocytic nevus or dysplastic nevus *(70,71)*. Lesions can be located on any anatomic site, although they most frequently appear on intermittently sun-exposed areas with the greatest density of nevi, such as the trunk and extremities in men and women, most commonly on the upper backs in men and on the legs of women. SSM is diagnosed most commonly in the fourth and fifth decades with a median age at diagnosis in the mid-40s. The usual history is that of a slowly evolving change of the precursor lesion over 1 to 5 yr (radial growth phase) before the vertical growth phase begins, in which a period of rapid growth may be observed months before the diagnosis.

At the time of diagnosis, SSM are smaller than lesions of LMM—approximately 2.5 cm in diameter or less. They typically present with the classic ABCD features of melanoma: an irregular lateral margin, irregular multicolored central pigmentation, and a history of growth of the lesion *(72)*. Initially, SSM appears as a deeply pigmented macule or barely raised plaque, with intact fine skin markings. In association with a preexisting nevus, it can appear as a focal, often eccentric area of darker pigmentation. As the dark areas expand, pigment variation may involve a mixture of colors ranging from dark brown to black to dark blue-gray to a pink or gray-white color. Areas of regression may present with a decrease or absence in pigmentation, which can be more readily identified with a Woods lamp (long-wave UV) as a hypopigmented area. As the lesion enlarges,

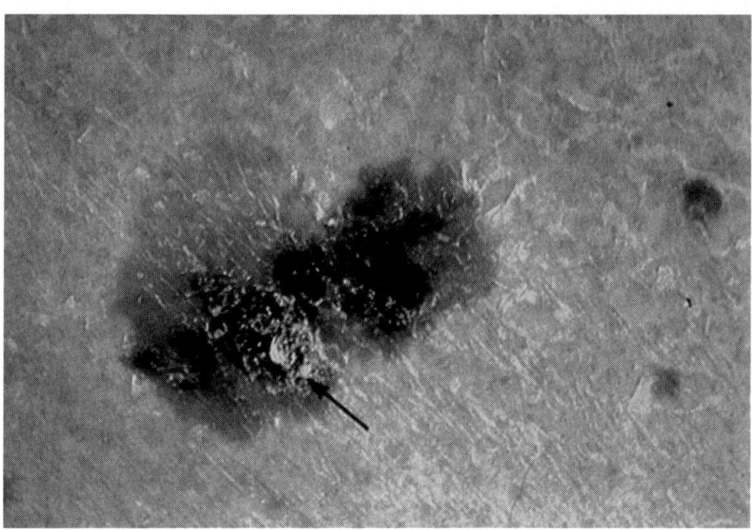

Fig. 2. Superficial spreading melanoma; the lesion demonstrates the classic clinical signs of asymmetry, border irregularity (notching), color variability (pink, brown, black, blue), and diameter (greater than 10 mm).

the surface may appear glossy, the borders may be irregular with angular indentations (notching) or scalloping, and the elevation may vary. The development of one or more nodules, or area of induration within the lesion usually heralds the vertical growth phase. The presence of these nodules does not represent conversion to nodular melanoma, but rather the fully evolved SSM, which is now in its vertical growth phase *(60)*.

4.1.3. Nodular Melanoma (Fig. 3; *see* Color Plate 3, ff. p. 176)

Nodular melanoma (NM) is the second most common type of melanoma, with a frequency of 15 to 30% of all types *(60)*. NM may arise from nevi or normal skin, but they lack an apparent radial growth phase. However, it is more common for NM to begin *de novo* in uninvolved skin than to arise in a preexisting nevus. The trunk, head, and neck are the most frequent anatomic sites for NM. It can occur at any age, but frequently arises in midlife, with a median age at onset of 53 yr *(73)*. NM is remarkable for its rapid evolution—about 16 to 18 mo on average *(62)*.

Nodular melanomas are usually 1 to 2 cm in diameter, but may be larger. They typically appear as a uniform blue-black, bluish-red, or amelanotic symmetrical papule or nodule, but can present as a polypoid lesion with a stalk. They may appear as a blueberry-shaped nodule with a thundercloud-gray appearance. NMs may be difficult to discriminate from pigmented basal cell carcinoma (BCC), pyogenic granuloma, hemangioma, hematoma, blue nevus, and eccrine

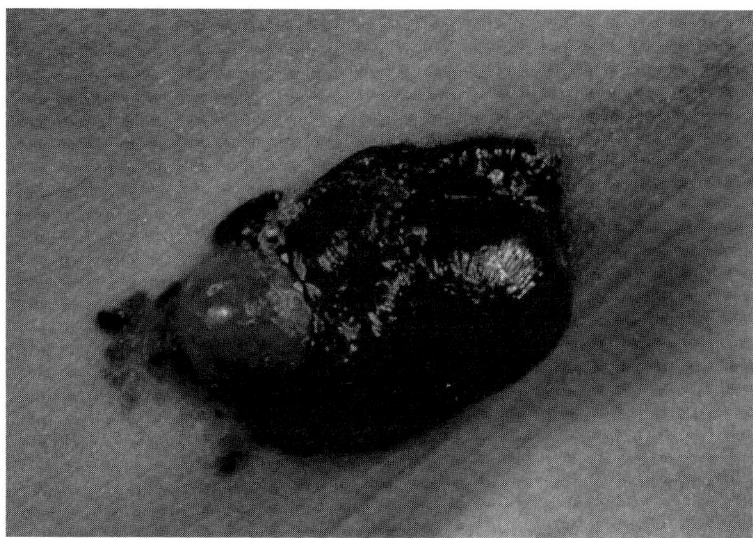

Fig. 3. Nodular melanoma.

poroma, because they lack many of the conventional clinical features of melanoma as previously outlined. Approximately 5% of nodular melanomas lack pigment altogether and have a fleshy appearance (amelanotic melanoma) *(60)*. Because NMs tend to be deep at the time of diagnosis, they often have a poor prognosis; however, the prognosis is similar to that associated with other types of melanoma of the same thickness. Polypoidal nodular melanomas, with a stalk or cauliflower appearance, are believed to behave in a particularly aggressive manner *(74)*, but this is likely the result of their substantial tumor thickness rather than their configuration *per se*.

4.1.4. Acral Lentiginous Melanoma (Fig. 4; *see* Color Plate 4, ff. p. 176)

Acral lentiginous melanoma (ALM) is relatively infrequent in light-skinned individuals (only 2 to 8% of melanomas), but represents the most common form in darker complected individuals (constitutes 60 to 72% in blacks and 29 to 46% in Asians) *(60)*. Although darker pigmented patients have a greater proportion of ALM than other types of melanoma, the site-specific incidence of melanoma is similar between ethnic groups *(75)*. ALM occurs on the palms, soles, or beneath the nail plate, with the sole being the most common site. Not all plantar or palmar melanomas are ALMs; a minority are SSMs or NMs *(62)*. ALM usually occurs in older persons, with patients being in their 60s, on average, at the time of diagnosis. It is believed that the evolution tends to be shorter than it tends to be for the case for SSM or LMM, ranging from a few months to several years, with an average of 2.5 yr. However, this supposition may be inaccurate and underes-

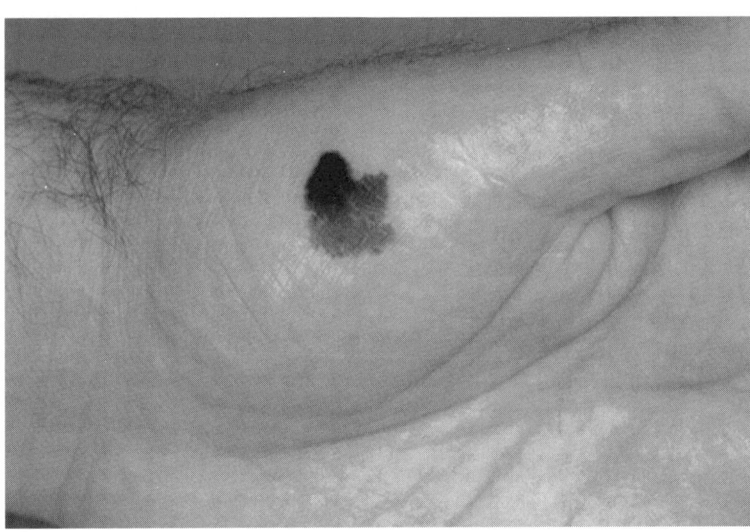

Fig. 4. Acral lentiginous melanoma.

timated, because ALM occurs at sites difficult to visualize, with an associated delay in diagnosis. ALM typically undergoes irregular horizontal spread during a radial growth phase lasting approximately 2 to 3 yr before the vertical growth phase begins.

As a result of delayed diagnosis, ALM often reach diameters of greater than 2 cm. Acquired melanocytic lesions of the sole that are 9 mm or more in diameter are likely to represent melanoma, however, especially in patients older than 50 yr of age *(76)*. Early ALM are characterized by macular lesions with variegated tan to black pigmentation and irregular and convoluted borders. Papules or nodules are often present. A few lesions have a flesh-colored appearance and can be misdiagnosed as a "corn", "wart", or pyogenic granuloma. The surface of an ALM can become hyperkeratotic. Ulceration is common in advanced lesions, and fungating masses can result from neglected lesions *(60)*. Because the diagnosis of ALM is often delayed, patients, therefore, frequently present with advanced disease and have a poor prognosis, which correlates with the increased tumor thickness *(77)*.

4.1.5. Subungual Melanoma (Fig. 5; *see* Color Plate 5, ff. p. 176)

Subungual melanoma is a rare form of cutaneous melanoma and is often classified as a variant of ALM *(60)*, although SSMs and NMs can occur at this site *(78)*. It represents 2 to 3% of melanomas in the light-skinned population, but a higher proportion in the dark-skinned population. The majority of subungual melanomas involve the great toe or the thumb. It occurs with equal frequency in men and women and is often found in older patients (median age 55 to 65 yr).

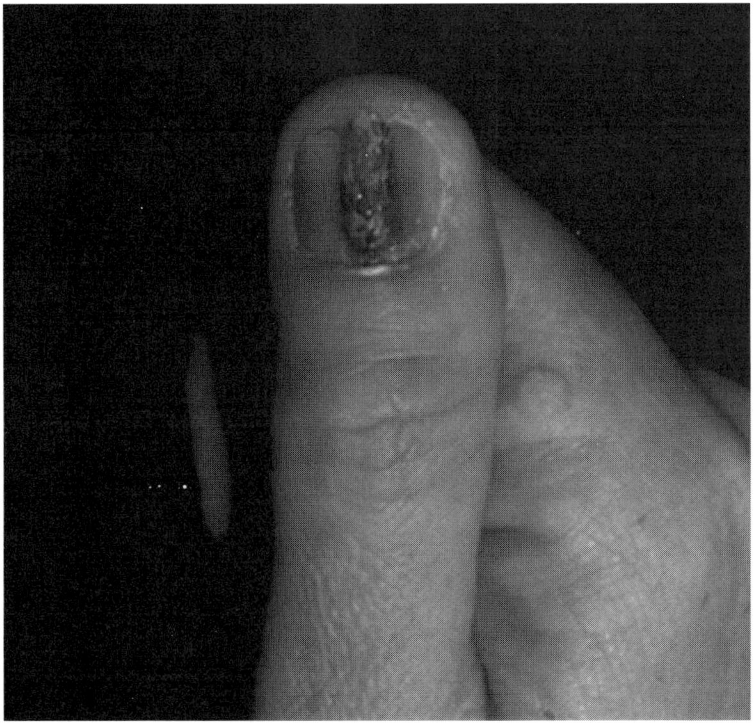

Fig. 5. Subungual melanoma.

An early subungual melanoma may be recognized as a brown to black discoloration in the nail bed, usually at a proximal location. Hutchinson's sign is the finding of pigmentation of the posterior nail fold and has been considered as an ominous finding associated with advance subungual melanoma *(62)*. Ten to fifteen percent of subungual melanomas may be nonpigmented and have a fleshy appearance. Benign lesions that can mimic subungual melanoma include subungual hematoma (most commonly), longitudinal melanonychia, onychomycosis, paronychia, ingrown toenail, nevus, or pyogenic granuloma. Traditionally, the poorer prognosis ascribed to this variant of melanoma may be due to late diagnosis of more advanced disease rather than a true difference in the biological nature of the tumor *(60)*.

5. ESTABLISHING A HISTOLOGIC DIAGNOSIS

Although the clinical history is crucial, it pales in comparison to the importance that an adequate sample for pathologic review will provide. Because early diagnosis is of paramount importance in reducing the mortality from melanoma, any patient presenting with a lesion suspected of being a melanoma should promptly be biopsied. An adequate sample should be submitted for histological interpretation and diagnosis, as this will determine the prognosis and plan of therapy. The NIH Consensus Conference on Early Melanoma *(79)* recommends an excisional biopsy with a narrow margin of normal appearing skin for any suspicious lesions whenever possible. The excisional biopsy specimen should include a portion of subcutaneous fat for accurate microstaging and may be obtained by elliptical excision, deep saucerization, and punch biopsy (if the lesion is small enough). A Woods light examination may aid in delineating margins of the suspicious pigmented lesion. An incisional biopsy technique is acceptable when the suspicion for melanoma is low, the lesion is large, or when it is impractical to perform an excisional biopsy *(80)*. This should entail removal of an ellipse or core of full thickness of skin and subcutaneous tissue at the most raised and irregular site or, if the lesion is flat, the darkest area of pigmentation. It may sometimes be necessary to sample several areas if the lesion is large and has morphologic variation *(81)*. Since an incisional biopsy samples only part of the tumor, a repeat biopsy must be performed if the histologic diagnosis does not correlate with the clinical impression. Furthermore, the diagnosis established by incisional biopsies must defer final determination of the final thickness and level of the tumor until the entire specimen has been excised and examined *(81)*. There is no evidence that biopsy or incision of a melanoma leads to "seeding" of tissue and metastasis *(62)*. Recognizing that the initial biopsy is the first step of a 2-step process, it is recommended that the orientation of the excisional biopsy be planned along the axis of anticipated lymphatic drainage, or for best cosmetic result upon re-excision *(80)*.

Shave biopsy and curettage specimens yield inadequate specimens, frequently disrupt the tumor, and preclude conventional microstaging *(62)* and, therefore, should not be submitted for histologic diagnosis of a suspicious lesion. Fine-needle aspiration cytology should not be used to assess the primary tumor *(80)*.

The diagnosis and microstaging of the suspicious lesion should be performed on fixed histologic specimens and interpreted by physicians experienced in the microscopic diagnosis of pigmented lesions. The role of frozen sections in the diagnosis of melanoma remains controversial. Current consensus seems to be that frozen section analysis is not as reliable as paraffin-embedded sections for the diagnosis of melanoma. There are some melanomas with subtle histomorphologic features that are difficult to diagnose by frozen section, and this requires some experience in interpretation. However, frozen section analysis may be useful for the evaluation of surgical margins for melanoma *(82)*.

5.1. Histopathologic Criteria for the Diagnosis of Melanoma

A lesion is diagnosed as melanoma when it exhibits sufficient architectural and cytologic atypia and when specific histopathologic changes correlate with the patient's biologic response *(83)*. Fully evolved cytologic atypia is considered necessary for the diagnosis of melanoma. This generally refers to pronounced cellular enlargement, nuclear enlargement, variations in nuclear size and shape (anisokaryosis), nuclear hyperchromasia with irregular lumping and distribution of chromatin, and enlarged nucleoli *(3)*. In melanoma, epithelioid and spindle cells are described. The former are characterized by abundant granular, eosinophilic, or "dusty" cytoplasm, and the latter have less cytoplasm, which is frequently basophilic or amphophilic, with high nuclear to cytoplasmic ratios.

Architectural features suggestive of melanoma include large size (greater than 5 to 6 mm), asymmetry, and pagetoid spread or intraepidermal upward migration of melanocytes. Also, there is loss of nevic growth pattern or loss of elongated epidermal rete, with variation in junctional nesting pattern and confluence of nests with dyshesion of cells in nests *(62)*.

5.2. Immunohistochemistry

Although not routinely used in the diagnosis of melanoma, immunohistochemistry may be important for diagnosis in certain situations. Most common uses include the diagnosis of melanoma in the following settings: in primary or metastatic poorly differentiated malignant neoplasms containing little or no pigment; in spindle cell tumors; in tumors with pagetoid epidermal patterns, but which are not obvious melanoma; and in small cell malignant tumors suggesting melanoma, lymphoma, or neuroendocrine carcinoma *(84–87)*. S-100 protein and HMB-45 are the antisera most often used for routine evaluation of paraffin-embedded specimens. S-100 protein is a sensitive immunohistochemical marker for pigmented neoplasms. It stains 96.4% of malignant melanomas and 98.4% of benign melanocytic nevi *(88)*, but also a variety of other tumors, such as peripheral nerve sheath tumors, cartilaginous tumors, osteosarcomas, eccrine and visceral carcinomas, and Langerhans cell tumors, among others *(84,85)*. HMB-45 is a sensitive and specific marker for malignant melanoma, however, it stains some benign neoplasms, including atypical nevi and occasional Spitz nevi *(88)*. In general, it is not immunoreactive with carcinomas, lymphomas, or sarcomas *(86,87)*. It is frequently negative in spindle cell and desmoplastic melanoma, however, these tumors commonly exhibit vimentin and s-100 positivity *(87)*. In general, it is recommended that these two reagents be used in concert with a panel of antibodies against other tumor markers, such as cytokeratins, vimentin, leukocyte common antigen, among others, depending on the clinical and histologic features.

5.3. Microstaging

Microstaging is defined as the use of microscopic measurements of malignant tumors for the purpose of predicting prognosis *(89)*.

5.3.1. Clark's Levels of Tumor Invasion

Anatomic level of invasion refers to progressive penetration of certain anatomic barriers in the skin by melanoma. Clark *(90)* designated the following five levels for measuring the depth of a malignant melanoma.

Level I: confinement of malignant melanoma cells to the epidermis and its appendages.
Level II: extension of tumor cells into the papillary dermis.
Level III: extension of tumor cells throughout the papillary dermis, up to but not invading the reticular dermis.
Level IV: involvement of the reticular dermis.
Level V: involvement of the subcutaneous fat.

Clark's levels of invasion constitute a good system for microstaging of malignant melanoma, but the reticular dermis is a thick portion of the skin and varies by anatomic site (e.g., acral skin). A limitation in the ease, reproducibility, and objectivity of measuring tumor depth has made Clark's levels less significant in the microstaging of melanoma.

5.3.2. Breslow's Tumor Thickness

Breslow *(91)* proposed that the thickness of a malignant melanoma be measured from the top of the granular cell layer of the epidermis to the deepest extension of the tumor. If the thickness is less than 0.76 mm, the malignant melanoma usually does not metastasize, and no lymph node excision is necessary. This has proved to be the single most important predictor of survival in primary cutaneous melanoma *(60,92)*. To avoid underestimation of thickness in the presence of ulceration, the Breslow thickness should be measured from the ulcer surface vertically to the point of deepest melanoma invasion. In general, there is a crudely linear relationship between thickness and survival. Therefore, early diagnosis and treatment are crucial.

6. SURGICAL MANAGEMENT OF PRIMARY MELANOMA

Following a histologic diagnosis of malignant melanoma, the treatment of choice is excision of any remaining tumor and the biopsy site, with a margin of clinically normal appearing skin along with the underlying subcutaneous tissue. Surgical excision remains the most effective treatment modality for melanoma. The primary goal of surgical treatment is to remove all melanoma cells at the primary site. Hopefully, this serves as a cure for those patients with early disease (and low risk of occult metastatic disease) or provides local control of the disease if there is little likelihood of a cure. An important secondary goal is to minimize the functional impairment and disfigurement of the patient. The width of excisional margin has been controversial during the last several decades.

As a result of randomized surgical trials, our guidelines for excision margins for melanoma have become more clearly defined.

6.1. Margins of Excision

Until the late 1970s, margins of 4 to 5 cm of normal skin were the standard of care for excising melanoma. The resulting defects were usually closed with a skin graft. The belief was that such a wide excision should remove any local micrometastases and local lymphatic spread of the primary tumor.

Several retrospective studies were undertaken in the late 1970s and early 1980s comparing wide and narrow excisions *(93–96)*. These reports showed that overall survival was not affected by narrower excision margins. However, increases in local recurrences were seen with narrow margins for thicker melanomas. These studies suggested that local recurrence was more likely due to factors attributable to the tumor itself rather than the width of margin of excision. Many of the local recurrences in these series were in patients who underwent very narrow excision margins, less than or equal to 0.5 cm, suggesting that recurrence is somewhat influenced by the surgical margin as well as the biologic behavior of melanoma *(95,96)*. These studies suggested that a more conservative (and less morbid) excision could be applied based on the risk of local recurrence.

Recently several prospective randomized trials evaluated margins for excision required for adequate local control, based on thickness of the melanoma. Compared in a World Health Organization (WHO) Melanoma Program trial were 1-cm vs 3-cm margins in 612 patients with melanomas <2 mm in thickness *(97,98)*. No local recurrences occurred with either margin in patients with melanomas <1 mm in thickness. There were six local recurrences in patients with tumors between 1 and 2 mm. Five of these six were in the group treated with the more conservative 1-cm margin. However, there was no statistically significant difference in the rate of local recurrence between the groups.

Studied in the Intergroup Melanoma Trial were 486 patients with intermediate thickness melanomas (1–4 mm) *(99)*. Patients were randomly assigned to have either a 2- or 4-cm margin. The rate of local recurrence was 0.8% for the 2-cm margin group compared with 1.7% for the 4-cm margin group. No difference in survival, local recurrence, in-transit, or distant metastases between the two groups was statistically significant. The rate of repair with skin grafts was more than 4 times greater (46% vs 11%) in the group that had wide (4 cm) excision, resulting in a longer hospital stay.

The excision margins of deeper melanomas (>4 mm) have not been studied by prospective randomized trials. Retrospectively reviewed were 250 patients with thick melanomas over a 10-yr period *(100)*. Mean follow-up was 28 mo. They demonstrated no increase in local recurrence and no decrease in overall survival in patients with margins of 2 cm or less, compared with more extensive excisions.

6.2. Recommendations

Current recommended margins for excision of melanoma, according to tumor thickness, are based on the previously mentioned clinical trials (*see* Table 1). A margin of 0.5 to 1 cm is recommended for *in situ* melanomas. Although by definition, they are not invasive, *in situ* melanomas do have a risk for local recurrence and potential for invasion and subsequent metastases. Given a location where primary closure can be accomplished, a 1-cm margin is preferred. For invasive melanomas less than 1 mm in thickness, the WHO study endorses a 1-cm margin as the standard of care.

The margins for melanomas between 1 and 2 mm are somewhat controversial. Although a difference in survival has not been shown for margins 1 cm versus greater, a narrow margin for these lesions is associated with a higher absolute risk for local recurrence. Several authors *(101–103)* recommend a 2-cm margin, particularly in areas where primary closure is feasible. Other prognostic factors may influence one to perform a wider (2 cm) excision. The presence of ulceration, for example, is associated with an increased risk of local recurrence *(101)*.

A 2-cm margin is recommended for melanomas between 2 and 4 mm based on results of several of the aforementioned studies. Low local recurrence rates and lower morbidity can be achieved as compared to traditional larger (4 to 5 cm) margins.

The recommended margins for melanomas >4 mm thick are less clear. These patients are at a relatively high risk for local recurrence (approximately 12%) and have a very high risk of distant metastases (60%) *(100,104,105)*. Based on the retrospective analysis by Heaton et al. *(100)*, it would seem appropriate to recommend a 2-cm margin for melanomas >4 mm. The local recurrence rate was approximately 11% and did not seem to be associated with a poorer overall prognosis compared with the same patient population without local recurrence. Patients with melanomas >4 mm thick have other tumor-related factors that influence their regional and distant metastases.

6.3. Surgical Technique

Because the recent recommendations for surgical margins have decreased, most patients undergoing excision of a primary melanoma can have a simple elliptical excision with primary closure using only local anesthesia. The long axis of the ellipse should be oriented in the direction of lymphatic drainage in an attempt to remove any microsatellites. If possible, the ellipse should also follow the resting skin tension lines (Langer's lines) to facilitate primary closure and optimize the aesthetic result of the scar.

Before measuring for margins, a Wood's light examination is helpful in determining if any residual tumor and/or pigment remains. The appropriate margin is then measured from the edge of the intact tumor or the scar from the previous excisional biopsy site. The depth of the excision is generally down to the underlying muscular fascia, and the specimen should be removed en bloc.

There may be exceptions for the recommended margins for excision based on the anatomic location and prognostic factors of the primary tumor. For example, melanomas on the face may have limited excision margins because of proximity to vital structures. There is less proven data regarding margins for melanomas of the face, because many of the major trials excluded melanomas in this region.

Hudson et al. *(106)* recently studied narrow excision margins in 106 patients with Stage I melanomas of the face. Thirty patients had margins <1 cm, 64 had margins between 1 and 2 cm, and 12 had margins >2 cm. Seven patients (7/106) developed local recurrences, which were not significantly related to the surgical margins.

Defects that can not be closed primarily, should be considered for local flaps or skin grafts. The appearance of local flaps is usually superior to grafts. Cuono and Ariyan *(107)* showed that flap closure does not increase the risk of local recurrence. Split- or full-thickness skin grafts are reasonable options for covering a defect that cannot otherwise be repaired. The disadvantages of skin grafts are often a poor cosmetic result and greater morbidity for the patient.

6.4. Sentinel Lymph Node Biopsy

The presence or absence of lymph node metastases is the most powerful predictor of survival in patients with malignant melanoma. The likelihood of regional lymph node involvement may be predicted by primary tumor variables such as Breslow thickness, ulceration, anatomic site, and sex or gender. However, once patients develop metastases to their regional nodes, their 5-yr survival decreases by approximately 40% (compared to those with no evidence of nodal metastases). Patients with palpable lymph nodes have a high likelihood of distant metastases (70–80%) and a 5-yr survival rate of approximately 30% *(108,109)*. Patients with occult disease (or micrometastases) have a better prognosis *(109)*.

Prior to the early 1990s, physicians had two options for managing patients with clinically negative lymph nodes: observation and elective lymph node dissection (ELND). ELND is the removal of clinically negative nodes for more accurate staging in patients considered at risk for micrometastases (T > 1 mm). Some proponents of ELND believe that removing micrometastases may prevent systemic spread. There is controversy as to whether ELND has a survival benefit for patients or acts solely as a staging procedure. ELND is associated with a relatively high degree of morbidity.

It is universally accepted that patients with primary melanomas <1 mm and >4 mm in thickness do not benefit from ELND. Several prospective randomized trials have shown no significant difference in survival comparing patients who underwent ELND and wide local excision (WLE) and those who had WLE alone *(110–113)*. Two large retrospective studies have shown a small but significant reduction in mortality in subpopulations of patients with intermediate to thick lesions *(108,114)*. The Intergroup Melanoma Surgical Trial prospectively randomized patients with intermediate thickness melanomas (1–4 mm) to ELND versus nodal observation. It was the first prospective trial to require preoperative lymphoscintigraphy to help identify all nodal basins at risk for metastases. Overall survival was not significantly different, but long-term results have shown a statistically significant survival benefit in patients with melanomas 1 to 2 mm thick, those with nonulcerated lesions, and those with melanomas of the extremities *(115)*.

Morton et al. in 1992 *(116,117)* introduced the concept of sentinel node biopsy for the staging of patients with malignant melanoma. The sentinel lymph node (SLN) is the first draining node between the primary tumor and the regional nodal basin. Theoretically, the metastatic status of the SLN should accurately predict the status of the remainder of the involved nodal basin. They injected vital (blue) dyes into the dermis at the site of the primary tumor. The dye is carried to corresponding regional nodes by lymphatic vessels. The regional lymph basin was surgically exposed, and the first blue node or nodes (sentinel nodes) were identified, excised, and sent for frozen section pathologic analysis. They reported identification of a SLN in 82% (194 of 237 lymphatic basins) with stage I disease. Eighteen percent of SLNs were positive by hematoxalin and eosin (H&E) or immunohistochemistry. All patients underwent complete lymphadenectomy following SLN biopsy. Non-SLNs were the exclusive site of metastases in only 2 of 3079 nodes from 194 dissections, for a false negative rate of <1% (0.1%). An analysis by patients showed that of 40 patients with histologically positive nodes, SLN mapping identified 38, for a 5% false negative rate. This technique accurately identified patients with occult lymph node metastases who may benefit from complete lymphadenectomy and adjuvant therapy.

Subsequent studies *(118–121)* confirmed Morton's success in identifying the sentinel lymph node and the prediction that the SLN is the first and favored site of metastatic disease. These studies showed that SLNs in the lymphatic basins could be individually identified and that they reflect the presence or absence of melanoma metastases in the remainder of the nodal basin *(122)*. Increasing experience and further improvements, specifically the incorporation of radiolabeled colloid as a tracer, have improved successful identification of SLNs *(121)*. The technique involves, first, injecting a radiolabeled colloid (Tc-sulfur colloid) intradermally around the site of the tumor. Lymphoscintography is done to approximate the location of the nodal basin (or identify any in-transit nodes), and then a handheld gamma probe is used intraoperatively to locate the sentinel node. A small incision is made over the "hot" node or nodes, which are then dissected and removed. The use of isosulfan blue dye in conjunction with radiolabeled colloid is complementary and permits successful localization of the SLN in almost 100% of patients *(121,123)*. The false negative rate has continued to be approximately 1% in most studies.

After the sentinel node(s) are removed, they are submitted to a pathologist for routine H&E and immunohistochemical stains (S-100, HMB45). Because only a small number of nodes (1–3) are sent for examination, serial sectioning can be done through the entire node; something that is too burdensome with the number of nodes removed with ELND. Other methods of examining lymph nodes are being studied. Polymerase chain reaction (PCR) analysis for tyrosinase messenger RNA has been shown to positively identify nodes that were previously negative with routine H&E and immunohistochemistry *(122,124)*.

6.5. Patient Selection

It is not known at this time whether SLN biopsy (SLNB) will be associated with improved survival in patients with melanoma. Patients who have negative SLN have a significantly reduced risk of regional and systemic involvement compared to those who are SLN positive. Regional recurrences have been documented in patients who have previously had a negative SLNB *(125)*. Retrospective analysis of these sentinel nodes using serial sectioning, immunohistochemical stains, or PCR for tyrosinase, revealed occult metastases that had previously been overlooked.

SLNB is an accurate and minimally invasive procedure for determining nodal status for patients with clinically negative lymph nodes. Patients with positive SLNBs are treated with a complete lymphadenectomy, with a reasonable expectation of survival benefit. Another advantage of identifying nodal status is that node-positive patients can be considered for adjuvant therapy, such as interferon α-2b, or ongoing clinical trials. The Multicenter Selective Lymphadenectomy Trial (MSLT) is an ongoing prospective randomized trial that will help to answer the question of whether the routine performance of SLNB will be associated with improved survival. The results will probably not be available until 2003.

SLNB is an option for patients with clinically node-negative melanoma who have a significant risk for micrometastatic nodal disease. Patients with primary tumors 1–4 mm in thickness, or Clark's Level IV or greater, are appropriate candidates *(108)*. These patients have greater than a 5% risk of occult nodal micrometastases. Patients with melanomas between 0.76 and 1.0 mm in thickness have approximately a 5% chance of having occult nodal micrometastases and may be given the option of having a SLNB. Female patients with melanoma <0.76 mm thickness have less than a 1% risk of having nodal micrometastases; therefore, SLNB would not be of additional benefit for this population. In contrast, however, males with melanoma of the trunk 0.76 mm or less have a 9% incidence of occult nodal metastases, which emphasizes the importance of gender and anatomic site in predicting occult nodal disease. Male patients with tumors that are Clark's Level III or greater, ulcerated primary lesions, regressed lesions, and axial melanomas have been shown to be at greater risk for metastases and death at 5 years (approximately 10%) *(126)*. Patients with these negative prognostic factors should consider SLN, even if their primary tumor is less than 0.76 mm in thickness *(122)*.

Patients with thick melanomas (>4 mm) are at a high risk for regional and systemic disease, and ELND is not recommended because of the lack of survival benefit. With the availability of effective adjuvant therapy, SLNB is indicated in order to identify the subset of patients who may benefit. Patients with thick melanomas, who have documented micrometastases, have a worse survival than patients with thick melanomas and no evidence of nodal spread *(127)*. These patients (T4N1) were in the subset of patients who benefited from high dose adjuvant interferon α-2b.

Patients who have already had WLE or other prior surgery may have unpredictable lymphatic drainage and should be excluded. SLNB should not be performed in these patients because the procedure and results are less reliable. Whenever possible the decision to perform SLNB should be made before WLE, so that the two procedures may be combined appropriately.

6.6. Patient (Staging) Work-Up and Follow-Up (Post-Treatment Surveillance)

The primary factors in the clinical and pathologic staging of primary melanoma are tumor thickness (pT) and level of invasion, nodal involvement (N), and distant metastases (M). Prognosis and survival probabilities can be estimated according to which stage grouping a patient falls into. The most recent AJCC (American Joint Committee on Cancer) TNM staging system for malignant melanoma of the skin is found in Table 2. In patients with localized node-negative disease, other characteristics of the primary tumor including ulceration, tumor location, and sex are useful predictors of survival.

Characteristics of the primary tumor assume less significance in patients with lymph node involvement. The presence of nodal metastases lowers the 5-yr survival rate by 40% compared to patients without nodal involvement *(128)*. The likelihood of nodal metastases for any tumor thickness can be estimated from studies of ELND and SLNB. Patients with primary melanomas between 1.5 and 4.0 mm (Stage II) in thickness have a 15–30% incidence of nodal metastases at the time of diagnosis *(129)*.

Less then 2% of melanoma patients initially present with distant metastases. These patients have a poor prognosis, with a 5-yr survival rate of 6% and a median survival of approximately 6 mo *(130)*. Review of Stage I/II and III patients treated in 14 centers suggest that up to 20% (early stage) and 65% (node-positive) of patients with melanoma may harbor asymptomatic distant metastases at the time of diagnosis *(131)*.

6.7. Proposed Changes to AJCC Staging

Several changes to the current AJCC staging system have been proposed for the next staging guidelines. Tumor thickness in millimeters, rather than level of invasion, will be used to determine the T classification. There is adequate data to support the conclusion that thickness, not level of invasion, is the more accurate and reproducible predictor of outcome *(108,131–136)*. The proposed breakpoints for the substages were chosen to represent the "best fit" between favorable and unfavorable prognosis. T1 tumors will include melanomas, ≥ 1.0 mm; T2 tumors, 1.01–2.0 mm; T3 tumors, 2.01–4.0 mm, and T4 tumors, >4.0 mm.

Ulceration will be included as a separate important prognostic variable within the T classification. Ulceration is determined by pathologic examination and defined by the absence of an intact epidermis overlying the primary tumor. Melanoma ulceration portends a significantly worse prognosis and higher risk of metastases compared to nonulcerative melanomas of equivalent thickness *(131–133,135,137–139)*. Patients will be designated according to absence(a) or presence(b) of ulceration. Patients with stage I, II, and III disease will be "upstaged" when their primary melanoma is ulcerated.

The N classification will be changed to reflect the number of positive lymph nodes rather than the size or diameter of lymph node metastases. In almost all studies analyzing prognosis, either the number or the percentage of positive lymph nodes was the strongest predictor of outcome *(109,131,133,140–147)*. Gross size of metastatic lymph nodes has little value as a prognostic factor other than the simple delineation of either microscopic or macroscopic lymph node metastases. Patients with 1 metastatic node did better than those with any combination of 2 or more *(131,135,141,142,145–147)*. The primary new N classification will group patients with 1 lymph node (N1) vs 2 to 3 nodes (N2) vs 4 or more metastatic nodes (N3).

The secondary criterion for patients in the N classification is the presence of micrometastases versus macrometastases. The increasing utilization of sentinel lymph node biopsy is identifying more patients with clinically occult lymph node metastases (micrometastases). The AJCC Melanoma Staging Committee felt it was important to identify these patients in the staging classification because of data demonstrating that patients with microscopic lymph node involvement fare better than those with clinically evident lymph node metastases *(142,146,148)*.

The presence of clinical or microscopic satellites around a primary melanoma and/or in-transit metastases between the primary melanoma and the regional lymph nodes will be assigned to a separate classification (N2c). Both represent intralymphatic metastases and portend an equally poor prognosis *(135)*. These patients' prognoses are equivalent to those with lymph node involvement and would be classified as stage IIIc. Patients with a combination of satellites or in-transit metastases and lymph node metastases have worse survival and/or outcomes than those with either finding alone. These patients are assigned to an N3 classification (stage III) regardless of the number of lymph nodes involved *(135,142)*.

The classification of metastases is divided into 3 subgroups (M1–3). In all studies evaluating the prognoses of patients with metastases, patients with distant metastases in the skin, subcutaneous tissue, or distant lymph nodes (M1) had better prognoses than those with metastases in any other sites *(149–152)*. In several studies *(150,151)*, patients with metastases to the lung had intermediate prognoses, compared with patients who had metastases to skin or subcutaneous sites (better) and all other visceral sites (worse prognoses). Therefore, patients with lung metastases are assigned to an M2 classification, while those with any other visceral metastases are assigned a M3 classification.

An increased serum lactate dehydrogenase (LDH) was one of the most predictive factors of poor outcome in all published studies in which it was analyzed, even after accounting for location and number of metastases *(149,152–156)*. Therefore, the committee recommended that patients with distant metastases at any site with a serum LDH above the upper limits of normal be assigned to the M3 classification as long as other causes of LDH elevation are excluded.

6.8. Work-Up for Melanoma Staging

The initial clinical evaluation of a patient with a primary melanoma consists of a thorough history and physical examination. The history should focus on prior personal or family history of melanoma, history of sun exposure, and review of symptoms focusing on pulmonary, gastrointestinal, neurological, musculoskeletal, and constitutional symptoms. A complete skin exam should be done looking for atypical pigmented lesions. Palpation of all regional lymph node basins is essential to account for aberrant lymphatic drainage. The skin surrounding the tumor site should also be palpated for satellite lesions or in-transit nodes. In the event of a clinically palpable lymph node, a fine-needle biopsy (FNB) is usually done. If the FNB is negative or equivocal, an open biopsy should be performed. Other suspicious findings by history or physical exam warrant further diagnostic testing using laboratory and imaging studies followed by histologic confirmation if positive.

Laboratory investigations and imaging studies are of low yield in asymptomatic patients with stage I to II melanoma *(130,157–159)*. Common laboratory screening tests such as a complete blood count (CBC) and liver function tests (LFTs) are controversial. There is not evidence that routine laboratory investigations are useful for screening or surveillance. Because of the relatively low cost, many practitioners will obtain at least a baseline LDH to help detect later liver metastases. A serum LDH of greater than 300 μ/L has been shown to be a sensitive marker for hepatic metastases *(159)*.

Chest radiographs (CXR) are probably the most common imaging study obtained in patients diagnosed with melanoma *(128,160)*. The lung is the most common site of isolated (solitary) visceral metastases. Although most studies have shown no benefit of screening CXRs, they are relatively inexpensive. Furthermore, surgical resection of isolated pulmonary metastases has been associated with prolonged survival *(161)*.

Although frequently obtained, the use of extensive radiological studies (computed tomography [CT], magnetic resonance imaging [MRI], and radionucleotide) in the asymptomatic patient to search for occult metastases is not warranted. The rate of detection of metastases is very low, and a high false positive rate (10–20%) leads to patient anxiety as well as further unnecessary and costly invasive procedures *(158,159,162–165)*. 18F-flluorodeoxyglucose positron emission tomography (FDG-PET) is a promising experimental imaging study for the staging and surveillance of patients with melanoma. Prospective studies have shown a sensitivity of 94–100% and a specificity of 83–94% *(166,167)*. FDG-PET was significantly better than CT at detecting regional and mediastinal lymph nodes, abdominal visceral, and soft tissue metastases. The false positive rate in these studies was <5%. Its use is currently limited because of high cost and limited availability, however, FDG-PET could potentially replace standard imaging for melanoma patients in the future.

7. POST-TREATMENT SURVEILLANCE

The goal in following patients after a diagnosis of malignant melanoma is to detect recurrences as early as possible, in order for treatment to have an impact on long-term survival. Unfortunately with melanoma, recurrence when detected is not always treatable, nor is treatment when possible necessarily curative. A direct relationship does not exist between the intensity of follow-up and overall survival in melanoma patients. Currently, there is no consensus regarding the frequency of follow-up or recommendations for surveillance testing for patients with melanoma. Guidelines for follow-up and surveillance are based on the risk of recurrence, pattern of relapse, and the treatment options available if a recurrence is detected.

There is a direct correlation between depth of invasion and the risk of recurrence. One in four patients with Stage I or II melanoma will develop a recurrence *(168)*. Patients with *in situ* melanomas and invasive melanomas <0.75 mm have a low risk of metastatic disease. Tumor ulceration, extremity location, increasing age (>60 yr), and male sex increase the risk of recurrence in early stage melanoma. Patients with Stage III melanoma have a high risk of recurrence (60–70%) *(142,169)*.

The time interval to recurrence varies inversely with tumor thickness and clinical stage at the time of diagnosis. The greatest annual risk of recurrence is during the first year following diagnosis, after which the risk steadily decreases over time. The majority of recurrences occur within 2 to 3 yr. Approximately 55 to 67% of recurrences become apparent within 2 yr and 65 to 85% within 3 yr of initial treatment. Few recurrences occur after 5 yr, however recurrences beyond 10 yr after treatment of primary melanoma are not uncommon *(168,170,171)*. Most patients with late recurrence had a thin (Stage I) primary melanoma at the time of diagnosis with clinically or pathologically negative lymph nodes *(168,171)*.

The majority of recurrences in patients with melanoma are locoregional. Regional lymph nodes are the most common initial site of recurrence in patients who did not undergo elective lymph node dissection as part of their primary treatment (50–60%) *(172)*. Visceral metastases are more common in patients who have undergone ELND, although regional node involvement is seen in 2 to 33% of these patients *(169,172,173)*. Local and in-transit recurrences are seen in 2 to 10% and 2 to 38% of melanoma patients, respectively *(129,172,174)*.

Visceral metastases are the initial site of relapse in approximately 20 to 26% of patients who develop a recurrence *(168,169,172,174,175)*. The most common sites of visceral metastases are the lung, brain, liver, and gastrointestinal tract. However, metastatic melanoma can be seen in almost any organ.

The majority of melanoma recurrences are symptomatic or are found during physical examination. Patients should be educated in regular self-examination of their skin and regional nodal basins, as well as signs and symptoms of systemic metastases. Alerting their physicians to new or unusual symptoms or findings can facilitate detection of locoregional recurrences and new primary melanomas at an early stage. Patients with a diagnosis of melanoma have a 5% risk of a second primary melanoma during their lifetime. Patients with multiple atypical nevi, a family history of melanoma, or multiple primary melanomas should be followed closely with full skin exams.

A history and physical examination are the cornerstones of follow-up and surveillance for patients with melanoma. A prospective study of Stage II and III melanoma patients by the North Central Cancer Treatment Group found a recurrence in 145 of 261 patients. Ninety-four percent of recurrences were detected by routine surveillance. Ninety-nine patients (68%) with a recurrence were symptomatic, while 37 (26%) were asymptomatic *(130)*. Only 9 of 145 (6%) were identified by an abnormal chest radiograph, and no recurrences were detected solely by abnormal laboratory exams. Mooney et al. *(176)* also studied the impact of a surveillance program using physical examination, chest radiographs and blood tests in patients with Stage I or II melanoma. Physical examination detected 72% of recurrences, patient symptoms indicated 17%, chest radiographs revealed 11% of recurrences, and blood tests did not identify any recurrence. In summary, a directed history and thorough physical examination can identify most recurrences during follow-up visits.

Extensive radiologic exams and laboratory studies for follow-up and surveillance of asymptomatic patients are generally not indicated. A posteroanterior chest radiograph is sufficiently sensitive and cost-effective to recommend for routine screening in asymptomatic patients. In the absence of symptoms or abnormal finding on physical examination, chest radiograph, or laboratory tests (i.e., LDH), the yield of CT scanning is too low for it to be recommended as a screening tool.

The sensitivity of serum LDH is low in asymptomatic patients with melanoma. Even so, an isolated elevation of this enzyme is considered by many to be evidence of metastatic disease. LDH levels greater than 300 U/L were found in all patients with radiologic evidence of chest, lung, bone, and visceral metastases in a study by Khansur et al. *(159)*. They concluded that serum LDH is a useful screening test for metastatic disease.

7.1. Current Practice

No consensus exists for surveillance of patients with Stage I and II melanoma. Most recommendations for follow-up are empiric and based on the risk of developing a recurrence or second primary melanoma. Patient anxiety and preference also influence the frequency and intensity of follow-up surveillance.

Several studies have addressed the frequency of follow-up and what should be included during follow-up examination in addition to history and physical examination. The National Cancer Institute (NCI) in 1991 published a consensus statement for the follow-up of patients with melanoma less than 1.0 mm in thickness *(177)*. Patients with *in situ* melanoma can be followed with only yearly skin examinations. Patients with thin melanoma (<1 mm) and no atypical nevi or family history of melanoma can be followed every 6 mo for 2 yr, and then yearly. Early melanoma patients with multiple atypical nevi and/or a positive family history of melanoma can be followed only by history and physical examination at 3- to 6-mo intervals for 2 yr. Education of all patients with regard to self-examination and sun avoidance is recommended.

More recently, the National Comprehensive Cancer Network (NCCN) proposed staging, treatment, and surveillance guidelines for all stages of melanoma *(178)*. Opinions on the appropriate follow-up for patients with melanoma varied widely, and the recommendations included a range of suggestions. Patients with melanomas <1.0 mm thick can be followed with history and physical examination alone every 6 mo for 2 yr, then annually. Patients with melanomas ≥ 1.0 mm should have a history and physical examination every 3 to 6 mo for the first 3 yr, then every 6 to 12 mo for yr 4 to 5, then annually. Routine use of liver function tests and chest radiographs were recognized as very low yield, but were recommended at 6- to 12-mo intervals at the discretion of the treating physician. Patients with Stage III melanoma were recommended to have a history and physical examination every 3 to 6 mo for the first 3 yr, every 4 to 12 mo for yr 4 and 5, then yearly thereafter. Chest radiographs, liver function tests, and CBCs were recommended every 3 to 12 mo at the discretion of the physician. The routine use of CT scans was considered inappropriate in the absence of abnormal findings on history, physical examination, laboratory tests, or chest radiograph.

A definitive program for staging and follow-up for melanoma can only be defined in the context of a prospective randomized trial. Until such a trial is completed, staging and surveillance strategies should be based on currently available data.

REFERENCES

1. Schaffer JV, Bolognia JL. The clinical spectrum of pigmented lesions. *Clin Plast Surg* 2000; 27: 391–408.
2. Slade J, Marghoob AA, Salopek TG, Rigel DS, Kopf AW, Bart RS. Atypical mole syndrome: risk factor for cutaneous malignant melanoma and implications for management. *J Am Acad Dermatol* 1995; 32: 479–494.
3. Graham S, Marshall J, Haughey B, et al. An inquiry into the epidemiology of melanoma. *Am J Epidemiol* 1985; 122: 606–619.
4. Beral V, Evans S, Shaw H, et al. Cutaneous factors related to the risk of malignant melanoma. *Br J Dermatol* 1983; 109: 165–172.
5. Dubin N, Moseson M, Pasternack BS. Epidemiology of malignant melanoma: pigmentary traits, ultraviolet radiation, and the identification of high-risk populations. *Recent Results Cancer Res* 1986; 102: 56–75.
6. Graham S, Marshall J, Haughey B, et al. Op cit.
7. Elwood JM, Gallagher RP, Hill GB, et al. Pigmentation and skin reaction to sun as risk factors for cutaneous melanoma: Western Canada Melanoma Study. *Br Med J* 1984; 288: 99–102.
8. Green A, Bain C, McLennan R, et al. Risk factors for cutaneous melanoma in Queensland. *Recent Results Cancer Res* 1986; 102: 76–97.
9. MacKie RM, Freudenberger T, Aitchison TC. Personal risk-factor chart for cutaneous melanoma. *Lancet* 1989; 2: 487–490.
10. Holman CDJ, Armstron BK, Heenan PJ. Relationship of cutaneous malignant melanoma to individual sunlight—exposure habits. *J Natl Cancer Inst* 1986; 76: 403–414.
11. Elwood JM, Williamson C, Stapleton PJ. Malignant melanoma in relation to moles, pigmentation, and exposure to fluorescent and other lighting sources. *Br J Cancer* 1986; 53: 65–74.
12. Titus-Ernstoff L. An overview of the epidemiology of cutaneous melanoma. *Clin Plast Surg* 2000; 27: 305–316.
13. Lancaster HO. Geographical aspects of melanoma. *Lancet* 1955; 2: 929.
14. Holman CDJ, Mulroney CD, Armstrong BK. Epidemiology of preinvasive and invasive malignant melanoma in Western Australia. *Int J Cancer* 1980; 25: 317–332.
15. Mack TM, Floderus B. Malignant melanoma risk by nativity, place of residence at diagnosis, and age at migration. *Cancer Causes Control* 1991; 2: 401–411.
16. Collins JJ, Devine N. Period and cohort factors in the incidence of malignant melanoma in the state of Connecticut. *Environ Health Perspect* 1984; 56: 255–259.
17. Roush GC, Schymura MJ, Holford TR, et al. Time period compared to birth cohort in Connecticut incidence rates for twenty-five malignant neoplasms. *J Natl Cancer Inst* 1985; 74: 779–788.
18. Thorn M, Bergstrom R, Adami HO, et al. Trends in the incidence of malignant melanoma in Sweden, by anatomic site, 1960–1984. *Am J Epidemiol* 1990; 132: 1066–1077.

19. Venzon DJ, Mootgavkar SH. Cohort analysis of malignant melanoma in five countries. *Am J Epidemiol* 1984; 119: 62–70.
20. Swerdlow AJ. International trends in cutaneous melanoma. *Ann NY Acad Sci* 1990; 609: 235–251.
21. Elwood JM, Jopson J. Melanoma and sun exposure: an overview of published studies. *Int J Cancer* 1997; 73: 198–203.
22. Kraemer KH, Lee MM, Andrews AD, et al. The role of sunlight and DNA repair in melanoma and nonmelanoma skin cancer. The xeroderma pigmentosum paradigm. *Arch Dermatol* 1994; 130: 1018–1021.
23. Swerdlow AJ, Weinstock MA. Do tanning lamps cause melanoma? An epidemiologic assessment. *J Am Acad Dermatol* 1998; 38: 89–98.
24. Stern RS, Nichols KT, Vakeva LH. Malignant melanoma in patients treated for psoriasis with methoxsalen (Psoralen) and ultraviolet A radiation (PUVA). *N Engl J Med* 1997; 336: 1041–1045.
25. Greene MH, Hoover RN, Fraumeni JF. Subsequent cancer in patients with chronic lymphocytic leukemia—a possible immunologic mechanism. *J Natl Cancer Inst* 1978; 61: 337–340.
26. Greene MH, Young TL, Clark WH. Malignant melanomas in renal transplant recipients. *Lancet* 1981; 1: 1196–1199.
27. Titus-Ernstoff L. op cit.
28. Clark WH Jr, Reimer RR, Greene M, et al. Origin of familial malignant melanomas from heritable melanocytic lesions: "the B-K mole syndrome." *Arch Dermatol* 1978; 114: 732–738.
29. Lynch HT, Frichot BC III, Lynch JF. Familial atypical multiple mole-melanoma syndrome. *J Med Genet* 1978; 15: 352–356.
30. Greene MH, Clark WH Jr, Tucker MA, et al. Precursor naevi in cutaneous malignant melanoma: a proposed nomenclature. *Lancet* 1980; 2: 1024.
31. Bondi EE, Clark WH Jr, Elder D, et al. Topical chemotherapy of dysplastic melanocytic nevi with 5% fluorouracil. *Arch Dermatol* 1981; 117: 89–92.
32. Nollet DJ. "Clark's nevus syndrome." *Am J Dermatopathol* 1986; 8: 367.
33. Consensus Development Panel on early melanoma. Diagnosis and treatment of early melanoma. *JAMA* 1992; 268: 1314–1319.
34. Kopf AW, Friedman RJ, Rigel DS. Atypical mole syndrome. *J Am Acad Dermatol* 1990; 22: 117–118.
35. Consensus Conference on Precursors to Malignant Melanoma. *J Dermatol Surg Oncol* 1985; 11: 537–542.
36. Consensus Development Panel on early melanoma. Op cit.
37. Lynch HT, Fusaro RM, Kimberling WJ, et al. Familial atypical multiple mole melanoma (FAMMM) syndrome: segregation analysis. *J Med Genet* 1983; 20: 342–344.
38. Bale SJ, Chakravanti A, Greene MH. Cutaneous malignant melanoma and familial dysplastic nevus: evidence for autosomal dominance and pleiotropy. *Am J Hum Genet* 1986; 38: 188–196.
39. Bergman W, Palan A, Went LN. Clinical and genetic studies in six Dutch kindred with the dysplastic naevus syndrome. *Ann Hum Genet* 1986; 50: 249–258.
40. Bale SJ, Dracopoli NC, Tucker MA, et al. Mapping the gene for hereditary cutaneous malignant melanoma—dysplastic nevus to chromosome 1p. *N Engl J Med* 1989; 320: 1367–1372.
41. Goldstein AM, Dracopoli NC, Ho EC, et al. Further evidence for a locus for cutaneous malignant melanoma—dysplastic nevus (CMM/DN) on chromosome 1p, and evidence for genetic heterogeneity. *Am J Hum Genet* 1993; 52: 537–550.
42. Cannon-Albright LA, Goldgar DE, Meyer LJ, et al. Assignment of a locus for familial melanoma, MLM, to chromosome 9p13-22. *Science* 1992; 258: 1148–1152.

43. Trent JM, Stanbridge EJ, McBride HL, et al. Tumorigenicity in human melanoma cell lines controlled by introduction human chromosome 6. *Science* 1990; 247: 568–571.
44. Koprowski H, Herlyn M, Balaban G, et al. Expression of the receptor for epidermal growth factor correlates with increased dosage of chromosome 7 in malignant melanoma. *Somat Cell Mol Genet* 1985; 11: 297–302.
45. Greene MH, Goldin RL, Clark WH Jr, et al. Familial cutaneous malignant melanoma: autosomal dominant trait possibly linked to the RH locus. *Proc Natl Acad Sci USA* 1983; 80: 6071–6075.
46. Goldstein AM, Dracopoli NC, Engelstein M, et al. Linkage of cutaneous malignant melanoma/dysplastic nevi to chromosome 9p, and evidence for genetic heterogeneity. *Am J Hum Genet* 1994; 54: 489–496.
47. Augustsson A, Steirner U, Rosdahl, I, et al. Common and dysplastic naevi as risk factors for cutaneous malignant melanoma in a Swedish population. *Acta Derm Venereol Suppl (Stockh)* 1991; 71: 518–524.
48. Tucker MA, Halpern A, Holly EA, et al. Clinically recognized dysplastic nevi: a central risk factor for cutaneous melanoma. *JAMA* 1997; 277: 1439–1444.
49. Whiteman D, Green A. Melanoma and sunburn. *Cancer Causes Control* 1994; 5: 564–572.
50. Beral V, Evans S, Shaw H, et al. Malignant melanoma and exposure to fluorescent lighting at work. *Lancet* 1982; 1: 290–293.
51. Weinstock MA. Do sunscreens increase or decrease melanoma risk: an epidemiologic evaluation. *J Invest Dermatol Symp Proc* 1999; 4: 97–100.
52. Vinceti M, Rothman KJ, Bergomi M, et al. Excess melanoma incidence in a cohort exposed to high levels of environmental selenium. *Epidemiol Biomarkers Prevent* 1998; 7: 853–856.
53. Bain C, Green A, Siskind V, et al. Diet and melanoma: an exploratory study. *Ann Epidemiol* 1993; 3: 235–238.
54. Kirkpatrick CS, White E, Lee JAH. Case-control study of malignant melanoma in Washington state. II. Diet, alcohol, and obesity. *Am J Epidemiol* 1994; 139: 869–879.
55. Beral V, Evans S, Shaw H, et al. Oral contraceptive use and malignant melanoma in Australia. *Br J Cancer* 1984; 50: 681–685.
56. Osterlind A. Hormonal and reproductive factors in melanoma risk. *Clin Dermatol* 1992; 10: 75–78.
57. Pfahlberg A, Hassan K, Wille L. Systematic review of case-control studies: oral contraceptives show no effect on melanoma risk. *Public Health Rev* 1997; 25: 309–315.
58. Austin DF, Reynolds PJ, Snyder MA, et al. Malignant melanoma among employees of Lawrence Livermore National Laboratory. *Lancet* 1981; 2: 712–716.
59. Antonelli NM, Dotters DJ, Katz VL, et al. Cancer in pregnancy: a review of the literature, Part I. *Obstet Gynecol Surv* 1996; 51: 125–134.
60. Langley RGB, Fitzpatrick TB, Sober AJ. Clinical characteristics. In: Balch CM, Houghton AN, Sober AJ, eds. *Cutaneous Melanoma, 3rd ed.* Quality Medical Publishing, St. Louis, 1998, pp. 82–101.
61. Langley RGB, Sober AJ. Causes for the delay in the diagnosis of melanoma. In: JJ Grob, RS Stern, RM Mackie, WA Weinstock, eds. *Epidemiology, Causes and Prevention of Skin Diseases.* Blackwell, Cambridge, UK, 1997, pp. 177–183.
62. Langley RGB, Barnhill RL, Mihm MC Jr, Fitzpatrick TB, Sober AJ. Neoplasms: cutaneous melanoma. In: Freedberg IM, Eisen AZ, Wolff K, et al., eds. *Fitzpatrick's Dermatology in General Medicine, 5th ed.* McGraw-Hill, New York, 1999, pp. 1080–1116.
63. Sober AJ, Burstein JM. Computerized digital image analysis: an aid for melanoma diagnosis—preliminary investigations and brief review. *J Dermatol* 1994; 21: 885–890.
64. Rajadhyaksha M, Grossman M, Esterowitz D, Webb RH, Anderson RR. In vivo confocal scanning laser microscopy of human skin: melanin provides strong contrast. *J Invest Dermatol* 1995; 104: 946–952.

65. Albert LS, Fewkes J, Sober AJ. Metastatic lentigo maligna melanoma. *J Dermatol Surg Oncol* 1990; 16: 56–58.
66. Pittelkow MR, Su WPD, Wick M, Sanchez N, Palestine R. Clinicopathologic study of lentigo malignant melanoma [abstract]. *J Cutan Pathol* 1986; 13: 75.
67. O'Donnel BF, Marsden JM, O'Donnel CA, et al. Does palpability of primary cutaneous melanoma predict dermal invasion? *J Am Acad Dermatol* 1995; 34: 923.
68. Su WPD. Malignant melanoma: basic approach to clinicopathologic correlation. *Mayo Clin Proc* 1997; 72: 267–272.
69. Weinstock MA, Sober AJ. The risk of progression of lentigo maligna to lentigo maligna melanoma. *Br J Dermatol* 1987; 116: 303–310.
70. Rhodes AR, Harrist TJ, Day CL Jr, et al. Dysplastic melanocytic nevi in histologic association with 234 cutaneous melanomas. *J Am Acad Dermatol* 1983; 9: 563–574.
71. Gruber SB, Barnhill RL, Stenn KS, et al. Nevomelanocytic proliferations in association with cutaneous malignant melanoma: a multivariate analysis. *J Am Acad Dermatol* 1989; 21: 773–780.
72. MacKie RM. Malignant melanoma: clinical variants and prognostic indicators. *Clin Exp Dermatol* 2000; 25: 471–475.
73. Clark WH Jr, Elder DE, Van Horn M. The biologic forms of malignant melanoma. *Hum Pathol* 1986; 17: 443–450.
74. Manci EA, Balch CM, Murad TM, et al. Polypoid melanoma, a virulent variant of the nodular growth pattern. *Am J Clin Pathol* 1981; 75: 810–815.
75. Stevens NG, Liff JM, Weiss NS. Plantar melanoma: is the incidence of melanoma of the sole of the foot really higher in blacks than in whites? *Int J Cancer* 1990; 45: 691–693.
76. Saida T, Yoshida N, Ikegawa S, et al. Clinical guidelines for the early detection of plantar malignant melanoma. *J Am Acad Dermatol* 1990; 23: 37–40.
77. Ridgeway CA, Hieken TJ, Ronan SG, et al. Acral lentiginous melanoma. *Arch Surg* 1995; 130: 88–92.
78. Blessing K, Kernohan NM, Park KGM. Subungual malignant melanoma: clinicopathological features of 100 cases. *Histopathology* 1991; 19: 425–429.
79. Consensus Development Panel on Early Melanoma. Diagnosis and treatment of early melanoma. *JAMA* 1992; 268: 1314–1319.
80. Sober AJ, et al. AAD Guidelines of Care for Primary Cutaneous Melanoma (draft). Dermatol World, May 2000.
81. Ho VC, Sober AJ, Balch CM. Biopsy techniques. In: Balch CM, Houghton AN, Sober AJ, eds. *Cutaneous Melanoma, 3rd ed.* Quality Medical Publishing, St. Louis, 1998, pp. 135–140.
82. Zitelli JA, Moy RL, Abell E. The reliability of frozen sections in the evaluation of surgical margins for melanoma. *J Am Acad Dermatol* 1991; 24: 102–106.
83. Barnhill RL, Mihm MC Jr. Histopathology and precursor lesions. In: Balch CM, Houghton AN, Sober AJ, eds. *Cutaneous Melanoma, 3rd ed.* Quality Medical Publishing, St. Louis, 1998, pp. 103–133.
84. Cochran AJ, Wen D-R. S-100 protein as a marker for melanocytic and other tumours. *Pathology* 1985; 17: 340–345.
85. Schmitt FC, Bacchi CE. S-100 protein: is it useful as a marker in diagnostic immunocytochemistry? *Histopathology* 1989; 15: 281–288.
86. Gown AM, Vogel AM, Hoak D, Gough F, McNutt MA. Monoclonal antibodies specific for melanocytic tumors distinguish subpopulations of melanocytes. *Am J Pathol* 1986; 123: 195–203.
87. Wick MR, Swanson PE, Rocamora A. Recognition of malignant melanoma by monoclonal antibody HMB-45: an immunohistochemical study of 200 paraffin-embedded cutaneous tumors. *J Cutan Pathol* 1988; 15: 201–207.

88. Smoller BR. Immunohistochemistry in the diagnosis of melanocytic neoplasms. *Pathol State Art Rev* 1994; 2: 371–383.
89. Daniel WP, Bradley RR. Amelanotic lentigo maligna. *Arch Dermatol* 1980; 116: 82–83.
90. Clark WH Jr. A classification of malignant melanoma in man correlated with histogenesis and biologic behavior. *Adv Biol Skin* 1967; 8: 621–647.
91. Breslow A. Thickness, cross sectional area and depth of invasion in the prognosis of cutaneous melanoma. *Ann Surg* 1970; 172: 902–908.
92. Barnhill RL. Malignant melanoma: pathology and prognostic factors. *Curr Opin Oncol* 1993; 5: 364–376.
93. Cosimi AB, Sober AJ, Mihm MC, Fitzpatrick TB. Conservative surgical management of superficially invasive cutaneous melanoma. *Cancer* 1984; 53: 1256–1259.
94. Kelly JW, Sagebiel RW, Calderon W, Murillo L, Dakin RL, Blois MS. The frequency of local recurrence and microsatellites as a guide to reexcision margins for cutaneous malignant melanoma. *Ann Surg* 1984; 200: 759–763.
95. O'Rourke MG, Altmann CR. Melanoma recurrence after excision. Is wide margin justified? *Ann Surg* 1993; 217: 2–5.
96. Milton GW, Shaw HM, McCarthy WJ. Resection margins of melanoma. *Aust NZ J Surg* 1985; 55: 225–226.
97. Veronesi U, Cascinelli N, Adamus J, et al. Thin primary cutaneous malignant melanoma: comparison of excision with margins of 1 or 3 cm. *N Engl J Med* 1988; 318: 1159–1162.
98. Veronesi U, Cascinelli N. Narrow excision (1 cm margin): a safe procedure for thin cutaneous melanoma. *Arch Surg* 1991; 126: 438–441.
99. Balch CM, Urist MM, Karakousis CP, et al. Efficacy of 2 cm surgical margins for intermediate-thickness melanomas (1 to 4 mm): results of a multi-institutional randomized surgical trial. *Ann Surg* 1993; 218: 262–267.
100. Heaton KM, Sussman JJ, Gershenwald JE, et al. Surgical margins and prognostic factors in patients with thick (>4 mm) primary melanoma. *Ann Surg Oncol* 1998; 5: 322–328.
101. Ross MI, Balch CM. Surgical treatment of primary melanoma. In: Balch CM, Houghton AN, Sober AJ, Soong SJ, eds. *Cutaneous Melanoma, 3rd ed.* Quality Medical Publishing, St. Louis, 1998; pp. 141–153.
102. Narayan D, Ariyan S. Surgical management of primary melanoma. *Clin Plast Surg* 2000; 27: 409–419.
103. Urist MM. Surgical management of primary cutaneous melanoma. *CA Cancer J Clin* 1996; 46: 217–224.
104. Schneebaum S, Briele HA, Walker MJ, et al. Cutaneous thick melanoma: prognosis and treatment. *Arch Surg* 1987; 122: 707–711.
105. Spellman JE Jr, Driscoll D, Velez A, Karakousis C. Thick cutaneous melanoma of the trunk and extremities: an institutional review. *Surg Oncol* 1994; 3: 335–343.
106. Hudson DA, Krige JE, Grobbelaar AO, Morgan B, Grover R. Melanoma of the face: the safety of narrow excision margins. *Scand J Plast Reconstr Hand Surg* 1998; 32: 97–104.
107. Cuono CB, Ariyan S. Versatility and safety of flap coverage for wide excision of cutaneous melanoma. *Plast Reconstr Surg* 1985; 76: 281–285.
108. Balch CM, Soong SJ, Milton GW, et al. A comparison of prognostic factors and surgical results in 1,786 patients with localized (stage I) melanoma treated in Alabama, USA, and New South Wales, Australia. *Ann Surg* 1982; 196: 677–684.
109. Balch CM, Soong SJ, Murad TM, Ingalls AL, Maddox WA. A multifactorial analysis of melanoma. III. Prognostic factors in melanoma patients with lymph node metastases (stage II). *Ann Surg* 1991; 193: 377–388.
110. Veronesi U, Adamus J, Bandiera DC, et al. Inefficacy of immediate node dissection in stage I melanoma of the limbs. *N Engl J Med* 1977; 297: 627–630.

111. Sim FH, Taylor WF, Pritchard DJ, Soule EH. Lymphadenectomy in the management of stage I malignant melanoma: a prospective randomized study. *Mayo Clin Proc* 1986; 61: 697–705.
112. Sim FH, Taylor WF, Ivins JC, Pritchard DJ, Soule EH. A prospective randomized study of the efficacy of routine elective lymphadenectomy in the management of malignant melanoma. Preliminary results. *Cancer* 1978; 41: 948–956.
113. Balch CM, Soong SJ, Bartolucci AA, et al. Efficacy of an elective regional lymph node dissection of 1 to 4 mm thick melanomas for patients 60 years of age and younger. *Ann Surg* 1996; 224: 255–263.
114. Reintgen DS, Cox EB, McCarthy KS Jr, Vollmer RT, Seigler HF. Efficacy of elective lymph node dissection in patients with intermediate thickness primary melanoma. *Ann Surg* 1983; 198: 379–385.
115. Balch CM, Soong S. Long-term results of a multi-institutional randomized trial comparing prognostic factors and surgical results for intermediate thickness melanomas (1.0 to 4.0 mm). Intergroup Melanoma Surgical Trial. *Ann Surg Oncol* 2000; 7: 87–97.
116. Morton DL, Wen DR, Cochran AJ. Management of early-stage melanoma by intraoperative lymphatic mapping and selective lymphadenectomy or "watch and wait." *Surg Oncol Clin North Am* 1992; 1: 247.
117. Morton DL, Wen DR, Wong JH, et al. Technical details of intraoperative lymphatic mapping for early stage melanoma. *Arch Surg* 1992; 127: 392–399.
118. Reintgen DS, Cruse CW, Wells K, et al.. The orderly progression of melanoma nodal metastases. *Ann Surg* 1994; 220: 759–767.
119. Thompson J, McCarthy WH, Bosch CM, et al. Sentinel lymph node status as an indicator of the presence of metastatic melanoma in regional lymph nodes. *Melanoma Res* 1995; 5: 255–260.
120. Ross MI, Reintgen DS, Balch CM. Selective lymphadenectomy: emerging role of lymphatic mapping and sentinel node biopsy in the management of early stage melanoma. *Semin Surg Oncol* 1993; 9: 219–223.
121. Krag DN, Meijer SJ, Weaver DL, et al. Minimal-access surgery for staging of melanoma. *Arch Surg* 1995; 130: 654–658.
122. Reintgen DS, Rapaport DP, Tanabe KK, Ross MI. Lymphatic mapping and sentinel lymphadenectomy. In: Balch CM, Houghton AN, Sober AJ, Soong SJ, eds. *Cutaneous Melanoma, 3rd ed.* Quality Medical Publishing, St. Louis, 1998; pp. 227–244.
123. Albertini JJ, Cruse CW, Rapaport D, et al. Intraoperative radiolymphoscintigraphy improves sentinel lymph node identification for melanoma patients. *Ann Surg* 1996; 223: 217–224.
124. Wang X, Heller R, VanVoorhis N, et al. Detection of submicroscopic lymph node metastasis with polymerase chain reaction in patients with malignant melanoma. *Ann Surg* 1994; 220: 768–774.
125. Gershenwald JE, Colome MI, Lee JE, et al. Patterns of recurrence following a negative sentinel lymph node biopsy in 243 patients with stage I or II melanoma. *J Clin Oncol* 1998; 16: 2253–2260.
126. Slingluff CL Jr, Vollmer RT, Reintgen DS, Seigler HF. Lethal "thin" malignant melanoma. Identifying patients at risk. *Ann Surg* 1988; 208: 150–161.
127. Balch CM, Buzaid AC. Finally a successful adjuvant therapy for high-risk melanoma [editorial]. *J Clin Oncol* 1996; 14: 1–3.
128. Provost N, Marghoob AA, Kopf AW, DeDavid M, Wasti Q, Bart RS. Laboratory tests and imaging studies in patients with cutaneous malignant melanomas: a survey of experienced physicians. *J Am Acad Dermatol* 1997; 36: 711–720.
129. Olson JA Jr, Jaques DP, Coit DG, Hwu WJ. Staging work-up and post-treatment surveillance of patients with melanoma. *Clin Plast Surg* 2000; 27: 377–390.

130. Weiss M, Loprinzi CL, Creagan ET, Dalton RJ, Novotny P, O'Fallon JR. Utility of follow-up tests for detecting recurrent disease in patients with malignant melanomas. *JAMA* 1995; 274: 1703–1705.
131. Balch CM. Cutaneous melanoma: prognosis and treatment results worldwide. *Semin Surg Oncol* 1992; 8: 400–414.
132. Balch CM, Murad TM, Soong SJ, Ingalls AL, Halpern NB, Maddox WA. A multifactorial analysis of melanoma: prognostic histopathological features comparing Clark's and Breslow's staging methods. *Ann Surg* 1978; 188: 732–742.
133. Balch CM, Soong SJ, Murad TM, Ingalls AL, Maddox WA. A multifactorial analysis of melanoma. II. Prognostic factors in patients with stage I (localized) melanoma. *Surgery* 1979; 86: 343–351.
134. Buttner P, Garbe C, Bertz J, et al. Primary cutaneous melanoma. Optimized cutoff points of tumor thickness and importance of Clark's level for prognostic classification. *Cancer* 1995; 75: 2499–2506.
135. Buzaid AC, Ross MI, Balch CM, et al. Critical analysis of the current American Joint Committee on Cancer staging system for cutaneous melanoma and proposal of a new staging system. *J Clin Oncol* 1997; 15: 1039–1051.
136. Schuchter L, Schultz DJ, Synnestvedt M, et al. A prognostic model for predicting 10-year survival in patients with primary melanoma. The Pigmented Lesion Group. *Ann Intern Med* 1996; 125: 369–375.
137. Gershenwald JE, Thompson W, Mansfield PF, et al. Multi-institutional melanoma lymphatic mapping experience: the prognostic value of sentinel lymph node status in 612 stage I or II melanoma patients. *J Clin Oncol* 1999; 17: 976–983.
138. Urist MM, Balch CM, Soong SJ, et al. Head and neck melanoma in 534 clinical Stage I patients. A prognostic factors analysis and results of surgical treatment. *Ann Surg* 1984; 200: 769–775.
139. Balch CM, Wilkerson JA, Murad TM, Soong SJ, Ingalls AL, Maddox WA. The prognostic significance of ulceration of cutaneous melanoma. *Cancer* 1980; 45: 3012–3017.
140. Buzaid AC, Tinoco LA, Jendiroba D, et al. Prognostic value of size of lymph node metastases in patients with cutaneous melanoma. *J Clin Oncol* 1995; 13: 2361–2368.
141. Drepper H, Biess B, Hofherr B, et al. The prognosis of patients with stage III melanoma. Prospective long-term study of 297 patients of the Frachklinik Hornheide. *Cancer* 1993; 71: 1239–1246.
142. Coit DG, Rogatko A, Brennan MF. Prognostic factors in patients with melanoma metastatic to axillary or inguinal lymph nodes. A multivariate analysis. *Ann Surg* 1991; 214: 627–636.
143. Karakousis CP, Hena MA, Emrich LJ, Driscoll DL. Axillary node dissection in malignant melanoma: results and complications. *Surgery* 1990; 108: 10–17.
144. Koh HK, Sober AJ, Day CL Jr, et al. Prognosis of clinical stage I melanoma patients with positive elective regional node dissection. *J Clin Oncol* 1986; 4: 1238–1244.
145. Morton DL, Wanek L, Nizze JA, Elashoff RM, Wong JH. Improved long-term survival after lymphadenectomy of melanoma metastatic to regional nodes. Analysis of prognostic factors in 1134 patients from the John Wayne Cancer Clinic. *Ann Surg* 1991; 214: 491–499.
146. Roses DF, Provet JA, Harris MN, Gumport SL, Dubin N. Prognosis of patients with pathologic stage II cutaneous malignant melanoma. *Ann Surg* 1985; 201: 103–107.
147. Cascinelli N, Vaglini M, Nava M, et al. Prognosis of skin melanoma with regional node metastases (stage II). *Surg Oncol* 1984; 25: 240–247.
148. Cascinelli N, Morabito A, Santinami M, et al. Immediate or delayed dissection of regional nodes in patients with melanoma of the trunk; a randomised trial. WHO Melanoma Programme. *Lancet* 1998; 351: 793–796.
149. Eton O, Legha SS, Moon TE, et al. Prognostic factors for survival of patients treated systemically for disseminated melanoma. *J Clin Oncol* 1998; 16: 1103–1111.

150. Balch CM, Soong SJ, Murad TM, Smith JW, Maddox WA, Durant JR. A multifactorial analysis of melanoma. IV. Prognostic factors in 200 melanoma patients with distant metastases (stage III). *J Clin Oncol* 1983; 1: 126–134.
151. Barth A, Wanek LA, Morton DL. Prognostic factors in 1,521 melanoma patients with distant metastases. *J Am Coll Surg* 1995; 181: 193–201.
152. Keilholz U, Conradt C, Legha SS, et al. Results of interleukin-2-based treatment in advanced melanoma: a case record-based analysis of 631 patients. *J Clin Oncol* 1998; 16: 2921–2929.
153. Deichmann M, Benner A, Bock M, et al. S100-Beta, melanoma-inhibiting activity, and lactate dehydrogenase discriminate progressive from non-progressive American Joint Committee on Cancer stage IV melanoma. *J Clin Oncol* 1999; 17: 1891–1896.
154. Agrawal S, Yao T-J, Coit DG. Surgery for melanoma metastatic to the gastrointestinal tract. *Ann Surg Oncol* 1999; 6: 336–344.
155. Franzke A, Probst-Kepper M, Buer J, et al. Elevated pretreatment serum levels of soluble vascular cell adhesion molecule 1 and lactate dehydrogenase as predictors of survival in cutaneous metastatic malignant melanoma. *Br J Cancer* 1998; 78: 40–45.
156. Sirott M, Bajorin D, Wong GY, et al. Prognostic factors in patients with metastatic malignant melanoma: a multivariate analysis. *Cancer* 1993; 72: 3091–3098.
157. Kuvshinoff BW, Kurtz C, Coit DG. Computed tomography in evaluation of patients with stage III melanoma. *Ann Surg Oncol* 1997; 4: 252–258.
158. Buzaid AC, Sandler AB, Mani S, et al. Role of computed tomography in the staging of primary melanoma. *J Clin Oncol* 1993; 11: 638–643.
159. Khansur T, Sanders J, Das S. Evaluation of staging workup in malignant melanoma. *Arch Surg* 1989; 124: 847–849.
160. Huang CL, Provost N, Marghoob AA, Kopf AW, Levin L, Bart RS. Laboratory tests and imaging studies in patients with cutaneous malignant melanoma. *J Am Acad Dermatol* 1998; 39: 451–463.
161. Coit DG. Role of surgery for metastatic malignant melanoma: a review. *Semin Surg Oncol* 1993; 9: 239–245.
162. Au F, Maier W, Malmud L, Goldman LI, Clark WH Jr. Preoperative nuclear scans in patients with melanoma. *Cancer* 1984; 53: 2095–2097.
163. Evans RA, Bland KI, McMurtrey MJ, Ballantyne AJ. Radionuclide scans not indicated for clinical stage I melanoma. *Surg Gynecol Obstet* 1980; 150: 532–534.
164. Roth JA, Eilber FR, Bennett LR, Morton DL. Radionuclide photoscanning: usefulness in preoperative evaluation of melanoma patients. *Arch Surg* 1975; 110: 1211–1212.
165. Zartman GM, Thomas MR, Robinson WA. Metastatic disease in patients with newly diagnosed malignant melanoma. *J Surg Oncol* 1987; 35: 163–164.
166. Holder WD Jr, White RL, Zuger JH, Easton EJ Jr, Greene FL. Effectiveness of positron emission tomography for the detection of melanoma metastases. *Ann Surg* 1998; 227: 764–769.
167. Rinne D, Baum RP, Hor G, Kaufmann R. Primary staging and follow-up of high risk melanoma patients with whole-body 18F-fluorodeoxyglucose positron emission tomography: results of a prospective study of 100 patients. *Cancer* 1998; 82: 1664–1671.
168. Slingluff CL Jr, Dodge RK, Stanley WE, Seigler HF. The annual risk of melanoma progression. Implications for the concept of cure. *Cancer* 1992; 70: 1917–1927.
169. Gadd MA, Coit DG. Recurrence patterns and outcome in 1019 patients undergoing axillary or inguinal lymphadenectomy for melanoma. *Arch Surg* 1992; 127: 1412–1416.
170. Koh HK, Sober AJ, Fitzpatrick TB. Late recurrence (beyond ten years) of cutaneous malignant melanoma. Report of two cases and a review of the literature. *JAMA* 1984; 251: 1859–1862.
171. Crowley NJ, Seigler HF. Late recurrence of malignant melanoma. Analysis of 168 patients. *Ann Surg* 1990; 212: 173–177.

172. McCarthy WH, Shaw HM, Thompson JF, Milton GW. Time and frequency of recurrence of cutaneous stage I malignant melanoma with guidelines for follow-up study. *Surg Gynecol Obstet* 1988; 166: 497–502.
173. Warso MA, Das Gupta TK. Melanoma recurrence in a previously dissected lymph node basin. *Arch Surg* 1994; 129: 252–255.
174. Fusi S, Ariyan S, Sternlicht A. Data on first recurrence after treatment for malignant melanoma in a large patient population. *Plast Reconstr Surg* 1993; 91: 94–98.
175. Reintgen DS, Cox C, Slingluff CL, Seigler HF. Recurrent malignant melanoma: the identification of prognostic factors to predict survival. *Ann Plast Surg* 1992; 28: 45–49.
176. Mooney MM, Kulas M, McKinley B, Michalek AM, Kraybill WG. Impact on survival by method of recurrence detection in stage I and II cutaneous melanoma. *Ann Surg Oncol* 1998; 5: 54–63.
177. Diagnosis and treatment of early melanoma. NIH Consensus Development Conference, January 27–29, 1992. *NIH Consensus Statement* 1992; 10: 1–25.
178. Houghton A, Coit DG, Bloomer W, et al. NCCN melanoma practice guidelines: National Comprehensive Cancer Network. *Oncology* 1998; 12: 153–177.

2 A Pathologist's Perspective on Prognostic Features of Malignant Melanoma

Ralph J. Tuthill, MD

Contents

1. INTRODUCTION

1.1. The Dysplasia-Melanoma Sequence and Borderline Melanocytic Neoplasia

Today, at the beginning of the twenty-first century, most dermatologists, surgeons, and oncologists that deal with melanoma patients have a simple view of pigment lesion pathology. It consists of benign nevus, including dysplastic nevus, *in situ* melanoma, and invasive melanoma. These are regarded as discrete entities with only minimal reference to a sequence of change from dysplasia to melanoma. Once invasive melanoma is diagnosed, the only additional necessary information is tumor thickness and the presence or absence of ulceration *(1,2)*.

From: *Current Clinical Oncology, Melanoma: Biologically Targeted Therapeutics*
Edited by: E. C. Borden © Humana Press Inc., Totowa, NJ

However, from a pathologist's point of view, the process of changing from a premalignant dysplasia to malignant melanoma is not that simple. A brief history of the past, present, and future of pigment lesion pathology is in order.

At the beginning of the twentieth century, patients, clinicians, and pathologists had two options for a pigmented lesion—either benign nevus or malignant melanoma. Granted that there were different types of benign nevus, but the decision would come down to either a benign nevus or a malignant melanoma. A diagnosis of malignant melanoma was followed by fear and radical surgery. It was not until the mid-twentieth century that pathologists began considering the possibilities of low-risk and high-risk melanoma. Borrowing from earlier work, pathologists developed the concepts of *in situ* and microinvasive melanomas that together constitute the so-called radial growth phase of melanoma *(3–6)*. Radial growth phase lesions are slowly enlarging and flat. Radial growth phase is qualified as nontumorigenic melanoma and considered low-risk disease with very little chance of metastasis. Metastasis and death is most consistently associated with the presence of so-called vertical growth, which is characterized by raised nodules of tumor.

The advent of the dysplastic nevus has changed the above categories of discrete entities to a continuum: the dysplasia–melanoma sequence. The dysplasia segment of the sequence begins with mild melanocytic dysplasia, progresses gradually to severe dysplasia, and ends with severe dysplasia and microinvasion, the so-called radial growth phase. Dysplasia and the radial growth phase become one and the same thing. In other words, radial growth phase is the end of the dysplasia segment of the dysplasia–melanoma sequence *(7–13)*.

The beginning of the melanoma segment of the dysplasia–melanoma sequence is best considered to reside in the beginning of vertical growth. There are two complementary ways of recognizing vertical growth: Clark's criteria *(14,15)* and Reed's criteria *(16,17)*.

Clark's criteria state that vertical growth is present when atypical melanocytes show that they can grow as an expansile aggregate in the dermis. Tumor cells are not merely dropping into the dermis as single cells and very small nests of cells, but are now characterized by nests that are larger than any in the overlying epidermis and measure 15 to 25 cells in diameter (Fig. 1; *see* Color Plate 6, following p. 176).

Reed's criteria are slightly different, but allow us to recognize vertical growth at an earlier stage of development.

Reed's criteria state that vertical growth is present when five or more nests of atypical melanocytes are present at two or more strata within the dermis. The melanocytes must show at least moderate cytologic atypia and occur within a preexisting dysplastic nevus showing moderate to severe melanocytic dysplasia (Fig. 2; *see* Color plate 7, following p. 176).

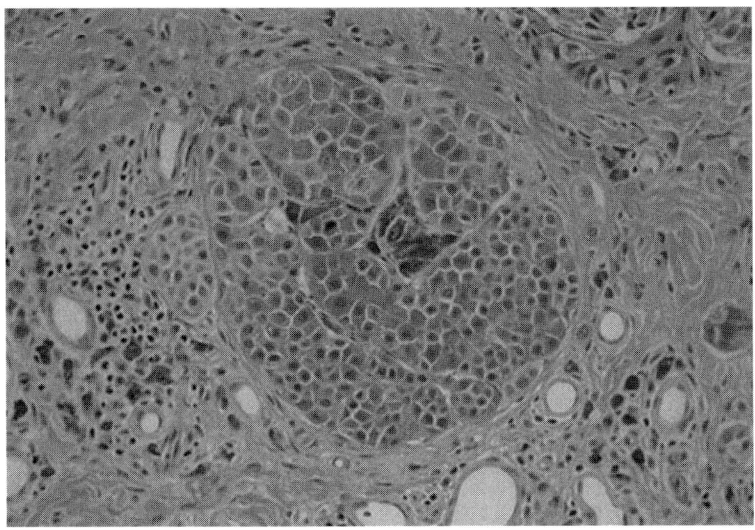

Fig. 1. Vertical growth. There is an expansile nest of cells in the dermis. It is 15 to 25 cells wide and larger than any nest in the overlying epidermis. This latter finding implies that the tumor cells have the ability to divide and multiply in the dermis, in contrast to simply dropping into the dermis.

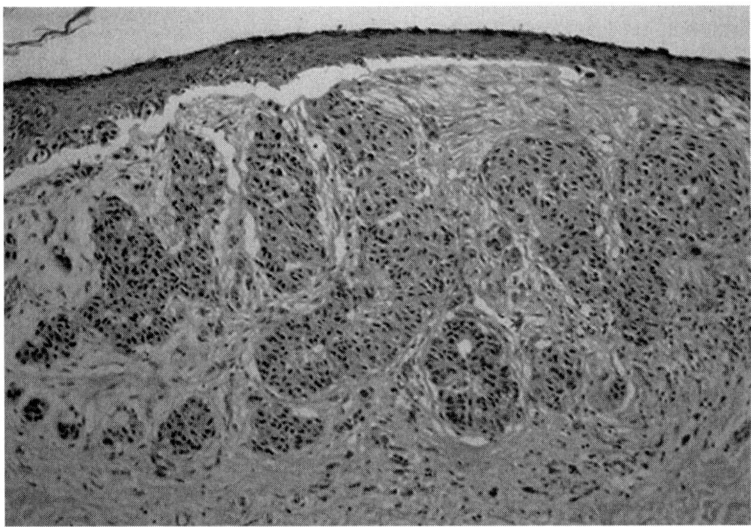

Fig. 2. Variant vertical growth. There are five or more nests of moderately atypical cells at two or more strata, which are separately and regularly spaced in the dermis. The individual nests do not need to meet the requirements of typical vertical growth. The stratification of the nests implies that the cells are being delivered to the dermis at an increased rate.

Table 1
Borderline Melanocytic Neoplasia

Borderline lesions: Dysplasia (radial growth) patterns:
Moderate to severe melanocytic dysplasia (melanoma *in situ*).
Severe melanocytic dysplasia (melanoma *in situ*; Pagetoid melanosis).
Compound melanocytic dysplasia (*in situ* and microinvasive melanoma).
Borderline lesions: Thin minimal deviation melanoma (vertical growth) patterns:
Arrested variant vertical growth.
Variant vertical growth.
Typical vertical growth (less than 1.0 mm thickness).

Any of the above borderline lesions may be seen with or without regression, and any of the above lesions may at times be associated with metastasis. Therefore, although the risk of recurrence and metastasis is low, none of the above lesions is without such risk, and the patient should be so advised.

These early steps of vertical growth are thin and measure less than 1.0 mm in vertical dimension. They are characteristically nevoid in appearance and are therefore referred to as minimal deviation. The biologic behavior of thin minimal deviation vertical growth is generally benign. Recurrence and metastasis are unlikely. However, as these lesions acquire more bulk and thickness that approaches 1.0 mm in vertical dimension, the risk for recurrence and metastasis increases. These early steps of vertical growth are in direct lineage with lesions that do metastasize.

The criteria for vertical growth of both Clark and Reed are not contradictory, but rather complementary.

2. BORDERLINE LESIONS (BORDERLINE MELANOCYTIC NEOPLASIA OF INDETERMINATE MALIGNANT POTENTIAL)

Borderline melanocytic neoplasms are those lesions of the dysplasia–melanoma sequence that are at the interface of premalignant dysplasia changing to malignant melanoma. The borderline lesions can be separated into dysplasia patterns and melanoma patterns (*see* Table 1). The dysplasia patterns include moderate to severe dysplasia, severe dysplasia, and *in situ* and microinvasive melanoma also known as radial growth phase. Melanoma patterns include the various patterns of thin minimal deviation vertical growth. Any of the above borderline lesions may be present with or without histologic regression. The presence of histologic regression adds an additional element of uncertainty, because the nature of the changes that have undergone regression cannot be determined. It is always possible that vertical growth with its risk of metastasis has regressed, but has metastasized before regressing.

Moderate to severe (Fig. 3; *see* Color Plate 8, following p. 176) and severe dysplasia (Fig. 4; *see* Color Plate 9, following p. 176) are patterns of atypical

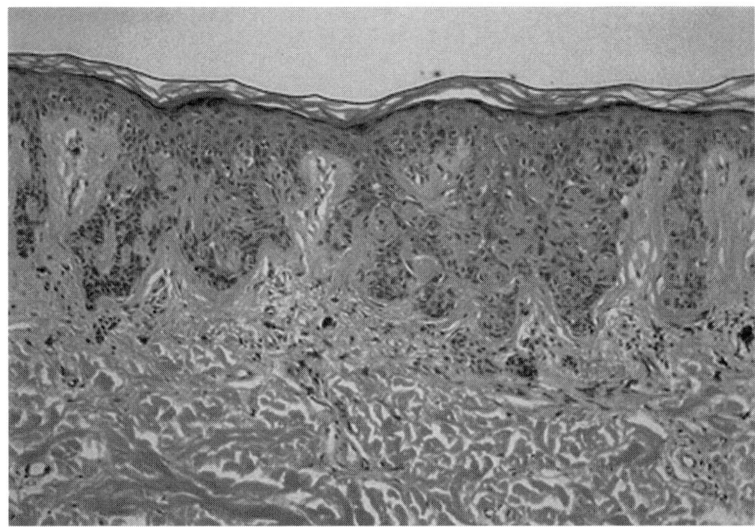

Fig. 3. Moderate to severe melanocytic dysplasia. There is elongation of the rete ridges with Pagetoid disarray in the lower half of the epidermis. Cytologic atypia of most of the melanocytes is moderate or severe. This pattern is equivalent to so-called melanoma *in situ*.

melanocytic proliferation within the epidermis and should be considered equivalent to melanoma *in situ*. They differ slightly, and moderate to severe dysplasia is a precursor step to severe dysplasia. Moderate to severe dysplasia is characterized by elongation of the rete ridges with lentiginous proliferation of atypical melanocytes. Pagetoid disarray is present but only in the lower half of the epidermis. Severe melanocytic dysplasia is characterized by extensive pagetoid disarray within the epidermis and reactive hyperplasia of the epidermis in the form of so-called acanthosis. This is the pattern that most pathologists and clinicians are familiar with as melanoma *in situ*.

When randomly scattered atypical melanocytes or small groups of melanocytes are present in the dermis, the lesion may be referred to as compound melanocytic dysplasia (Fig. 5; *see* Color Plate 10, following p. 176). When the pattern in the epidermis is that of moderate to severe or severe dysplasia, and there are similar appearing atypical melanocytes in the dermis, the compound dysplasia is currently considered *in situ* and microinvasive melanoma. Also, *in situ* and microinvasive melanoma is currently qualified as nontumorigenic melanoma with very little risk of metastasis. However, because we now have a dysplasia–melanoma sequence, the so-called *in situ* and microinvasive melanoma is best considered the end of the dysplasia segment of the sequence, rather than the beginning of the melanoma (vertical growth) segment.

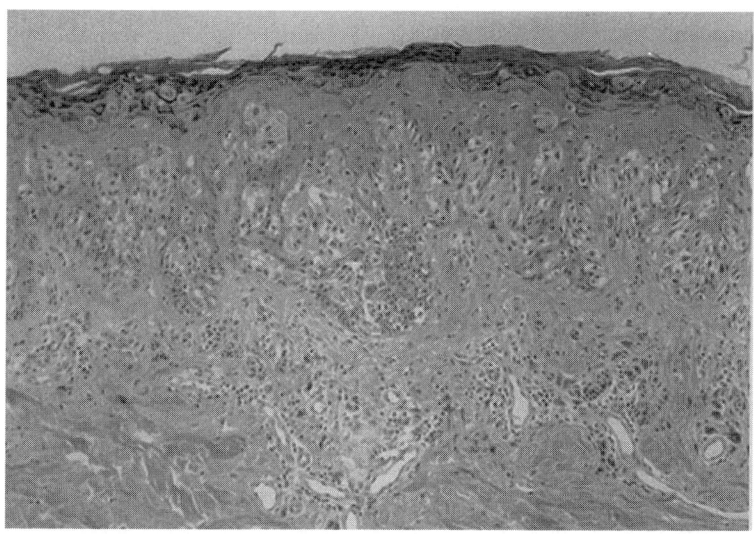

Fig. 4. Severe melanocytic dysplasia. There is extensive Pagetoid melanosis accompanied by broad acanthosis in the epidermis. This pattern is equivalent to so-called melanoma *in situ*.

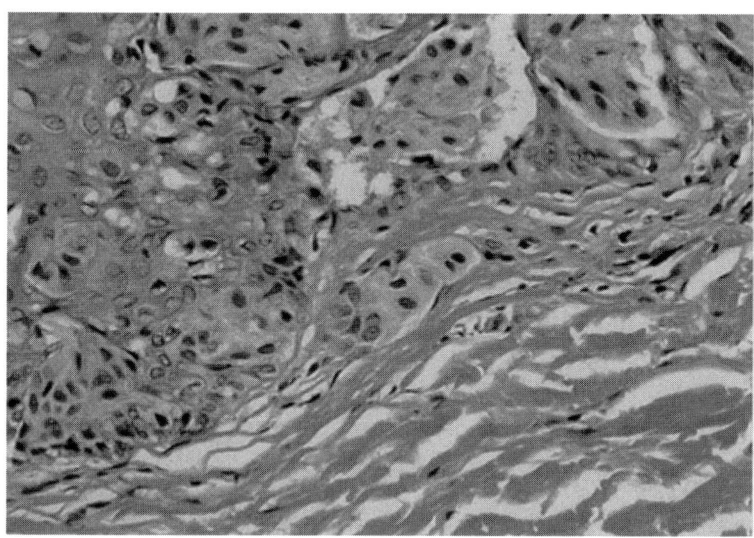

Fig. 5. Severe compound melanocytic dysplasia. There is Pagetoid growth of atypical melanocytes in the epidermis and a single nest of similar appearing atypical melanocytes in the papillary dermis. Synonyms are radial growth phase dysplasia (level II pattern) and nontumorigenic melanoma. This pattern is not associated with recurrence and metastasis, unless there is regression present or occult vertical growth elsewhere in the lesion.

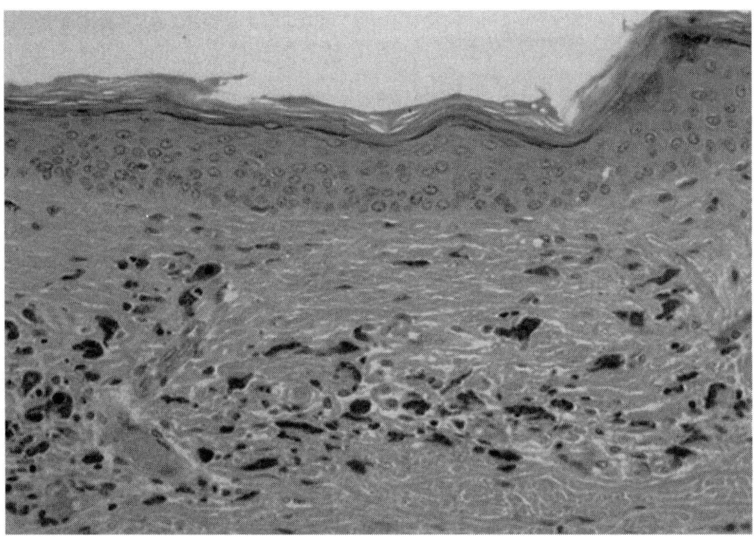

Fig. 6. Histology of regression. There is absence of atypical melanocytes in the epidermis and dermis accompanied by mild chronic inflammation and melanoderma. The nature of the changes that have undergone regression cannot be determined.

Therefore, borderline dysplasia patterns include moderate to severe dysplasia, severe dysplasia, and even those patterns that most pathologists consider *in situ* and microinvasive disease *(7–9)*. There are two caveats to remember. One is that histologic interpretation is always subject to sampling error. When a specimen is submitted for histologic examination, it is bisected or serial sectioned at 2- to 3-mm intervals. In other words, each piece of tissue measures 2 to 3 mm in thickness. Melanomatous vertical growth of a millimeter or less in thickness may be in the tissue, but not examined histologically. Fortunately, this is a rare event. The second caveat is that when histologic regression (Fig. 6; *see* Color Plate 11, following p. 176) is present, we can only comment on what is seen and not what may have been present before regression occurred. Therefore, any interpretation, which includes the presence of regression, must be considered a conservative estimate of risk. Again, fortunately, there are few adverse outcomes when regression is present in a pattern of dysplasia.

Borderline melanoma patterns are vertical growth patterns that measure less than 1.0 mm in vertical dimension (thickness). Nests of atypical melanocytes separated by bands of fibrous tissue characterize the earliest pattern of thin minimal deviation vertical growth (Fig. 2). The nests are nevoid in appearance but at least moderately atypical in cytology. When separated in this fashion, they are referred to as early variant vertical growth. If the fibrous tissue is dense and hyalinized, the variant vertical growth is further qualified as arrested variant

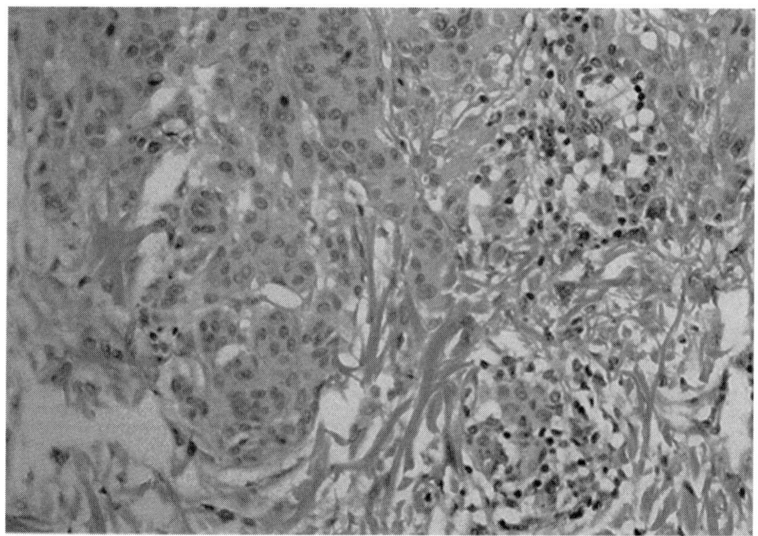

Fig. 7. Thin (0.76 mm) level IV vertical growth with subsequent metastasis and death. Thin metastasizing melanoma has vertical growth, occult vertical growth elsewhere in the lesion, or regression. Level IV involvement implies migratory behavior by the tumor cells.

vertical growth. Variant vertical growth is a precursor step to typical vertical growth (Fig. 1) characterized by closely spaced nests and sheets of tumor cells. Typical vertical growth is usually characterized by high-grade cytology, measures 1.0 mm or greater in thickness, and is no longer a borderline lesion. It is important to stress that we are talking about evolutionary steps of vertical growth toward malignancy and not the magic of one cell crossing a basement membrane.

3. A CAVEAT—THIN METASTASIZING LEVEL IV MELANOMA

We are all aware of the thin metastasizing primary melanomas. Usually they are vertical growth phase melanoma and show migrant or infiltrative growth into the reticular dermis (Fig. 7; *see* Color Plate 12, following p. 176). If they do not show vertical growth, they show regression or are incomplete biopsies of larger lesions. The recent staging committee of the American Joint Committee on Cancer (AJCC) has wisely chosen to include Level IV and Level V lesions in the T1b category along with ulceration for lesions that are 1.0 mm in thickness or less *(1)*.

4. HISTOPATHOLOGIC FACTORS RELEVANT TO PROGNOSIS IN VERTICAL GROWTH PHASE MELANOMA

Once a lesion of the dysplasia–melanoma sequence has acquired vertical growth and is 1.0 mm or greater in vertical dimension, the lesion has entered a phase of development that is associated with greater risk of metastasis. For years, pathologists and clinicians have been looking a various attributes of primary localized melanoma in order to predict which patients will have metastasis either at initial diagnosis or in the future.

4.1. Thickness

The value of tumor thickness in risk assessment has been confirmed over and over again since it was first proposed in 1970 *(1,18–22)*. This is for two reasons. First, tumor thickness is directly proportional to the number of cells present in a vertical growth nodule and, therefore, proportional to the risk that the nodule of melanoma has given rise to the one cell that can go through the complicated steps of successful metastasis. Melanoma cells must not only survive at the primary site but also travel and survive at a distant site, and not every melanoma cell has that ability. Second, tumor thickness is proportional to the amount of time that has passed *(23)*. It takes time for the dysplasia–melanoma sequence to evolve the cells that can successfully metastasize. Therefore, tumor thickness is not just another way of expressing invasiveness. Thickness or bulk is a different attribute than invasiveness.

Tumor thickness is most appropriately applied to lesions of the dysplasia–melanoma sequence that are in vertical growth. The method for obtaining tumor thickness has been clearly defined by Breslow *(20)*. The key is to select the area for measurement that most appropriately reflects tumor bulk (Fig. 8; *see* Color Plate 13, following p. 176). The Breslow tumor thickness is not a measure of invasiveness, but rather tumor bulk. The pathologist should avoid measuring sections that are tangential sections and should avoid measuring areas that may represent growth from an adjacent skin appendage, which might give an unfairly thick measurement. The recently proposed new AJCC staging system for cutaneous melanoma has reviewed 22 studies that used the Cox model to assess prognostic factors. The authors concluded that in virtually all the studies, tumor thickness and ulceration are the strongest predictors *(1)*. Similarly, in 54 multivariate studies, tumor thickness was the strongest predictor *(21)*. In a recently completed Southwest Oncology Group (SWOG) multivariate Cox regression study of vertical growth phase melanoma, tumor thickness was one of three independent predictive factors *(24)*.

Tumor thickness is often separated into categories of different thickness or so-called breakpoints. At times, investigators have tried to define natural breakpoints, implying different risks or stages of disease. Various mathematical models of risk assessment have used various thickness categories to assess risk. However, melanoma thickness has no natural breakpoints for risk, and survival in melanoma has a continuous curved line relationship to tumor thickness (Fig. 9). An equation for an exponential transformation of thickness into a continuous variable, which can be used in Cox model regression analysis to predict survival, has been developed *(25)*. This transformation of thickness has been

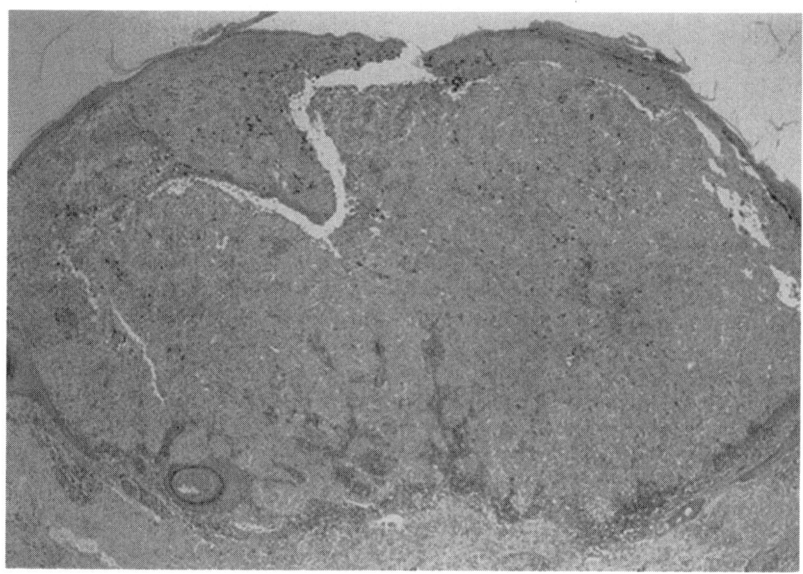

Fig. 8. Breslow's tumor thickness measurement. Vertical dimensions of a tumor nodule are measured at a right angle to the surface of the epidermis. The measurement is taken from the top of the granular layer to the deepest tumor cell. Angio-lymphatic spread and satellitosis are not used in obtaining the measurement. If ulceration is present as in this case, the measurement uses the top of the base of the ulcer and includes the fibrinopurulent exudate.

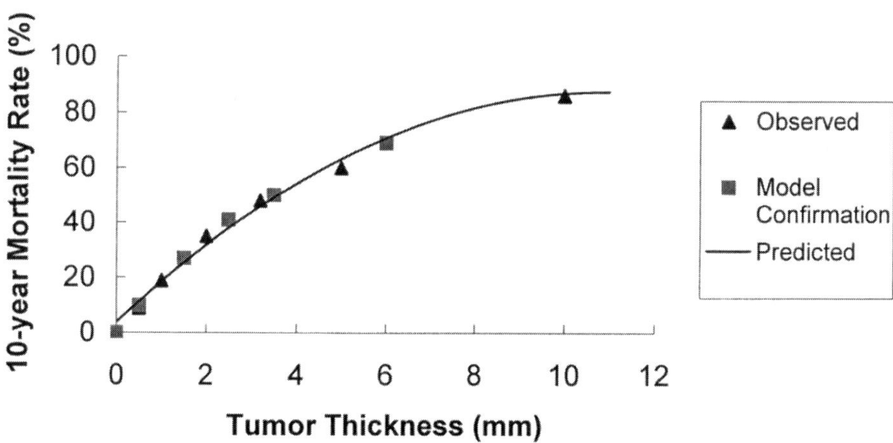

Fig. 9. Stadelmann curve of tumor thickness and survival. The 10-yr mortality in 2627 patients with melanoma related to tumor thickness is a gentle curve without any natural breakpoints. (From Balch CM, Houghton AN, Sober AJ, Soon S-J, Cutaneous Melanoma, 3rd edition. St. Louis, Quality Medical Publishing, 1999.)

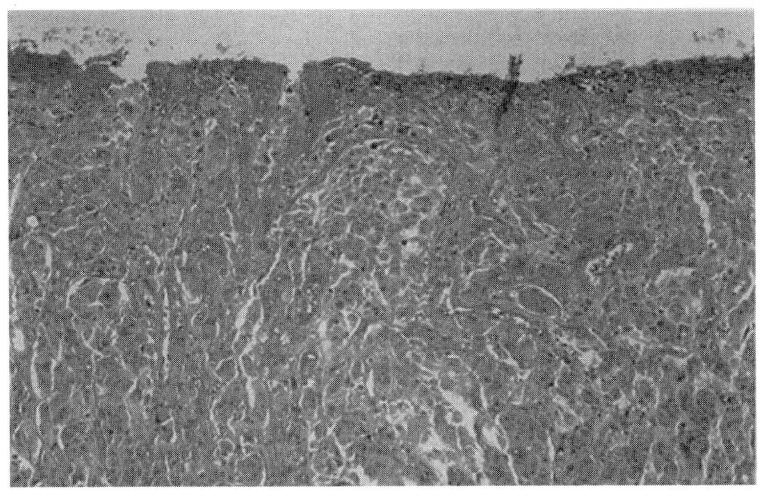

Fig. 10. Ulceration. There is absence of the epidermis with a fibrino-purulent exudate. Ulceration, as well as tumor thickness, is important in risk assessment of primary localized melanoma.

evaluated in 1910 of their patients and found that it can be used without re-sorting to artificial cut points *(26)*. This transformation avoids the problem of small changes in tumor thickness becoming large changes in a hazard score for survival.

Finally, it is appropriate to stress that Breslow's tumor thickness is not just another way of expressing invasiveness. Some melanomas are pedunculated and do not invade the reticular dermis or subcutis, but are thick tumors with significant risk of metastasis proportionate to their thickness.

4.2. Ulceration

Ulceration is defined as absence of intact epidermis overlying a vertical growth phase nodule or plaque (Fig. 10; *see* Color Plate 14, following p. 176). It is important to identify a fibrino-purulent exudate on the surface as evidence of real ulceration and not simply an artifact of the laboratory technique. The AJCC Melanoma Staging Committee reviewed 13 Cox regression analysis studies of melanoma, which included ulceration, and found that in virtually every study in which ulceration was associated with, a worse prognosis existed compared to melanomas of similar thickness that were not ulcerated *(1)*. In the 54 studies, ulceration was important in 20 studies, not significant in 25 studies, and not evaluated in 9 studies *(21)*. Ulceration was independently predictive of survival in a recent multivariate study of 1910 patients *(26)*. In the recently completed SWOG study, the presence or absence of ulceration was marginally predictive of survival with $P = 0.06$ *(24)*.

4.3. Clark's Levels of Invasion and Radial Growth Versus Vertical Growth

In the mid-twentieth century, it became apparent to many that prognosis in melanoma varied with depth of penetration by the melanoma, and many began talk of superficial forms of the disease in contrast to more deeply penetrating melanomas. Levels of invasion consisting of *in situ*, papillary dermis, reticular dermis, and subcutaneous tissue was proposed *(27)*. In 1969, Clark modified these levels into 5 levels and, in 1975, defined radial growth phase and vertical growth phase melanoma *(3,28)*. It is unfortunate that Clark did not modify his levels of invasion to fit better with the concept of radial growth and vertical growth. Many pathologist now use a modification of Clark's levels, because it seems quite natural and appropriate to equate levels I and II with radial growth and levels III, IV, and V with vertical growth *(8,9)*.

Levels of invasion and growth phase assess different aspects of tumor biology than tumor thickness. Levels of invasion and growth phase assess patterns of biologic growth and stages of tumor progression, whereas tumor thickness assesses tumor bulk. They are quite different aspects of tumor biology. Tumor thickness has less to do with invasiveness than levels of invasion and growth phase. Level IV invasion retains some usefulness in risk assessment, particularly in thin lesions, and has been retained by the AJCC staging committee for cutaneous melanoma for use in lesions that measure less than 1.0 mm *(1)*. For lesions that are greater than 1.0 mm in thickness, the level of invasion gives no statistically significant information relative to prognosis.

4.4. Tumor Infiltrating Lymphocytes

Pathologists in the past have noticed that the presence or absence of a host response in the form of lymphocytic inflammation may correlate with biologic outcome, but none have attempted to grade it into categories and evaluate it statistically until Clark et al. *(14)*. Clark et al. defined three categories of tumor infiltrating lymphocytes (TIL). A brisk host response of TIL was present when a band of lymphocytes completely surrounded a vertical growth phase nodule or plaque (Fig. 11; *see* Color Plate 15, following p. 176). The lymphocytes may also infiltrate throughout the vertical growth, but may be restricted to the periphery. Even if restricted to the periphery, the lymphocytes should show close relationship with tumor cells, by at least partially infiltrating the vertical growth. If there was a defect in this band-like quality, the TILs were classified as nonbrisk, and if lymphocytes were present but infiltrating the tumor, e.g., perivascular, TILs were classified as absent. Clark et al. found TIL an independent predictor of survival with $P = 0.0015$. Using the same categories of tumor infiltrating lymphocytes and analyzing patient survival with the Cox regression model, the

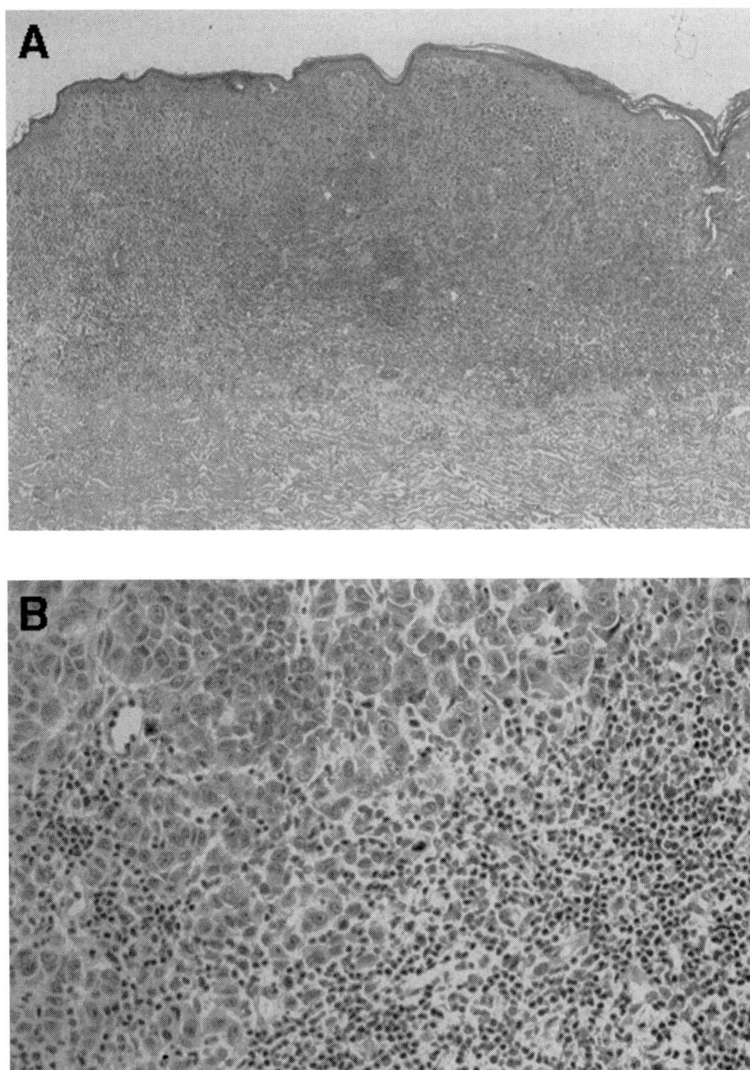

Fig. 11. TILs. **(A)** A dense band of lymphocytes surrounds the vertical growth phase nodule (low magnification). **(B)** Lymphocytes surround individual tumor cells as well as small groups of cells (intermediate magnification).

presence of tumor infiltrating lymphocytes was found to be an independent positive predictive factor *(29)*. And similarly, the SWOG study found TIL to significant predictor with $P = 0.005$ *(24)*. Vollmer did not include host response in his review of studies *(21)*.

4.5. Mitotic Activity and Rate of Proliferation

Most studies, which have looked at mitotic rate and survival in melanoma, show that survival is inversely related to mitotic activity. However, it is not consistently found to be an independent predictor of survival *(21,24)*. The mitotic rate is recorded differently from study to study. In some studies, it is simply grades of low, medium, or high mitotic activity based upon the number of mitoses per a specified number of high power fields. Not all microscopes are the same, and field size may vary from scope to scope and, therefore, from study to study. The best way to count mitoses is per square millimeter using a micrometer to calculate the area of one high power field. Schmoeckel and Braun-Falco published a method and index, in which they counted at least 1.5 mm^2, converted the count to mitoses per 1.0 mm^2, and multiplied the result by the tumor thickness *(30)*. This product was called the prognostic index. The index was divided into categories of low risk for values of 0 to 6.0, intermediate risk for values of 6.1 to 12.0, and high risk for values of 12.1 or above. Some melanomas are early and thin, and it is difficult to count even 1 mm^2 without going to step sections or otherwise extrapolating.

Proliferation rates can be estimated by other means. DNA flow cytometry of cells removed from paraffin-embedded sections can be used to estimate the proliferation rate via the Hedley technique *(31)*. However, estimation of the proliferative or S-phase fraction is plagued by problems of contamination by normal cells and variability from laboratory to laboratory *(32)*. Proliferation may be estimated by using immunohistology and antibodies to Ki-67, a nuclear protein elevated in cells that are cycling through phases of replication and cell division. Using the MIB-1 antibody to Ki-67, many groups have found decreased survival in patients with tumors that express high levels of MIB-1 immunoreactivity *(33–36)*.

4.6. Regression

Regression is defined histologically as complete absence of atypical melanocytes in the epidermis and dermis following a host response of inflammation. Fibrosis and chronic inflammation with melanoderma as evidence of a prior melanocytic proliferation is characteristically present (Fig. 6). Regression may be focal and measure no more than 0.30 mm in radial extent, or it may be extensive and measure up to a centimeter or greater in extent. If the area of regression is large, it is more likely to be recognized clinically. If regression is present, neither pathologist nor clinician can determine with certainty the nature of the changes that have undergone regression. Both radial growth dysplasia and vertical growth melanoma patterns may have undergone regression. Therefore, the presence of regression adds uncertainty to risk assessment, and any interpretation must be accepted as a conservative estimate of risk. Clark et al. found that the

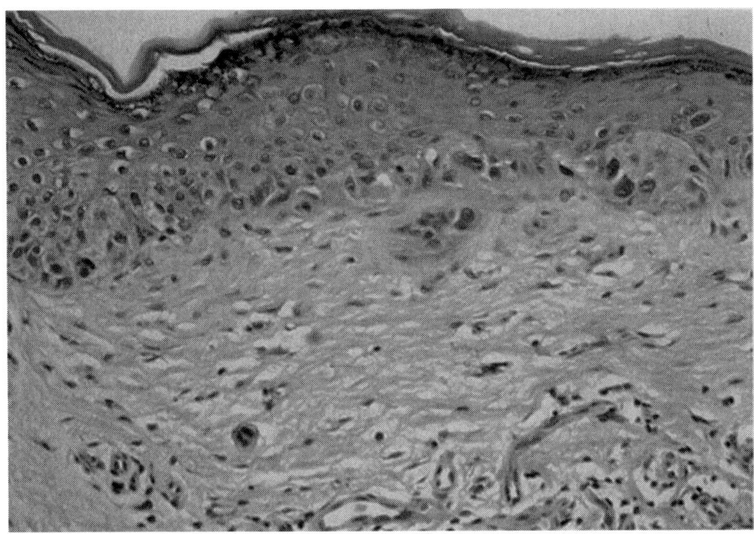

Fig. 12. Immune-reactive stroma (incomplete regression). Tumor cells are present in the epidermis and in the dermis as small groups and single cells. There is prominent fibrosis, chronic inflammation, and new blood vessel formation. All of this indicates that there has been prolonged interaction between the dysplastic process and the patient's tissues. A vertical growth phase nodule may have occurred and disappeared. Risk assessment must be considered a conservative estimate.

presence or absence of regression was an independent predictive factor and used it along with other factors in developing a predictive model *(14)*. However, the predictive validity waxed and waned as they followed the outcome of the patients in their cohort. In the SWOG study, regression was not an independent predictive factor *(24)*. In Vollmer's review of multivariate studies, regression was significant in 3 studies, not significant in 21 studies, and not evaluated in 30 studies *(21)*. In summary, although the presence of regression cannot be used to predict outcome, its presence adds an element of uncertainty.

4.7. Immune-Reactive Stroma (Incomplete Regression)

Although there have been no thorough studies, and definition for incomplete regression is not clearly delineated, a similar element of uncertainty must arise when a lesion shows unusually prominent chronic inflammation, fibrosis, and new blood vessel formation without complete absence of tumor cells in the epidermis and dermis (Fig. 12; *see* Color Plate 16, following p. 176). We must assume that there has been a prolonged interaction between the neoplasm and the patient's immune response and that there is a history we can no longer see in the lesion being examined. That past history may include vertical growth, even though all that is seen is radial growth dysplasia or thin minimal deviation vertical growth. It is difficult to define the immune-reactive stroma as separate from the reactive changes that occur in the lateral junctional spread of atypical nevi but should, in part, consist of fibrosis in the papillary dermis, which is not specifically related to the rete ridges. The fibrosis expands the papillary dermis in a manner very similar to that commonly seen in regression. However, a few surviving atypical melanocytes are present in the dermis and epidermis. When such a stroma is present, it is justification for qualifying the interpretation of risk as being a conservative estimate.

4.8. Angio-Lymphatic Spread and Localized Satellitosis

Angio-lymphatic spread and localized satellitosis are closely related entities. Vascular involvement implies a recognizable vascular structure with intravascular tumor. The pathologist must look for evidence of organization, such as adherence to endothelial lining cells with fibrin and growth of endothelium over the aggregate of tumor. This is in order to exclude technical artifact of tissue carry-over from tumor elsewhere in the specimen. Similarly, localized satellitosis must be distinguished from tissue carry-over. Also, the satellites, if close to the main tumor, may simply be the advancing edge of infiltrative growth and not true discontinuous groups of tumor cells. Clark et al. looked at both angio-lymphatic spread and satellitosis and found that neither was an independent predictor of survival *(14)*. Although both were associated with poor survival, neither was an independent predictor. The SWOG study did not evaluate either finding. In Vollmer's review, satellites were significant in 3 of 11 studies, and vascular invasion was significant in 3 of 10 studies *(21)*. These changes were not evaluated in 41 studies. Therefore, neither angio-lymphatic spread and satellitosis can be used as an independent predictor, but both are associated with an adverse outcome, and both imply greater likelihood of failure to control local recurrence if re-excision of the primary site is not performed.

4.9. Desmoplastic Growth Patterns

Rare melanomas are pure desmoplastic melanomas and, as such, are often very interesting in that a precursor radial growth dysplasia is not seen. Sometimes, this can be explained by the history of a prior excision, biopsy, or electrodesiccation without histologic examination. But some patients with pure desmoplastic melanomas give no such history, and there is very little evidence of a precursor lesion. Desmoplastic patterns are usually accompanied by chronic inflammation, and if no precursor lesion or other common pattern of melanoma is present, the lesion is unfortunately misdiagnosed as chronic inflammation without recognizing the malignant qualities present. More commonly, desmoplastic patterns arise in lentigo maligna melanoma or superficial spreading melanoma, and if they are small and limited in extent, they may be overlooked by the pathologist. These small focal desmoplastic patterns, if overlooked, probably do not make a significant difference to the patient as long as the lesion is completely excised. However, desmoplastic melanomas that are extensive and close to the margins of excision are likely to be problems of local recurrence. Therefore, these patterns should be highlighted by the pathologist, and the clinicians should modify their plans for local control of the melanoma accordingly.

4.10. Neurotropic Spread

Neurotropic spread is a rare phenomenon that, when present, is usually associated with desmoplastic vertical growth. Both desmoplastic and neurotropic patterns of spread represent a heteromorphism or change in the appearance and biologic behavior of the melanoma. Vollmer did not mention finding any studies to evaluate neurotropism, and the Clark study and SWOG study did not evaluate neurotropic growth *(21)*. Nevertheless, when identified in a primary melanoma, it should be considered a warning sign for increased risk of local recurrence, particularly if the neurotropic spread is at a distance from the primary tumor. Patients with neurotropic spread can be very uncomfortable with pain, if the involvement is advanced and widespread.

4.11. Angioplasia

The vertical growth phase nodule of melanoma is the perfect example of Juda Folkman's tumor with neovascularization. There have been some attempts at relating angiogenesis to survival in melanoma with varied results. Clark et al. showed that grading the amount of vascular proliferation as absent or sparse versus moderate or brisk had no predictive value at all *(14)*. More recently, Neitzel et al. compared primaries from patients with and without metastasis *(37)*. They used immunostaining with antibodies to factor VIII-related antigen and counted vessels in a specified area. The results showed increased numbers of positive staining vessels in patients with metastasis, and interestingly, those patients with distant metastasis had more vessels in the primary tumor than patients with only lymph node metastasis. There is currently a great deal of interest in the vascularity of solid tumors such as melanoma, and clinicians are beginning to evolve therapeutic trials of anti-angiogenesis agents. However, there is very little past experience in counting vessels as an aid in risk assessment.

4.12. Histologic Subtype

Histologic subtypes such as nodular melanoma, superficial spreading melanoma, and lentigo maligna melanoma are based upon the character of the precursor severe dysplasia or radial growth phase and not on the nature of the melanomatous or vertical growth phase. It should be no surprise, then, that survival in these categories of melanoma relates more to the nature of the vertical growth than the radial growth. Studies have confirmed that thickness for thickness, these categories of melanoma have similar survival *(21,38)*. However, these categories probably have different pathways of etiology. For instance, superficial spreading and nodular melanoma characteristically arise from the common dysplastic nevus and are more commonly seen in patients with the dysplastic nevus syndrome. Whereas lentigo maligna melanoma evolves from sun-damaged skin and the precursor dysplasia, which is referred to as lentigo maligna. Similarly, acral lentiginous melanomas and mucosal lentiginous melanomas arise from precursor dysplasias unique to the site and probably involve pathways of evolution separate from the dysplastic nevus syndrome and chronic actinic damage.

4.13. Pigmentation

The presence or absence of pigmentation or the amount of pigmentation have absolutely nothing to do with survival in melanoma of any site or type. Further, it is difficult to grade the degree of melanin pigmentation or to say that it is completely absent, because melanin is very effective in producing clinically apparent pigmentation when very little is present histologically.

5. PREDICTING SURVIVAL (RISK ASSESSMENT) USING STATISTICAL–MATHEMATICAL MODELS

A diagnosis of malignant melanoma implies a risk of recurrence, metastasis, and death. In the early twentieth century, that risk was not qualified as low or high, and any diagnosis of melanoma was followed by fear and radical surgery. Now, with organized data and follow-up information, we can refine the risks for patients. The simplest way is to look at the survival after a diagnosis of melanoma without any other qualification. In this simple manner, survival is 78.4% at 10 yr. If one excludes the dysplasia patterns (radial growth phase), the survival drops to 71.2% at 8 yr, and 55% at 10 yr in selected studies. Tumor thickness remains the strongest single attribute to further refine risk assessment. If tumor thickness is stratified or broken down into breakpoints, survival is noted to vary as follows: <0.76 mm, 91.75%; 0.76–1.49 mm, 81.13%; 1.50–2.49 mm, 66.5%; 2.50–3.99 mm, 56.75%; 4.00–7.99 mm, 56.5%; and ≥8.00 mm, 25%. It is currently believed to be most practical to have the following breakpoints with corresponding survival: ≤1.00 mm, 91.2%; 1.1–2.0 mm, 74.5%; 2.10–4.00 mm, 57.2%; and >4.00 mm, 44.00% *(1,2,22)*.

Within the last 10 to 15 yr, there have been several attempts to increase the accuracy of predicting survival in localized primary cutaneous melanoma by combining additional clinical and pathologic variables with tumor thickness. The result is usually expressed by plugging the variables into a mathematical equation that is then solved. The solved product may be either a percentage estimate of survival at a certain time point or a number that is used as an index to define low-risk or high-risk disease. For such a probability model to be useful in risk assessment for an individual patient, several criteria must be satisfied: (*i*) the patient under consideration and the patients in the study from which the model was derived must be comparable; (*ii*) the clinical state predicted by the model must be relevant to the clinical situation of the patient under consideration; (*iii*) all of the input variables used by the model must be available for the patient under consideration; (*iv*) the calculated result of the model must useful to the clinician and patient; (*v*) the degree of uncertainty in the result must be small enough to be useful to the clinician and patient; (*vi*) the outcome probabilities determined by the model must be close to the outcomes actually observed in the study patients from which the model was derived; and (*vii*) the model must be validated and compared to traditional methods using a separate population of patients from which it was derived *(39)*.

There are several models published in the literature that may meet the above criteria. Clark et al. published a study in 1989 that provided both a mathematical equation and a table for use in risk assessment of individual patients *(14)*. Six factors or attributes were the independent variables used to arrive at the dependent variable of survival prediction in the form of a percentage probability of survival at 8 yr. Eight-year survival was justified, because most survival failures occur within an 8-yr follow-up. Presenting the probabilities as 2 tables makes the model easy for a clinician to use without having to use a computer or calculator. Clark et al. validated their model using a separate population of patients and compared the results to survival probabilities obtained by tumor thickness alone. The McNemar's test was used to compare the number of correct predictions. Their model was found to have an error rate of 16.9% when validated. This compared to an error rate of 15.9% in the population of patients used to derive the model and was significantly better than 24.2% error rate of thickness alone.

There have been several attempts to test or validate the Clark model using patients in different databases. Fifty-three patients with a 10-yr follow-up were used in one test of the Clark model to predict survival *(40)*. It is not clear from the published report whether the Clark model was correct 75.5 or 58.5% of the time in their group of patients. It is also not clear whether or not radial growth phase lesions were included or excluded. It appears that they included radial growth phase lesions. Clearly, the authors did not count mitoses in the same way as did Clark et al. Therefore, it is doubtful that this report can support or question the usefulness of the Clark model. Fifty-five patients with an 8-yr follow-up were rigorously studied with the same criteria as Clark et al. Radial growth phase was separated from vertical growth and mitoses counted *(41)*. The authors were 85.1% correct in predicting survival among those patients with vertical growth phase melanoma. Eight of eight patients with radial growth phase melanomas survived as predicted by the Clark model. In 259 patients enrolled in a SWOG study of vitamin A, of the patients with localized melanoma and a minimum follow-up of 10 yr, all had vertical growth phase tumors *(24)*. Accuracy of the model using the McNemar test was only 62.5%. This finding in a large group of patients leaves in doubt the usefulness of the Clark model.

A 4-variable model was developed using a database of 488 patients *(42,43)*. The goal of the model was to predict survival at 10 yr using variables that are commonly available in pathology reports and not restricted to reports from specialists in pigment lesion pathology. They chose 6 variables (tumor thickness, age, site, gender, histologic subtype, and level of invasion) for univariate analysis. Four of these were significantly associated with outcome and were entered into a multivariate logistic regression model. Point estimates with corresponding confidence intervals were then generated for patients within the various strata of the 4 variables. Thus, a table similar to that of the Clark model was generated. They used a separate population of 142 patients to validate the model. The model correctly predicted survival in 74% of the original 488 patients, but only 69% of the validation sample. This latter value is essentially identical to prediction accuracy of 68% by tumor thickness alone. This data was subsequently studied and, in a limited fashion, corroborated *(44)*. Those studied were 780 patients using multivariate logistic regression to create a similar model and table *(44)*. Upon comparison, both tables showed similar point estimates and confidence intervals *(43,44)*. However, gender was not an independent variable in the second study *(44)*.

The Scottish Melanoma Group database of 1978 patients was used to derive a prediction model *(45)*. In 1991, a study determined that there was no evidence for breakpoints in tumor thickness related to prognosis. In 1995, a proportional hazards model was developed relating 5-yr survival to gender, ulceration, site, mitoses, Clark's levels, and thickness as a continuous variable. The model was successful with 1128 new patients *(46)*. Tumor thickness was analyzed at 1.0, 3.0, and 5.0 mm, but remained a continuous variable in the mathematical equation used to derive the predictors. Survival at any one tumor thickness could vary markedly depending on the other variables *(46)*. For instance, a woman with a nonulcerated 1.0 mm primary has predicted 5-yr survival of 94%, whereas a man with an ulcerated, level 3, 4, or 5 primary of 1.0 mm thickness has only a 51% predicted survival *(46)*.

The above model was transformed into 4 figures called "prognostic trees" based upon log rank tests at each step of the tree, with at least 50 patients at each node *(47)*. New branches of the diagnostic tree were formed until no further prognostic information could be obtained from the data. Each of the final branches gives probability of survival at 2 and 5 yr. The authors evaluated the performance of the prognostic trees by using data from 300 new patients and found the observed survival to be essentially the same as the predicted survival.

Several versions of prognostic models beginning in 1985 have been evolved from the University of Alabama database *(48–51)*. These models, using Cox's proportional hazards regression model, are based upon data obtained from patients of both the University of Alabama in Birmingham and the Sydney Melanoma Unit (Australia). It began in 1985 with a combined data set of 1096 patients. The patient characteristics, methods of data collection, and patient management and follow-up were virtually the same for both groups of patients. The original model published in 1985 required the use of unique software written specifically for the task of assessing risk in melanoma patients. The software was run on either a microcomputer or mainframe computer used on a time-share basis. The result was a probability of survival at that changed at yearly intervals from diagnosis to 10 yr. The probability of survival at 10 yr was then called a clinical score that could be ranked into categories or stages of risk and, thereby, used in making patient management decisions.

In 1992, a more user-friendly model using Cox's method, but expressed as tables, which could be used without special software or a computer, was published *(49,50)*. Predicted survival at 5 and 10 yr was given in a single table, which included input variables of thickness, site, ulceration, Clark's level, and gender. The point estimates of probability were not accompanied by confidence intervals. Four tables were devised that gave survival probability estimates at disease-free intervals of 2, 5, 10, 15, and 20 yr. The input variables included thickness, ulceration, and site. Thickness, ulceration, and site were important in estimating 2- and 5-yr survival. Tumor thickness and site were important for 10-yr estimates, and tumor thickness alone for survival beyond 10 yr. Therefore, it seems that different attributes are important at different time intervals of survival. A subsequent report on this model had no important changes *(51)*.

With the recent interest in sentinel lymph node sampling, the above methods of risk analysis will lose even the limited interest that was given to them before. There may still, however, be a place for statistical risk assessment before sentinel lymph node examination *(52)*. In assessment of 573 patients, a mathematical model was developed predicting the finding of a positive lymph node in lymph node dissections performed within 1 yr of excising the primary. This was an attempt to simulate the current sentinel lymph node procedure, but used patients having complete lymph node dissections before the sentinel lymph procedure was available. Among the pretest variables available, thickness, ulceration, and site were statistically significant and used in the mathematical model to predict lymph node status at dissection. The rationale for this exercise was to refine decision making before performing sentinel lymph node examination. For some patients, the risk of finding a positive lymph is too low to justify the procedure. For other patients, the risk is so great and follow-up survival so poor that the patient should be treated aggressively even if the sentinel lymph nodes are negative. And Patients with a positive reverse transcription polymerase chain reaction (RT-PCR) tyrosinase assay but negative histology and immunohistology and low pretest prediction of positive lymph node may be considered a lower risk for recurrence than the so-called lymph node status might indicate.

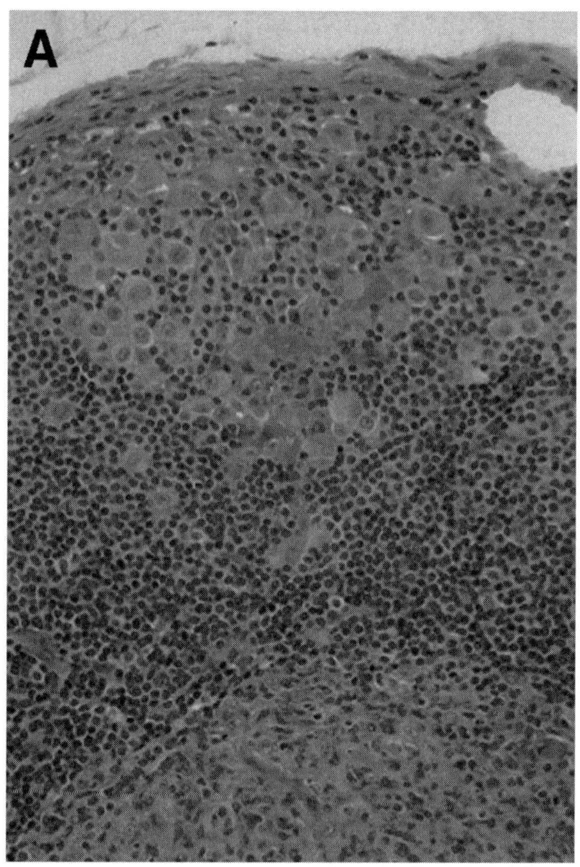

Fig. 13. Micrometastasis in a sentinel lymph node. H&E stain shows a small group of atypical cells of uncertain nature **(A)**. Immunostaining with antibodies to Melan-A (Mart-1) supports the interpretation of micrometastasis of malignant melanoma **(B)**.

6. SENTINEL LYMPH NODE EXAMINATION

The above statistical models were developed in the era before sentinel lymph node examination and were primarily envisioned as ways of advising patients with localized melanoma about the predicted survival and perhaps intervening with surgery, immunotherapy, or chemotherapy. The models predicted survival at 5 or 10 yr or predicted lymph node metastasis at similar intervals. Currently, sentinel lymph node examination is popular in staging patients that appear to have localized melanoma. It began as an attempt by surgeons to identify patients who would benefit from a formal lymph node dissection. It soon became apparent to oncologists that it was also an excellent way to stage patients with localized melanoma, i.e., to identify those patients that were really stage II patients. There

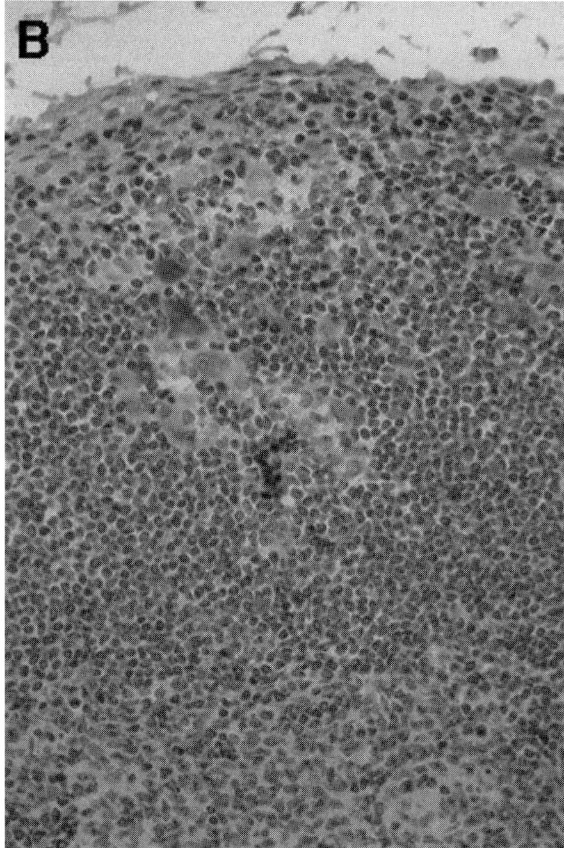

Fig. 13. *(continued).*

are now many studies with enough follow-up to see a definite benefit in survival for those patients that are sentinel lymph node negative compared to those that are sentinel lymph node positive. Sentinel lymph nodes are positive in breast cancer patients in approximately 34% of cases and positive in melanoma patients in approximately 17% of cases *(53)*.

Not all pathology laboratories are studying the sentinel lymph node in the same manner *(53–57)*. Initially, laboratories simply bisected the lymph node and stained one representative section with hematoxylin and eosin (H&E). In one study, 235 sentinel lymph nodes from 94 patients, which were originally examined by bisection, were submitted to multiple additional levels and immunostaining. Additional micrometastases (Fig. 13; *see* Color Plate 17, following p. 176) were discovered in 12% of the cases. Clearly, additional sections and immunostains are essential in the pathologic evaluation of sentinel lymph nodes for melanoma. In both breast cancer and melanoma, there appears to be a limit to the number of sections and immunostains needed to discover the majority of micrometastases. The only way to discover 100% of the micrometastases is to study the node in its entirety with step sections and immunostains, which not practical. It appears that 3 step sections, taken at 50- to 100-µm intervals, is enough to find 70 to 90% of the micrometastases present. It also appears that most micrometastases are located in the subcapsular sinuses of the hilar region of the lymph node *(54,57)*. Thus, it is sufficient to simply bisect the lymph node along the long axis. Frozen sections should be discouraged, because trimming or facing the block may destroy centrally located micrometastases *(54,57)*.

The Surgical Pathology Committee of the College of American Pathologists has proposed a standard for breast and melanoma that, with modifications, may become the standard for pathologic examination of sentinel lymph nodes *(58)*. In summary, the lymph node may be bisected along the long axis or serial sectioned in bread-loaf fashion, if it is large enough. Each section should be approximately 2.0 mm in thickness. Frozen sections for melanoma patients should be discouraged, although acceptable for breast cancer patients. After paraffin embedding, sections are taken in serial fashion from the block. The total number may vary from 10 to 20 depending upon the number of immunostains including controls that may be performed. The interval between sections may remain unspecified or specified at 50- to 100-µm intervals. Three of the step sections are stained with H&E and examined before performing immunostains. If positive for melanoma, the pathologic procedure is complete. If negative, the laboratory may proceed with immunostains using antibodies to S100 protein, HMB-45, Melan-A (Mart-1), and NK1/C3. The antibodies to be used are determined by the pathologist interpreting the sections. A positive immunoreaction must be confirmed by morphology, either in the H&E-stained section or, at times, on the immunostained section itself, if the histologic detail is clear enough for interpretation.

Along with histology and immunohistology, the sentinel lymph node tissue is being submitted for reverse transcriptase polymerase reaction assay for tyrosinase messenger RNA, the so-called RT-PCR assay *(59,60)*. Even when histologically and immunohistologically negative, nodal tissue may be interpreted as positive for metastatic melanoma when the assay is positive. There are several caveats to keep in mind. A positive reaction is not verifiable with accompanying morphology and may be a false positive secondary to benign nevus inclusions within the lymph node capsule or because of a positive reaction associated with benign nerve tissue within the sample *(53)*. In spite of these precautions, it seems that patients with negative histology and immunohistology but positive tyrosinase RT-PCR assays have a higher rate of subsequent recurrence of melanoma.

With the recent interest in sentinel lymph node sampling, the previously discussed statistical methods of risk analysis will lose even the limited interest that was given to them to date. There may still be a place, however, for statistical risk assessment before sentinel lymph node examination *(52)*. A mathematical model predicting the finding of a positive lymph node was developed based upon 573 patients in whom lymph node dissections were performed within 1 yr of excising the primary. It was an attempt to simulate the current sentinel lymph node procedure, but using patients having complete lymph node dissections before the sentinel lymph procedure was available. Among the pretest variables available, thickness, ulceration, and site were statistically significant and used in the mathematical model to predict lymph node status at dissection. The rationale for this exercise was to refine decision making before performing sentinel lymph node examination. For some patients, the risk of finding a positive lymph node is too low to justify the procedure. For other patients, the risk is so great and follow-up survival so poor that the patient should be treated aggressively even if the sentinel lymph nodes are negative. Patients with a positive RT-PCR tyrosinase assay, but negative histology and immunohistology, and low pretest prediction of positive lymph node may be considered a lower risk for recurrence than the so-called lymph node status might indicate.

7. SPECIAL TECHNIQUES THAT MAY BE PERFORMED ON PRIMARY MELANOMAS TO ASSESS PROGNOSIS

7.1. DNA Flow Cytometry

In the mid-80s, there was a lot of interest among pathologists in using flow cytometry to evaluate any and all tumors for aneuploidy and s-phase fraction. In flow cytometry, the solid tumor must be broken up into individual cells in a solution that can then be passed through a device to measure the cells for DNA content and other features. Melanoma was not excluded from these studies, and in general, the presence of aneuploidy and an increased s-phase fraction correlated with an adverse outcome. There are several problems with doing these studies on melanoma. First, the primary or part of the primary must be sacrificed to the technique, and the more important information of tumor thickness may be compromised. Small tumors would have to be sacrificed in total. Large tumors may be sampled—can the pathologist be sure that the thickest portion is saved for histologic examination? Second, fresh tissue is best for use in flow cytometry. In melanoma, most primaries are excised and placed in formalin or other fixative. Pathologists began using the Hedley technique, which allowed use of formalin-fixed and paraffin-embedded tissue sections, but the quality of the data was not as good. Interest in flow cytometry on solid tumors has essentially ended, although it is pursued very actively in lymphomas and leukemias using fluorescence staining and a variety of antibodies.

7.2. Image Analysis Cytometry

Image analysis cytometry was derived from flow cytometry. Instead of a solution of cells flowing through an aperture, cells were smeared or touched onto a glass slide, and special computerized imaging equipment was used to analyze the cells for DNA content and s-phase fraction. In spite of computerization, the technique was laborious, time-consuming, and did not provide the accuracy needed for clinical decision making. Newly defined ploidy related parameters have been correlated with survival in 106 patients with primary melanoma *(61)*.

7.3. Structural Cytogenetics

Cytogenetic studies looking for structural abnormalities of chromosomes, such as rearrangements and deletions, have been performed on melanoma tissue since the 1970s, and a variety of findings have been found. Most of these studies are primarily in reference to the possible etiology of melanoma and are not applicable to prognosis. One study of 158 patients with metastatic melanoma evaluated statistical methods that correlate survival with chromosome band regions *(62,63)*.

7.4. Fluorescence In Situ *Hybridization*

Fluorescence *in situ* hybridization (FISH) is a technique that may be applied to sections of tissue obtained from the paraffin block. Therefore, it can be applied to sections of a primary melanoma without destroying the tissue and without requiring fresh tissue. The technique allows determination of the presence, or possibly the absence, of specific segments of DNA or RNA. Probes to these segments can be fluorescently labeled for detection.

7.5. Microdissection of Tissue from Paraffin-Embedded Tissue Blocks

Microdissection of small groups of tumor cells for study with advanced techniques is now available in pathology laboratories associated with teaching and research hospitals. The pathologist can now identify small groups of cells within a radial growth dysplasia or vertical growth melanoma and remove them from the section for analysis. The technique was first developed using a small 26-gauge hypodermic needle used to scrape and, then by vacuum pressure, extract the cells of interest. Currently, laboratories are using laser method of removing or capturing the cells. Adjacent step sections are used, one stained with H&E and the other stained with eosin alone. The H&E-stained section is used to identify the cells of interest. The eosin-stained section is used for the microdissection, because hematoxylin damages DNA and makes molecular studies difficult. The laser capture method uses a transparent film that is applied to the area of interest under direct visualization by the pathologist. Laser light is then used to make only the cells of interest adhere to the transparent film. The film with the cells attached is removed from the eosin-stained slide and placed in a buffered solution that allows the cells of interest to detach from the transparent film. The cells are now ready for processing in the molecular laboratory.

7.6. Comparative Genomic Hybridization and Array-Based Comparative Genomic Hybridization

Comparative genomic hybridization (CGH) is a technique that can be applied to microdissected tissue from paraffin blocks as describe above *(64)*. Once the cells are extracted from the tissue, they are amplified via PCR and then digested with a proteinase that breaks the DNA into segments of 150 to 2000 bps, which can be labeled with a fluorescent die of one color such as green. Normal reference DNA is treated in a similar manner, but labeled with a different die such as red. The test DNA and reference DNA are allowed to hybridize with normal metaphase chromosomes that have been applied to a glass slide. The different colors allow comparison of the amount of hybridization that occurs to the normal chromosomes. An increase in hybridization appears green, and a relative decrease in hybridization appears red. The pathologist can then localize increased DNA copy numbers and decreased DNA copy numbers to specific loci on specific chromosomes. As such, this technique allows for discovery of genetic abnormalities that might relate to the etiology and progression of melanoma, but not specifically to risk assessment.

Risk assessment accompanied by CGH may be realized when the technique is modified by using DNA and protein array chips. The DNA-array chip is the counterpart of the chromosome spread above. The difference is that the chip can be manufactured to include gene segments of interest. The pathologist can then identify groups of cells in melanomatous vertical growth phase nodules, which have or lack specific genetic changes that may relate to metastasis and survival. The same can be applied to micrometastases found in sentinel lymph nodes. Protein arrays are just beginning to be produced, but offer the promise of screening tumor cells' cytoplasmic constituents for the presence of proteins that might relate to invasiveness and metastasis.

7.7. Gene Expression Profiling

Microarrays can now be produced that include thousands of segments of gene-specific targets for hybridization. This allows investigators to identify those genes that are overexpressed or underexpressed relative to the reference DNA. This characteristically leads to identifying 30 or so genes, which, as a group, are uniquely over- or underexpressed in aggressive or nonaggressive tumors and are, thereby, referred to as the gene expression profile of the respective tumor type in melanoma *(65,66)* and breast cancer *(67)*.

Using a variation of microarray-based CGH has been studied in 31 melanomas *(66)*. Messenger RNA was isolated from the tumors and prepared as fluorescently labeled complementary DNA, which was then hybridized to a microarray containing 8150 cDNAs representing 6971 unique genes. Obtained were both quantitative and comparative information on the relative expression of each gene included in the microarray. Some genes are overexpressed, and others are underexpressed. Using this information, the authors were able to characterize the tumors into groups with different expression patterns, which in the limited number of cases studied, appeared to correlate with survival. Their study also appears to highlight genes that may be important in producing invasive and metastasizing tumors *(66)*.

A variation of microarray-based CGH was used to study human and mouse cultured melanoma cells *(65)*. In this study, the authors studied colonies of poorly metastatic melanoma cells derived from both human and mouse tumors. They showed that they could select for metastasizing clones of cells and produce highly metastatic tumor cells. Both nonmetastasizing and metastasizing tumors grew the same when injected subcutaneously into experimental animals. Using the microarray-based CGH they compared the poorly metastatic melanoma cells with the highly metatstatic melanoma cells and could detect different gene expression patterns. The microarrays had 7070 human genes and 6347 mouse genes. Interestingly, several genes in both the human and mouse metastasizing melanomas were the same. Out of the 13,000 genes, they found 32 genes and expressed sequence tags that were associated with the metastasizing melanomas.

7.8. Genes of Interest Relative to Melanoma Behavior

Although primary melanoma is diagnosed when vertical growth phase is present, only 1 out of 3 or 4 tumors actually metastasizes and leads to the death of the patient. Pathologists have tried to improve our ability to predict which ones will metastasize by looking at characteristics such as tumor thickness, ulceration, mitoses, etc. We are still left with occasional thin lesions that unexpectedly metastasize and occasional thick lesions that do not. The above techniques will soon be available in many laboratories and will be applicable to sections taken from a paraffin block. This will be ideal for combining histologic interpretation with various molecular studies in order to improve our ability to predict which lesions will be most likely to metastasize.

The above studies provide a good review of genes currently known to be relevant to risk of metastasis *(65,66)*. The extracellular matrix appears to be important for invasive behavior and the ability of a tumor to set up foci of tumorous growth at distant sites. Therefore, identification of tumor cells, which can produce greater amounts of such constituents, may be a marker of increased risk for local recurrence and metastasis. Fibronectin is an extracellular glycoprotein that has been correlated with invasive and metastatic behavior in melanoma.

Fibronectin is a ligand for cell adhesion receptors such as integrin β-1, β-3, and α-1. Collagen subunits α-2(I) and α-1(III) have been associated with metastasis. Fibromodulin, a matrix G1a protein, and biglycan, a proteoglycan that regulates collagen fibril formation, were associated with metastatic phenotype *(65)*. Many of the genes identified in the metastatic phenotype are related to the structure and function of the cytoskeleton. Thymosin β-4 expression was enhanced in the metastatic phenotype. Thymosin β-4 is an actin-sequestering protein that regulates actin polymerization and, which along with thymosin β-10 and β-15, has now been associated with metastatsis. α-Actin 1, α-catenin, and α-centractin also function as regulators of cytoskeleton function and showed enhance expression in the metastatic phenotype. Much attention was focused on RhoC, a member of the GTPase family, which regulates cytoskeletal function in response to extracellular factors *(65)*. RhoC may enhance migratory and invasive aspects of tumor cells. By introducing the RhoC gene into poorly metastatic tumors, they became highly metastatic *(65)*. The RhoC gene could be inhibited when present and resulted in poorly metastatic tumors. The integrins β-1, β-3, and α-1 are cell adhesion receptors that may interact with fibronectin and when present in tumor cells, is associated with the metastatic phenotype.

7.9. Telomerase

Telomerase is an enzyme that protects chromosomal telomeres from degradation during repeated cell division and, as such, would be expected to protect actively proliferating tumor cells from degeneration and cell death. It has been shown that immunohistologic staining with antibodies to telomerase reveals increased positivity with progression from dysplasia and may correlate with survival *(68–71)*.

7.10. Angiogenesis and Vasculogenic Mimicry

There is renewed interest in angiogenesis and an entirely new concept of vasculogenic mimicry. Several investigators have shown correlation with vascular endothelial growth factor and other growth factors, tumor progression, and survival in melanoma *(72,73)*. Some investigators suggest that tumor cells produce factors that stimulate vascular growth *(74)*. Various vascular endothelial growth factors (VEGF) have been discovered and are referred to as VEGF-D, VEGF-2, and VEGF-3.

Vasculogenic mimicry is a new and somewhat controversial discovery in which tumor cells themselves are believed to be providing channels for blood flow in nodules of vertical growth phase melanoma. Vasculogenic mimicry was described in tumors of the uveal tract of the eye *(75)*. The tumors were highly aggressive metastasizing tumors, and gene expression profiles showed a reversion to a pluripotent embryonic-like genotype. Some similarity of gene expression profiling was also found in cutaneous melanomas in a separate unrelated study *(66)*. In one study of vascular growth factors and related growth factors, correlation with clinical outcome could not be confirmed *(76)*. Chaplain has reported a mathematical model of angiogenesis that may improve our ability to study and quantitate tumor related angiogenesis *(77)*.

7.11. Melastatin

Melastatin is a gene believed to be specific for melanocytes *(78)*. When down-regulated in melanoma, it correlates with aggressive behavior and metastasis *(79,80)*. FISH can be used to detect the presence or absence of melastatin within sections obtained from paraffin blocks *(79)*.

8. SUMMARY AND CONCLUSIONS

1. The dysplastic nevus logically implies a dysplasia–melanoma sequence.
2. Borderline melanocytic neoplasia are transitional lesions on the continuum of the dysplasia–melanoma sequence and are at the interface of dysplasia changing to melanoma. Borderline melanocytic neoplasia include moderate to severe melanocytic dysplasia (radial growth) and thin minimal deviation melanoma (vertical growth).
3. Borderline melanocytic neoplasia may be seen with or without regression. The presence of regression implies that the pathologic interpretation is a conservative estimate of risk.
4. Risk assessment in primary localized melanoma remains best correlated with tumor thickness. The presence or absence of ulceration is an important additional factor. For lesions that measure 1.0 mm or less in vertical dimension, level IV invasion is an important factor.
5. Tumor thickness has been commonly broken into categories separated by break points. However, tumor thickness is a continuous variable, and, using the Stadelmann transformation, tumor thickness can be used in mathematical models *(26)*.
6. Sentinel lymph node sampling and staging have made the existing mathematical prognostic models obsolete. However, new models may be created to address issues of who should get sentinel lymph node examination and what are the survival probabilities after sentinel lymph node information is available.
7. Pathologists have several new techniques available to study primary melanoma tissues without destroying the tissue. These techniques include FISH, microdissection, and comparative genomic hybridization. In particular, gene expression profiling may add important information relative to survival in primary localized cutaneous melanoma.

REFERENCES

1. Balch CM, et al. A new American Joint Committee on Cancer staging system for cutaneous melanoma. *Cancer* 2000; 88: 1484–1491.
2. Buzaid A, et al. Critical analysis of the current American Joint Committee on Cancer Staging System for cutaneous melanoma and proposal of a new staging system. *J Clin Oncol* 1997; 15: 1039–1051.

3. Clark WH Jr, et al. The developmental biology of primary human malignant melanomas. *Semin Oncol* 1975; 2: 83–103.
4. Clark WH Jr, et al. A study of tumor progression: the precursor lesions of superficial spreading and nodular melanoma. *Hum Pathol* 1984; 15: 1147–1165.
5. Clark WH Jr, Elder DE, Van Horn M. The biologic forms of malignant melanoma. *Hum Pathol* 1986; 17: 443–450.
6. Elder D, et al. Invasive malignant melanomas lacking competence for metastasis. *Am J Dermatopathol* 1984; 6(Suppl 1): 55–61.
7. Reed RJ. A classification of melanocytic dysplasias and malignant melanomas. *Am J Dermatopathol* 1984; 6(Suppl): 195–206.
8. Reed RJ. Melanoma in situ: images, segments, appellations, and implications. *Hum Pathol* 1998; 29: 1–3.
9. Reed RJ. Dimensionalities: borderline and intermediate melanocytic neoplasia. *Hum Pathol* 1999; 30: 521–524.
10. Reed R. The Reed patch, whither part 1, real and virtual images. *World Wide Web* 1999; October (http://www.xmission.com/~bweems/rjrpatch2.htm).
11. Reed R. The Reed patch, whither, part 2, the soil. *World Wide Web* 1999; November (http: //www.xmission.com/~bweems/whither11025.html).
12. Reed R. The Reed patch, whither, part 3, the nature of seeds, anatomic boundaries, and taking root. *World Wide Web* 2000; January (http://www.xmission.com/~bweems/whither31130.htm).
13. Reed RJ. The Reed patch (a neglected garden). *World Wide Web* 2000 (http://www. xmission.com/~bweems/rjrpatch2.htm).
14. Clark W Jr, et al. Model predicting survival in stage I melanoma based on tumor progression. *J Natl Cancer Inst* 1989; 81: 1893–1904.
15. McDermott N, et al. Identification of vertical growth phase in malignant melanoma. A study of interobserver agreement. *Am J Clin Pathol* 1998; 110: 753–757.
16. Reed RJ. Minimal deviation melanoma. *Monogr Pathol* 1988: 110–152.
17. Reed R. Minimal deviation melanoma. *Hum Pathol* 1990; 21: 1206–1211.
18. Breslow A. Thickness, cross-sectional areas and depth of invasion in the prognosis of cutaneous melanoma. *Ann Surg* 1970; 172: 902–908.
19. Breslow A. Tumor thickness, level of invasion and node dissection in stage I cutaneous melanoma. *Ann Surg* 1975; 182: 572–575.
20. Breslow A. Prognosis in cutaneous melanoma: tumor thickness as a guide to treatment. *Pathol Annu* 1980; 15: 1–22.
21. Vollmer R. Malignant melanoma. A multivariate analysis of prognostic factors. *Pathol Annu* 1989; 24: 383–407.
22. Balch CM, et al. Long-term results of a multi-institutional randomized trial comparing prognostic factors and surgical results for intermediate thickness melanomas (1.0 to 4.0 mm). *Ann Surg Oncol* 2000; 7: 87–97.
23. Reed R. Nevoid melanoma and index. Morphologic ambiguities: their impact on the interpretation of histologic patterns of melanocytic lesions. 2000; (http://www.pathology-skin-rjreed.com/mihm1.html).
24. Tuthill R, et al. Risk assessment in localized primary cutaneous melanoma: a Southwest Oncology Group study evaluating nine factors and a test of the Clark logistic regression prediction model. *Mod Pathol* 2000; 13: 69a.
25. Stadelmann W, et al. Prognostic factors that influence melanoma outcome. In: Balch CM, et al., eds., *Cutaneous Melanoma*, Quality Medical Publishing, St. Louis, MO, 1998, pp. 11–35.
26. Vollmer RT, Seigler HF. Using a continuous transformation of the Breslow thickness for prognosis in cutaneous melanoma. *Am J Clin Pathol* 2001; 115: 205–212.

27. Menhert J, Heard J. Staging of malignant melanomas by depth of invasion. *Am J Surg* 1965; 110: 168.
28. Clark WH Jr, et al. The histogenesis and biologic behavior of primary human malignant melanomas of the skin. *Cancer Res* 1969; 29: 705.
29. Clemente C, et al. Prognostic value of tumor infiltrating lymphocytes in the vertical growth phase of primary cutaneous melanoma. *Cancer* 1996; 77: 1303–1310.
30. Schmoeckel C, Braun-Falco O. Prognostic index in malignant melanoma. *Arch Dermatol* 1978; 114: 871–873.
31. Alvarez-Mendoza A, et al. Malignant melanoma in children and congenital melanocytic nevi: DNA content and cell cycle analysis by flow cytometry. *Pediatr Dev Pathol* 2001; 4: 73–81.
32. Coon J, Weinstein R. Evaluation of solid tumors by flow cytometry: methods and interpretation. In: Coon J, Weinstein R, eds., *Diagnostic Flow Cytometry*, Williams & Wilkins, Baltimore, 1991, pp. 115–134.
33. Henrique R, et al. Prognostic value of Ki-67 expression in localized cutaneous malignant melanoma. *J Am Acad Dermatol* 2000; 43: 991–1000.
34. Moretti S, et al. Correlation of Ki-67 expression in cutaneous primary melanoma with prognosis in a prospective study: different correlation according to thickness. *J Am Acad Dermatol* 2001; 44: 188–192.
35. Ramsay JA, et al. MIB-1 proliferative activity is a significant prognostic factor in primary thick cutaneous melanomas. *J Invest Dermatol* 1995; 105: 22–26.
36. Vuhahula E, Straume O, Akslen LA. Frequent loss of p16 protein expression and high proliferative activity (Ki-67) in malignant melanoma from black Africans. *Anticancer Res* 2000; 20: 4857–4862.
37. Neitzel L, et al. Angiogenesis correlates with metastasis in melanoma. *Ann Surg Oncol* 1999; 6: 70–74.
38. Weyers W, et al. Classification of cutaneous malignant melanoma—a reassessment of histopathologic criteria for the distinction of different types. *Cancer* 1999; 86: 288–299.
39. Braitman L, Davidoff F. Predicting clinical states in individual patients. *Ann Intern Med* 1996; 125: 406–412.
40. Rowley M, Cockerell C. Reliability of prognostic models in malignant melanoma. *Am J Dermatopathol* 1991; 13: 431–437.
41. Schmoeckel C, Braun-Falco O. Prognostic index in malignant melanoma. *Arch Dermatol* 1978; 114: 871–873.
42. Schuchter L, et al. A prognostic model for predicting 10-year survival in patients with primary melanoma. *Ann Intern Med* 1996; 125: 369–375.
43. Halpern A, Schuchter L. Prognostic models in melanoma. *Semin Oncol* 1997; 24(Suppl 4): S4-2–S4-7.
44. Sahin S, et al. Predicting ten-year survival of patients with primary cutaneous melanoma. Corroboration of a prognostic model. *Cancer* 1997; 80: 1426–1431.
45. MacKie R, et al. Prognostic models for subgroups of melanoma patients from the Scottish melanoma group database 1979–86, and their subsequent validation. *Br J Cancer* 1995; 71: 173–176.
46. MacKie RM. Malignant melanoma: clinical variants and prognostic indicators. *Clin Exp Dermatol* 2000; 25: 471–475.
47. Aitchison T, et al. Prognostic trees to aid prognosis in patients with cutaneous malignant melanoma. *Br Med J* 1995; 311: 1536–1539.
48. Soong S-J. A computerized mathematical model and scoring system for predicting outcome in melanoma patients. In: Balch CM, et al., eds., *Cutaneous Melanoma*, J.B. Lippincott, Philadelphia, 1985, pp. 353–367.
49. Soong S-J, et al. Predicting survival and recurrence in localized melanoma: a multivariate approach. *World J Surg* 1992; 16: 191–195.

50. Soong S-J. A computerized mathematical model and scoring system for predicting outcome in patients with localized melanoma. In: Balch CM, Houghton A, Sober AJ, eds., *Cutaneous Melanoma*, J.B. Lippincott, Philadelphia, 1992, pp. 200–212.
51. Soong S-J, Weiss H. Predicting outcome in patients with localized melanoma. In: Balch CM, et al., eds., *Cutaneous Melanoma*, Quality Medical Publishing, Inc, St. Louis, MO, 1998.
52. Vollmer RT, Seigler HF. A model for pretest probability of lymph node metastasis from cutaneous melanoma. *Am J Clin Pathol* 2000; 114: 875–879.
53. Treseler P, Tauchi P. Sentinel lymph node hypotheses and the role of pathologic analysis. *Surg Clin North Am* 2000; 80: 1695–1719.
54. Yu LL, et al. Detection of microscopic melanoma metastases in sentinel lymph nodes. *Cancer* 1999; 86: 617–627.
55. Messina JL, et al. Pathologic examination of the sentinel lymph node in malignant melanoma. *Am J Surg Pathol* 1999; 23: 686–690.
56. Cochran AJ. Surgical pathology remains pivotal in the evaluation of "sentinel" lymph nodes. *Am J Surg Pathol* 1999; 23: 1169–1172.
57. Cochran AJ. Melanoma metastases through the lymphatic system. *Surg Clin North Am* 2000; 80: 1683–1693.
58. Cibull M. Handling sentinel lymph node biopsy specimens. A work in progress. *Arch Pathol Lab Med* 1999; 123: 620–621.
59. Blaheta HJ, et al. Detection of melanoma micrometastasis in sentinel nodes by reverse transcription-polymerase chain reaction correlates with tumor thickness and is predictive of micrometastatic disease in the lymph node basin. *Am J Surg Pathol* 1999; 23: 822–828.
60. McMasters K, et al. Clinical relevance of molecular staging for melanoma—comparison of RT-PCR and immunohistochemistry staining in sentinel lymph nodes of patients with melanoma—discussion. *Ann Surg* 2000; 231: 801–803.
61. Korabiowska M, et al. Prognostic significance of newly defined ploidy related parameters in melanoma. *Anticancer Res* 2000; 20: 1685–1690.
62. Haybittle J, Yuen P, Machin D. Multiple comparisons in disease mapping. *Stat Med* 1995; 14: 2503–2505.
63. Nelson MA, et al. Chromosome abnormalities in malignant melanoma: clinical significance of nonrandom chromosome abnormalities in 206 cases. *Cancer Genet Cytogenet* 2000; 122: 101–109.
64. Wiltshire R, et al. Direct visualization of the clonal progression of primary cutaneous melanoma: application of tissue microdissection and comparative genomic hybridization. *Cancer Res* 1995; 55: 3954–3957.
65. Clark E, et al. Genomic analysis of metastasis reveals an essential role for RhoC. *Nature* 2000; 406: 532–535.
66. Bittner M, et al. Molecular classification of cutaneous malignant melanoma by gene expression profiling. *Nature* 2000; 406: 536–540.
67. Hedenfalk I, et al. Gene-expression profiles in hereditary breast cancer. *N Engl J Med* 2001; 344: 539–548.
68. Miracco C, et al. Detection of telomerase activity and correlation with mitotic and apoptotic indices, Ki-67 and expression of cyclins D1 and A in cutaneous melanoma. *Int J Cancer* 2000; 88: 411–416.
69. Glaessl A, et al. Increase in telomerase activity during progression of melanocytic cells from melanocytic naevi to malignant melanomas. *Arch Dermatol Res* 1999; 291: 81–87.
70. Rudolph P, et al. Telomerase activity in melanocytic lesions—a potential marker of tumor biology. *Am J Pathol* 2000; 156: 1425–1432.
71. Yang P, Becker D. Telomerase activity and expression of apoptosis and anti-apoptosis regulators in the progression pathway of human melanoma. *Int J Oncol* 2000; 17: 913–919.

72. Rofstad EK, Halsor EF. Vascular endothelial growth factor, interleukin 8, platelet-derived endothelial cell growth factor, and basic fibroblast growth factor promote angiogenesis and metastasis in human melanoma xenografts. *Cancer Res* 2000; 60: 4932–4938.
73. Vacca A, et al. Angiogenesis and anti-angiogenesis in human neoplasms. Recent developments and the therapeutic prospects. *Ann Ital Med Int* 2000; 15: 17–19.
74. Achen MG, et al. Localization of vascular endothelial growth factor-D in malignant melanoma suggests a role in tumour angiogenesis. *J Pathol* 2001; 193: 147–154.
75. Maniotis AJ, et al. Vascular channel formation by human melanoma cells in vivo and in vitro: vasculogenic mimicry. *Am J Pathol* 1999; 155: 739–752.
76. Lin EY, et al. Angiogenesis and vascular growth factor receptor expression in malignant melanoma. *Plast Reconstr Surg* 1999; 104: 1666–1674.
77. Chaplain MAJ. Mathematical modelling of angiogenesis. *J Neurooncol* 2000; 50: 37–51.
78. Hunter J, et al. Chromosomal localization and genomic characterization of the mouse melastatin gene (MLSN-1). *Genomics* 1998; 54: 116–123.
79. Duncan LM, et al. Melastatin expression and prognosis in cutaneous malignant melanoma. *J Clin Oncol* 2001; 19: 568–576.
80. Duncan LM, et al. Down-regulation of the novel gene melastatin correlates with potential for melanoma metastasis. *Cancer Res* 1998; 58: 1515–1520.

3 Clinical Prognostic Factors and Staing

Hamed Daw, MD *and Thomas Olencki,* DO

Contents

1. INTRODUCTION

While it is not difficult to ascertain the prognosis for patients with metastatic melanoma, the outcome of the majority of patients with clinically localized melanoma is far less clearly defined. Prognostic variables help make rationale patient care decisions and guides the design and evaluation of clinical trials. Determining the prognosis of a patient with a diagnosis of melanoma is an evolving field. Prognostic criteria, once limited to clinical characteristics, have been augmented by a better understanding of melanoma histology and sentinel lymph node status. Investigation of lymph node and circulating melanoma antigens by reverse transcription polymerase chain reaction (RT-PCR) may further clarify a patient's prognosis.

From: *Current Clinical Oncology, Melanoma: Biologically Targeted Therapeutics*
Edited by: E. C. Borden

2. PATIENT CHARACTERISTICS

2.1. Sex

Women with melanoma generally fare better than men. Melanoma in women presents more frequently on the extremities and is less likely to be ulcerated. However, multivariate analysis suggests that even when thickness and ulceration are accounted for, gender continues to correlate with survival.

A retrospective review from the Duke University Melanoma Clinic, with a database of 1489 patients, noted a significantly favorable influence of gender, with multivariate analysis demonstrating a significant survival benefit of women ($p = 0.005$) predominantly in the 40–89 yr age range *(1)*. This favorable status could not be explained by any other variable such as thickness or location.

An evaluation of 780 stage I/II patients from the Sydney Hospital Melanoma Clinic found that women presented with statistically thinner melanoma lesions than men ($p < 0.001$) *(2)*. They also had a superior 5-yr overall survival rate at 83 vs 67% ($p < 0.001$), which extended throughout the thickness range and was greatest among lesions >3.1 mm (no p value given). Later that year, they noted 5-yr survival rates significantly greater for women up to 49 yr of age (43 vs 33%, $p < 0.005$), regardless of thickness and site *(3)*. For women over 50, survival dropped markedly and paralleled that of men, which could not be explained by tumor thickness alone. The authors questioned whether a beneficial premenopausal effect was detected. Later, with a larger database of 2669 patients, the same group confirmed the survival drop for women over 50, but stated that women still had a better survival than that in men in all age groups *(4)*.

A review from the University of Edinburgh, Scotland, suggested that prognostic data might vary with geographic location *(5)*. The male to female ratio (1:2) of their 356 patients was unlike regions of higher risk, which commonly have a ratio of 1:1. Despite an increased incidence in women, they noted that overall survival was similar for men and women until age 50, at which point men had significantly higher ($p = 0.001$) melanoma mortality. A comparable increase in mortality did not occur for women until after 80 yr of age. The higher survival of women between 50–80 yr was attributed to women presenting with thinner melanomas, which where more often on extremity sites, relative to men.

Confirming the findings of the Edinburgh group, the Arizona Cancer Center found on multivariate analysis of 440 stage I patients, a survival drop for men and women over 50, but also noted a better prognosis for younger women ($p = 0.002$) *(6,7)*. They termed this the "age/sex interaction" which they hoped would replace both age and sex as separate prognostic variables.

The combined database of the Sidney Melanoma Unit and the University of Alabama at Birmingham, consisting of 8500 patients accrued between 1955 and 1986, was recently reviewed *(8)*. While the tendency for women to present with extremity lesions, thinner melanomas, and less ulceration was acknowledged, female sex still retained a survival advantage after multivariate analysis (p = 0.00014).

Recently, a retrospective review of 9223 patients treated at Duke University from 1970 to 1997 noted a significantly shorter median disease-free period (0.4 yr) in men than in women ($p = 0.0163$) *(9)*. The Memorial Sloan-Kettering Cancer Center also noticed a worse prognosis for men compared to women (p = 0.029) in the group of 284 patients retrospectively reviewed *(10)*. Others have reached similar conclusions *(11–15)*. Alternatively, others have noted no influence of sex on prognosis *(16–19)*. Overall, women may have a better prognosis than men, but while this difference may be statistically significant, it is not clinically relevant (outside of a stratification factor in a clinical trial) and should not affect clinical decisions.

2.2. Location

Most studies indicate anatomic location of the primary melanoma to be an important factor. In 1982, the Melanoma Cooperative Group reported that melanoma primaries of 0.76 to 1.69 mm thickness in the upper back, posterior arms, posterior and lateral neck, and posterior scalp (BANS) region had a 15% inferior 5-yr survival relative to other locations *(20)*. While this was borne out by some *(21)*, others did not encounter the same statistical unfavorable prognosis of the BANS location *(6,22–24)*. In a retrospective review of 156 consecutive patients by Massachusetts General Hospital, a greater death rate was noted among primaries in the BANS region, but this did not reach statistical significance *(25)*. As the absence of effect may have been due to insufficient patient numbers for adequate power, a meta-analysis was performed by the same group using data from 5 other trials (1458 patients), excluding the original paper by Day et al. *(20)*. With this pooled data, a significant ($p = 0.002$) relative risk of mortality of 1.6 (60% increased risk of death) was associated with a primary in the BANS location. More recently, the acronym TANS (thorax, upper arm, neck and scalp) has been coined to describe the anterior area outlined by the BANS region, with inclusion of the thorax *(9,26,27)*. Multivariate analysis suggests that there may be more of a consensus of increased risk represented by this region. Whether a particular region may be "high risk" in the era of the sentinel lymph node biopsy may be a moot point, as the BANS/TANS region may simply be one of occult and unpredictable lymphatic drainage. Alternatively, as more sentinel lymph node data accumulates, this region may truly be one of high risk.

Noncutaneous melanoma, including mucosa of the head and neck, vulvar, penile, and anal subtypes, have a poorer prognosis than cutaneous primaries. In a large retrospective review, a Swedish investigator *(28)* evaluated all patients in Sweden found to have vulvar melanoma from 1960 to 1984. In the 25-yr period, 219 patients were diagnosed, but sufficient data were available on only 198 (90.4% of the total). Complete follow-up was until 1994. In multivariate analysis, stage ($p < 0.001$) and tumor thickness ($p = 0.009$) were independent predictors of survival. For stage I (localized disease) patients, tumor thickness ($p = 0.003$), ulceration ($p = 0.034$), and clinical amelanosis ($p = 0.052$) were adverse for survival. The authors commented that while the 5-yr relative survival for this study was 47%, the survival for cutaneous primaries in Sweden during the same time period went from 50% in the 1960s to 80% in the 1990s. This has been the largest and most complete study demonstrating the poorer prognosis of mucosal melanomas.

Some of the reasons cited for the poorer prognosis of mucosal melanomas have been reviewed *(29,30)*. These include: (*i*) the patient may have nonspecific symptoms that result in a delay in seeking treatment; (*ii*) physicians may fail to recognize the rare subtype of melanoma; (*iii*) patients with these lesions tend to be older than those with cutaneous melanoma and, thus, may have poor immune systems; (*iv*) anatomic constraints often preclude surgery with generous margins, which may result in a subsequent local recurrence; and (*v*) mucosal melanoma tends to be histologically more aggressive than cutaneous forms and develops in sites rich in blood and lymphatic vessels.

In general, the leg is considered a good prognostic location. However, a recent review suggests that melanoma arising on the foot has a particularly poor prognosis *(31)*. Appropriate controls for tumor thickness and acral lentiginous histology revealed that those variables were not responsible for the poor outcome *(31)*.

2.3. Age

Melanoma is generally considered a disease of adults. A review of 4246 melanoma patients from the Duke University Melanoma Clinic database was undertaken to determine the incidence and characteristics of melanoma in the young *(32)*. Seventy-eight patients, 1.8%, were found to be younger than 20 yr of age. All patients were Caucasian with equal numbers of males and females. The age range was 1.5 to 19.9 yr, with a mean of 16.3 yr. The distribution of primary sites and histologic subtypes with associated risk factors occurred in a pattern similar to that seen in adults. While a trend for a decreased 5-yr disease-free survival was noted for young patients (57%) relative to adults (65%) ($p = 0.16$), overall survival was similar at 11.9 and 12.9 yr, respectively. Multiple regression analysis in this review confirmed that young age in and of itself does not alter the overall prognosis of melanoma in terms of disease-free and overall survival.

Using a similar database to examine prognosis in the elderly, others studied 3872 melanoma patients registered in the Duke University Melanoma Clinic *(33)*. The patients ranged in age from 11 to 100 yr old and reflected an age pattern similar to that in the U.S. at large. The median age and disease distribution at presentation were similar in both sexes. While trunk and extremities predominated as the primary site up to age 70, after age 81, trunk sites decreased, and the head and neck sites increased in frequency. Breslow thickness increased with age from a mean of 1.76 mm, for those less than 20 to 4.70 mm, in patients over 90 yr old. To evaluate the effect of age on prognosis, 1489 patients with stage I/II disease underwent multivariate analysis. This revealed that advancing age alone was a significant poor prognostic variable ($p = 0.008$). The following conclusions were reached: (*i*) older patients tend to present with thicker melanoma primaries; (*ii*) the increase in thickness with age cannot solely be accounted for by a delay in diagnosis, as there was no increase in nodal or metastatic disease with age; and (*iii*) despite correction for thickness, other factors must cause the poorer prognosis of the older melanoma patient. This year, an update of this database of 9223 patients confirmed that those patients less than 30 fared significantly better than those over 70 ($p = 0.0001$) *(9)*. Similar conclusions were reached by those at the H. Lee Moffitt Cancer Center *(34)* and the Pigmented Lesion group at the University of Pennsylvania *(15)*.

The Intergroup Melanoma Surgical Trial *(18)* randomized 740 stage I/II patients to elective lymph node dissection (ELND) or observation with additional randomization for width of excision margin. Although not initially part of the original stratification process, on multifactorial analysis age of 60 or less was found to be a significant favorable prognostic factor ($p = 0.019$). Later, updated with a median 10-yr follow up, this study continued to find age greater than 60 to be a significant variable, especially in those with nonulcerated primaries ($p = 0.009$) *(35)*.

Others have noted no influence of age on prognosis *(36,37)* or have stated that when thickness and ulceration are corrected for, age drops out as a poor prognostic factor *(38)*. Age in the setting of metastatic melanoma has received only sporadic comment. Two groups found no influence of age on response rate or on overall survival *(39,40)*. Taken as a whole, very young patients with stage I/II melanoma have a prognosis comparable to the average, whereas the older patient, may have a poorer prognosis.

3. CHARACTERISTICS OF PRIMARY

3.1. Histology

Anecdotally, nodular melanoma has been associated with a poorer overall survival than superficial spreading or lentigo maligna melanoma. However, once tumor thickness is corrected for, histologic subtype drops out as a prognostic factor *(41)*. In contradistinction, a large tree-based method evaluated over 5000 patients and calculated a comparable prognosis for superficial spreading and lentigo maligna melanoma with a worsening prognosis for nodular and then acral melanoma *(42)*. Others are in general agreement *(19,43)*.

3.2. Thickness and Clark Level of Invasion

One of the most important determinants of outcome in melanoma is the degree of cutaneous microinvasion. In 1969, a system of microinvasion based on anatomic–histologic levels of the skin was devised *(44)*. The greater the level (level I–V), the greater the melanoma penetration into the skin. The system suggested a correlation with biologic behavior. Levels I and II are in the radial growth phase with rare systemic metastasis, and levels III–V are in vertical growth phase with an increased risk of metastasis. Issues that complicate use of this system involve varying skin thickness, the lack of clear papillary-reticular dermis interface in some regions of the body and poor intra- and inter-pathologist reproducibility *(45–48)*. One year later in 1970, a system using an oculometer to measure overall contiguous melanoma thickness in millimeters was developed *(49)*. This system was straightforward and objective. In comparison to Clark's level of invasion, Breslow thickness was found to be significantly more reproducible among practicing pathologists and a more indicative prognostic indicator than Clark's level *(7,47,48,50,51)*.

A variety of breakpoints have been developed and used over the years. Initially, Breslow used cut off points of <0.76, 0.76–1.50, and >1.50 mm *(49,52)*. In 1982, an alternate set of breakpoints, <0.85, 0.85–1.69, 1.70–3.59, and >3.60 mm, were thought to have greater prognostic accuracy *(53)*. However, others disagreed and preferred the original Breslow values *(54,55)*.

Breslow's original cut off points were modified in 1983 and 1988 by the American Joint Committee on Cancer (AJCC) to <0.75, 0.76–1.50, 1.51–4.0, and >4.0 mm *(56)*. According to the system, Clark's level of invasion was an integral part of the staging, but should there be a discrepancy between tumor thickness and level of invasion, then thickness should take precedence. The staging system was again modified in 1992. If a discrepancy developed, the post surgical or pathologic T category (pT) would be based on the less favorable criteria. This had the effect of overstaging patients relative to actual survival data *(57)*. Recently, a massive data review of 4688 patients noted a tighter fit of actual survival with breakpoints at 1, 2, and 4 mm *(57)*. Significantly, Buttner's group found that the level of invasion did not add prognostic significance except in the <1.0 mm subgroup. Patients with level III or IV had a 3.5 times poorer 10-yr survival than those with level II or I. They concluded that in the <1.0 mm patient subgroup, the level of invasion adds biologic information regarding the aggressiveness of the tumor.

Others, including Clark, have come to similar conclusions *(58–60)*. The John Wayne Cancer Center remains the only group with data suggesting the utility of the Clark's level for the full range of tumor thickness *(61)*. Largely as a result of the work outlined by Buttner, use of even integers as cut off points and the use of level of invasion in <1.0-mm tumors have been proposed for the new melanoma staging system *(62,63)*.

One of the more perplexing issues in melanoma prognostication is why 10–15% of patients with melanoma of ≤0.76 mm develop recurrent disease at 10-yr follow-up. This has been explored in a preliminary fashion *(64)*. Antibodies against factor VIII and CD34 were used to determine mean vessel count in 10 Spitz nevi (benign) and 37 melanoma specimens, which included 12 matched pairs (five ≤ 0.75 mm and seven ≥5.5 mm). They found no difference in mean vessel count of Spitz nevi versus melanoma ($p = 1.00$). In reviewing the 37 melanomas and specifically the melanomas ≥5.5 mm in thickness, the mean vessel count had no predictive value. But the 5 matched pairs ≤0.75 mm in thickness demonstrated a significant ($p = 0.035$) correlation of mean vessel count and subsequent metastasis. Additionally, 13 of 14 melanomas ≤0.95 mm thick were noted to have evidence of histologic regression. Seven of that group who developed metastasis had aggregations of vessels associated with the regression. The authors stated that others reported a similar finding in thin melanomas *(65)*. While suggesting a possible correlation of increased vascularity and regression as a poor prognostic factor for thin melanomas, the authors readily acknowledged the need to reproduce this work in larger numbers of patients.

A similar retrospective study was performed in Norway. Nodular melanoma taken from 102 patients was stained with factor VIII antibody *(66)*. On multivariate analysis, vascular invasion proved to be a significant poor prognostic sign.

One of the new concepts, which has developed largely over the past 5 yr, is that of evaluating the prognosis of the primary in the context of the regional lymph nodes. In the past, current tumor thickness staging, regardless of cut off points, has been based on recurrence risk of the primary. The lymph node status of a clinically negative draining region had not yet become an integral part of microstaging. As the most predictive factor for outcome is the regional lymph node status, more careful staging with lymphoscintography and the sentinel lymph node biopsy has resulted in patients being upstaged, thus improving the prognosis of those patients remaining in the original clinical stage. Therefore, the prognosis for a pathologically staged nonulcerated T4 N0 melanoma primary has a markedly better prognosis than that listed in the staging system.

3.3. Ulceration

The presence of ulceration suggests a much more aggressive melanoma with a propensity for local invasion and metastasis. In retrospective reviews of large databases *(7,9,67)* and in a prospective randomized study *(18)*, ulceration has been shown to be a powerful poor prognostic indicator. Five- and ten-yr overall survival rates were calculated for all tumor thickness values with and without ulceration, and ulceration was found to have significant deleterious impact at all values. On the basis of these findings, the MD Anderson Melanoma group recommended that ulceration be included in the upcoming revision of the staging system *(62)*.

3.4. Mitotic Rate

The determination of mitotic activity is fraught with difficulty and interobserver differences among pathologists. The mitosis can be quantitated per high-powered field or square millimeter and evaluated in a region of greatest activity or in random fields. Thus, mitotic activity in and of itself may be a poor correlate of survival *(17,41)*. Others have found mitotic activity to be significant on multivariate review *(17,68)*. Mitotic activity has also been integrated into a predictive model quantitating the probability of 8-yr survival of a patient with a cutaneous primary *(60)*. In that model, mitotic activity was a stratified variable with adjusted odds ratio for survival of 11.7, 3.5, and 1.0 for mitotic rates of 0.0/mm^2, 0.1–6.0/mm^2, >6.0/mm^2, respectively *(69)*.

3.5. Regression

Regression, explained in detail in Chapter 2, remains an area of investigation. The major issue remains the inability to develop clear reproducible objective criteria that define the finding. Although generally considered today to be a poor prognostic factor *(60,70)*, it has also been an equivocal *(71,72)* or favorable criteria *(41)* in the past.

4. LYMPH NODE STATUS

The lymph node status of a patient at presentation is the single most important prognostic factor known. For this reason, evaluation of lymph node status has had the greatest technologic evolution recently.

Prior to the sentinel lymph node biopsy era, a surgical review from Memorial Sloan Kettering Cancer Center *(73)* evaluated prognostic indicators for melanoma patients presenting with clinical lymph node involvement. The review reinforced the general agreement that once lymph nodes are involved, traditional prognostic factors normally used to evaluate cutaneous primaries drop out. Of critical concern were the clinical absence or presence of lymphadenopathy, the number of lymph nodes, the degree of tumor involvement within the lymph node, and whether extranodal extension occurred. Of particular importance, lymph node number proved to be a continuous variable with no cut off points or plateau of risk for recurrence. On the other hand, lymph node size, site, and status of the highest node proved to be of minimal value.

Recently, concern has been expressed regarding the lack of prognostic benefit associated with the use of lymph node size as a variable in melanoma staging *(74)*. The 1983 AJCC staging system had cut off points of ≤5 and >5 cm for N1 and N2 lymph node status, respectively. This was later revised in the 1988 system to ≤3 and >3 cm for N1 and N2, respectively. Critical review of the MD Anderson Cancer Center 442 patient database revealed that lymph node size, with either 3- or 5-cm breakpoints, to have no prognostic value. Rather, a clear correlation of disease-free and overall survival with lymph node number was found, as has been noted by others *(67,73,75,76)*. The MD Anderson group found that using lymph node subgroups of 1, 2 to 4, and ≥5 nodes provided the best fit with clearly delineated survival curves. Ten-year overall patient survival was plotted at 60, 35, and 25%, respectively.

In 1997, the same MD Anderson melanoma group presented a critical review and proposal for a completely revised melanoma staging system *(62)*. In addition to lymph node size and number, they evaluated in-transit metastases, micro- and macrosatellitosis, and local recurrence. As these terms are all descriptors on a continuum of cutaneous lymphatic drainage and as the 10-yr overall survival was superimposible to that seen with lymph node-positive patients, the suggestion was made that patients with these findings should be placed in the stage III category. Additionally, as patients with both lymph node-positive disease and in-transit disease were in a particularly high-risk group (28–35% 10-yr overall survival compared to 41–56% for lymph node only disease), the recommendation was made that these patients should be placed in a separate subcategory in stage III.

A landmark study comparing sentinel lymph node status through the use of routine hematoxylin and eosin (H&E) and RT-PCR for tyrosinase was released in 1998 by the H Lee Moffitt Cancer Center *(77)*. RT-PCR is a sensitive technique capable of detecting one melanoma cell in one million normal nucleated cells. Patients were followed for a mean of 28 mo and then evaluated for disease recurrence and death. The 114 patients were divided into 3 groups based on their lymph node status. Group I (H&E negative, RT-PCR negative), group II (H&E negative, RT-PCR positive), and group III (H&E positive, RT-PCR positive) had a recurrence rate of 2, 13, and 61%, respectively. No deaths were seen in the double negative group I, but patients in group III had only a 45% chance of survival at follow-up. Those in group II had a survival midway between groups III and I. This study suggests that RT-PCR of the sentinel lymph node may be more sensitive and predictive for overall survival than routine H&E or immunohistochemistry staining. This hypothesis is currently undergoing rigorous evaluation in the multicenter Sunbelt Melanoma Trial that is using the markers tyrosinase, gp-100, Mart-1, and MAGE-3.

One year later, a similar but smaller study had comparable findings *(78)*. Seventy-two consecutive patients were divided into the same three groups, as described above, after sentinel lymph node biopsy. At a mean of 1-yr follow-up, recurrence rates were 0, 15, and 31% for Groups I, II, and III, respectively. Multiple mRNA markers MAGE-3, MART-1, and tyrosinase were used which, in this study, had greater sensitivity and specificity than tyrosinase alone.

5. GENETIC FACTORS

At least 40 million individuals globally are at risk for development of melanoma because of genetic factors. Individuals with the dysplastic nevus syndrome or atypical mole syndrome, both familial and sporadic, whose skin has multiple irregular nevi, particularly over the trunk and arms, are at high risk for primary disease developments. This risk substantially increases if the dysplastic nevus syndrome is familial *(79)*. Dysplastic nevi or atypical moles are characterized by size of >5 mm, variable pigmentation, irregular, asymmetric outline, and indistinct borders. Dysplastic nevi operate independently of other identifiable melanoma risk factors, such as hair and eye color, complexion, and history of sun exposure.

A dominant mode of inheritance for melanoma and dysplastic nevi, when occurring in familial aggregates, has been identified *(80)*. Cytogenetic studies have pointed to chromosome 9p as an area of frequent abnormality *(80,81)*. These studies have now been refined to locate a specific region of 9p21 as a cutaneous melanoma locus. Genes at this location have been identified as an inhibitor of cyclin-dependent kinases 4 and 6. The inhibitory protein is designated P16^{INK}4A *(82)*. When cyclin-dependent kinases 4 and 6 are active and not under suppression by p16, they phosphorylate the retinoblastoma protein, allowing resting cells to proliferate. Thus, mutations at this locus result in unchecked melanocyte proliferation. Mutations have been defined in 33 of 36 melanoma patients from nine different families *(83)*. Overall, 18% of families with cutaneous melanoma carry germ line mutations of this gene *(84)*.

6. PROGNOSIS OF METASTATIC DISEASE

The length of the disease-free interval from diagnosis of primary cutaneous melanoma to the development of metastatic disease suggests a favorable prognosis *(9)*. In 1975, Morton's group at the John Wayne Cancer Center published a remarkable paper with the data of 1521 patients with metastatic disease *(85)*. Notable was the lack of improvement in survival since 1971. On multivariate analysis, the initial site of metastasis; soft tissue versus lung versus liver/brain/bone ($p < 0.0001$), stage prior to progression; I/II versus III ($p = 0.0001$), and disease-free interval of >72 mo for initial stage I/II, and >18 mo for initial stage III ($p = 0.0001$) were all significant variables for survival. Also remarkable was that there was a 5-yr survival of 14, 4, and 3%, respectively, for soft tissue, lung, and liver/brain/bone sites of disease.

The Memorial Sloan-Kettering Cancer Center developed a model of prognostic factors in metastatic disease. In a retrospective review of 284 patients treated on in-house protocols, serum lactate dehydrogenase (LDH) ($p = 0.0001$), and albumin ($p = 0.0035$) were determined to be powerful prognostic indicators. Those with a normal LDH and albumin had a mean survival of 11.8 mo, whereas an LDH greater than twice normal and low albumen resulted in a 3.6-mo survival. Patients who were expected to do poorly, those with a performance status equal to or less than 50%, and those with CNS disease, were excluded from protocol entry and were not included in the analysis *(10)*.

The MD Anderson Cancer Center performed a similar retrospective review of 318 patients *(86)*. As with the Sirott study, serum LDH on multivariate analysis proved to be the most powerful prognostic indicator ($p = 0.0001$). Other factors found to be significant were soft tissue or one visceral metastasis ($p = 0.01$), female sex ($p = 0.02$), and serum albumin ($p = 0.03$).

Recently a prognostic factor analysis reviewed 8 Eastern Cancer Oncology Group (ECOG) trials that had been completed over the prior 25 yr *(87)*. Both clinical- and laboratory-based criteria were evaluated by multivariate and landmark analysis on the 1362 patients for which there was complete data. Using clinical data, tumor burden as defined by performance status ≥1, number of metastatic sites, and response to treatment were the most significant factors. Whereas with the use of laboratory parameters, LDH elevated by more than 10% over normal, number of metastatic sites, and response to treatment were the most significant. The authors and others *(88)* have noted an apparent survival increase in patients treated more recently on protocols compared to those treated in the 1970s and early 1980s. Careful examination suggests that more recent laboratory and radiologic staging has excluded those patients with subclinical poor prognosis who may have been entered on the study in the early years.

Prognostic factors remain useful in the setting of metastatic disease, as they are valuable for patient stratification in studies, assist patient's life planning with greater accuracy, and permit timely institution of palliative care. Because of the above reviews, the serum LDH will be incorporated into the upcoming revision of the melanoma staging system as one of the factors used to differentiate M1 from M2 disease.

7. SERUM MARKERS

Better methods of identifying patients with cutaneous primaries at high risk of relapse continues to be a pressing need. Additionally, the allure of a simple accurate serum prognostic marker continues to drive research. Serum levels of S-100β (to detect occult circulating melanoma cells) in 266 patients with resected stage I to III melanoma were tested *(89)*. Both the immunoradiometric and the immunoluminometric assay of S-100β were drawn in the first 3 mo post surgery. While the sensitivity was only 43.2%, ±12.4, the specificity was 92%. When detected in the serum, both assays in combination detected a 2.5-fold increase in recurrence ($p = 0.018$). This concurred with findings of others *(90,91)*. The authors stated that the S-100β, with its low sensitivity and high specificity, may be appropriate to combine with the serum RT-PCR assay for tyrosinase and MART-1, which have a higher sensitivity but lower specificity.

Tyrosinase alone or in combination with MART-1, MAGE-3, and gp-100, have been used as serum markers to assess for occult circulating melanoma cells. To date, a wide range of detection rates (0–100%) have been published. In some series, the procedure has been of little value in stage I patients *(92–94)*. In stage IV patients, detection rates from 100% *(93,95–97)* to less than 50% *(98–102)* have been noted. False positive rates may come from the use of contamination *(99,101,102)* and the use of more than 30 cycles in the PCR procedure *(93,103,104)*. False negative results may be seen with tyrosinase as a single marker, because tyrosinase may be decreased in amelanomatic melanoma *(105)*, and a decreased chance of detection may be seen secondary to low copy number secondary or to tumor heterogeneity *(104,105)*, or the release of the marker may be transient and random *(94,102)*.

Additionally, there are differences of opinion as to whether whole blood methods *(106)* or density gradient methods *(102)* produce more accurate results *(107)*. The sensitivity and specificity of serum markers is being assessed further in the Sunbelt Melanoma Trial. This trial, which will have at least 3000 enrolled patients, should have sufficient power to determine the role of these serum markers in the setting of early melanoma.

In the setting of metastatic melanoma, additional serum markers with greater specificity and sensitivity have been sought. Serum levels of S100β and melanoma inhibiting activity (MIA) were assessed for their discriminating ability in the setting of tumor-free individuals and patients with metastatic melanoma *(108)*. Unexpectedly, LDH was discovered to have greater specificity, minimally less sensitivity, and, hence, greater discriminating ability than either the S100β or MIA markers individually or together. The erythrocyte sedimentation rate (ESR) was of little value in predicting progressive disease.

8. STAGING SYSTEMS

A system using primarily clinical factors, mitosis, and ulceration was discussed in 1972 *(109)*. Thickness of the primary and Clark's level were not criteria in the prognostic scoring system. With accuracy rates of 80% in Scotland and much less in Australia, that particular system never came into widespread use.

In 1989, a landmark model for predicting survival in stage I melanoma was developed. The model integrated factors shown by multifactorial analysis to have significance, including mitotic rate, tumor infiltrating lymphocyte presence, tumor thickness anatomic site, sex, and evidence of regression *(60)*. These risk factors were placed in tabular form, which permitted the pathologist and clinician to refine the patients risk of 8-yr survival.

Despite the increased accuracy rendered by the above model, it became apparent that the vast number of pathology reports lacked information regarding mitotic rate, tumor infiltrating lymphocytes, and evidence of regression. A more clinically-based model was developed using variables of tumor thickness, site of primary (axial vs extremity), age, and sex of the patient *(15)*. Subsequent validation of this model demonstrated its ease of use and improved prognostic information over tumor thickness alone for those patients with a primary over 0.76 mm.

The John Wayne Cancer Center utilized a model to individualize prognosis *(110)*. Site, gender, age, Breslow thickness, and ulceration were all found to be significant. These factors were integrated into two slightly different formulas to produce likelihood of recurrence and death at 3-, 5-, and 10-yr follow-up.

A number of tree-based methods in survival analytic schemas have been developed to more accurately predict an individual patient's overall survival. This method has the theoretical advantage of being applicable to more situations than the Cox regression model. Two different schemas *(19,42)* have been proposed.

As accurate as these prognostic models may have been, they have been rendered obsolete by the development of the sentinel lymph node biopsy staging.

9. NEW AJCC MELANOMA STAGING SYSTEM

The first draft of the revised melanoma staging system was released in early 2000 *(63)*. As discussed above, the cut off points for the T category have been changed to ≤1.0, 1.01–2.0, 2.01–4.0, and >4.0 mm for T1, T2, T3, and T4, respectively. A descriptor for the absence or presence or of ulceration will follow the T with "a" or "b" respectively. Additionally, the T1 category will have Clark's level of invasion listed if the primary involves level IV or the rare V due to the poor prognosis. Such primaries will designated T1b.

The N category will be was follows: N1, one lymph node; N2, 2 to 3 lymph nodes; and N3, ≥4 lymph nodes, matted lymph nodes, any number of lymph nodes with either in-transit metastasis–satellitosis, or an ulcerated primary. Patients with in-transit metastasis–satellitosis and no lymph node involvement will be N2c. A descriptor will follow the N for macrometastasis (nonpalpable lymphadenopathy) or for macrometastasis (palpable lymphadenopathy) of "a" or "b," respectively. Metastatic disease will be divided into two groups of M1 and M2. The M1 category will have patients with distant skin, subcutaneous, or lymph node disease. The M2 category will be for patients with an LDH > 10% over the laboratory normal irrespective of tumor burden or for those with visceral disease. Initially, the lung was to have been a separate subcategory, but it has now been placed in M2 *(111)*.

The actual stage groupings, as outlined in Table 1 and Table 2, are in the process of being finalized and, in all probability, will be different than listed in this first draft *(112)*.

Addendum: The final version of the updated melanoma staging system has been published *(113)*.

Table 1
Definition of TNM

Type	*Stage*	*Criteria*
Primary tumor	T1a	≤1.0 mm
a, Without ulceration	T1b*	
b, With ulceration	T2a	1.01–2.0 mm
T1b, with ulceration *or* level IV–V	T2b	
	T3a	2.0–4.0 mm
	T3b	
	T4a	>4.0 mm
	T4b	
Regional lymph nodes	N1a	1 Lymph node
a, Micrometastasis (detected	N1b	
on pathologic review only)	N2a	2–3 Lymph nodes
b, Macrometastasis	N2b	
(clinically palpable) *or* gross extracapsular extension	N2c	In-transit mets or satellitosis without lymph node involvement.
	N3	≥4 Lymph nodes *or*, N2c and N1/N2 *or*, ulcerated melanoma and N1/N2
Distant metastasis	M1a	Distant skin, SQ *or* lymph node metastasis with normal LDH.
	M1b	Lung metastasis.
	M1c	All other visceral metastasis, or any metastasis with an elevated LDH.

Table 2
Pathologic Staging

0	Tis	N0	M0
IA	T1a	N0	M0
IB	T1b	N0	M0
	T2a	N0	M0
IIA	T2b	N0	M0
	T3a	N0	M0
IIB	T3b	N0	M0
	T4a	N0	M0
IIC	T4b	N0	M0
IIIA	T1-4a	N1a	M0
IIIB	T1-4a	N1b	M0
	T1-4a	N2a	M0
IIIC	any T	N2b, N2c	M0
	any T	N3	M0
IV	any T	any N	any M

10. CONCLUSIONS

Conclusions that can be drawn based on prognostic variables include:

1. Women do fare better than men, but the reason for this is unknown.
2. Axial primaries (head, neck, trunk, palm of hand, and sole of foot) tend to do worse, but this maybe due to clinically occult and unpredictable lymphatic drainage.
3. Older patients tend to do worse, but the reason for this also remains unknown.
4. Tumor thickness and ulceration are the most critical prognostic variables of the primary.
5. The single most important predictor of clinical outcome is the patient's lymph node status.
6. Evaluation of the sentinel lymph node and serum with melanoma differentiation markers for use in patient prognosis is still considered investigational.
7. Prognostic models based on characteristics of the cutaneous primary have been supplanted by the technology of sentinel lymph node evaluation.

REFERENCES

1. Reintgen DS, Paull DE, Seigler HF, et al. Sex related survival differences in instances of melanoma. *Surg Gynecol Obstet* 1984; 159: 367–372.
2. Shaw HM, McGovern VJ, Milton GW, et al. Histologic features of tumors and the female superiority in survival from malignant melanoma. *Cancer* 1980; 45: 1604–1608.
3. Shaw HM, McGovern VJ, Milton GW, et al. Malignant melanoma: influence of site of lesion and age of patient in the female superiority in survival. *Cancer* 1980; 46: 2731–2735.
4. Shaw HM, McCarthy WH, Milton GW. Melanoma: differing clinical patterns in older men and women. *Geriatr Med Today* 1985; 4: 31–43.
5. O'Doherty CJ, Prescott RJ, White H, et al. Sex differences in presentation of cutaneous malignant melanoma and in survival from stage I disease. *Cancer* 1986; 58: 788–792.
6. Meyskens FL, Berdeaux DH, Parks B, et al. Cutaneous malignant melanoma (Arizona Cancer Center experience): I Natural history and prognostic factors influencing survival in patients with stage I disease. *Cancer* 1988; 62: 1207–1214.
7. Berdeaux DH, Meyskens FL, Parks B, et al. Cutaneous malignant melanoma. II The natural history and prognostic factors influencing the development of stage II disease. *Cancer* 1989; 63: 1430–1436.
8. Stadelman WK, Raport DR, Soong SJ, et al. Prognostic clinical and pathologic features. In: Balch CM, Houghton AN, Sober AJ, Soong SJ, eds., *Cutaneous Melanoma*, 3rd ed., Quality Medical Publishing, St. Louis, MO, 1998.
9. Dong XD, Tyler D, Johnson JL, DeMatos P, Seigler HF. Analysis of prognosis and disease progression after local recurrence of melanoma. *Cancer* 2000; 88: 1063–1071.
10. Sirott MN, Bajorin DF, Wong GC, et al. Prognostic factors in patients with metastatic malignant melanoma. *Cancer* 1993; 72: 3091–3098.
11. Blois MS, Sagebiel RW, Tuttle MS, et al. Judging prognosis in malignant melanoma of the skin. *Ann Surg* 1983; 198: 200–206.
12. Sondergaard, K, Schou G. Therapeutic and clinico-pathological factors in the survival of 1,469 patients with primary cutaneous malignant melanoma in clinical stage I. *Virchows Arch (Pathol Anat)* 1985; 408: 249–258.

13. Johnson OK, Emrich LJ, Karakousis CP, et al. Comparison of prognostic factors for survival and recurrence in malignant melanoma of the skin clinical stage I. *Cancer* 1985; 55: 1107–1117.
14. Karjalainen S, Hakulin T. Survival and prognostic factors of patients with skin melanoma. *Cancer* 1988; 62: 2274–2280.
15. Schuchter L, Schultz DJ, Synnestvedt M, et al. A prognostic model for predicting 10-year survival in patients with primary melanoma. *Ann Intern Med* 1996; 125: 369–375.
16. Sober AJ, Day CL, Fitzpatrick TB, et al. Early death from clinical stage I melanoma. *J Invest Dermatol* 1983; 80: 505–525.
17. Barnhill RL, Fine JA, Rousch GC, et al. Predicting five-year outcome for patients with cutaneous melanoma in a population-based study. *Cancer* 1996; 78: 427–432.
18. Balch CM, Soong SJ, Bartolucci AA, et al. Efficacy of an elective regional lymph node dissection of 1 to 4 mm thick melanomas for patients 60 years of age and younger. *Ann Surg* 1996; 224: 255–266.
19. Huang X, Soong SJ, McCarthy WH, et al. Classification of localized melanoma by the exponential survival trees method. *Cancer* 1997; 79: 1122–1128.
20. Day CL JR, Sober AJ, Kopf AW, et al. A prognostic model for clinical stage I melanoma of the upper extremity: the importance of anatomic subsites in predicting recurrent disease. *Ann Surg* 1981; 193: 436–440.
21. Bernengo MG, Reali UM, Doveil GC, et al. BANS: a discussion of the problem. *Melanoma Res* 1992; 2: 157–162.
22. Cascinelli N, Vaglini M, Bufalino R, et al. BANS: a cutaneous region with no prognostic significance in patients with melanoma. *Cancer* 1986; 57: 441–444.
23. Woods JE, Taylor WF, Pritchard DJ, et al. Is the BANS concept for malignant melanoma valid? *Am J Surg* 1985; 150: 452–455.
24. Rogers GS, Kopf AW, Rigel DS, et al. Influence of anatomic location on prognosis of malignant melanoma: attempt to verify the BANS model. *J Am Acad Dermatol* 1986; 15: 231–237.
25. Weinstock MA, Morris BT, Lederman JS, et al. Effects of BANS location of clinical Stage I melanoma: new data and meta-analysis. *Br J Dermatol* 1988; 119: 559–565.
26. Garbe C, Buttner P, Bertz J, et al. Primary cutaneous melanoma. Prognostic classification of anatomic location. *Cancer* 1995; 75: 2492–2498.
27. Balch CM, Soong S, Ross MI, et al. Long term results of a multi-institutional randomized trial comparing prognostic factors and surgical results for intermediate thickness melanomas (1.0 to 4.0mm). *Ann Surg Oncol* 2000; 7: 87–97.
28. Ragnarsson-Olding, BK, Nilsson BR, Kanter-Lewensohn LR, et al. Malignant melanoma of the vulva in a nationwide, 25-year study of 219 Swedish females. *Cancer* 1999; 96: 1285–1293.
29. Milton GW, Shaw HM. Rare variants of malignant melanoma. *World Surg* 1992; 16: 173–178.
30. Kilpatrick SE, White WL, Browne JD. Desmoplastic malignant melanoma of the oral mucosa. An underrecognized diagnostic pitfall. *Cancer* 1996; 78: 383–389.
31. Talley LI, Soong SJ, Harrison RA, et al. Clinical outcomes of localized melanoma of the foot: a case control study. *J Clin Epidemiol* 1998; 51: 853–857.
32. Reintgen DS, Vollmer R, Seigler HF. Juvenile malignant melanoma. *Surg Gynecol Obstet* 1989; 168: 249–253.
33. Cohen HJ, Cox E, Manton K, et al. Malignant melanoma in the elderly. *J Clin Oncol* 1987; 5: 100–106.
34. Austin PF, Cruse CW, Lyman G, et al. Age as a prognostic factor in the malignant melanoma population. *Ann Surg Oncol* 1994; 1: 487–494.

35. Balch CM, Soong S, Ross MI, et al. Long term results of a multi-institutional randomized trial comparing prognostic factors and surgical results for intermediate thickness melanomas (1.0 to 4.0 mm). *Ann Surg Oncol* 2000; 7: 87–97.
36. Sober AJ, Day CL, Fitzpatrick TB, et al. Early death from clinical stage I melanoma. *J Invest Dermatol* 1983; 80: 505–525.
37. Barnhill RL, Fine JA, Rousch GC, et al. Predicting five-year outcome for patients with cutaneous melanoma in a population-based study. *Cancer* 1996; 78: 427–432.
38. Shaw HM, McCarthy WH, Milton GW. Melanoma: Differing clinical patterns in older men and women. *Geriatr Med Today* 1985; 4: 31–43.
39. Falkson CI, Falkson HC. Prognostic factors in metastatic malignant melanoma. *Oncology* 1998; 55: 59–64.
40. Hena MA, Emrich LJ, Nabisan RN, et al. Effect of surgical treatment on stage IV melanoma. *Am J Surg* 1987; 153: 270–275.
41. McGovern VJ, Shaw HM, Milton GW, et al. Prognostic significance of the histological features of malignant melanoma. *Histopathology* 1979; 3: 385–393.
42. Garbe CG, Buttner P, Bertz J, et al. Primary cutaneous melanoma. Identification of prognostic groups and estimation of individual prognosis for 5093 patients. *Cancer* 1995; 75: 2484–2491.
43. Sober AJ, Day, CL, Fitzpatrick TB, et al. Early death from clinical stage I melanoma. *J Invest Dermatol* 1983; 80: 505–525.
44. Clark WH, From L, Bernardino EA, et al. The histogenesis and biologic behavior of primary human malignant melanomas of the skin. *Cancer Res* 1969; 29: 705–726.
45. Cohen MH, Ketcham AS, Felix EL, et al. Prognostic factors in patients undergoing lymphadectomy for malignant melanoma. *Ann Surg* 1977; 186: 635–642.
46. Breslow A, Macht S. Evaluation of prognosis in stage I cutaneous melanoma. *Plast Reconstr Surg* 1978; 61: 342–346.
47. Prade M, Sancho-Garnier H, Cesari JP, et al. Difficulties encountered in the application of the Clark's classification and the Breslow thickness measurement in cutaneous malignant melanoma. *Eur J Cancer* 1980; 26: 159–163.
48. Lock-Anderson J, Hou-Jensen K, Hansen J, et al. Observer variation in histologic classification of cutaneous malignant melanoma. *Scand J Plast Reconstr Surg Hand Surg* 1995; 29: 141–148.
49. Breslow A. Thickness, cross-sectional areas and depth of invasion in the prognosis of cutaneous melanoma. *Ann Surg* 1970; 172: 902–908.
50. Veronesi U, Cascinelli N, Morabito A, et al. Prognosis of stage I melanoma of the skin. *Int J Cancer* 1980; 26: 733–739.
51. Heenan PJ, Matz LR, Blackwell JB, et al. Inter-observer variation between pathologists in the classification of cutaneous malignant melanoma in Western Australia. *Histopathology* 1984; 8: 717–729.
52. Breslow A. Tumor thickness, level of invasion and node dissection in stage I cutaneous melanoma. *Ann Surg* 1975; 182: 572–575.
53. Day CL, Lew RA, Mihm MC Jr, et al. The natural break points for primary-tumor thickness in clinical stage I melanoma. *N Engl J Med* 1981; 305: 1155.
54. Mackie RM. Tumor thickness in melanoma. *N Engl J Med* 1982; 306: 1179–1180.
55. Kuehnl-Petzoldt C, Wiebelt H, Berger H. In what sense are breakpoints prognostic in malignant melanoma? *Am J Dermatopathol* 1984; 6(1 Suppl): 349–350.
56. American Joint Committee on Cancer. *Manual for Staging of Cancer, 3rd ed.* JB Lippincott, Philadelphia, 1988.
57. Buttner P, Garbe C, Bertz J, et al. Primary cutaneous melanoma. Primary cutoff points of tumor thickness and importance of Clark's level for prognostic classification. *Cancer* 1995; 75: 2499–2506.

58. Kelly JW, Sagebiel RW, Clyman S, et al. Thin level IV malignant melanoma. *Ann Surg* 1985; 202: 98–103.
59. Shaw HM, McCarthy WH, McCarthy SW, et al. Thin malignant melanomas and recurrence potential. *Arch Surg* 1987; 122: 1147–1150.
60. Clark WH, Elder DE, Guerry D, et al. Model predicting survival in stage I melanoma based on tumor progression. *J Natl Cancer Inst* 1989; 81: 1893–1904.
61. Morton DL, Davtyan DG, Wanek LA, et al. Multivariate analysis of the relationship between survival and the microstage of primary melanoma by Clark level and Breslow thickness. *Cancer* 1993; 71: 3737–3743.
62. Buzaid AC, Ross MI, Balch CM, et al. Critical analysis of the current American Joint Committee on Cancer staging system for cutaneous melanoma and proposal of a new staging system. *J Clin Oncol* 1997; 15: 1039–1051.
63. Balch CM, Buzaid AC, Atkins MB, et al. A new American Joint Committee on Cancer staging system for cutaneous melanoma. *Cancer* 2000; 88: 1484–1491.
64. Graham CH, Rivers J, Kerbel RS, et al. Extent of vascularization as a prognostic indicator in thin (<0.76 mm) malignant melanomas. *Am J Pathol* 1994; 145: 510–514.
65. Barnhill RL, Levy MA. Regressing thin cutaneous malignant melanomas (less than or equal to 1.00 mm) are associated with angiogenesis. *Am J Pathol* 1993; 143: 99–104.
66. Straume O, Akslen LA. Independent prognostic importance of vascular invasion in nodular melanomas. *Cancer* 1996; 78: 1211–1219.
67. Balch C. Cutaneous melanoma: prognosis and treatment results worldwide. *Semin Surg Oncol* 1992; 8: 400–414.
68. Schmoeckel C, Braun-Falco O. Prognostic index in malignant melanoma. *Arch Dermatol* 1978; 144: 871–873.
69. Halpern AC, Schuchter LM. Prognostic models in melanoma. *Semin Oncol* 1997; 24: S4-2–S4-7.
70. Vollmer RT. Malignant melanoma: a multivariate analysis of prognostic factors. *Pathol Annu* 1989; 24: 383–407.
71. Kelly JW, Sagebiel RW, Blois MS, et al. Regression in malignant melanoma: a histologic feature without independent prognostic significance. *Cancer* 1985; 56: 2287–2291.
72. Heenan PJ, English DR, D'Arcy C, et al. Survival among patients with clinical stage I cutaneous malignant melanoma diagnosed in western Australia in 1975/1976 and 1980/1981. *Cancer* 1991; 68: 2079–2087.
73. Coit DG. Prognostic factors in patients with melanoma metastatic to regional nodes. *Surg Oncol Clin N Am* 1992; 1: 281–295.
74. Buzaid AC, Tinoco LA, Jendiroba D, et al. Prognostic value of size of lymph node metastases in patients with cutaneous melanoma. *J Clin Oncol* 1995; 13: 2361–2368.
75. Bevilacqua R, Coit D, Rogatka A, et al. Axillary dissection in melanoma: prognostic variables in node-positive patients. *Ann Surg* 1990; 212: 125–131.
76. Drepper H, Bieb B, Hofherr B, et al. The prognosis of patients with stage III melanoma. *Cancer* 1993; 71: 1239–1246.
77. Shivers SC, Wang X, Li W, et al. Molecular staging of malignant melanoma. Correlation with clinical outcome. *JAMA* 1998; 280: 1410–1415.
78. Bostick PJ, Morton Dl, Turner RR, et al. Prognostic significance of occult metastasis detected by sentinel lymphadenectomy and reverse transcriptase-polymerase chain reaction in early-stage melanoma patients. *J Clin Oncol* 1999; 17: 3238–3244.
79. Hayward N. New developments in melanoma genetics. *Curr Oncol Rep* 2000; 2: 300–306.
80. Greene MH. The genetics of hereditary melanoma and nevi. *Cancer* 1999; 86: 2464–2477.
81. Cowan JM, Halaban R, Francke U. Cytogenetic analysis of melanocytes from premalignant nevi and melanomas. *J Natl Cancer Inst* 1988; 80: 1159–1164.

82. Kamb A, Gruis NA, Weaver-Feldhaus J, et al. A cell cycle regulator potentially involved in genesis of many tumor types. *Science* 1994; 264: 436–440.
83. Hussussian CJ, Struewing JP, Goldstein AM, et al. Germline p16 mutations in familial melanoma. *Nat Genet* 1994; 8: 15–21.
84. Haluska FG, Hodi FS. Molecular genetics of familial cutaneous melanoma. *J Clin Oncol* 1998; 16: 670–682.
85. Barth A, Wanek L, Morton DL. Prognostic factors in 1,521 melanoma patients with distant metastasis. *J Am Coll Surg* 1995; 181: 193–201.
86. Eton O, Legha SS, Moon TE, et al. Prognostic factors for survival of patients treated systemically for disseminated melanoma. *J Clin Oncol* 1998; 16: 1103–1111.
87. Manola J, Atkins M, Ibrahim J, et al. Prognostic factors in metastatic melanoma: a pooled analysis of Eastern Cooperative Oncology Group trials. *J Clin Oncol* 2000; 18: 3782–3793.
88. Ryan L, Kramar A, Borden E. Prognostic factors in metastatic melanoma. *Cancer* 1993; 71: 2995–3005.
89. Curry BJ, Farrelly M, Hersey P. Evaluation of S-100β assays for the prediction of recurrence and prognosis in patients with AJCC stage I-III melanoma. *Melanoma Res* 1999; 9: 557–567.
90. von Schoultz E, Hansson LO, Djureen E, et al. Prognostic value of serum analysis of S-100β protein in malignant melanoma. *Melanoma Res* 1993; 6: 133–137.
91. Bonfer JMG, Korse CM, Nieweg OE, Rankin EM. The luminescence immunoassay S-100: a sensitive test to measure circulating S-100β: its prognostic value in malignant melanoma. *Br J Cancer* 1998; 77: 2210–2214.
92. Battayani Z, Grob JJ, Xerri L, et al. Polymerase chain reaction detection of circulating melanocytes as a prognostic marker in patients with melanoma. *Arch Dermatol* 1995; 131: 443–447.
93. Mellado B, Colomer D, Castel T, et al. Detection of circulating neoplastic cells by reverse-transcriptase polymerase chain reaction in malignant melanoma: association with clinical stage and prognosis. *J Clin Oncol* 1996; 14: 2091–2097.
94. Reinhold U, Ludtke-Handjery HC, Schnautz S, et al. The analysis of tyrosinase-specific mRNA in blood samples of melanoma patients by RT-PCR is not a useful test for metastatic tumor progression. *J Invest Dermatol* 1997; 108: 166–169.
95. Brossart P, Keilholz U, Willchauk M, et al. Hematogenous spread of malignant melanoma cells in different stages of disease. *J Invest Dermatol* 1993; 101: 887–889.
96. Brossart P, Schmier J, Kruger S, et al. A polymerase chain reaction-based semi-quantitative assessment of malignant melanoma cells in peripheral blood. *Cancer Res* 1995; 55: 4065–4068.
97. Hoon D, Wang Y, Dale P, et al. Detection of occult melanoma cells in blood with a multiple-marker polymerase chain reaction assay. *J Clin Oncol* 1995; 13: 2109–2116.
98. Battayani Z, Xerri L, Hassoun J, et al. Tyrosine gene expression in human tissues. *Pigment Cell Res* 1993; 6: 400–405.
99. Foss A, Guille M, Occleston N, et al. The detection of melanoma cells in peripheral blood by reverse transcription-polymerase chain reaction. *Br J Cancer* 1995; 72: 155–159.
100. Kunter U, Buer J, Probst M, et al. Peripheral blood tyrosinase messenger RNA detection and survival in malignant melanoma. *J Natl Cancer Inst* 1996; 88: 590–594.
101. Pittman K, Burchill S, Smith B, et al. Reverse transcriptase-polymerase chain reaction for expression of tyrosinase to identify malignant melanoma cells in peripheral blood. *Ann Oncol* 1996; 7: 297–301.
102. Jung FA, Buzaid AC, Ross MI, et al. Evaluation of tyrosinase as a tumor marker in the blood of melanoma patients. *J Clin Oncol* 1997; 15: 2826–2831.
103. Smith B, Shelby P, Southgate J, et al. Detection of melanoma cells in peripheral blood by means of reverse transcriptase and polymerase chain reaction. *Lancet* 1991; 338: 1227–1229.

104. Palmieri G, Strazzullo M, Ascierto PA, et al. Polymerase chain reaction-based detection of circulation melanoma cells as an effective marker of tumor progression. *J Clin Oncol* 1999; 17: 304–311.
105. Hoon, DS, Bostick P, Kuo C, et al. Molecular markers in blood as surrogate prognostic indicators of melanoma recurrence. *Cancer Res* 2000; 60: 2253–2257.
106. Keilholz U. Diagnostic PCR in melanoma, methods and quality assurance. *Eur J Cancer* 1996; 32: 1661–1663.
107. Keilholz U. Reliability of reverse transcription-polymerase chain reaction (RT-PCR)-based assays for the detection of circulating tumor cells: a quality-assurance initiative of the EORTC Melanoma Cooperative Group. *Eur J Cancer* 1998; 34: 750–753.
108. Deichmann M, Benner A, Bock M, et al. S100-beta, melanoma-inhibiting activity, and lactate dehydrogenase discriminate progressive from nonprogressive American Joint Committee on Cancer stage IV melanoma. *J Clin Oncol* 1999; 17: 1891–1896.
109. Mackie RM, Carfrae DC, Cochran AJ. Assessment of prognosis in patients with malignant melanoma. *Lancet* 1972; 2: 455–4546.
110. Cochran AJ, Elashoff D, Morton DL, et al. Individualized prognosis for melanoma patients. *Hum Pathol* 2000; 31: 327–331.
111. Gershenwald JE. Pittsburgh Perspective in Melanoma Meeting, Pittsburgh, PA, June 1–2, 2000.
112. Melanoma Consensus Conference, Atlanta Georgia, April 1–2, 2000.
113. Balch CM, Bozaid AC, Soong SJ, et al. Final version of the American Joint Committee on Cancer Staging system for cutaneous melanoma. *J Clin Oncol* 19:3635-3648, 2001.

II Biological and Targeted Therapeutics

4 Principles of Antitumor Immunity and Tumor-Mediated Immunosuppression

Peter A. Cohen, MD, *Suyu Shu,* PhD, *and James H. Finke,* PhD

Contents

From: *Current Clinical Oncology, Melanoma: Biologically Targeted Therapeutics*
Edited by: E. C. Borden

1. INTRODUCTION

A quarter of a century ago, a series of discoveries alerted investigators to the possibility that the immune system could be successfully harnessed to cure cancer. Intratumor injection of bacterial extracts such as Bacille Calmette-Guérin (BCG) or *Corynebacterium parvum* proved sufficient to induce local rejection of mouse tumors, and, in some cases, led to systemic acquisition of specific antitumor immunity *(1,2)*. Melanoma patients whose tumor nodules were injected with such bacterial adjuvants frequently experienced local tumor regressions, sometimes with downstream tumor regressions at sites of lymphatic drainage and, rarely, even distant metastases *(1,3–6)*. At approximately the same time, it was discovered that individual melanoma patients had evidence of peripheral blood T cells that could directly kill their own tumor cells in culture, and such in vitro killer T cell reactivity sometimes correlated to spontaneous clinical remissions *(7)*. Furthermore, with the discovery of interleukin (IL)-2 (also known as a T cell growth factor) in the late 1970s, the prospect of raising vast numbers of antitumor killer T cells for therapeutic reinfusion appeared imminent and inevitable *(8)*.

A quarter of a century later, we appreciate the excitement experienced by immunotherapists in the late 1970s, but we can also see much more clearly that there existed tremendous gaps in knowledge that would doom or severely limit the outcome of translational efforts in that era and for many years thereafter. In the year 2000, we experience the same sense of optimism that immunotherapists did in the late 1970s, but it is now fortunately coupled with even more substantive evidence, both in animal tumor models and in recent patient trials, that T cell-mediated tumor rejection has a complicated but consistent physiology, which can be successfully harnessed for clinical translation.

We now recognize that the immune system has a plethora of mechanisms available besides T cells to identify tumor cells for elimination. Not all such mechanisms require that tumor antigens (Ag) be expressed on the tumor cell surface, or that a tumor even express unique antigens. Nonetheless, the participation of Ag-specific T cells can demonstrably galvanize the tumor rejection process and can lead both to highly selective rejection of established tumors and to long-term protective "memory" against tumor recurrence. When optimally implemented, T cell-mediated tumor rejection may be an ideal form of cancer treatment, since tumors at multiple anatomic sites can be uniformly eliminated with minimum toxicity to normal bystander tissues, just as the immune system often successfully eradicates disseminated infectious pathogens. Although this ideal outcome remains uncommon to date in cancer patients treated with immunotherapy, tremendous progress has recently been achieved in animal tumor models, clarifying the T cell characteristics which can and must be elicited to achieve consistently effective immunotherapy *(9,10)*. Furthermore, increasing numbers of responses have recently been observed in cancer patients receiving certain novel forms of immunotherapy, substantiating the basis for optimism among immunotherapists *(11,12)*.

While our ability to implement effective T cell-mediated tumor rejection in animal models continues to advance, the ability of many tumors to withstand immunotherapy has also been increasingly appreciated and respected. The capacity of tumors to suppress, evade, and/or eliminate an antitumor immune response is a consequence of the tumor cell's innate capacity to secrete and/or express immunosuppressive factors, also produced by normal tissues such as placenta, coupled with the tumor's additional random acquisition of serviceable mutations such as down-regulated major histocompatibility complex (MHC) expression *(13,14)*.

Nonetheless, despite the formidable ability of tumors to resist immune recognition and rejection, current animal and human evidence indicates that optimized vaccine strategies and T cell generation can lead to tumor rejection even in the face of such tumor resistance. Even in such favorable circumstances, it remains likely that adjunct treatments, which specifically counteract tumor-mediated immunosuppression, will help to sustain effector T cell activity and potentiate the outcome of immunotherapy. The main objective of this chapter is, therefore, to review and consider the immunotherapist's dual need to optimize T cell function and to anticipate and continually address the impact of tumor-mediated immunosuppression.

2. ANTIGENIC MECHANISMS BY WHICH THE IMMUNE SYSTEM DISTINGUISHES TUMOR CELLS

2.1. T Cell Reactivities with Tumor: Target Lysis, Proliferation, and Cytokine Secretion

Tumor cells frequently express molecules which are recognized by the immune system as "antigenic". Such antigenicity is typically demonstrated by the presence of antibodies (Ab) or T cells within a tumor host, which react with tumor cells and/or tumor-derived molecules. The reactivity of extracorporealized T cells with tumor Ag can be demonstrated by a variety of in vitro assays, including the capacity of T cells to kill radiolabeled or fluorescently labeled tumor targets (lytic assays), the capacity of radiolabeled or fluorescently labeled T cells to replicate in the presence of tumor (proliferation assays), and the capacity of T cells to secrete a variety of cytokines such as interferon-γ (IFN-γ) or granulocyte-macrophage colony-stimulating factor (GM-CSF) in the presence of tumor *(15,16)*.

Ag-specific T cell reactivity to tumor in vitro has frequently proved predictive for therapeutic responses (e.g., tumor regressions) when the T cells are reinfused into the tumor host, both in animal models and in melanoma patients *(9,10,15,17)*.

Just as importantly, an absence of Ag-specific T cell reactivity to tumor in vitro is often predictive for treatment failure when T cells are reinfused *(9,10,15)*. Specific T cell cytokine production is frequently observed in vitro in the absence of specific T cell proliferation or tumor target lysis, whereas it is uncommon to observe specific T cell proliferation or target killing in the absence of T cell cytokine production *(15,17,18)*. It is, therefore, generally accepted that T cell cytokine secretion is the most sensitive current in vitro assay of antigenic specificity. Furthermore, an inability of cytokine-producing T cells to lyse tumors in vitro is not a negative predictor for subsequent tumor rejection, and T cells can acquire the capacity for tumor lysis after reinfusion and subsequent activation within the tumor host *(17)*.

2.2. Tumor Ag May Be Uniquely Expressed by Tumor or also Expressed by Normal Tissues

Tumor-associated Ag recognized by T cells are, in some cases, uniquely expressed by the tumor cell (e.g., mutated oncogenes), enabling exquisitely specific T cell reactivity with a low prospect for "autoimmune" reactivity with normal host tissues *(19)*. Alternatively, the tumor-associated Ag recognized by T cells may be concomitantly expressed by a portion of normal host tissues, providing only a relatively specific pattern of reactivity. When sensitized T cells react with Ag expressed by both tumor and normal tissues, the potential for autoimmune toxicity is apparent, and this epiphenomenon is, in fact, observed both in animals and in humans. For example, the natural host response to melanoma frequently invokes T cell sensitization to melanin pigment-associated proteins such as tyrosinase, which are expressed both by melanoma cells and by normal melanocytes *(20–22)*. Not surprisingly, patchy vitiligo (depigmentation of normal tissues) is frequently observed in melanoma patients and animals who are responders to immunotherapy *(21,22)*. It is not currently understand why this autoimmune epiphenomenon is incomplete (i.e., why patients fail to develop total body vitiligo, since all normal melanocytes express the antigenic pigment proteins). However, since complete and permanent regression of the patients' melanomas seldom accompany such immunotherapy, the patchiness of the observed vitiligo may correlate to the indecisiveness of current immunotherapy.

Such observations suggest that more potent immunotherapy directed against Ag shared by tumor and normal tissues might well be accompanied by more extensive and frequently unacceptable autoimmune complications. For example, escalated immunotherapy targeting normal melanocyte proteins may, in theory, cause blindness by destroying retinal melanocytes. Therefore, it is widely considered preferable, when possible, to target tumor-specific Ag not shared by normal tissues, or, if unavoidable, shared tissue Ag, which are only expressed by host organs nonessential to survival. Examples of such "expendable" shared tissue Ag include prostate-specific Ag and prostatic acid phosphatase, each of which is expressed only by malignant prostate cancer and by normal prostate, a nonessential organ *(23)*. Similarly, the expression of several Ag is limited to tumors and to normal testes (e.g., RAGE and MAGE), again a theoretically expendable organ, which is, furthermore, absent in females *(24–26)*.

2.3. T Cells Recognize Tumor Ag as Peptides in MHCs

Ag recognition by T cells normally employs an interaction between the T cell receptor (TCR) of T cells and the MHC molecules on the surface of other cells. Two types of MHC complexes, MHC class I and MHC class II, may be expressed by somatic and tumor cells. The majority of peripheral (mature) T cells express either CD4 or CD8 molecules, which are appositional ligands for MHC class II and I molecules, respectively. Once juxtaposed with an MHC class II or I molecule, the T cell's TCR can accomplish a sweeping probe of the MHC cleft, permitting identification of antigenic peptides transported to the cleft from the inside of the cell. If the T cell's particular TCR has a high affinity for the particular contacted peptide-MHC complex, the process of T cell activation can be initiated *(27,28)*.

The typical studied tumor cell expresses MHC class I molecules, but displays a more variable or absent expression of MHC class II molecules *(28)*. Such observations led almost 25 yr ago to a hypothesis, still prevalent today, that T cell-mediated tumor rejection must primarily be mediated by $CD8^+$ killer T cells capable of direct interaction with the MHC class I-expressing tumor cells *(7)*. A corollary prevalent hypothesis is that $CD8^+$ killer T cells are sensitized primarily by direct contact with MHC class I-expressing tumor cells. In the past 25 yr, an ever-increasing body of evidence has rendered these hypotheses untenable *(9,28)*. Although the participation of killer $CD8^+$ T cells in the rejection of many tumors is undoubted, it is now also apparent that "killer $CD8^+$ T cells" represent merely one of many available mechanisms for successful tumor rejection.

2.4. T Cell Sensitization to Tumor Ag Requires Contact with Normal Host Ag-Presenting Cells Rather than Tumor Cells

Even when sensitized killer $CD8^+$ T cells are involved in rejection of an individual tumor, it is now clear that the initial sensitization of both $CD4^+$ and $CD8^+$ T cells typically requires contact with host Ag presenting cells (APC), which present scavenged tumor Ag, rather than contact with tumor cells themselves *(27,28)*. Host stromal cells such as macrophages and dendritic cells (DCs) are adept at ingesting ambient (exogenous) proteins to derive peptides for presentation in both MHC class II and MHC class I complex clefts, supporting sensitization of $CD4^+$ and $CD8^+$ T cells, respectively *(27,29,30)*. Therefore, extracellular tumor products, whether leached debris from apoptotic or dead tumor cells or secretions by viable and proliferating tumor cells, are locally available for macrophage and DC scavenging via exogenous processing pathways. The ability of host stromal cells such as macrophages and DCs to present exogenous tumor Ag to T cells provides many advantages to the host's immune system: (*i*) because tumor cells typically lack expression of co-stimulatory molecules such as intercellular adhesion molecule (ICAM)-1 and B7, they are unlikely to provide maximal activation of T cells, even if the tumor cells are able to present Ag via MHC molecules on their surface *(28,31,32)*. Furthermore, MHC presentation of Ag in the absence of co-stimulation can induce T cell tolerance rather than T cell activation *(33)*; (*ii*) DCs, which scavenge exogenous tumor Ag for presentation, have the capacity to migrate out of the tumor environment and transport the Ag downstream to draining lymph nodes, an undoubtedly superior environment in which to accomplish T cell sensitization and/or restimulation of memory T cell responses *(34,35)*; and (*iii*) spontaneous mutation by tumor cells frequently deletes their expression of functional MHC class I molecules and/or particular Ag, making them, at best, unreliable APC *(14,36)*.

2.5. Intratumoral Activation of Effector T Cells Is More Reliably Achieved by Contact with Normal Host Ag-Presenting Cells than by Tumor Cells

Once sensitized, antitumor effector T cells must recirculate until they become activated by encounters with relevant tumor Ag, ideally both at macrometastases and at micrometastases. Even at this stage of differentiation, current evidence suggests that both $CD4^+$ and $CD8^+$ T cells are more likely to be activated to effector function when exogenous tumor-derived peptides are presented by stromal host APC (e.g., macrophages) rather than by tumor cells themselves *(9,10,37)*.

It is possible to study the interactions of sensitized effector T cells with the tumor environment by enzymatically digesting solid tumors to yield a single-cell suspension of viable cells. Lineage analyses confirm that such tumor digests are typically composed of both neoplastic cells and normal host stromal cells, including macrophages, DCs, fibroblasts, endothelial cells, T cells, B cells, and other constituents *(38)*. Culture of in vitro-activated effector T cells with relevant tumor digests typically results in production of cytokine production such as IFN-γ *(10)*. Since many tumor cells do not constitutively express MHC class II molecules, it is not surprising that antitumor $CD4^+$ effector T cells are typically activated not by direct tumor cell contact, but rather by specific contact with MHC class II-expressing macrophages intercalated among the tumor cells *(10)*. It has additionally been observed, however, that even $CD8^+$ effector T cells are more consistently reactive with macrophages derived from relevant tumor than with MHC class I-expressing tumor cells *(10)*. Therefore, as in the case of their initial sensitization, both $CD4^+$ and $CD8^+$ effector T cells appear to benefit from the superior co-stimulatory properties of professional host APC, which process and present exogenous tumor Ag within the tumor bed.

2.6. T Cell-Mediated Tumor Rejection Can Proceed Even in the Absence of Direct Killer Cell Contact with Tumor Cells

If T cell-mediated tumor rejection absolutely required $CD8^+$ killer T cells to recognize and lyse each and every single tumor cell, it would render every tumor with a subpopulation of MHC class I nonexpressing tumor cells flatly resistant to immunotherapy *(39,40)*. Furthermore, when subjugated to $CD8^+$ killer T cell attack, even tumors with initially uniform MHC class I expression experience a potent selection pressure, which favors mutations resulting in nonexpression of MHC class I or of tumor Ag itself *(39–41)*. Fidler et al. first demonstrated in the 1970s the ease with which tumor cells developed complete resistance to specific lysis when exposed to $CD8^+$ killer T cells for several in vitro passages *(39,40)*. Similar selection pressure leading in vivo to tumor cell deletion of functional MHC class I expression resistance and/or resistance to $CD8^+$ killer T cells has also been described both in animal models and in melanoma patients following indecisive immunotherapy maneuvers *(14,41)*.

Fortunately for the tumor host, knock-out mouse studies have clearly indicated that no single T cell-mediated mechanism is absolutely essential for tumor rejection. For example, when $CD8^+$ T cells are sensitized to tumor in perforin knock-out mice, they retain the capacity to secrete cytokines, but are unable to lyse tumor targets due to their inability to produce the pore-punching molecule perforin. Nonetheless, perforin knock-out (i.e., nonlytic) antitumor $CD8^+$ retain their capacity to reject tumor challenges, although higher doses of T cells must sometimes be infused to achieve maximal efficacy *(17,42)*.

That tumor rejection can proceed in the complete absence of direct contact between T cells and tumor cells was recently confirmed. Plautz et al. *(37)* sensitized T cells in bone marrow-transplanted chimeric mice to switch their recognition of tumor Ag to an MHC restriction different from that expressed by the tumor cells themselves. When such T cells were then transferred into tumor-bearing mice, tumor rejection was only successful in hosts whose native APC expressed the switched MHC restriction, but not in hosts whose APC expressed the same MHC restriction as the tumor cells. These studies proved that tumor rejection could totally bypass direct interactions with tumor cells in favor of Ag recognition via normal host APC *(37)*.

3. NONANTIGENIC MECHANISMS BY WHICH THE IMMUNE SYSTEM DISTINGUISHES TUMOR CELLS

The fact that tumor-specific T cells can totally avoid direct tumor cell contact during rejection indicates that secondary rejection mechanisms must be triggered after T cells identify relevant tumor-derived peptides on the surfaces of normal host APC. It will be apparent to the reader that secretion of cytokines and chemokines within a tumor is likely to have a similar impact whether the secretion is triggered by T cell contact with a tumor cell or by T cell contact with an adjacent host APC. Therefore, it is not surprising that currently identified "secondary" rejection mechanisms may largely arise as a consequence of cytokine and chemokine secretion. These mechanisms include the anti-angiogenic and apoptotic effects of cytokines themselves, as well as cytokine-induced activation of accessory (non-T) cells. In addition, activated T cells and cytokine-activated natural killer cells (lymphokine-activated killer [LAK] cells) acquire the capacity to mediate FAS ligand (APO-1 ligand)-dependent apoptosis of many tumor cells, which requires reciprocal tumor cell expression of FAS instead of Ag or MHC molecules *(43–47)*.

3.1. Direct Antitumor Effects of Cytokines

In certain animal models, biologic agents such as tumor necrosis factor (TNF)-α display an anti-angiogenic effect on the tumor vascular bed, which itself is sufficient to cause tumor rejection *(48–50)*. Such anti-angiogenic activity has been exploited in patients by directly infusing TNF-α into the tumor blood supply *(51)*. In addition, agents such as IFN and/or TNF-α can directly induce apoptosis of individual tumor cells *(52–56)*. Systemic treatment with anti-TNF-α or anti-IFN-γ Ab can in certain tumor models fully abrogate the therapeutic effect of adoptively transferred T cells, and administration of recombinant TNF-α alone (without T cells) is sufficient to cure certain established animal tumors *(18,48–50)*. In such instances, no cellular participation beyond that of cytokine-secreting T cells may be necessary to explain tumor rejection.

Direct effects of cytokines on tumor cells may also render them more susceptible to other mechanisms of tumor rejection. For example, exposure of tumor cells to IFN and/or TNF-α can up-regulate tumor cell expression of MHC class II and/or class I molecules, potentially rendering them more recognizable for direct contacts with T cells, including killer T cells. In addition, exposure to IFN can increase tumor cell transcription of phospholipid scramblase, leading to translocation of phosphatidylserine lipid to the outer cell membrane *(57)*. Such elevated target cell surface phosphatidylserine has been implicated both in macrophage-mediated phagocytosis of apoptotic cells *(58)* and in the binding of tumoricidal macrophages to the tumor cell surface (see next section) *(59)*.

3.2. Cytokine Activate Accessory Cells Which Kill Tumor Cells Nonantigenically

In most instances, it is likely that cytokine-induced tumor rejection involves activation of many host cells in additional to T lymphocytes. A seemingly interchangeable array of cytokines secreted by either $CD4^+$ or $CD8^+$ T cells, including

INF-γ, IL-2, IL-4, and GM-CSF, leads to accumulation and/or activation of natural killer (NK) lymphocytes, monocytes, and neutrophils *(60–72)*. Under the influence of such cytokines, NK and other lymphocytes including T cells can differentiate into LAK cells *(73,74)*, while monocytes and tissue macrophages can differentiate into tumoricidal macrophages (TMϕ) *(75)*.

Besides their role in tumor rejection, LAK cells and TMϕ each play a recognized prominent role in the physiological control of infectious pathogens such as bacterial, viruses, and parasites. TMϕ have an increased ability to phagocytize bacteria, including non-opsonized bacteria, as well as an augmented lysosomal machinery capable of lysing bacteria resistant to normal macrophage digestion *(75)*; LAK cells (i.e., cytokine-activated NK cells) display similar antibacterial activities *(76–79)*. In addition, both TMϕ and LAK cells can often distinguish infected host cells from normal host cells and kill the former *(75,80–82)*. Recognizable infected targets include not only virally transformed cells, but also host cells infected by microbial parasites such as *toxoplasma gondii* and *listeria monocytogenes (83–85)*.

In addition to their abilities to distinguish and destroy infected host cells, both TMϕ and LAK cells can each distinguish and kill transformed host cells (i.e., tumor cells) that contain no identifiable pathogen. Although their killing mechanisms are different (e.g., LAK cells kill targets within hours, whereas TMϕ often require several days) *(75,82)*, LAK cells or TMϕ prepared from a particular mouse or human are capable of recognizing and killing tumor cells not only from that individual, but also tumor cells from unrelated donors of the same species (allogenic) and even tumor cells from other species (xenogenic) *(80,81)*. Thus, this pattern of tumor killing is totally non-MHC restricted and does not involve any identifiable tumor Ag *(75,81,82)*. While nonactivated NK cells themselves have an ability to recognize and kill tumor targets with down-regulated MHC expression *(86–89)*, they acquire the ability to recognize and kill a vastly wider panoply of tumor cell targets after they experience LAK differentiation *(82)*. Similarly, monocytes typically do not recognize and kill tumor targets unless differentiated by cytokine exposure to become TMϕ *(75)*.

The mechanisms by which LAK cells and TMϕ identify that a target is transformed and needs to be destroyed is one of the great persistent enigmas of tumor immunology, because it implies there is a fundamental difference between transformed and normal cells which is independent of antigenicity. It is likely that the surface membranes of transformed cells display generic physicochemical properties which markedly increase their affinity for LAK cells and TMϕ. Such properties may include a chronically high density of exposed carbohydrates, linked to a diminished presence of differentiation elements, which may normally mask such carbohydrates *(59,90)*. Increased tumor surface exposure of such carbohydrates has been positively correlated with a variety of tumor characteristics, including ras mutations and invasive or metastatic behavior *(91–95)*.

In contrast, such carbohydrates are densely exposed on nontransformed cells only during mitosis *(91)*. Plant-derived lectin proteins, which specifically agglutinate such carbohydrates, typically display a much higher affinity for transformed cells and mitosing normal cells than for quiescent normal cells *(90–101)*. Consistent with the hypothesis that such exposed carbohydrates provide a basis for TMϕ interaction with tumor cells, lectin-like molecules have recently been isolated from TMϕ which can competitively block the binding of tumor cells by macrophages *(102–104)*. It is, therefore, possible that lectin-like molecules, which facilitate the binding of macrophages to bacterial carbohydrates, also provide a basis for affinity between TMϕ and tumor targets. Interestingly, expulsion of lysosomes from TMϕ into bound tumor cells—a kind of regurgitant phagocytosis that may persist for days—is a likely mechanism by which TMϕ kill tumor targets *(105,106)*.

Just as remarkable as their ability to identify and kill tumor cells, however, is the ability of TMϕ to spare normal cells. Even more remarkable is the fact that such sparing involves an active process of recognition rather than simply a lack of detection. TMϕ display a high binding affinity for replicating and/or activated cells, whether normal or transformed, but secondarily distinguish those bound cells that are transformed and suitable candidates for destruction. Classic target cell competition studies by Hamilton et al. demonstrated that activated normal lymphoblasts and growing cultured normal cells (but not resting lymphocytes) bound competitively to TMϕ and prevented their killing of tumor targets *(107–110)*. Nonetheless, normal lymphoblasts and growing normal cells proved markedly less susceptible than tumor cells to lysis by TMϕ, despite their shared high binding capacity *(107–110)*. The basis by which TMϕ form strong contacts with normal growing cells, but generally fail to kill them is unknown. It must be stressed, however, that a small fraction of such normal cells does display in vitro susceptibility to TMϕ-mediated killing *(107,111–113)*. Whether this susceptible fraction represents cells with a transiently elevated lectin agglutinability (such as those actively engaged in M phase of cell division) has not been elucidated *(91)*.

Prior to LAK differentiation, resting NK cells utilize a sophisticated battery of surface receptors, such as killer-cell immunoglobulin-like receptor(s) (KIR), to identify infected and transformed host cells with down-regulated MHC class I expression *(86–89)*. Recent data indicate that individual NK clones recognize specific combinations of hypoexpressed and normal MHC class I elements, enabling detection of tumor cells which hypoexpress MHC molecules to escape direct T cell recognition *(87)*. Not unexpectedly, the majority of tested tumors exhibit complete or heterogeneous resistance to such NK cell recognition *(114–117)*. Therefore, it is not surprising that, in addition to direct lysis of recognized target cells *(118–121)*, the NK response includes production of cytokines such as IFN-γ, GM-CSF, and TNF-α *(67,122)*, which enable NK cells themselves to acquire the extended tumor-recognizing capacity of LAK cells *(123–125)*.

Similar to TMϕ, the LAK cell interaction with potential targets appears to involve a generic affinity for replicating and/or activated cells, followed by a relatively specific recognition of the transformed state. Recent evidence suggests that LAK cells may utilize carbohydrate contacts for tumor recognition similar to those utilized by TMϕ *(126,127)*. The role of phosphatidylserine in LAK cell target recognition has not been studied. In contrast to the slow expulsion of lysosomes observed during the interaction between TMϕ and tumor cells, target killing by LAK cells is rapid and depends upon several mechanisms, including production of the pore punching protein perforin, Fas ligand expression, and TNF-α secretion *(128)*. Therefore, following activation by T cell- or NK cell-produced cytokines, LAK cells can perform Ag-nonrestricted, MHC-nonrestricted, direct tumor cell lysis even when such tumor cells escape direct NK or $CD8^+$ T cell recognition.

The likelihood that LAK cells and TMϕ utilize chronically dedifferentiated features of the transformed cell membrane for recognition may explain the observed inability of LAK- or TMϕ-challenged tumor lines to develop resistance to these mechanisms of killing. In classic murine studies performed by Fidler et al., it was demonstrated that B16 melanoma tumor cells remained susceptible to killing by TMϕ after repetitive co-culture with "sublethal" numbers of TMϕ in vitro, while in contrast, the same melanoma cell line rapidly developed resistance to killing by antitumor $CD8^+$ T cells following similar co-culture *(81,129)*. A similar failure of tumor cells to develop resistance to killing by LAK cells has also been described *(60)*. However, recent experiments indicate that malignant cells of various tissue derivations treated with differentiating retinoids display a reduced susceptibility to LAK lysis, despite their continued high binding affinity for LAK cells *(130)*. Other reports indicate that individual tumor lines may display constitutive resistance to LAK- or TMϕ-mediated killing even in the absence of in vitro challenges with LAK or TMϕ *(131–139)*. Such constitutively resistant tumor lines demonstrate decreased binding affinity for LAK cells or TMϕ, which may correlate to low surface expression of adhesion molecules and/or carbohydrate *(131,135)*. Nonetheless, tumor cell modulations which decrease their susceptibility to LAK- or TMϕ-mediated killing have been shown to reciprocally increase their susceptibility to NK-mediated killing, as well as *vice versa (135,136)*, suggesting that host mechanisms may already successfully anticipate such avenues of tumor escape.

3.3. T Cell Directed "Team Approach" to Tumor Rejection

As reviewed above, current evidence indicates that the immune system exploits, but does not rely solely upon, Ag and MHC expression by tumor cells to achieve tumor rejection. Since T cells entering a tumor bed can initially recognize relevant tumor-derived peptides on ambient host APC, there is no requirement for uniform MHC or Ag expression by tumor cells themselves. Thus, activated T cells can provide a cytokine-secreting catalyst to recruit and activate a wide spectrum of host attacks, including not only TCR/MHC restricted tumor cell lysis, but also Fas-mediated target killing, NK cell recognition of MHC hypoexpression, LAK cell and TMϕ recognition of nonantigenic physicochemical variances, and cytokine-mediated anti-angiogenesis and pro-apoptotic effects. Animal knock-out studies confirm that perforin-dependent (killer) T cell lysis can be a significant event in tumor rejection *(17)*, but other coincidental rejection events fully bypass the need for tumor cell MHC or Ag expression. When this spectrum of attacks is forcefully implemented, an individual tumor cell is less likely to escape immune recognition due to modulations in MHC or Ag expression, or otherwise acquired resistance to a particular attack mechanism (see above).

It is likely that intralesional injection of immune adjuvants such as BCG or *C. parvum* engages a similar activation of host recognition elements at the local injection site, often leading to successful tumor rejection even in the absence of tumor-specific T cells *(1,2,140–148)*. Such intralesional treatment apparently sensitizes host T cells to adjuvant-derived peptides, and their presentation by host APC within the injected tumor bed triggers T cell cytokine production *(144,145)*, activating host cells, such as TMϕ, which can directly contact, recognize, and kill tumor cells *(2)*. While intralesional BCG is currently instilled in this manner with considerable success to treat locally confined bladder cancer *(142,143)*, it is impossible to deliver such adjuvants to widely disseminated and/or poorly visualized cancers, which is why BCG therapy ultimately proved to be an ineffective treatment for metastatic melanoma. In contrast, effector T cells, which can recirculate and enter tumor deposits at any anatomic site, recognize tumor Ag bed, and initiate a cytokine/chemokine cascade similar to that induced by intralesional BCG, have the potential to catalyze systemically useful antitumor responses. Hence, properly functioning antitumor T cells are nature's own, frankly superior, immunologic "adjuvant".

4. MOUSE MODELS OF ANTITUMOR IMMUNITY

Great progress has been achieved in recent years, demonstrating for the first time that intravenously administrated T cells can in fact mediate rejection of poorly immunogenic and advanced tumors at all tested anatomic locations, including the brain. The earliest successful studies of T cell-mediated antitumor therapy had required that T cells be sensitized in animals that were not bearing progressive tumors *(149–151)*. This was accomplished by vaccinating healthy mice with lethally irradiated tumor cells, or by challenging healthy mice with tumor cells admixed with adjuvant such as *C. parvum* to ensure tumor rejection. T cells derived from such animals could often be adoptively transferred to cure syngeneic mice bearing the relevant progressive tumor. However, such studies did not establish whether similarly effective T cells could be derived from animals or patients already burdened by progressive tumors.

It became possible during the mid 1980s to propagate specific antitumor CD8+ T cells from the lymph nodes, spleens, and even tumor beds of mice bearing progressive tumors. These T cells were called "in vitro-sensitized" T cells or tumor-infiltrating lymphocytes (TILs) depending upon their method of preparation *(141,152–159)*. Such T cells frequently were tumor-specific, producing cytokines upon in vitro exposure to the relevant tumor and/or lysing the relevant tumor cells in vitro *(18)*. However, when these T cells were adoptively transferred into mice bearing the relevant tumor, the observed therapeutic effects were disappointing compared to T cells from immunized nontumor-bearing mice. In the latter instance, adoptively transferred T cells were effective for the treatment of tumors at multiple anatomic sites, and co-administration of recombinant IL-2 (rIL-2) was unnecessary for tumor rejection. In contrast, the CD8+ T cells propagated from tumor-bearing mice were typically ineffective therapy for tumors at extrapulmonary sites such as the skin and typically required co-administration of recombinant IL-2 to achieve therapeutic effects against pulmonary tumors *(9,38,155,160–162)*.

Investigators began to report the occurrence of TCR signal transduction abnormalities in tumor-bearing hosts, rendering more comprehensible the difficulties encountered in rendering such T cells therapeutically effective *(163–166)*. These reports kept alive the hope that naturally sensitized CD4+ and CD8+ pre-effector T cells existed in tumor-bearing hosts whose function had not yet been successfully activated and demonstrated.

To address this possibility, T cell cultures were modified by incorporating novel activation stimuli, such as immobilized anti-CD3 Ab or bacterial superantigens (sAg) *(166–187)*, and succeeded in reversing tumor-induced T cell signaling abnormalities *(166)*. For the first time in adoptive immunotherapy experiments, T cells cultured from tumor-bearing mice displayed a therapeutic potency equivalent to fresh T cells from immunized, non tumor-bearing mice (Fig. 1) *(168,188,189)*. Anti-CD3 or sAg-activated T cells derived from tumor-draining lymph nodes (TDLN) could be adoptively transferred to cure tumor established not only at the pulmonary location, but even at extrapulmonary locations such as the skin and even the brain, a location notorious as an immunotherapy-resistant relapse site in cancer patients (Figs. 2–4) *(189,190)*. Despite their being derived from tumor-bearing mice, T cells activated by these novel culture methods did not require co-administration of rIL-2 for their therapeutic effect.

An additional major result of these culture improvements was the first successful in vitro propagation of both antitumor CD4+ T cells and helper-independent CD8+ T cells from tumor-bearing mice *(10,189)*. These two distinct subpopulations had already proven to contain the most therapeutically potent

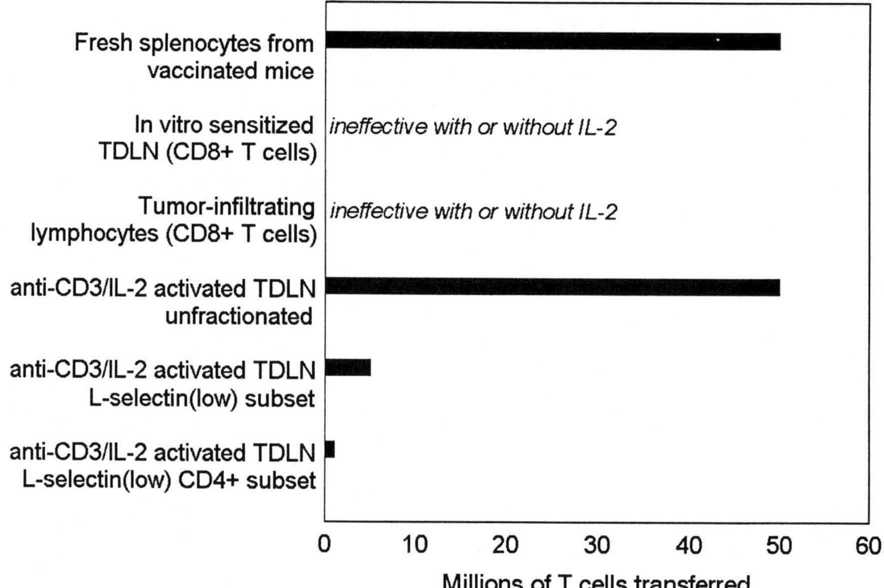

Fig. 1. Relative efficacy trends of different T cell preparations for the treatment of subcutaneous (s.c.) tumors. In many murine models, established s.c. tumors have the lowest susceptibility to adoptive therapy *(9)*. For purposes of historical comparison, the typical results of numerous experiments are compiled and represented graphically. Serially passed weakly immunogenic methylcholanthrene (MCA) sarcomas (203, 205, or 207) were implanted s.c. in syngeneic C57BL/6 mice. Mice received 500R of immunosensitizing whole body irradiation either prior to tumor implantation or prior to adoptive therapy with identical results. Adoptive therapy consisted of administration of syngeneic T cells through the tail vein. Dose of T cells displayed for each treatment is the number of T cells typically required for consistent and complete rejection of established s.c. tumors without co-administration of rIL-2. Treatment groups shown are "Fresh splenocytes from vaccinated mice" (mice induced to reject syngeneic tumor challenge by vaccination with tumor cells plus *C. parvum*, sacrificed after third tumor challenge is rejected, and immune splenocytes immediately given in adoptive transfer to syngeneic mice bearing the relevant 3-d s.c. tumor) *(9,38)*; "in vitro-sensitized TDLN" (TDLN harvested from tumor-bearing mice, then $CD8^+$ T cells expanded in vitro by in vitro sensitization method prior to use as adoptive therapy) *(155)*; "Tumor-infiltrating lymphocytes" ($CD8^+$ T cells expanded in vitro from whole cell digests of tumors prior to use as adoptive therapy) *(9,155)*; "Anti-CD3/IL-2-activated TDLN, unfractionated" (TDLN harvested from tumor-bearing mice, then T cells expanded in vitro by anti-CD3/IL-2 method prior to use as adoptive therapy) *(188)*; "Anti-CD3/IL-2-activated TDLN, L-selectin(low) subset" (L-selectin^{low} subset of TDLN harvested and isolated from tumor-bearing mice, then expanded in vitro by anti-CD3/IL-2 method prior to use as adoptive therapy) *(10)*; "Anti-CD3/IL-2-activated TDLN, L-selectin(low) $CD4^+$ subset" (L-selectin^{low} $CD4^+$ subset of TDLN harvested and isolated from tumor-bearing mice, then expanded in vitro by anti-CD3/IL-2 method prior to use as adoptive therapy) *(10)*.

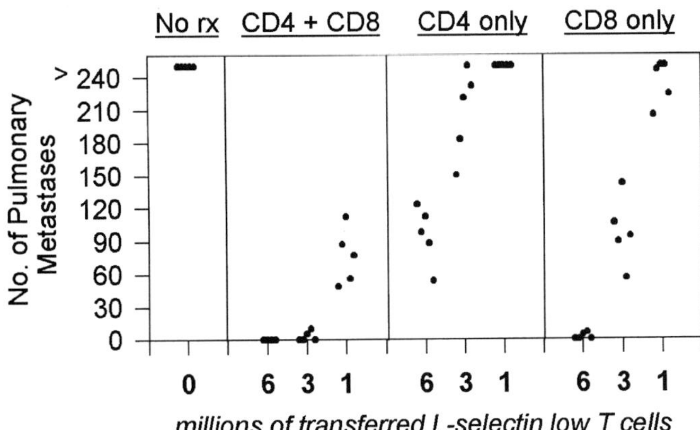

Fig. 2. Successful treatment of 10-d pulmonary metastases with L-selectin^{low} TDLN T cell subsets. Syngeneic C57BL/6 (B6) mice were injected with viable MCA-205 cells and TDLN harvested on d 12. L-selectin^{low} TDLN T cells containing both CD4^{+} and CD8^{+} cells ("CD4 + CD8"), as well as individual L-selectin^{low} CD4^{+} and CD8^{+} subsets ("CD4","CD8") were isolated for a 5-d culture-activation with anti-CD3/rIL-2, as described in ref. *10*. Each cultured T cell group was harvested and adoptively transferred into syngeneic mice with 10-d established MCA-205 pulmonary metastases. Recipient mice received sublethal irradiation (500R) prior to adoptive transfer. Mice received 1 milli on (1E6), 3E6, or 6E6 T cells. Ordinate shows number of pulmonary metastases observed in mice sacrificed 11 d after adoptive therapy. Each point represents a single mouse (5 mice per treatment group). Mice received no rIL-2 treatment during adoptive therapy. Modified from ref. *10*.

T cells in vaccinated (nontumor-bearing) mice *(9,191,192)*. Now, for the first time, it was apparent that these highly potent T cell subsets were also naturally sensitized even in mice bearing aggressive, progressively growing tumors (Figs. 2–4) *(10,189)*. Although the CD4^{+} and helper-independent CD8^{+} T cell subsets required ex vivo activation to unmask their effector potency, both subsets proved to be easily purified from TDLN, due to their phenotypically distinct low expression of the surface protein L-selectin (CD62L) *(9,10,189)*.

L-selectin is a cell surface molecule involved in the extravasation of cells from the bloodstream, displaying a strong lectin-like affinity for the postcapillary venules of peripheral lymph nodes *(193)*. With such a homing affinity, it is not surprising that the majority of T cells present in peripheral lymph nodes express high levels of L-selectin. However, since down-regulated expression of L-selectin is commonly observed in T cells following activation stimuli *(194–197)*, it is also not surprising that the TDLN T cell subset with low L-selectin expression includes T cells specifically sensitized to tumor in vivo *(9)*. Since the L-selectin down-regulated T cell's affinity for peripheral lymph node post-capillary venules is decreased, the results appears to be greater trafficking free-

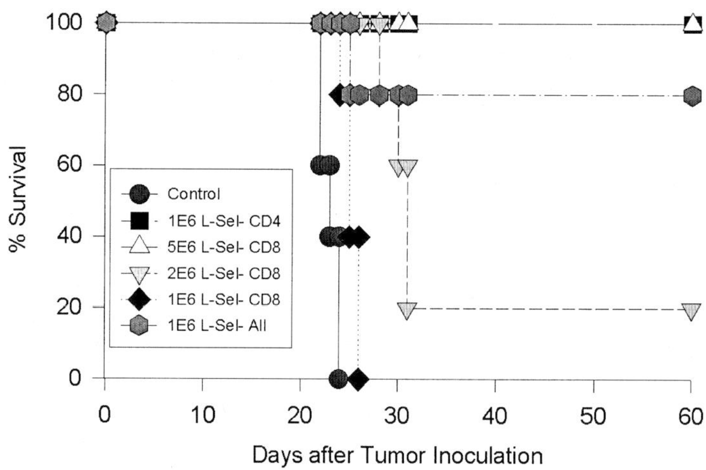

Fig. 3. Successful treatment of d 3 intracranial L-selectin^{low} TDLN T cell subsets. L-selectin^{low} T cells unfractionated for CD4 and CD8, L-selectin^{low} CD4^{+} T cells, and L-selectin^{low} CD8^{+} T cells were each prepared from freshly harvested TDLN cells of B6 mice bearing syngeneic 12-d MCA-205 tumors as described in ref. *10*. Following a 5-d culture-activation with anti-CD3/IL-2, each T cell group was harvested and administered to sublethally irradiated (500R) B6 mice bearing d 3 intracranial tumors. The future shows long-term survival of mice with intracranial MCA-205 treated with 1 million (1E6) L-selectin^{low} T cells unfractionated for CD4 and CD8 ("L-Sel-All"), 1E6 L-selectin^{low} CD4^{+} T cells ("L-Sel-CD4"), or 1E6, 2E6, or 5E6 L-selectin^{low} CD8^{+} T cells ("L-Sel-CD8)." Historically, mice surviving symptom-free at d 60 are cured in this model. Mice received no rIL-2 treatment during adoptive therapy. Modified from ref. *10*.

dom when it recirculates in the bloodstream, thus increasing its random likelihood of entering tumor beds at diverse anatomic locations. This as yet unproven hypothesis is strongly supported by the observed traffic patterns of adoptive transferred L-selectin^{low} T cells, which enter tumors at all tested anatomic locations at a much higher frequency than L-selectin^{high} T cells regardless of their Ag specificity *(193)*.

As observed for L-selectin^{high} T cells, accessory cells such as LAK and TMϕ also appear to have a limited capacity to traffick into tumors, at least in the absence of supervisory signals from T cells *(60)*. Such observations underscore the possibility that many components of cell-mediated immunity depend upon the superior initial capacity of L-selectin^{low} T cells to randomly enter tumor beds, react with tumor Ag, and launch a cytokine-chemokine cascade to recruit and activate the other cellular elements. An additional remarkable property of L-selectin^{low} T cells is their ability to sustain and augment an antitumor response even when their initial presence in a tumor is scant. In fact, a tumor may continue to grow progressively for several weeks before L-selectin^{low} T cell-

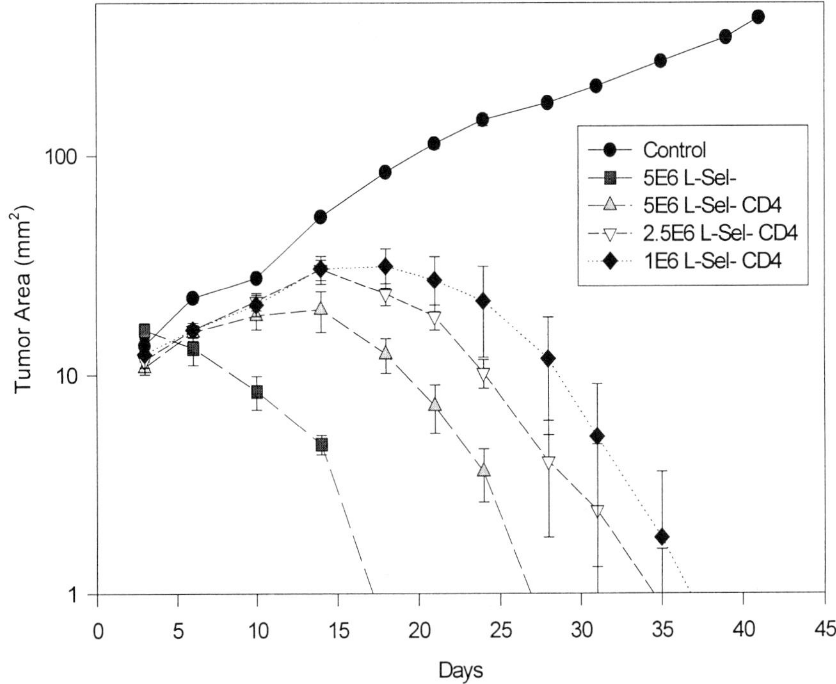

Fig. 4. Dose dependence of T cell adoptive therapy of 3-d s.c. metastases with CD4$^+$ L-selectin^{low} TDLN T cells. Syngeneic C57BL/6 (B6) mice were injected with viable MCA-205 cells and TDLN harvested on d 9 to prepare purified L-selectin^{low} T cells, either unfractionated for CD4 and CD8 or purified L-selectin^{low} CD4$^+$ T cells. On d 5 after anti-CD3/IL-2 culture-activation, T cell groups were harvested and adoptively transferred to treat syngeneic mice with 3-d established s.c. tumors. Recipient mice received 500R prior to adoptive transfer. Subsequent growth of the s.c. tumors was serially evaluated. Ordinate displays tumor area determined by two perpendicular caliper measurements; abscissa displays the day following tumor inoculation. Symbols on each line display average tumor measurement of each treatment group at particular time points, 5 mice per treatment group, with standard deviation (SD) displayed. Data are shown in log scale to facilitate visualization of differences between groups at early timepoints. Each treatment group received adoptive transfer of either L-selectin^{low} T cells unfractionated for CD4 and CD8 ("L-selectin low [CD4 + CD8]") or purified L-selectin^{low} CD4$^+$ T cells ("L-selectin low CD4"). Mice received no rIL-2 treatment during adoptive therapy. Modified from ref. *10*.

initiated tumor rejection becomes detectable *(10)*. The surprising capacity of L-selectin^{low} T cells to proliferate within the tumor bed suggests that they are able to augment their own presence as an initial effector tactic *(193)*.

It must be stressed, however, that despite the superior attributes of L-selectin^{low}-sensitized T cells, many tumor models remain incompletely susceptible to T cell-mediated immunotherapy. For example, tumors implanted at the subcutaneous location in syngeneic mice remain insusceptible to T cell adoptive immunotherapy, unless the tumor hosts also receive immunosensitizing sublethal irradiation or cyclophosphamide *(188,198)*. Interestingly, such adjunct irradiation can be administered to mice even prior to tumor inoculation (i.e., tumor cells themselves need not be irradiated), indicating that normal host cells such as Ag-presenting macrophages, rather than tumor cells themselves, are the probable therapeutic target of adjunct irradiation *(188,198)*. Such findings reinforce the concern that even optimally activated T cells can be subverted by immunosuppressive features of the tumor environment, which are reviewed in detail under Subheading 6.

5. CANCER PATIENTS AND IMMUNOTHERAPY

Attempts during the 1980s and 1990s to obtain clinical responses in cancer patients by preparing and adoptively transferring autologous LAK cells, TMϕ, or TIL yielded disappointing results. For example, although treatment of melanoma patients with TIL plus recombinant IL-2 (rIL-2) increased the total objective response rate compared to rIL-2 treatment alone (36% vs 20%), the underlying complete response (CR) rate with either treatment group remained 7% *(199)*. Similar 7% CR rates were obtained when patients were vaccinated with melanoma-associated peptide (modified GP-100 peptide) plus rIL-2 *(200)*, or whole cell allogenic melanoma cells without rIL-2 *(201)*. Such results suggested that approximately one fourteenth (7%) of melanoma patients were exceptionally responsive to a wide variety of therapies, but that the great majority of melanoma patients did not benefit, since even partial responses (PRs) were not clearly associated with improved survival. Furthermore, in the case of modified GP-100 peptide vaccination, demonstrable sensitization of patient T cells, specific T cell accumulation in metastatic nodules, and even intratumoral IFN-γ production were demonstrable even in the absence of detectable tumor regression *(200,202)*.

Clinical responses to LAK cells, TMϕ, and TIL therapy have led to continued efforts in animal models to improve efficacy of adoptive therapies (see above). Efforts to purify the human equivalent of the highly efficient L-selectin^{low} effector T cells obtainable in murine tumors are ongoing. In addition, several recent clinical trials have demonstrated the possibility of increasing the CR/PR rate to immunotherapy in patients with kidney cancer and melanoma.

Patients with metastatic kidney cancer, who underwent nonmyeloablative conditioning and received human leukocyte antigen (HLA)-compatible sibling bone marrow and T cells, achieved a 55% total response rate, including a 16% CR rate *(203)*. Patients with metastatic kidney cancer, who received vaccines of their own tumor cells electrofused to normal donor (allogenic) DCs, could achieve a 25% CR rate even without allogenic bone marrow transplant *(11)*. With either treatment, laboratory evidence supported *de novo* T cell sensitization as one of the primary events of treatment, but it remains to be confirmed that T cells form the basis of tumor rejection. From the clinical point of view, these trials are remarkable, because patient responses, both CRs and PRs, appear to be associated with prolongation of survival, and the response rates observed are superior to previous immunotherapy (i.e., for kidney cancer, the total response [CR + PR] to conventional rIL-2 therapy is ≤20%, with a CR rate ≤9%). Although such dramatic increases in response rate have not yet been observed in the immunotherapy of melanoma, a recent and ongoing trial has demonstrated an increased CR rate (13%) with a suggestion also of sustained PRs in patients who received repeated vaccination with autologous DCs pulsed with a variety of melanoma Ag *(12)*. Furthermore, a 13% CR rate in patients with in-transit melanoma lesions who were vaccinated with whole cell allogenic melanoma cells has been reported *(204)*.

Is there a unifying element to the improved response rates in these recent studies? We know from earlier clinical studies, as well as from animal studies, that three different types of responses are typically observed following successful T cell sensitization to tumor Ag: (*i*) complete tumor regression without recurrence, as observed following successful adoptive therapy with L-selectin^{low} T cells in mouse tumor models *(10)*; (*ii*) transient tumor regression followed by tumor regrowth, as observed following certain vaccine maneuvers *(205)*; and (*iii*) no clinical response despite successful T cell sensitization, as observed in the case of modified GP-100 peptide vaccination (without rIL-2) *(200)*. In the case of transient tumor regressions, there is evidence that interval booster revaccination can produce repetitive temporary regressions, suggesting that the problem is an inadequately sustained effector T cell response, rather than apoptosis (i.e., cloncal deletion) of the T cell response or changed Ag/MHC expression by tumor cells themselves *(205)*. Whereas such findings would seem to mandate frequent repetitive treatments, kidney cancer patients in the Kugler et al. study obtained sustained CRs merely with infrequent (every 3 mo) vaccine boosts, and the majority of CRs were obtained even before the first booster, suggesting that truly effective immunotherapy can be self-sustaining, even in patients with advanced disease *(11)*.

What enables an immunotherapy stimulus to become a self-sustaining response? It has repeatedly been observed that CD4$^+$ T cell responses are frequently necessary or at least helpful for sustaining CD8$^+$ T cell responses, and that in at least certain circumstances such CD4$^+$ T cell responses can themselves be self-sustaining. The ability of CD4$^+$ T cells to condition DCs to promote CD8$^+$ T cell responses, in part through CD40 ligation, is well established *(206)*. It is noteworthy that each of the above-described vaccination treatments with heightened clinical responses employed whole-cell tumor materials rather than purified MHC class I-binding peptides, increasing the likelihood of generating both $CD4^+$ and $CD8^+$ responses *(11,12,204)*. In addition, the inclusion of allogenic stimuli in many of these trials (e.g., allogenic tumor cells, allogenic DCs, or allogenic donor T cells) may increase DC conditioning through a potent $CD4^+$ T cell anti-allogenic response, ultimately facilitating the sensitization of both $CD8^+$ and $CD4^+$ tumor-specific T cells *(11,203,204)*.

Current evidence suggests that T cell sensitization to Ag can be accompanied by several different types of functional specialization. For example, "T1" specialization results in T cells that preferentially secrete biologic factors involved in cell-mediated immunity and generation of complement-fixing Ab (e.g., IFN-γ, perforin, IL-2). In contrast, "T2" specialization results in T cells that preferentially secrete biologic factors involved in generation of neutralizing Ab, IgA, and IgE (e.g., IL-4, IL-5, and IL-10), and such responses may sometimes down-regulate cell-mediated immunity *(207)*. T1 vs T2 specialization may be modulated by specialized DCs deemed "DC1" and "DC2" *(208)*. Mice successfully vaccinated against tumor contain committed T1-type antitumor $CD4^+$ T cells *(38,209)*, and recent data appear to confirm that T cell responses biased in favor of T1 specialization may more efficiently promote tumor rejection *(207)*. It is, therefore, apparent that immunotherapy strategies, which specifically promote DC1 function, hence, T1 function, may be highly desirable.

6. IMMUNOSUPPRESSION AS A NORMAL (PHYSIOLOGIC) EVENT

If effective antitumor immunity consists of a T1-type sustained response against tumor Ag, it is apparent that a tumor may successfully subvert the immune response in a variety of ways, including induction of a T1→T2 (or DC1→DC2) shift, induction of T cell tolerance (nonsustained response), or clonal deletion of antitumor T cells (e.g., apoptosis). However, such subversion is not unique to tumors. To the contrary, there are many circumstances in which immunosuppression is necessary to maintain normal tissue function, as in the cases of alloantigenic placenta and bacterially-commensualized large intestine. Substances within these tissues, such as prostaglandins (PGs), IL-10, vascular endothelial growth factor (VEGF), transforming growth factor beta (TGFβ), and glucocorticoids, each display distinctive immunosuppressive effects on T lymphocytes and/or APC *(13,210,211)*. Such factors may be secreted by several cell types within each tissue, including parenchymal cells *(212–216)*, fibroblasts *(217)*, endothelial cells *(218,219)*, macrophages *(220,221)*, and lymphocytes *(222,223)*. The abundance of cyclooxygenase-2 (COX-2)-derived cAMP-elevating PG, as well as IL-10 and TGFβ in colonic mucosa and placenta, suggest that these agents significantly contribute to the chronic immunosuppression exemplified by these tissues *(212,216,221,223–236)*. This is corroborated by findings that IL-10 deficient mice, anti-TGFβ1-treated mice, and COX-2-inhibited rats each display heightened tissue injury during experimental inflammatory bowel disease *(237–243)*. In addition, placental trophoblasts can express a variety of surface molecules such as Fas/Apo-1 ligand and TNF receptor p55 to induce apoptosis of activated maternal T cells *(244–247)*.

The next sections describe in detail several well-studied molecular mechanisms of immunosuppression, which appear to be highly relevant to tumor escape.

7. EVIDENCE FOR IMMUNE DYSFUNCTION IN T CELLS FROM PATIENTS WITH TUMORS

Within many solid tumors, there is typically a significant infiltrate of mononuclear cells consisting primarily of T lymphocytes and variably of macrophages, with little accumulation of NK, B cells, or granulocytes *(248)*. The T cell population is composed of CD4$^+$ and CD8$^+$ subsets containing clones capable of preferentially recognizing autologous as well as nonspecific effector cells *(249,250)*. However, despite this infiltrate, there is little compelling data to suggest the development of a Th1-type response in the tumor bed. Analysis of cytokine gene expression by reverse transcription-polymerase chain reaction (RT-PCR) indicates variable, but typically low percentage, of infiltrating lymphocytes that express mRNA for IL-2 and IFN-γ *(251,252)*. These findings are similar to those reported for other tumor types *(253)*. Moreover, less than 5% of TILs express IL-2 receptor (IL-2R)α (mRNA or surface protein), which is up-regulated on activated T cells *(254)*.

There is also data showing that freshly isolated TILs demonstrate a selective unresponsive state in vitro suggesting a defect in immunological competence in vivo. TILs are impaired in their proliferative capacity irrespective of the stimuli used, which is a common feature of infiltrating cells from a variety of tumor types *(254–256)*. Defective proliferation may be partly linked to altered signaling through the IL-2R. The addition of exogenous IL-2 to in vitro-activated TILs expressing IL-2Rα and IL-2Rβ chains did not result in cell cycle progression from G0 through G1 (Kolenko and Finke, unpublished data). The inducible cytolytic capacity of TILs is also diminished.

There is also evidence for immune dysfunction in vivo. Delayed type hypersensitivity is impaired in a subset of cancer patients challenged with common recall Ag (purified protein derivative [PPD], mumps, and Candida) *(257)*. Furthermore, the response rate to PPD skin testing with stage I renal cell carcinoma (RCC) was significantly higher than that of patients with stage IV disease *(258)*.

8. ALTERED SIGNAL TRANSDUCTION IN CANCER PATIENT T CELLS

Impairment in signal transduction pathways may contribute to the immune dysfunction observed in T cells from tumor-bearing host. Decreased expression of signaling elements linked to TCR have been reported to be depressed in certain murine tumor models and in patients with cancer *(164,259–261)*. This includes the ζ chain of the TCR as well as the expression of associated tyrosine kinases, $p56^{lck}$, $p59^{fyn}$, and ZAP-70 *(164,259–261)*. Several different mechanisms have been proposed to account for the defect in ζ chain expression. Two different groups showed that hydrogen peroxide produced by tumor-associated macrophages down-regulates ζ chain expression and inhibits tumor specific T cell and NK cell-mediated cytotoxicity *(262,263)*. Chronic Ag stimulation has been suggested as another means of down-regulating the ζ chain *(264)*. Additional data suggest that the ζ chain is degraded by activated caspase-3 and caspase-7 in T cells as a consequence of apoptosis *(265)*.

There is also evidence that activation of the transcription factor nuclear factor (NF)κB is impaired in T cells from tumor-bearing host, which may contribute to the immune dysfunction *(266–268)*. The nuclear translocation of NFκB regulates the transcription of genes involved in the development of T cell immunity. Animal studies have demonstrated impairment in NFκB translocation during tumor progression, which appears to precede the alteration in the ζ chain expression of T cells *(266,267)*. Furthermore, the decrease in NFκB activation coincided with reduced expression of IL-2 and IFN-γ production *(266,267)*. We have demonstrated impaired activation of NFκB in T cells derived from RCC patients *(268)*. The major problem is the normal nuclear accumulation of NFκB after activation *(269)*. Gangliosides shed from RCC may be partially responsible for this defect in NFκB activation *(270)*.

There are several lines of evidence to suggest that alteration in NFκB activation in RCC patient T cells increases their sensitivity to apoptosis. We have observed T cells in the tumor bed with evidence of DNA breaks as defined by the terminal deoxynucleotidyl transferase-mediated dUTP-X nick end-labeling (TUNEL) assay *(271)*. In addition, peripheral blood T cells from 30% of RCC patients, but not normal individuals, display an early marker of apoptosis, the externalization of phosphatidyl serine *(271)*.

9. SOLUBLE PRODUCTS PRODUCED BY TUMORS MAY INHIBIT T CELL ANTITUMOR ACTIVITY

Tumor cells are known to produce a variety of biologically active substances that may contribute to their proliferation and survival either directly, by autocrine or paracrine effects on transformed cells, or indirectly, by muting the normal immune cellular response to foreign cellular proteins. A cell, which has been transformed, may, therefore, continue to produce substances it generated before oncogenesis, albeit in a manner that may differ quantitatively or qualitatively. In addition, new or mutated cellular proteins, such as tumor suppressor gene products, may also contribute to the unregulated growth that is characteristic of malignant cells.

Table 1
Immunosuppressive Molecules
Produced by the Tumor and/or Associated Stroma

Products	*Potential signaling targets*
PGE2	NFκB, JAK3
H_2O_2	TCRζ
TGFβ	IL-2R signaling
IL-10	NFκB
Gangliosides	NFκB
Soluble Fas-L	Fas-death pathway

Inadequate function of T-TILs may be attributable in part to a variety of immunosuppressive molecules produced by the tumor and/or its associated stroma (Table 1). These products, including cytokines such as IL-10 and TGFβ, PGs and tumor-derived gangliosides, may serve as paracrine mediators to diminish effective cellular antitumor immunity via their effects on T cell surface molecules, signaling events and ultimately, effector function.

9.1. IL-10

The complex relationship between cytokines and cancer is poorly understood. Under the best conditions, local production of cytokines and chemokines within the tumor bed would result in recruitment and activation of tumor-associated inflammatory cells capable of initiating an effective antitumor response *(272,273)*. However, there is little evidence for this type of effective orchestrated cytokine activity within the bed of most solid tumors. Instead, the predominant cytokine expressed in the tumor, including RCC, appears to be the T2 cytokine IL-10 *(251,252)*. The biologic properties of IL-10 may counteract both specific and nonspecific T cell-mediated immunity, primarily due to its ability to downregulate MHC class II expression on monocytes and/or DCs leading to impaired Ag presentation *(274)*. IL-10 also has direct inhibitory effects on T cell growth *(275)*, which may be related to its known ability to inhibit the transcription factor NFκB *(276)*. IL-10 can further reduce antitumor immunity by suppressing the secretion of other pro-inflammatory cytokines such as IL-1, IL-6, IL-8, and TNF-α *(277)*. Expression of IL-10 has been attributed both to primary tumor cells *(278)* and to inflammatory cells, such as activated monocytes and helper T cells *(251,252)*. The relative contribution of each of these sources of IL-10 within the tumor bed and its implication for alterations in T cell activity remain to be determined. Recent findings provide in vivo evidence for IL-10-mediated suppression of antitumor responses, which may promote tumor progression. The injection of a murine bladder tumor (MB49) into IL-10 knock-out mice did prime T cells for an Ag-specific T cell response. In addition, IL-10 knock-out mice showed prolonged survival and an increased capacity to reject tumors when compared to normal mice *(279)*. However, these findings differ from those of others who showed transfection of tumor with the IL-10 gene leads to an increased antitumor immune response and decreased tumorigenicity *(280,281)*. It may be that different tumors are inherently different in their response to IL-10. It is also noted that most of the studies correlating IL-10 with decreased tumorigenicity used IL-10-transfected tumor cells, which may not reflect the natural production of IL-10 in the tumor microenvironment. Nevertheless, under the right conditions IL-10 can either suppress or enhance the development of antitumor immunity.

9.2. TGFβ

A second immunosuppressive cytokine that may reduce effective T cell function in RCC is TGFβ. TGFβ can inhibit lymphocyte proliferation at very low (fentomolar) concentrations, suggesting that it is more potent than even the T cell-specific immunosuppressant cyclosporin A in diminishing the T cell response *(282,283)*. Such low levels of TGFβ are almost certainly attainable within the tumor microenvironment. The primary effect of TGFβ appears to be reduction of T cell proliferation by inhibiting both TCR and IL-2R-mediated tyrosine phosphorylation, which affects subsequent downstream signaling events central to the control of cell cycle progression, such as phosphorylation of the Rb protein *(282)*. These antiproliferative effects appear to involve both helper and cytotoxic T cells *(284)*.

9.3. Immunosuppressive PGs

Prostaglandin E_2 (PGE_2) can also inhibit T cell activation *(285,286)* and may functionally diminish immune cellular responsiveness in the tumor bed of cancer patients. The mechanism of T cell suppression by PGE_2 appears to be through increasing the levels of the intracellular second messenger, cyclic adenosine monophosphate (cAMP) *(286)*. PGE_2 is also known to inhibit the DNA binding activity of the transcriptional factor, NFκB, to the IL-2 transcriptional start site, thereby blocking production of IL-2 *(287)*. More recent studies indicate that PGE_2-induced inhibition of T cell proliferation is mediated through blocking IL-2-dependent G1-S transition *(288)*. This defect may be due to down-regulation of Janus Kinase (JAK)3 expression, resulting in impaired phosphorylation and DNA binding activity of signal transducer and activator of transcription (STAT5) *(289)*. Moreover, NK cell function may also be suppressed by PGs present within the tumor environment. Macrophages from mice bearing the Renca renal carcinoma were found to suppress the generation of LAK and NK cells in vitro through the synthesis of immunosuppressive PGs.

9.4. Immunosuppressive Gangliosides

A fourth important class of soluble mediators that may inhibit the host immune response is tumor-derived gangliosides. These glycosphingolipids are over-expressed in several tumor types, including melanoma, neuroblastoma, and RCC *(290–292)*, and may inhibit several steps critical to effective cellular immunity including Ag presentation or processing *(293)*, lymphocyte clonal expansion *(294)*, and cytotoxic effector function *(295)*. Purified bovine brain gangliosides have also been shown to suppress NFκB-specific binding activity in T cells and inhibit transcription of IL-2 and IFN-γ without affecting IL-4 or IL-10 production, suggesting they may contribute to a functional T1 to T2 cytokine shift *(296)*.

Gangliosides contribute to the immune suppression observed in tumor-bearing hosts. Select gangliosides are increased in expression and shed into the tumor microenvironment *(291)*. For example, in malignant melanomas and neuroblastomas, there is overexpression of the gangliosides GD3, GD2, and GM2 *(291)*. Rapid progression of tumor and lower survival rate was related to higher GD2 levels in patients with neuroblastoma *(297)*. Recent findings also show increased expression of GD1a, GM1, and GM2 in RCCs as compared to normal kidney tissue *(292)*. Tumor gangliosides isolated from different tumor sources, such as neuroblastoma, lymphoma, and melanoma, all can inhibit immune responses *(291)*. These gangliosides suppress T cell proliferation and T1 cytokine production in vitro *(296)*. Recent animal studies have shown that the administration of tumor-derived GM1b inhibited the in vivo development of antitumor immunity and promoted malignant growth *(298)*. Moreover, data from our laboratory indicates that select gangliosides render peripheral blood T cells sensitive to activation-induced cell death (Finke unpublished). Animal studies have also demonstrated that brain gangliosides (GM1, GD1a, GD1b) increased T cell susceptibility to activation-induced cell death (AICD) *(299)*. The increased sensitivity of the murine T cells to AICD correlated with ganglioside-mediated induction of mRNA encoding BAX, a pro-apoptotic Bcl-2 family member *(299)*.

We have recently identified tumor-derived gangliosides as one metabolically active component of crude tumor supernatant from RCC explants. Gangliosides have been isolated from RCC tumor and supernatant, but not from that of adjacent normal kidney, and are capable of inhibiting NFκB activation in normal T cells. The suppression of κB binding activity occurred in the setting of normal upstream signaling events such as degradation of the cytoplasmic inhibitor of NFκB activation, IκBα.

10. REDUCED EXPRESSION OF AG PRESENTATION MACHINERY IN TUMORS CONTRIBUTES TO IMMUNE DYSFUNCTION

Down-regulation of components of Ag processing and presenting machinery has been identified in human malignant cells, including RCC, which may blunt endogenous antitumor immunity *(300)*. This defect includes reduced or absent expression of MHC class I heavy and light chains, diminished levels of transporters associated with Ag processing (TAP) proteins, as well as deficient expression of latent membrane protein (LMP) = proteosomal complexes *(301)*. Down-regulation of the components of cellular Ag processing and presentation have been identified in a number of other solid tumors, including lesions of the lung, liver, prostate, colon, cervix, skin, and breast. Such TAP and MHC defects may provide malignant cells with a mechanism for escaping cytotoxic T lymphocyte (CTL)-mediated recognition and destruction.

11. TUMOR INDUCTION OF APOPTOSIS IN T CELL DIMINISHES EFFECTIVE ANTITUMOR IMMUNITY

Recent studies suggest that cell-mediated immunity may be down-regulated through apoptotic pathways *(302,303)*. Interactions between the Fas receptor (Apo-1/CD95) and its ligand (Fas-L/CD95-L) have been implicated in a number of normal and pathological processes regulating T cell function. Fas-L is used by lymphocytes not only as a cytotoxic effector mechanism to induce apoptosis in Fas-expressing targets *(304–306)*, but also to diminish the immune response once the targeted Ag has been eliminated *(307,308)*. Fas/Fas-L-mediated induction of apoptosis is, therefore, an effective mechanism of T cell homeostasis, whereby self-reactive clones can be eliminated *(307)*, conditions of tolerance *(309)* and immune sanctuaries can be achieved *(310,311)*, and overexuberance of the immune response can be prevented *(312)*. However, tumor cells may take advantage of these mechanisms to escape immune detection and destruction.

Malignant cells from a number of solid tumors including renal cell carcinoma *(271,302,313)* have been shown to express Fas-L and T-TILs are potential targets for these Fas-L-expressing tumor cells *(314)*. Fas-L expression on tumors has been detected by a variety of techniques. mRNA of Fas-L transcripts have been identified in short- and long-term tumor cell lines by RT-PCR. Fas-L protein expression as measured by Western blotting of whole cell lysates, cytospins of short-term tumor culture, *in situ* immunohistochemistry of fresh-fixed tumor specimens, and immunocytometry of tumor cell suspensions has been reported *(271,302,313)*. Moreover, T cells derived from the peripheral blood, as well as those infiltrating the tumor, have been shown to express Fas receptor *(271,315,316)*. These cells are, therefore, potential targets for apoptosis mediated by Fas-L expressing tumor. When preactivated allogenic T cells or the Jurkat T cell line are co-cultured with tumors expressing Fas-L, they exhibit DNA breaks as measured by TUNEL assay. This lethal interaction is partially blocked by antibodies against Fas-L, supporting its role in T cell death *(271,317)*. However, the role of Fas-L expression on tumors, in causing destruction of immune T cells, is controversial, since a recent paper suggest that melanomas do not express Fas-L *(318)*. Thus, additional studies are needed to clearly define the contribution Fas-L expression on tumor cells makes to tumor escape mechanisms.

A second potential mechanism whereby tumor-induced T cell deletion may occur via apoptosis is through the process of AICD. The process of AICD is critical to the down-regulation and termination of a completed immune response. Ordinarily, when T cells are stimulated multiple times, they undergo apoptosis so as to prevent overexuberance of the T cell response. In contrast, activation of resting or naive T cells does not result in AICD. However, peripheral blood T cells from patients with RCC appear susceptible to AICD upon initial activation with various stimuli, including the phorbol ester phorbol myristate acetate (PMA) in combination with the calcium ionohore ionomycin, as well as by stimulators of the TCR, and TNF-R *(271)*. This finding suggests that when T cells are stimulated by tumor Ag, they may undergo cell death rather than cell activation. Consistent with these emerging data is the finding of increased constitutive expression of the early apoptotic marker, phosphatidyl serine (detected by Annexin V staining) on the surface of T cells isolated from patients with RCC. This view is also further supported by the finding that melanoma-specific T lymphocytes undergo apoptotic death after MHC-restricted TCR recognition of tumor Ag. In this study, T cell death could be blocked by the addition of a specific antibody to Fas *(319)*. Thus, Fas-L expressed on activated T cells after tumor recognition and TCR signaling may cause apoptosis of the same T cells or other bystander T cells expressing Fas *(319)*. Recent work has demonstrated that tumor-specific T cells isolated from the peripheral blood of patients with melanoma using peptide-specific tetramers were found to be selectively non-responsive. It may be that these tumor-specific T cells are more sensitive to AICD and undergo apoptosis upon Ag recognition *(320)*. The precise mechanism of this unresponsive state needs to be defined.

12. CONCLUSIONS

A mechanistic overview of significant mechanisms of tumor-mediated immunosuppression is shown in Fig. 5. Understanding these mechanisms of defective cellular signaling and their relationship to induction of apoptosis in T cells is critical for designing strategies to overcome tumor-induced immune suppression. Implementation of therapies to counteract specific mediators of immunosuppression can, in certain cases, be implemented readily (e.g., treatment with conventional "anti-inflammatory" drugs to block secretion of immunosuppressive PGs). Other mediators (e.g., gangliosides) may be less readily neutralized, but T cells may ultimately be modifiable genetically to render them insusceptible when their molecular points of vulnerability are sufficiently delineated. Finally, understanding the mechanisms by which T cells successfully sustain effector function even within the tumor environment, as epitomized in

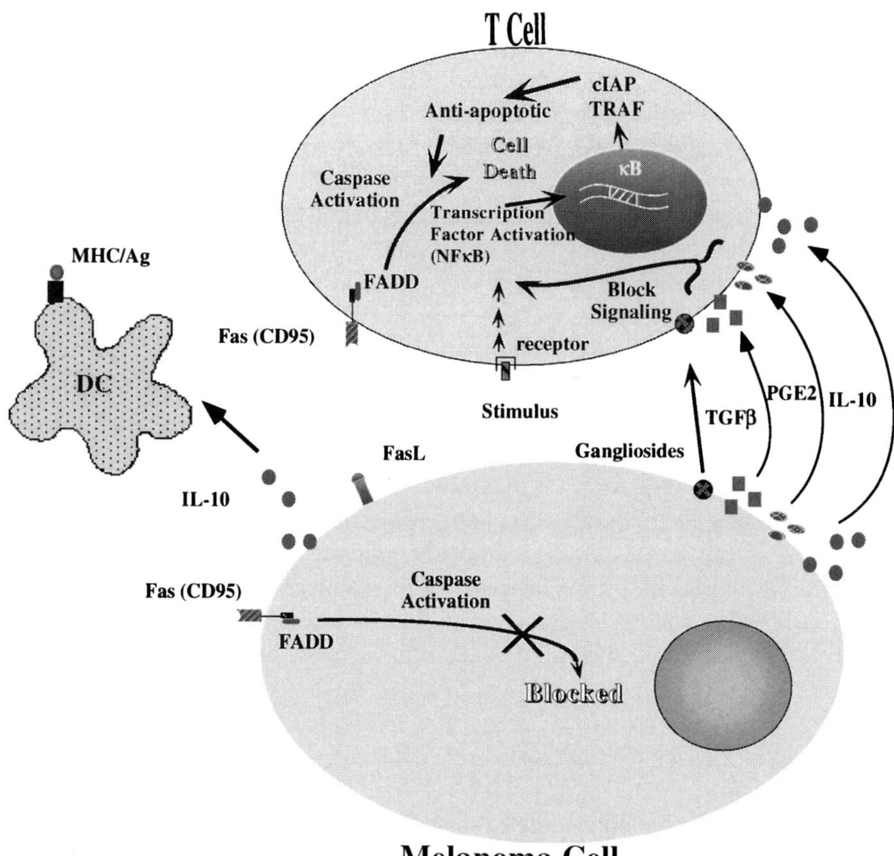

Fig. 5. Putative mechanisms by which tumor cells can induce immune dysfunction in T cells and dendritic cells. Tumor cells can produce a variety of immunosuppressive products that include IL-10, gangliosides, TGFβ, and PGs. These products can affect T cell signaling and can suppress activation of transcription factors such as NFκB. Blocking NFκB may also reduce expression of certain anti-apoptotic genes that would render T cells more sensitive to apoptosis. IL-10 can also inhibit the Ag-presenting function of DCs. Moreover, some tumors express Fas ligand (Fas-L) that can induce apoptosis in T cells that express Fas receptor. At the same time, some tumor cells, which express Fas receptor, may themselves be resistant to apoptosis induced by Fas-L expression on the activated T cells. Such resistance, in some cases, appears related to the tumor cells' reduced expression of molecules, such as caspase, that are essential for activation of apoptotic pathways.

mouse models by activated L-selectin^{low} effector T cells, may provide the physiological basis for arming T cells to resist many forms of tumor-mediated immunosuppression.

REFERENCES

1. Bast RC Jr, Zbar B, Borsos T, Rapp HJ. BCG and cancer (first of two parts). *N Engl J Med* 1974; 290: 1413.
2. Keller R. Abrogation of antitumor effects of *Corynebacterium parvum* and BCG by antimacrophage agents: brief communication. *J Natl Cancer Inst* 1977; 59: 1751.
3. Paterson AH, Willans DJ, Jerry LM, Hanson J, McPherson TA. Adjuvant BCG immunotherapy for malignant melanoma. *Can Med Assoc J* 1984; 131: 744.
4. Mastrangelo MJ, Bellet RE, Berkelhammer J, Clark WH Jr. Regression of pulmonary metastatic disease associated with intralesional BCG therapy of intracutaneous melanoma metastases. *Cancer* 1975; 36: 1305.
5. Lieberman R, Wybran J, Epstein W. The immunologic and histopathologic changes of BCG-mediated tumor regression in patients with malignant melanoma. *Cancer* 1975; 35: 756.
6. Morton DL, Eilber FR, Holmes EC, et al. BCG immunotherapy of malignant melanoma: summary of a seven-year experience. *Ann Surg* 1974; 180: 635.
7. Maurer H, McIntyre OR, Rueckert F. Spontaneous regression of malignant melanoma. Pathologic and immunologic study in a ten year survivor. *Am J Surg* 1974; 127: 397.
8. Poiesz BJ, Ruscetti FW, Mier JW, Woods AM, Gallo RC. T-cell lines established from human T-lymphocytic neoplasias by direct response to T-cell growth factor. *Proc Natl Acad Sci USA* 1980; 77: 6815-6819.
9. Cohen PA, Peng L, Plautz GE, Kim KK, Weng DE, Shu S. $CD4^+$ T cells in adoptive immunotherapy and the indirect mechanism of tumor rejection. *Crit Rev Immunol* 2000; 20: 17.
10. Peng L, Kjaergaard J, Weng DE, Plautz GE, Shu S, Cohen PA. Helper-independent $CD8^+$/CD62L low T cells with broad anti-tumor efficacy are naturally sensitized during tumor progression. *J Immunol* 2000; 165: 5738.
11. Kugler A, Stuhler G, Walden P, et al. Regression of human metastatic renal cell carcinoma after vaccination with tumor cell-dendritic cell hybrids. *Nat Med* 2000; 6: 332.
12. Nestle FO, Alijagic S, Gilliet M, et al. Vaccination of melanoma patients with peptide- or tumor lysate-pulsed dendritic cells. *Nat Med* 1998; 4: 328.
13. Wojtowicz-Praga S. Reversal of tumor-induced immunosuppression: a new approach to cancer therapy. *J Immunother* 1997; 20: 165.
14. Ferrone S, Marincola FM. Loss of HLA class I antigens by melanoma cells: molecular mechanisms, functional significance and clinical relevance. *Immunol Today* 1995; 16: 487.
15. Schwartzentruber DJ, Hom SS, Dadmarz R, et al. In vitro predictors of therapeutic response in melanoma patients receiving tumor-infiltrating lymphocytes and interleukin-2. *J Clin Oncol* 1994; 12: 1475.
16. Disis ML, Schiffman K, Gooley TA, McNeel DG, Rinn K, Knutson KL. Delayed-type hypersensitivity response is a predictor of peripheral blood T-cell immunity after HER-2/neu peptide immunization. *Clin Cancer Res* 2000; 6: 1347–1350.
17. Peng L, Krauss JC, Plautz GE, Mukai S, Shu S, Cohen PA. T-cell mediated rejection of established tumors displays a varied requirement for perforin and IFN-gamma expression which is not predicted by in vitro lytic capacity. *J Immunol* 2000; 165: 7116.
18. Barth RJ Jr, Mule JJ, Spiess PJ, Rosenberg SA. Interferon gamma and tumor necrosis factor have a role in tumor regressions mediated by murine $CD8^+$ tumor-infiltrating lymphocytes. *J Exp Med* 1991; 173: 647.
19. Yanuck M, Carbone DP, Pendleton CD, Tsukui T, Winter SF, Minna JD, Berzofsky JA. A mutant p53 tumor suppressor protein is a target for peptide-induced $CD8^+$ cytotoxic T-cells. *Cancer Res* 1993; 53: 3257.
20. Bakker AB, Schreurs MW, de Boer AJ, et al. Melanocyte lineage-specific antigen gp100 is recognized by melanoma-derived tumor-infiltrating lymphocytes. *J Exp Med* 1994; 179: 1005.

21. Rosenberg SA, White DE. Vitiligo in patients with melanoma: normal tissue antigens can be targets for cancer immunotherapy. *J Immunother Emphasis Tumor Immunol* 1996; 19: 81.
22. Overwijk WW, Lee DS, Surman DR, et al. Vaccination with a recombinant vaccinia virus encoding a "self" antigen induces autoimmune vitiligo and tumor cell destruction in mice: requirement for CD4(+) T lymphocytes. *Proc Natl Acad Sci USA* 1999; 96: 2982.
23. Murphy GP, Tjoa BA, Simmons SJ, et al. Phase II prostate cancer vaccine trial: report of a study involving 37 patients with disease recurrence following primary treatment. *Prostate* 1999; 39: 54.
24. Neumann E, Engelsberg A, Decker J, et al. Heterogeneous expression of the tumor-associated antigens RAGE-1, PRAME, and glycoprotein 75 in human renal cell carcinoma: candidates for T-cell-based immunotherapies? *Cancer Res* 1998; 58: 4090.
25. van der Bruggen P, Bastin J, Gajewski T, et al. A peptide encoded by human gene MAGE-3 and presented by HLA-A2 induces cytolytic T lymphocytes that recognize tumor cells expressing MAGE-3. *Eur J Immunol* 1994; 24: 3038.
26. Chaux P, Vantomme V, Stroobant V, et al. Identification of MAGE-3 epitopes presented by HLA-DR molecules to CD4(+) T lymphocytes. *J Exp Med* 1999; 189: 767.
27. Huang AY, Bruce AT, Pardoll DM, Levitsky HI. In vivo cross-priming of MHC class I-restricted antigens requires the TAP transporter. *Immunity* 1996; 4: 349.
28. Armstrong TD, Clements VK, Ostrand-Rosenberg S. MHC class II-transfected tumor cells directly present antigen to tumor-specific $CD4^+$ T lymphocytes. *J Immunol* 1998; 160: 661.
29. Kleijmeer MJ, Ossevoort MA, van Veen CJ, et al. MHC class II compartments and the kinetics of antigen presentation in activated mouse spleen dendritic cells. *J Immunol* 1995; 154: 5715.
30. Michalek MT, Grant EP, Gramm C, Goldberg AL, Rock KL. A role for the ubiquitin-dependent proteolytic pathway in MHC class I-restricted antigen presentation. *Nature* 1993; 363: 552.
31. Sule-Suso J, Arienti F, Melani C, Colombo MP, Parmiani G. A B7-1-transfected human melanoma line stimulates proliferation and cytotoxicity of autologous and allogeneic lymphocytes. *Eur J Immunol* 1995; 25: 2737,
32. Anichini A, Mortarini R, Alberti S, Mantovani A, Parmiani G. T-cell-receptor engagement and tumor ICAM-1 up-regulation are required to by-pass low susceptibility of melanoma cells to autologous CTL-mediated lysis. *Int J Cancer* 1993; 53: 994.
33. Matzinger P. Graft tolerance: a duel of two signals. *Nat Med* 1999; 5: 616.
34. Cruz PD, Bergstresser PR. Antigen processing and presentation by epidermal Langerhans cells, induction of immunity or unresponsiveness. *Dermatol Clin* 1990; 8: 633.
35. Girolomoni G, Simon JC, Bergstresser PR, Cruz PD. Freshly isolated spleen dendritic cells and epidermal Langerhans cells undergo similar phenotypic and functional changes during short term culture. *J Immunol* 1990; 145: 2820.
36. Cormier JN, Hijazi YM, Abati A, et al. Heterogeneous expression of melanoma-associated antigens and HLA-A2 in metastatic melanoma in vivo. *Int J Cancer* 1998; 75: 517.
37. Plautz GE, Mukai S, Cohen PA, Shu S. Cross presentation of tumor antigens to effector T cells is sufficient to mediate effective immunotherapy of established intracranial tumors. *J Immunol* 2000; 165: 3656.
38. Cohen PA. $CD4^+$ T cells in tumor rejection: past evidence and current prospects. In: Chang AE, Shu S, eds., *Immunotherapy of Cancer with Sensitized T Lymphocytes*. J.B. Lippincott, Philadelphia, 1994.
39. Fidler IJ. Recognition and destruction of target cells by tumoricidal macrophages. *Isr J Med Sci* 1978; 14: 177.
40. Fidler IJ, Bucana C. Mechanism of tumor cell resistance to lysis by syngeneic lymphocytes. *Cancer Res* 1977; 37: 3945.

41. Cohen EP, Kim TS. Neoplastic cells that express low levels of MHC class I determinants escape host immunity. *Semin Cancer Biol* 1994; 5: 419.
42. Winter H, Hu HM, Urba WJ, Fox BA. Tumor regression after adoptive transfer of effector T cells is independent of perforin or Fas ligand (APO-1L/CD95L). *J Immunol* 1999; 163: 4462.
43. Rosen D, Li J-H, Keidar S, Markon I, Orda R, Berke G. Tumor immunity in perforin-deficient mice: a role for CD95 (Fas/APO-1). *J Immunol* 2000; 164: 3229.
44. Berke G. The Fas-based mechanism of lymphocytotoxicity. *Hum Immunol* 1997; 54: 1.
45. Berke G. The CTL's kiss of death. *Cell* 1995; 81: 9.
46. Nagata S, Golstein P. The Fas death factor. *Science* 1995; 267: 1449.
47. Henkart PA. Lymphocyte-mediated cytotoxicity: two pathways and multiple effector molecules. *Immunity* 1994; 1: 343.
48. Asher AL, Mule JJ, Kasid A, et al. Murine tumor cells transduced with the gene for tumor necrosis factor-alpha. Evidence for paracrine immune effects of tumor necrosis factor against tumors. *J Immunol* 1991; 146: 3227.
49. Asher AL, Mule JJ, Rosenberg SA. Recombinant human tumor necrosis factor mediates regression of a murine sarcoma in vivo via Lyt-2^+ cells. *Cancer Immunol Immunother* 1989; 28: 153.
50. Mule JJ, Asher A, McIntosh J, et al. Antitumor effect of recombinant tumor necrosis factor-alpha against murine sarcomas at visceral sites: tumor size influences the response to therapy. *Cancer Immunol Immunother* 1988; 26: 202.
51. Bartlett DL, Ma G, Alexander HR, Libutti SK, Fraker DL. Isolated limb reperfusion with tumor necrosis factor and melphalan in patients with extremity melanoma after failure of isolated limb perfusion with chemotherapeutics. *Cancer* 1997; 80: 2084.
52. Koshiji M, Adachi Y, Sogo S, et al. Apoptosis of colorectal adenocarcinoma (COLO 201) by tumour necrosis factor-alpha (TNF-alpha) and/or interferon-gamma (IFN-gamma), resulting from down-modulation of Bcl-2 expression. *Clin Exp Immunol* 1998; 111: 211.
53. Spets H, Georgii-Hemming P, Siljason J, Nilsson K, Jernberg-Wiklund H. Fas/APO-1 (CD95)-mediated apoptosis is activated by interferon-gamma and interferon- in interleukin-6 (IL-6)-dependent and IL-6-independent multiple myeloma cell lines. *Blood* 1998; 92: 2914.
54. Burke F, East N, Upton C, Patel K, Balkwill FR. Interferon gamma induces cell cycle arrest and apoptosis in a model of ovarian cancer: enhancement of effect by batimastat. *Eur J Cancer* 1997; 33: 1114.
55. Tamura T, Ueda S, Yoshida M, Matsuzaki M, Mohri H, Okubo T. Interferon-gamma induces Ice gene expression and enhances cellular susceptibility to apoptosis in the U937 leukemia cell line. *Biochem Biophys Res Commun* 1996; 229: 21.
56. Yeung MC, Liu J, Lau AS. An essential role for the interferon-inducible, double-stranded RNA-activated protein kinase PKR in the tumor necrosis factor-induced apoptosis in U937 cells. *Proc Natl Acad Sci USA* 1996; 93: 12451.
57. Zhou Q, Zhao J, Al-Zoghaibi F, et al. Transcriptional control of the human plasma membrane phospholipid scramblase 1 gene is mediated by interferon-alpha. *Blood* 2000; 95: 2593–2599.
58. Krahling S, Callahan MK, Williamson P, Schlegel RA. Exposure of phosphatidylserine is a general feature in the phagocytosis of apoptotic lymphocytes by macrophages. *Cell Death Differ* 1999; 6: 183.
59. Utsugi T, Schroit AJ, Connor J, Bucana CD, Fidler IJ. Elevated expression of phosphatidylserine in the outer membrane leaflet of human tumor cells and recognition by activated human blood monocytes. *Cancer Res* 1991; 51: 3062.
60. Mule JJ, Ettinghausen SE, Spiess PJ, Shu S, Rosenberg SA. Antitumor efficacy of lymphokine-activated killer cells and recombinant interleukin-2 in vivo: survival benefit and mechanisms of tumor escape in mice undergoing immunotherapy. *Cancer Res* 1986; 46: 676.

61. Ettinghausen SE, Lipford EH III, Mule JJ, Rosenberg SA. Recombinant interleukin 2 stimulates in vivo proliferation of adoptively transferred lymphokine-activated killer (LAK) cells. *J Immunol* 1985; 135: 3623,
62. Ettinghausen SE, Lipford EH III, Mule JJ, Rosenberg SA. Systemic administration of recombinant interleukin 2 stimulates in vivo lymphoid cell proliferation in tissues. *J Immunol* 1985; 135: 1488.
63. Fidler IJ, Fogler WE, Kleinerman ES, Saiki I. Abrogation of species specificity for activation of tumoricidal properties in macrophages by recombinant mouse or human interferon-gamma encapsulated in liposomes. *J Immunol* 1985; 135: 4289.
64. Saiki I, Sone S, Fogler WE, Kleinerman ES, Lopez-Berestein G, Fidler IJ. Synergism between human recombinant gamma-interferon and muramyl dipeptide encapsulated in liposomes for activation of antitumor properties in human blood monocytes. *Cancer Res* 1985; 45: 6188.
65. Koff WC, Fogler WE, Gutterman J, Fidler IJ. Efficient activation of human blood monocytes to a tumoricidal state by liposomes containing human recombinant gamma interferon. *Cancer Immunol Immunother* 1985; 19: 85,
66. Mule JJ, Smith CA, Rosenberg SA. Interleukin 4 (B cell stimulatory factor 1) can mediate the induction of lymphokine-activated killer cell activity directed against fresh tumor cells. *J Exp Med* 1987; 166: 792.
67. Stewart-Akers AM, Cairns JS, Tweardy DJ, McCarthy SA. Effect of granulocyte-macrophage colony-stimulating factor on lymphokine-activated killer cell induction. *Blood* 1993; 81: 2671.
68. Ferrante A. Activation of neutrophils by interleukins-1 and -2 and tumor necrosis factors. *Immunol Ser* 1992; 57: 417.
69. Katayama H, Kitagawa S, Masuyama J, Yaoita H. Polymorphonuclear leukocyte-induced detachment of cultured epidermal carcinoma cells from the substratum. *J Invest Dermatol* 1991; 97: 949.
70. Barton DP, Blanchard DK, Duan C, et al. Interleukin-12 synergizes with interleukin-2 to generate lymphokine-activated killer activity in peripheral blood mononuclear cells cultured in ovarian cancer ascitic fluid. *J Soc Gynecol Invest* 1995; 2: 762.
71. Lindgren CG, Thompson JA, Robinson N, Keeler T, Gold PJ, Fefer A. Interleukin-12 induced cytolytic activity in lymphocytes from recipients of autologous and allogeneic stem cell transplants. *Bone Marrow Transplant* 1997; 19: 867.
72. Salvucci O, Mami-Chouaib F, Moreau JL, Theze J, Chehimi J, Chouaib S. Differential regulation of interleukin-12- and interleukin-15-induced natural killer cell activation by interleukin-4. *Eur J Immunol* 1996; 26: 2736.
73. Yang JC, Mule JJ, Rosenberg SA. Murine lymphokine-activated killer (LAK) cells: phenotypic characterization of the precursor and effector cells. *J Immunol* 1986; 137: 715.
74. Phillips JH, Lanier LL. Dissection of the lymphokine-activated killer phenomenon. Relative contribution of peripheral blood natural killer cells and T lymphocytes to cytolysis. *J Exp Med* 1986; 164: 814.
75. Fidler IJ. Macrophages and metastasis—a biological approach to cancer therapy. *Cancer Res* 1985; 45: 4714.
76. Toren A, Gadish M, Fabian I, Nagler A. The putative role of arylsulfatase in interleukin-2-mediated cytotoxicity and interleukin-7-mediated bactericidal activity of natural killer cells. *Ann Hematol* 1997; 74: 83.
77. Garcia-Penarrubia P, Bankhurst AD, Koster FT. Prostaglandins from human T suppressor/cytotoxic cells modulate natural killer antibacterial activity. *J Exp Med* 1989; 170: 601.
78. Garcia-Penarrubia P, Koster FT, Kelley RO, McDowell TD, Bankhurst AD. Antibacterial activity of human natural killer cells. *J Exp Med* 1989; 169: 99.

79. Abo T, Sugawara S, Amenomori A, et al. Selective phagocytosis of gram-positive bacteria and interleukin 1-like factor production by a subpopulation of large granular lymphocytes. *J Immunol* 1986; 136: 3189.
80. Henkart PA, Yue CC, Yang J, Rosenberg SA. Cytolytic and biochemical properties of cytoplasmic granules of murine lymphokine-activated killer cells. *J Immunol* 1986; 137: 2611.
81. Fogler WE, Fidler IJ. Nonselective destruction of murine neoplastic cells by syngeneic tumoricidal macrophages. *Cancer Res* 1985; 45: 14.
82. Rayner AA, Grimm EA, Lotze MT, Wilson DJ, Rosenberg SA. Lymphokine-activated killer (LAK) cell phenomenon. IV. Lysis by LAK cell clones of fresh human tumor cells from autologous and multiple allogeneic tumors. *J Natl Cancer Inst* 1985; 75: 67.
83. Subauste CS, Dawson L, Remington JS. Human lymphokine-activated killer cells are cytotoxic against cells infected with *Toxoplasma gondii*. *J Exp Med* 1992; 176: 1511.
84. Dannemann BR, Morris VA, Araujo FG, Remington JS. Assessment of human natural killer and lymphokine-activated killer cell cytotoxicity against *Toxoplasma gondii* trophozoites and brain cysts. *J Immunol* 1989; 143: 2684.
85. Gregory SH, Jiang X, Wing EJ. Lymphokine-activated killer cells lyse Listeria-infected hepatocytes and produce elevated quantities of interferon-gamma. *J Infect Dis* 1996; 174: 1073.
86. Moretta A, Sivori S, Ponte M, Mingari MC, Moretta L. Stimulatory receptors in NK and T cells. *Curr Top Microbiol Immunol* 1998; 230: 15.
87. Moretta A, Parolini S, Castriconi R, et al. Function and specificity of human natural killer cell receptors. *Eur J Immunogenet* 1997; 24: 455.
88. Moretta A, Biassoni R, Bottino C, et al. Major histocompatibility complex class I-specific receptors on human natural killer and T lymphocytes. *Immunol Rev* 1997; 155: 105.
89. Lopez-Botet M, Moretta L, Strominger J. NK-cell receptors and recognition of MHC class I molecules. *Immunol Today* 1996; 17: 212.
90. Rapin AM, Burger MM. Tumor cell surfaces: general alterations detected by agglutinins. *Adv Cancer Res* 1974; 20: 1.
91. Schwarz RE, Wojciechowicz DC, Park PY, Paty PB. Phytohemagglutinin-L (PHA-L) lectin surface binding of N-linked beta 1-6 carbohydrate and its relationship to activated mutant ras in human pancreatic cancer cell lines. *Cancer Lett* 1996; 107: 285.
92. Cornil I, Kerbel RS, Dennis JW. Tumor cell surface beta 1-4-linked galactose binds to lectin(s) on microvascular endothelial cells and contributes to organ colonization. *J Cell Biol* 1990; 111: 773.
93. Lotan R, Raz A. Endogenous lectins as mediators of tumor cell adhesion. *J Cell Biochem* 1988; 37: 107.
94. Raz A, Meromsky L, Zvibel I, Lotan R. Transformation-related changes in the expression of endogenous cell lectins. *Int J Cancer* 1987; 39: 353.
95. Woynarowska B, Skrincosky DM, Haag A, Sharma M, Matta K, Bernacki RJ. Inhibition of lectin-mediated ovarian tumor cell adhesion by sugar analogs. *J Biol Chem* 1994; 269: 22797.
96. Mitchell BS, Schumacher U. The use of the lectin Helix pomatia agglutinin (HPA) as a prognostic indicator and as a tool in cancer research. *Histol Histopathol* 1999; 14: 217.
97. Schumacher U, Adam E, Brooks SA, Leathem AJ. Lectin-binding properties of human breast cancer cell lines and human milk with particular reference to Helix pomatia agglutinin. *J Histochem Cytochem* 1995; 43: 275.
98. Devine PL, Harada H. Reactivity of mucin-specific lectin from Sambucus sieboldiana with simple sugars, normal mucins and tumor-associated mucins. Comparison with other lectins. *Biol Chem Hoppe Seyler* 1991; 372: 935.

99. Altevogt P, Fogel M, Cheingsong-Popov R, Dennis J, Robinson P, Schirrmacher V. Different patterns of lectin binding and cell surface sialylation detected on related high- and low-metastatic tumor lines. *Cancer Res* 1983; 43: 5138.
100. Andre S, Unverzagt C, Kojima S, Dong X, Fink C, Kayser K, Gabius HJ. Neoglycoproteins with the synthetic complex biantennary nonasaccharide or its alpha 2,3/alpha 2,6-sialylated derivatives: their preparation, assessment of their ligand properties for purified lectins, for tumor cells in vitro, and in tissue sections, and their biodistribution in tumor-bearing mice. *Bioconjug Chem* 1997; 8: 845.
101. Gabius HJ, Gabius S. Detection of tumor-associated expression of carbohydrate-binding proteins (lectins). The use of neoglycoproteins and neoglycoenzymes in glycohistochemical and glycocytological studies. *Methods Mol Biol* 1993; 14: 263.
102. Yamamoto K, Ishida C, Shinohara Y, et al. Interaction of immobilized recombinant mouse C-type macrophage lectin with glycopeptides and oligosaccharides. *Biochemistry* 1994; 33: 8159.
103. Oda S, Sato M, Toyoshima S, Osawa T. Binding of activated macrophages to tumor cells through a macrophage lectin and its role in macrophage tumoricidal activity. *J Biochem (Tokyo)* 1989; 105: 1040.
104. Imamura T, Toyoshima S, Osawa T. Lectin-like molecules on the murine macrophage cell surface. *Biochim Biophys Acta* 1984; 805: 235.
105. Bucana CD, Hoyer LC, Schroit AJ, Kleinerman E, Fidler IJ. Ultrastructural studies of the interaction between liposome-activated human blood monocytes and allogeneic tumor cells in vitro. *Am J Pathol* 1983; 112: 101.
106. Key ME, Hoyer L, Bucana C, Hanna MG Jr. Mechanisms of macrophage-mediated tumor cytolysis. *Adv Exp Med Biol* 1982; 146: 265.
107. Hamilton TA, Fishman M. Characterization of the recognition of target cells sensitive or resistant to cytolysis by activated rat peritoneal macrophages. *J Immunol* 1981; 127: 1702.
108. Hamilton TA, Fishman M. Characterization of the recognition of target cells sensitive to or resistant to cytolysis by activated macrophages. II. Competitive inhibition of macrophage-dependent tumor cell killing by mitogen-induced, nonmalignant lymphoblasts. *Cell Immunol* 1982; 68: 155.
109. Hamilton TA, Fishman M, Crawford G, Look AT. Sensitivity to macrophage-mediated cytostasis is cell cycle dependent. *Cell Immunol* 1982; 69: 363.
110. Hamilton TA, Fishman M. Activated macrophages selectively bind both normal and neoplastic lymphoblasts but not quiescent lymphocytes. *Cell Immunol* 1982; 72: 332.
111. Lohmann-Matthes ML, Kolb B, Meerpohl HG. Susceptibility of malignant and normal target cells to the cytotoxic action of bone-marrow macrophages activated in vitro with the macrophage cytotoxicity factor (MCF). *Cell Immunol* 1978; 41: 231.
112. Zambello R, Trentin L, Enthammer C, Cipriani A, Agostini C, Semenzato G. Lysis of pulmonary fibroblasts by lymphokine (IL-2)-activated killer cells—a mechanism affecting the human lung microenvironment? *Clin Exp Immunol* 1996; 105: 383.
113. Zambello R, Trentin L, Feruglio C, et al. Susceptibility to lysis of pulmonary alveolar macrophages by human lymphokine-activated killer cells. *Cancer Res* 1990; 50: 1768.
114. Martiniello R, Burton RC, Smart YC. Ly-6C$^+$ natural T (NT) cells mediate immune surveillance against NK-sensitive and NK-resistant transplantable tumours in certain strains of mice. *Int J Cancer* 1996; 66: 532.
115. Tran AC, Zhang D, Byrn R, Roberts MR. Chimeric zeta-receptors direct human natural killer (NK) effector function to permit killing of NK-resistant tumor cells and HIV-infected T lymphocytes. *J Immunol* 1995; 155: 1000.
116. Agah R, Malloy B, Kerner M, et al. Potent graft antitumor effect in natural killer-resistant disseminated tumors by transplantation of interleukin 2-activated syngeneic bone marrow in mice. *Cancer Res* 1989; 49: 5959.

117. Sarzotti M, Klimpel GR, Baron S. Long-term killing of natural killer-resistant target cells by interferon-alpha-, interferon-gamma-, and interleukin-2-activated natural killer cells. *Nat Immun Cell Growth Regul* 1989; 8: 66.
118. Bradley M, Zeytun A, Rafi-Janajreh A, Nagarkatti PS, Nagarkatti M. Role of spontaneous and interleukin-2-induced natural killer cell activity in the cytotoxicity and rejection of Fas^+ and Fas^- tumor cells. *Blood* 1998; 92: 4248.
119. Furuke K, Shiraishi M, Mostowski HS, Bloom ET. Fas ligand induction in human NK cells is regulated by redox through a calcineurin-nuclear factors of activated T cell-dependent pathway. *J Immunol* 1999; 162: 1988.
120. Sayers TJ, Brooks AD, Lee JK, et al. Molecular mechanisms of immune-mediated lysis of murine renal cancer: differential contributions of perforin-dependent versus Fas-mediated pathways in lysis by NK and T cells. *J Immunol* 1998; 161: 3957.
121. Halaas O, Vik R, Espevik T. Induction of Fas ligand in murine bone marrow NK cells by bacterial polysaccharides. *J Immunol* 1998; 160: 4330.
122. Kamamura Y, Takahashi K, Komaki K, Monden Y. Effects of interferon-alpha and gamma on development of LAK activity from mononuclear cells in breast cancer patients. *J Med Invest* 1998; 45: 71.
123. Fehniger TA, Shah MH, Turner MJ, et al. Differential cytokine and chemokine gene expression by human NK cells following activation with IL-18 or IL-15 in combination with IL-12: implications for the innate immune response. *J Immunol* 1999; 162: 4511.
124. Mohan K, Moulin P, Stevenson MM. Natural killer cell cytokine production, not cytotoxicity, contributes to resistance against blood-stage *Plasmodium chabaudi* AS infection. *J Immunol* 1997; 159: 4990,
125. Salazar-Mather TP, Ishikawa R, Biron CA. NK cell trafficking and cytokine expression in splenic compartments after IFN induction and viral infection. *J Immunol* 1996; 157: 3054.
126. Zhu HG, Voetsch W, Hauer J, Anderer FA. Chemospecificity and cross-reactivity of target cell recognition by human $CD56^+$ NK and LAK cells. *Scand J Immunol* 1995; 41: 545.
127. Steinmassl M, Anderer FA. Structural specificity of MHC-unrestricted recognition of HCMV-infected target cells by human $CD56^+$NK and LAK cells. *Scand J Immunol* 1994; 40: 665.
128. Lee RK, Spielman J, Zhao DY, Olsen KJ, Podack ER. Perforin, Fas ligand, and tumor necrosis factor are the major cytotoxic molecules used by lymphokine-activated killer cells. *J Immunol* 1996; 157: 1919.
129. Fidler IJ. Recognition and destruction of target cells by tumoricidal macrophages. *Isr J Med Sci* 1978; 14: 177.
130. Chao TY, Jiang SY, Shyu RY, Yeh MY, Chu TM. All-trans retinoic acid decreases susceptibility of a gastric cancer cell line to lymphokine-activated killer cytotoxicity. *Br J Cancer* 1997; 75: 1284.
131. Komatsu F, Kajiwara M. A lymphokine-activated killer (LAK)-resistant cell line, and low expression of adhesion molecules LFA-3 and VCAM-1 on its cell surface. *Oncol Res* 1998; 10: 263.
132. Rosenkrans CF Jr, Chapes SK. Macrophage binding of cells resistant and sensitive to contact-dependent cytotoxicity. *Cell Immunol* 1991; 133: 187.
133. Chapes SK, Duffin D, Paulsen AQ. Characterization of macrophage recognition and killing of SV40-transformed tumor cells that are "resistant" or "susceptible" to contact-mediated killing. *J Immunol* 1988; 140: 589.
134. Chapes SK, O'Neill AE, Flaherty L, Gooding LR. Macrophage-resistant murine simian virus 40 tumors express a retroviral type-specific gp70. *J Virol* 1987; 61: 928.
135. Pohajdak B, Lee KC, Sugawara I, Miller V, Wright JA, Greenberg AH. Comparative analysis of natural killer cell and macrophage recognition of concanavalin A-resistant Chinese hamster ovary cells: role of membrane oligosaccharides. *J Natl Cancer Inst* 1986; 76: 257.

136. Nestel FP, Casson PR, Wiltrout RH, Kerbel RS. Alterations in sensitivity to nonspecific cell-mediated lysis associated with tumor progression: characterization of activated macrophage- and natural killer cell-resistant tumor variants. *J Natl Cancer Inst* 1984; 73: 483.
137. Urban JL, Schreiber H. Selection of macrophage-resistant progressor tumor variants by the normal host. Requirement for concomitant T cell-mediated immunity. *J Exp Med* 1983; 157: 642.
138. Fady C, Gardner A, Gera JF, Lichtenstein A. Resistance of HER2/neu-overexpressing tumor targets to lymphokine-activated-killer-cell-mediated lysis: evidence for deficiency of binding and post-binding events. *Cancer Immunol Immunother* 1993; 36: 307.
139. Bean P, Mazumder A. Resistance of different tumor cells to lysis by lymphokine activated killer cells can be mediated by distinct mechanisms. *Immunobiology* 1992; 185: 63,
140. Bast RC Jr, Zbar B, Borsos T, Rapp HJ. BCG and cancer. *N Engl J Med* 1974; 290: 1458.
141. Sakai K, Chang AE, Shu S. Effector phenotype and immunologic specificity of T-cell-mediated adoptive therapy for a murine tumor that lacks intrinsic immunogenicity. *Cell Immunol* 1990; 129: 241.
142. Ratliff TL, Ritchey JK, Yuan JJ, Andriole GL, Catalona WJ. T-cell subsets required for intravesical BCG immunotherapy for bladder cancer. *J Urol* 1993; 150: 1018.
143. Gan YH, Mahendran R, James K, Lawrencia C, Esuvaranathan K. Evaluation of lymphocytic responses after treatment with Bacillus Calmette-Guerin and interferon-alpha 2b for superficial bladder cancer. *Clin Immunol* 1999; 90: 230.
144. Luo Y, Chen X, Downs TM, DeWolf WC, O'Donnell MA. IFN-alpha 2B enhances Th1 cytokine responses in bladder cancer patients receiving Mycobacterium bovis bacillus Calmette-Guerin immunotherapy. *J Immunol* 1999; 162: 2399.
145. Zlotta AR, Drowart A, Van Vooren JP, et al. Evolution and clinical significance of the T cell proliferative and cytokine response directed against the fibronectin binding antigen 85 complex of bacillus Calmette-Guerin during intravesical treatment of superficial bladder cancer. *J Urol* 1997; 157: 492.
146. Patard JJ, Muscatelli-Groux B, Saint F, et al. Evaluation of local immune response after intravesical bacille Calmette-Guerin treatment for superficial bladder cancer. *Br J Urol* 1996; 78: 709.
147. Sarica K, Baltaci S, Beduk Y, et al. Evaluation of cellular immunity following bacillus Calmette-Guerin therapy in patients with superficial bladder cancer. *Urol Int* 1995; 54: 137.
148. Ratliff TL. Role of the immune response in BCG for bladder cancer. *Eur Urol* 1992; 21(Suppl 2): 17.
149. Fernandez-Cruz E, Woda BA, Feldman JD. Elimination of syngeneic sarcomas in rats by a subset of T lymphocytes. *J Exp Med* 1980; 152: 823.
150. Greenberg PD, Cheever MA, Fefer A. Eradication of disseminated murine leukemia by chemoimmunotherapy with cyclophosphamide and adoptively transferred immune syngeneic Lyt-1$^+$2-lymphocytes. *J Exp Med* 1981; 154: 952.
151. Dunussi-Joannopoulos K, Krenger W, Weinstein HJ, Ferrara JL, Croop JM. CD8$^+$ T cells activated during the course of murine acute myelogenous leukemia elicit therapeutic responses to late B7 vaccines after cytoreductive treatment. *Blood* 1997; 89: 2915.
152. Shu S, Chou T, Rosenberg SA. In vitro sensitization and expansion with viable tumor cells and interleukin 2 in the generation of specific therapeutic effector cells. *J Immunol* 1986; 136: 3891.
153. Shu S, Chou T, Rosenberg SA. In vitro differentiation of T-cells capable of mediating the regression of established syngeneic tumors in mice. *Cancer Res* 1987; 47: 1354.
154. Shu SY, Chou T, Rosenberg SA. Generation from tumor-bearing mice of lymphocytes with in vivo therapeutic efficacy. *J Immunol* 1987; 139: 295.

155. Chou T, Bertera S, Chang AE, Shu S. Adoptive immunotherapy of microscopic and advanced visceral metastases with in vitro sensitized lymphoid cells from mice bearing progressive tumors. *J Immunol* 1988; 141: 1775.
156. Shu SY, Chou T, Sakai K. Lymphocytes generated by in vivo priming and in vitro sensitization demonstrate therapeutic efficacy against a murine tumor that lacks apparent immunogenicity. *J Immunol* 1989; 143: 740.
157. Spiess PJ, Yang JC, Rosenberg SA. In vivo antitumor activity of tumor-infiltrating lymphocytes expanded in recombinant interleukin-2. *J Natl Cancer Inst* 1987; 79: 1067.
158. Muul LM, Spiess PJ, Director EP, Rosenberg SA. Identification of specific cytolytic immune responses against autologous tumor in humans bearing malignant melanoma. *J Immunol* 1987; 138: 989.
159. Rosenberg SA, Spiess P, Lafreniere R. A new approach to the adoptive immunotherapy of cancer with tumor-infiltrating lymphocytes. *Science* 1986; 233: 1318.
160. Cohen PA. Role of T cell subsets in tumor immunity. In: DeVita VT, Hellman S, Rosenberg SA, eds., *Biologic Therapy of Cancer Updates*, Lippincott, Philadelphia, 1994.
161. Shu S, Rosenberg SA. Adoptive immunotherapy of a newly induced sarcoma: immunologic characteristics of effector cells. *J Immunol* 1985; 135: 2895.
162. Shu SY, Rosenberg SA. Adoptive immunotherapy of newly induced murine sarcomas. *Cancer Res* 1985; 45: 1657.
163. Correa MR, Ochoa AC, Ghosh P, Mizoguchi H, Harvey L, Longo DL. Sequential development of structural and functional alterations in T cells from tumor-bearing mice. *J Immunol* 1997; 158: 5292.
164. Mizoguchi H, O'Shea JJ, Longo DL, Loeffler CM, McVicar DW, Ochoa AC. Alterations in signal transduction molecules in T lymphocytes from tumor-bearing mice. *Science* 1992; 258: 1795.
165. Wang Q, Stanley J, Kudoh S, et al. T cells infiltrating non-Hodgkin's B cell lymphomas show altered tyrosine phosphorylation pattern even though T cell receptor/CD3-associated kinases are present. *J Immunol* 1995; 155: 1382.
166. Liu J, Finke J, Krauss JC, Shu S, Plautz GE. Ex vivo activation of tumor-draining lymph node T cells reverses defects in signal transduction molecules. *Cancer Immunol Immunother* 1998; 46: 268.
167. Arca MJ, Krauss JC, Aruga A, Cameron MJ, Shu S, Chang AE. Therapeutic efficacy of T cells derived from lymph nodes draining a poorly immunogenic tumor transduced to secrete granulocyte-macrophage colony-stimulating factor. *Cancer Gene Ther* 1996; 3: 39.
168. Kagamu H, Touhalisky JE, Plautz GE, Krauss JC, Shu S. Isolation based on L-selectin expression of immune effector T cells derived from tumor-draining lymph nodes. *Cancer Res* 1996; 56: 4338.
169. Plautz GE, Barnett GH, Miller DW, et al. Systemic T cell adoptive immunotherapy of malignant gliomas. *J Neurosurg* 1998; 89: 42.
170. Plautz GE, Touhalisky JE, Shu S. Treatment of murine gliomas by adoptive transfer of ex vivo activated tumor-draining lymph node cells. *Cell Immunol* 1997; 178: 101.
171. Shu S, Krinock RA, Matsumura T, et al. Stimulation of tumor-draining lymph node cells with superantigenic staphylococcal toxins leads to the generation of tumor-specific effector T cells. *J Immunol* 1994; 152: 1277.
172. Krauss JC, Shu S. Secretion of biologically active superantigens by mammalian cells. *J Hematother* 1997; 6: 41.
173. Chang AE, Aruga A, Cameron MJ, et al. Adoptive immunotherapy with vaccine-primed lymph node cells secondarily activated with anti-CD3 and interleukin-2. *J Clin Oncol* 1997; 15: 796,
174. Inoue M, Plautz GE, Shu S. Treatment of intracranial tumors by systemic transfer of superantigen-activated tumor-draining lymph node T cells. *Cancer Res* 1996; 56: 4702.

175. Plautz GE, Inoue M, Shu S. Defining the synergistic effects of irradiation and T-cell immunotherapy for murine intracranial tumors. *Cell Immunol* 1996; 171: 277.
176. Wahl WL, Strome SE, Nabel GJ, et al. Generation of therapeutic T-lymphocytes after in vivo tumor transfection with an allogeneic class I major histocompatibility complex gene. *J Immunother Emphasis Tumor Immunol* 1995; 17: 1.
177. Krauss JC, Strome SE, Chang AE, Shu S. Enhancement of immune reactivity in the lymph nodes draining a murine melanoma engineered to elaborate interleukin-4. *J Immunother Emphasis Tumor Immunol* 1994; 16: 77.
178. Sussman JJ, Shu S, Sondak VK, Chang AE. Activation of T lymphocytes for the adoptive immunotherapy of cancer. *Ann Surg Oncol* 1994; 1: 296.
179. Matsumura T, Sussman JJ, Krinock RA, Chang AE, Shu S. Characteristics and in vivo homing of long-term T-cell lines and clones derived from tumor-draining lymph nodes. *Cancer Res* 1994; 54: 2744.
180. Wahl WL, Sussman JJ, Shu S, Chang AE. Adoptive immunotherapy of murine intracerebral tumors with anti-CD3/interleukin-2-activated tumor-draining lymph node cells. *J Immunother Emphasis Tumor Immunol* 1994; 15: 242.
181. Shu S, Krinock RA, Matsumura T, et al. Stimulation of tumor-draining lymph node cells with superantigenic staphylococcal toxins leads to the generation of tumor-specific effector T cells. *J Immunol* 1994; 152: 1277.
182. Shu S, Sussman JJ, Chang AE. In vivo antitumor efficacy of tumor-draining lymph node cells activated with nonspecific T-cell reagents. *J Immunother* 1993; 14: 279.
183. Matsumura T, Krinock RA, Chang AE, Shu S. Cross-reactivity of anti-CD3/IL-2 activated effector cells derived from lymph nodes draining heterologous clones of a murine tumor. *Cancer Res* 1993; 53: 4315.
184. Geiger JD, Wagner PD, Cameron MJ, Shu S, Chang AE. Generation of T-cells reactive to the poorly immunogenic B16-BL6 melanoma with efficacy in the treatment of spontaneous metastases. *J Immunother* 1993; 13: 153.
185. Geiger JD, Wagner PD, Shu S, Chang AE. A novel role for autologous tumour cell vaccination in the immunotherapy of the poorly immunogenic B16-BL6 melanoma. *Surg Oncol* 1992; 1: 199.
186. Sondak VK, Tuck MK, Shu S, Yoshizawa H, Chang AE. Enhancing effect of interleukin 1 alpha administration on antitumor effector T-cell development. *Arch Surg* 1991; 126: 1503.
187. Yoshizawa H, Chang AE, Shu S. Specific adoptive immunotherapy mediated by tumor-draining lymph node cells sequentially activated with anti-CD3 and IL-2. *J Immunol* 1991; 147: 729.
188. Peng L, Shu S, Krauss JC. Treatment of subcutaneous tumor with adoptively transferred T cells. *Cell Immunol* 1997; 178: 24,
189. Kagamu H, Shu S. Purification of L-selectin(low) cells promotes the generation of highly potent CD4 antitumor effector T lymphocytes. *J Immunol* 1998; 160: 3444.
190. Mitchell MS. Relapse in the central nervous system in melanoma patients successfully treated with biomodulators. *J Clin Oncol* 1989; 7: 1701.
191. Greenberg P, Klarnet J, Kern D, Okuno K, Riddell S, Cheever M. Requirements for T cell recognition and elimination of retrovirally-transformed cells. *Princess Takamatsu Symp* 1988; 19: 287.
192. Klarnet JP, Kern DE, Dower SK, Matis LA, Cheever MA, Greenberg PD. Helper-independent $CD8^+$ cytotoxic T lymphocytes express IL-1 receptors and require IL-1 for secretion of IL-2. *J Immunol* 1989; 142: 2187.
193. Kjaergaard J, Shu S. Tumor infiltration by adoptively transferred T cells is independent of immunologic specificity but requires down-regulation of L-selectin expression. *J Immunol* 1999; 163: 751.

194. Jung TM, Dailey MO. Rapid modulation of homing receptors (gp90MEL-14) induced by activators of protein kinase C. Receptor shedding due to accelerated proteolytic cleavage at the cell surface. *J Immunol* 1990; 144: 3130.
195. Jung TM, Gallatin WM, Weissman IL, Dailey MO. Down-regulation of homing receptors after T cell activation. *J Immunol* 1988; 141: 4110.
196. Jung TM, Dailey MO. Reversibility of loss of homing receptor expression following activation. *Adv Exp Med Biol* 1988; 237: 519.
197. Bradley LM, Duncan DD, Tonkonogy S, Swain SL. Characterization of antigen-specific $CD4^+$ effector T cells in vivo: immunization results in a transient population of MEL-14-, CD45RB-helper cells that secretes interleukin 2 (IL-2), IL-3, IL-4, and interferon gamma. *J Exp Med* 1991; 174: 547.
198. Chang AE, Shu S, Chou T, Lafreniere R, Rosenberg SA. Differences in the effects of host suppression on the adoptive immunotherapy of subcutaneous and visceral tumors. *Cancer Res* 1986; 46: 3426.
199. Rosenberg SA, Yannelli JR, Yang JC, et al. Treatment of patients with metastatic melanoma with autologous tumor-infiltrating lymphocytes and interleukin2. *J Natl Cancer Inst* 1994; 86: 1159.
200. Rosenberg SA, Yang JC, Schwartzentruber DJ, et al. Immunologic and therapeutic evaluation of a synthetic peptide vaccine for the treatment of patients with metastatic melanoma. *Nat Med* 1998; 4: 321.
201. Morton DL, Foshag LJ, Hoon DS, et al. Prolongation of survival in metastatic melanoma after active specific immunotherapy with a new polyvalent melanoma vaccine. *Ann Surg* 1992; 216: 463.
202. Kammula US, Lee K, Riker AI, et al. Functional analysis of antigen-specific T lymphocytes by serial measurement of gene expression in peripheral blood mononuclear cells and tumor specimens. *J Immunol* 1999; 163: 6867.
203. Childs RW. Nonmyeloablative allogeneic peripheral blood stem-cell transplantation as immunotherapy for malignant diseases. *Cancer J Sci Am* 2000; 6: 179–187.
204. Hsueh EC, Nathanson L, Foshag LJ, et al. Active specific immunotherapy with polyvalent melanoma cell vaccine for patients with in-transit melanoma metastases. *Cancer* 1999; 85: 2160.
205. Speiser DE, Miranda R, Zakarian A, et al. Self antigens expressed by solid tumors do not efficiently stimulate naive or activated T cells: implications for immunotherapy. *J Exp Med* 1997; 186: 645.
206. Lu Z, Yuan L, Zhou X, Sotomayor E, Levitsky HI, Pardoll DM. CD40-independent pathways of T cell help for priming of CD8(+) cytotoxic T lymphocytes. *J Exp Med* 2000; 191: 541–550.
207. Hu HM, Urba WJ, Fox BA. Gene-modified tumor vaccine with therapeutic potential shifts tumor-specific T cell response from a type 2 to a type 1 cytokine profile. *J Immunol* 1998; 161: 3033.
208. Liu YJ, Kadowaki N, Rissoan MC, Soumelis V. T cell activation and polarization by DC1 and DC2. *Curr Top Microbiol Immunol* 2000; 251: 149.
209. Cohen PA, Fowler DJ, Kim H, et al. Propagation of murine and human T cells with defined antigen specificity and function. In: Frazer I, Chadwick D, Marsh J, eds., *Ciba Foundation Symposium No. 187: vaccines against virally induced cancers*, Wiley & Sons, Ltd, Chichester, 1994, p. 179.
210. Gabrilovich D, Ishida T, Oyama T, et al. Vascular endothelial growth factor inhibits the development of dendritic cells and dramatically affects the differentiation of multiple hematopoietic lineages in vivo. *Blood* 1998; 92: 4150.
211. Kavanaugh DY, Carbone DP. Immunologic dysfunction in cancer. *Hematol Oncol Clin North Am* 1996; 10: 927.

212. Slater D, Allport V, Bennett P. Changes in the expression of the type-2 but not the type-1 cyclo-oxygenase enzyme in chorion-decidua with the onset of labour. *Br J Obstet Gynaecol* 1998; 105: 745.
213. Ishihara O, Numari H, Saitoh M, et al. Prostaglandin E2 production by endogenous secretion of interleukin-1 in decidual cells from term fetal membrane. *Adv Exp Med Biol* 1997; 433: 419.
214. Imseis HM, Zimmerman PD, Samuels P, Kniss DA. Tumour necrosis factor-alpha induces cyclo-oxygenase-2 gene expression in first trimester trophoblasts: suppression by glucocorticoids and NSAIDs. *Placenta* 1997; 18: 521.
215. Singer II, Kawka DW, Schloemann S, Tessner T, Riehl T, Stenson WF. Cyclooxygenase 2 is induced in colonic epithelial cells in inflammatory bowel disease. *Gastroenterology* 1998; 115: 297.
216. Trautman MS, Collmer D, Edwin SS, White W, Mitchell MD, Dudley DJ. Expression of interleukin-10 in human gestational tissues. *J Soc Gynecol Investig* 1997; 4: 247.
217. Kim EC, Zhu Y, Andersen V, et al. Cytokine-mediated PGE2 expression in human colonic fibroblasts. *Am J Physiol* 1998; 275: C988.
218. Tonai T, Taketani Y, Ueda N, et al. Possible involvement of interleukin-1 in cyclooxygenase-2 induction after spinal cord injury in rats. *J Neurochem* 1999; 72: 302.
219. Cao C, Matsumura K, Ozaki M, Watanabe Y. Lipopolysaccharide injected into the cerebral ventricle evokes fever through induction of cyclooxygenase-2 in brain endothelial cells. *J Neurosci* 1999; 19: 716.
220. Wetzka B, Clark DE, Charnock-Jones DS, Zahradnik HP, Smith SK. PGE2 and TXA2 production by isolated macrophages from human placenta. *Adv Exp Med Biol* 1997; 433: 403.
221. Kelly RW, Critchley HO. A T-helper-2 bias in decidua: the prostaglandin contribution of the macrophage and trophoblast. *J Reprod Immunol* 1997; 33: 181.
222. Kelly RW, Critchley HO. T-cell modulation in decidua. *Immunol Today* 1998; 19: 142.
223. Braunstein J, Qiao L, Autschbach F, Schurmann G, Meuer S. T cells of the human intestinal lamina propria are high producers of interleukin-10. *Gut* 1997; 41: 215.
224. Hendel J, Nielsen OH. Expression of cyclooxygenase-2 mRNA in active inflammatory bowel disease. *Am J Gastroenterol* 1997; 92: 1170.
225. Terzioglu T, Yalti T, Tezelman S. The effect of prostaglandin E1 on experimental colitis in the rat. *Int J Colorectal Dis* 1997; 12: 63.
226. Schmidt C, Baumeister B, Kipnowski J, Schiermeyer-Dunkhase B, Vetter H. Alteration of prostaglandin E2 and leukotriene B4 synthesis in chronic inflammatory bowel disease. *Hepatogastroenterology* 1996; 43: 1508.
227. Duchmann R, Schmitt E, Knolle P, Meyer zum Buschenfelde KH, Neurath M. Tolerance towards resident intestinal flora in mice is abrogated in experimental colitis and restored by treatment with interleukin-10 or antibodies to interleukin-12. *Eur J Immunol* 1996; 26: 934.
228. Charpigny G, Reinaud P, Tamby JP, Creminon C, Guillomot M. Cyclooxygenase-2 unlike cyclooxygenase-1 is highly expressed in ovine embryos during the implantation period. *Biol Reprod* 1997; 57: 1032.
229. Swaisgood CM, Zu HX, Perkins DJ, et al. Coordinate expression of inducible nitric oxide synthase and cyclooxygenase-2 genes in uterine tissues of endotoxin-treated pregnant mice. *Am J Obstet Gynecol* 1997; 177: 1253.
230. Wetzka B, Nusing R, Charnock-Jones DS, Schafer W, Zahradnik HP, Smith SK. Cyclooxygenase-1 and -2 in human placenta and placental bed after normal and pre-eclamptic pregnancies. *Hum Reprod* 1997; 12: 2313.
231. Dudley DJ, Edwin SS, Dangerfield A, Jackson K, Trautman MS. Regulation of decidual cell and chorion cell production of interleukin-10 by purified bacterial products. *Am J Reprod Immunol* 1997; 38: 246.

232. Lim H, Paria BC, Das SK, et al. Multiple female reproductive failures in cyclooxygenase 2-deficient mice. *Cell* 1997; 91: 197.
233. Eckmann L, Stenson WF, Savidge TC, et al. Role of intestinal epithelial cells in the host secretory response to infection by invasive bacteria. Bacterial entry induces epithelial prostaglandin h synthase-2 expression and prostaglandin E2 and F2alpha production. *J Clin Invest* 1997; 100: 296.
234. Hancock WW, Polanski M, Zhang J, Blogg N, Weiner HL. Suppression of insulitis in non-obese diabetic (NOD) mice by oral insulin administration is associated with selective expression of interleukin-4 and -10, transforming growth factor-beta, and prostaglandin-E. *Am J Pathol* 1995; 147: 1193.
235. Neurath MF, Fuss I, Kelsall BL, Presky DH, Waegell W, Strober W. Experimental granulomatous colitis in mice is abrogated by induction of TGF-beta-mediated oral tolerance. *J Exp Med* 1996; 183: 2605.
236. Ando N, Hirahara F, Fukushima J, et al. Differential gene expression of TGF-beta isoforms and TGF-beta receptors during the first trimester of pregnancy at the human maternal-fetal interface. *Am J Reprod Immunol* 1998; 40: 48.
237. Kullberg MC, Ward JM, Gorelick PL, et al. Helicobacter hepaticus triggers colitis in specific-pathogen-free interleukin-10 (IL-10)-deficient mice through an IL-12- and gamma interferon-dependent mechanism. *Infect Immun* 1998; 66: 5157.
238. Davidson NJ, Hudak SA, Lesley RE, Menon S, Leach MW, Rennick DM. IL-12, but not IFN-gamma, plays a major role in sustaining the chronic phase of colitis in IL-10-deficient mice. *J Immunol* 1998; 161: 3143.
239. Reuter BK, Asfaha S, Buret A, Sharkey KA, Wallace JL. Exacerbation of inflammation-associated colonic injury in rat through inhibition of cyclooxygenase-2. *J Clin Invest* 1996; 98: 2076.
240. Lane JS, Todd KE, Lewis MP, et al. Interleukin-10 reduces the systemic inflammatory response in a murine model of intestinal ischemia/reperfusion. *Surgery* 1997; 122: 288.
241. Strober W, Kelsall B, Fuss I, et al. Reciprocal IFN-gamma and TGF-beta responses regulate the occurrence of mucosal inflammation. *Immunol Today* 1997; 18: 61.
242. Powrie F, Carlino J, Leach MW, Mauze S, Coffman RL. A critical role for transforming growth factor-beta but not interleukin 4 in the suppression of T helper type 1-mediated colitis by CD45RB(low) $CD4^+$ T cells. *J Exp Med* 1996; 183: 2669.
243. Giladi E, Raz E, Karmeli F, Okon E, Rachmilewitz D. Transforming growth factor-beta gene therapy ameliorates experimental colitis in rats. *Eur J Gastroenterol Hepatol* 1995; 7: 341.
244. Weetman AP. The immunology of pregnancy. *Thyroid* 1999; 9: 643.
245. Guller S, LaChapelle L. The role of placental Fas ligand in maintaining immune privilege at maternal-fetal interfaces. *Semin Reprod Endocrinol* 1999; 17: 39.
246. Jerzak M, Kasprzycka M, Wierbicki P, Kotarski J, Gorski A. Apoptosis of T cells in the first trimester human decidua. *Am J Reprod Immunol* 1998; 40: 130.
247. Payne SG, Smith SC, Davidge ST, Baker PN, Guilbert LJ. Death receptor Fas/Apo-1/CD95 expressed by human placental cytotrophoblasts does not mediate apoptosis. *Biol Reprod* 1999; 60: 1144.
248. Finke JH, Tubbs R, Connelly B, Pontes E, Montie J. Tumor-infiltrating lymphocytes in patients with renal-cell carcinoma. *Ann NY Acad Sci* 1988; 532: 387.
249. Finke JH, Rayman P, Hart L, et al. Characterization of tumor-infiltrating lymphocyte subsets from human renal cell carcinoma: specific reactivity defined by cytotoxicity, interferon-gamma secretion, and proliferation. *J Immunother Emphasis Tumor Immunol* 1994; 15: 91.
250. Schendel DJ, Oberneder R, Falk CS, et al. Cellular and molecular analyses of major histocompatibility complex (MHC) restricted and non-MHC-restricted effector cells recognizing renal cell carcinomas: problems and perspectives for immunotherapy. *J Mol Med* 1997; 75: 400.

251. Wang Q, Redovan C, Tubbs R, et al. Selective cytokine gene expression in renal cell carcinoma tumor cells and tumor-infiltrating lymphocytes. *Int J Cancer* 1995; 61: 780.
252. Nakagomi H, Pisa P, Pisa EK, et al. Lack of interleukin-2 (IL-2) expression and selective expression of IL-10 mRNA in human renal cell carcinoma. *Int J Cancer* 1995; 63: 366.
253. Pisa P, Halapi E, Pisa EK, et al. Selective expression of interleukin 10, interferon gamma, and granulocyte-macrophage colony-stimulating factor in ovarian cancer biopsies. *Proc Natl Acad Sci USA* 1992; 89: 7708.
254. Alexander JP, Kudoh S, Melsop KA, et al. T-cells infiltrating renal cell carcinoma display a poor proliferative response even though they can produce interleukin 2 and express interleukin 2 receptors. *Cancer Res* 1993; 53: 1380.
255. Tartour E, Latour S, Mathiot C, et al. Variable expression of CD3-zeta chain in tumor-infiltrating lymphocytes (TIL) derived from renal-cell carcinoma: relationship with TIL phenotype and function. *Int J Cancer* 1995; 63: 205.
256. Miescher S, Whiteside TL, Moretta L, von Fliedner V. Clonal and frequency analyses of tumor-infiltrating T lymphocytes from human solid tumors. *J Immunol* 1987; 138: 4004.
257. Klugo RC. Diagnostic and therapeutic immunology of renal cell cancer. *Henry Ford Med J* 1979; 27: 106.
258. Amano T, Koshida K, Nakajima K, Naito K, Hisazumi H. PPD, PHA and Su-PS skin tests in genitourinary malignancies. *Hinyokika Kiyo* 1985; 31: 2107.
259. Salvadori S, Gansbacher B, Pizzimenti AM, Zier KS. Abnormal signal transduction by T cells of mice with parental tumors is not seen in mice bearing IL-2-secreting tumors. *J Immunol* 1994; 153: 5176.
260. Nakagomi H, Petersson M, Magnusson I, et al. Decreased expression of the signal-transducing zeta chains in tumor-infiltrating T-cells and NK cells of patients with colorectal carcinoma. *Cancer Res* 1993; 53: 5610.
261. Zea AH, Curti BD, Longo DL, et al. Alterations in T cell receptor and signal transduction molecules in melanoma patients. *Clin Cancer Res* 1995; 1: 1327.
262. Kono K, Salazar-Onfray F, Petersson M, et al. Hydrogen peroxide secreted by tumor-derived macrophages down-modulates signal-transducing zeta molecules and inhibits tumor-specific T cell-and natural killer cell-mediated cytotoxicity. *Eur J Immunol* 1996; 26: 1308.
263. Otsuji M, Kimura Y, Aoe T, Okamoto Y, Saito T. Oxidative stress by tumor-derived macrophages suppresses the expression of CD3 zeta chain of T-cell receptor complex and antigen-specific T-cell responses. *Proc Natl Acad Sci USA* 1996; 93: 13119.
264. Ohcoa A, Longo DL. Alteration of signal transduction in T cells from cancer patients. In: DeVita V, Hellman S, Rosenberg SA, eds., *Important Advances in Oncology*. J.B. Lippincott, Philadelphia, 1995.
265. Rabinowich H, Reichert TE, Kashii Y, Gastman BR, Bell MC, Whiteside TL. Lymphocyte apoptosis induced by Fas ligand-expressing ovarian carcinoma cells. Implications for altered expression of T cell receptor in tumor-associated lymphocytes. *J Clin Invest* 1998; 101: 2579.
266. Ghosh P, Sica A, Young HA, et al. Alterations in NF kappa B/Rel family proteins in splenic T-cells from tumor-bearing mice and reversal following therapy. *Cancer Res* 1994; 54: 2969.
267. Ghosh P, Komschlies KL, Cippitelli M, et al. Gradual loss of T-helper 1 populations in spleen of mice during progressive tumor growth. *J Natl Cancer Inst* 1995; 87: 1478.
268. Li X, Liu J, Park JK, et al. T cells from renal cell carcinoma patients exhibit an abnormal pattern of kappa B-specific DNA-binding activity: a preliminary report. *Cancer Res* 1994; 54: 5424.
269. Xu J, Ling EA. Upregulation and induction of major histocompatibility complex class I and II antigens on microglial cells in early postnatal rat brain following intraperitoneal injections of recombinant interferon-gamma. *Neuroscience* 1994; 60: 959.
270. Uzzo RG, Rayman P, Kolenko V, et al. Renal cell carcinoma-derived gangliosides suppress nuclear factor-kappaB activation in T cells. *J Clin Invest* 1999; 104: 769.

271. Uzzo RG, Rayman P, Kolenko V, et al. Mechanisms of apoptosis in T cells from patients with renal cell carcinoma. *Clin Cancer Res* 1999; 5: 1219.
272. Pardoll DM. Cancer vaccines. *Nat Med* 1998; 4: 525.
273. Pardoll DM. Cancer vaccines. *Immunol Today* 1993; 14: 310.
274. de Waal Malefyt R, Haanen J, Spits H, et al. Interleukin 10 (IL-10) and viral IL-10 strongly reduce antigen-specific human T cell proliferation by diminishing the antigen-presenting capacity of monocytes via downregulation of class II major histocompatibility complex expression. *J Exp Med* 1991; 174: 915.
275. Taga K, Mostowski H, Tosato G. Human interleukin-10 can directly inhibit T-cell growth. *Blood* 1993; 81: 2964.
276. Romano MF, Lamberti A, Petrella A, et al. IL-10 inhibits nuclear factor-kappa B/Rel nuclear activity in CD3-stimulated human peripheral T lymphocytes. *J Immunol* 1996; 156: 2119.
277. Fiorentino DF, Zlotnik A, Mosmann TR, Howard M, O'Garra A. IL-10 inhibits cytokine production by activated macrophages. *J Immunol* 1991; 147: 3815.
278. Gastl GA, Abrams JS, Nanus DM, et al. Interleukin-10 production by human carcinoma cell lines and its relationship to interleukin-6 expression. *Int J Cancer* 1993; 55: 96.
279. Halak BK, Maguire HC Jr, Lattime EC. Tumor-induced interleukin-10 inhibits type 1 immune responses directed at a tumor antigen as well as a non-tumor antigen present at the tumor site. *Cancer Res* 1999; 59: 911.
280. Allione A, Consalvo M, Nanni P, et al. Immunizing and curative potential of replicating and nonreplicating murine mammary adenocarcinoma cells engineered with interleukin (IL)-2, IL-4, IL-6, IL-7, IL-10, tumor necrosis factor alpha, granulocyte-macrophage colony-stimulating factor, and gamma-interferon gene or admixed with conventional adjuvants. *Cancer Res* 1994; 54: 6022.
281. Kundu N, Beaty TL, Jackson MJ, Fulton AM. Antimetastatic and antitumor activities of interleukin 10 in a murine model of breast cancer. *J Natl Cancer Inst* 1996; 88: 536.
282. Ahuja SS, Paliogianni F, Yamada H, Balow JE, Boumpas DT. Effect of transforming growth factor-beta on early and late activation events in human T cells. *J Immunol* 1993; 150: 3109.
283. Kehrl JH, Wakefield LM, Roberts AB, et al. Production of transforming growth factor beta by human T lymphocytes and its potential role in the regulation of T cell growth. *J Exp Med* 1986; 163: 1037.
284. Stoeck M, Miescher S, MacDonald HR, von Fliedner V. Transforming growth factors beta slow down cell-cycle progression in a murine interleukin-2 dependent T-cell line. *J Cell Physiol* 1989; 141: 65.
285. Rappaport RS, Dodge GR. Prostaglandin E inhibits the production of human interleukin 2. *J Exp Med* 1982; 155: 943.
286. Minakuchi R, Wacholtz MC, Davis LS, Lipsky PE. Delineation of the mechanism of inhibition of human T cell activation by PGE2. *J Immunol* 1990; 145: 2616.
287. Chen D, Rothenberg EV. Interleukin 2 transcription factors as molecular targets of cAMP inhibition: delayed inhibition kinetics and combinatorial transcription roles. *J Exp Med* 1994; 179: 931.
288. Lingk DS, Chan MA, Gelfand EW. Increased cyclic adenosine monophosphate levels block progression but not initiation of human T cell proliferation. *J Immunol* 1990; 145: 449.
289. Kolenko V, Rayman P, O'Shea J, Tubbs R, Bukowski R, Finke J. Downregulation of Jak3 protein levels in T lymphocytes by prostaglandin E2 and other cyclic AMP-elevanting agents: impact on IL2 receptor signaling pathway. *Blood* 1999; 93: 2308.
290. Hakomori S. Bifunctional role of glycosphingolipids. Modulators for transmembrane signaling and mediators for cellular interactions. *J Biol Chem* 1990; 265: 18713.
291. Ritter G, Livingston PO. Ganglioside antigens expressed by human cancer cells. *Semin Cancer Biol* 1991; 2: 401.

292. Hoon DS, Okun E, Neuwirth H, Morton DL, Irie RF. Aberrant expression of gangliosides in human renal cell carcinomas. *J Urol* 1993; 150: 2013.
293. Ladisch S, Ulsh L, Gillard B, Wong C. Modulation of the immune response by gangliosides. Inhibition of adherent monocyte accessory function in vitro. *J Clin Invest* 1984; 74: 2074.
294. Lengle EE. Increased levels of lipid-bound sialic acid in thymic lymphocytes and plasma from leukemic AKR/J mice. *J Natl Cancer Inst* 1979; 62: 1565.
295. Bergelson LD, Dyatlovitskaya EV, Klyuchareva TE, et al. The role of glycosphingolipids in natural immunity. Gangliosides modulate the cytotoxicity of natural killer cells. *Eur J Immunol* 1989; 19: 1979.
296. Irani DN, Lin KI, Griffin DE. Brain-derived gangliosides regulate the cytokine production and proliferation of activated T cells. *J Immunol* 1996; 157: 4333.
297. Valentino L, Moss T, Olson E, Wang HJ, Elashoff R, Ladisch S. Shed tumor gangliosides and progression of human neuroblastoma. *Blood* 1990; 75: 1564.
298. McKallip R, Li R, Ladisch S. Tumor gangliosides inhibit the tumor-specific immune response. *J Immunol* 1999; 163: 3718.
299. Irani DN. The susceptibility of mice to immune-mediated neurologic disease correlates with the degree to which their lymphocytes resist the effects of brain-derived gangliosides. *J Immunol* 1998; 161: 2746.
300. Seliger B, Maeurer MJ, Ferrone S. TAP off—tumors on. *Immunol Today* 1997; 18: 292.
301. Seliger B, Hohne A, Knuth A, et al. Analysis of the major histocompatibility complex class I antigen presentation machinery in normal and malignant renal cells: evidence for deficiencies associated with transformation and progression. *Cancer Res* 1996; 56: 1756.
302. O'Connell J, O'Sullivan GC, Collins JK, Shanahan F. The Fas counterattack: Fas-mediated T cell killing by colon cancer cells expressing Fas ligand. *J Exp Med* 1996; 184: 1075.
303. Saas P, Walker PR, Hahne M, et al. Fas ligand expression by astrocytoma in vivo: maintaining immune privilege in the brain? *J Clin Invest* 1997; 99: 1173.
304. Lowin B, Hahne M, Mattmann C, Tschopp J. Cytolytic T-cell cytotoxicity is mediated through perforin and Fas lytic pathways. *Nature* 1994; 370: 650.
305. Kagi D, Vignaux F, Ledermann B, et al. Fas and perforin pathways as major mechanisms of T cell-mediated cytotoxicity. *Science* 1994; 265: 528.
306. Walker PR, Saas P, Dietrich PY. Role of Fas ligand (CD95L) in immune escape: the tumor cell strikes back. *J Immunol* 1997; 158: 4521.
307. Alderson MR, Tough TW, Davis-Smith T, et al. Fas ligand mediates activation-induced cell death in human T lymphocytes. *J Exp Med* 1995; 181: 71.
308. Daniel PT, Krammer PH. Activation induces sensitivity toward APO-1 (CD95)-mediated apoptosis in human B cells. *J Immunol* 1994; 152: 5624.
309. Mountz JD, Zhou T, Bluethmann H, Wu J, Edwards CK III. Apoptosis defects analyzed in TcR transgenic and fas transgenic lpr mice. *Int Rev Immunol* 1994; 11: 321.
310. Griffith TS, Brunner T, Fletcher SM, Green DR, Ferguson TA. Fas ligand-induced apoptosis as a mechanism of immune privilege. *Science* 1995; 270: 1189.
311. French LE, Hahne M, Viard I, et al. Fas and Fas ligand in embryos and adult mice: ligand expression in several immune-privileged tissues and coexpression in adult tissues characterized by apoptotic cell turnover. *J Cell Biol* 1996; 133: 335.
312. Nagata S, Suda T. Fas and Fas ligand: lpr and gld mutations. *Immunol Today* 1995; 16: 39.
313. Hahne M, Rimoldi D, Schroter M, et al. Melanoma cell expression of Fas(Apo-1/CD95) ligand: implications for tumor immune escape. *Science* 1996; 274: 1363.
314. Zeytun A, Hassuneh M, Nagarkatti M, Nagarkatti PS. Fas-Fas ligand-based interactions between tumor cells and tumor-specific cytotoxic T lymphocytes: a lethal two-way street. *Blood* 1997; 90: 1952.

315. Cardi G, Heaney JA, Schned AR, Ernstoff MS. Expression of Fas(APO-1/CD95) in tumor-infiltrating and peripheral blood lymphocytes in patients with renal cell carcinoma. *Cancer Res* 1998; 58: 2078.
316. Saito T, Dworacki G, Gooding W, Lotze MT, Whiteside TL. Spontaneous apoptosis of $CD8^+$ T lymphocytes in peripheral blood of patients with advanced melanoma. *Clin Cancer Res* 2000; 6: 1351.
317. Gastman BR, Johnson DE, Whiteside TL, Rabinowich H. Tumor-induced apoptosis of T lymphocytes: elucidation of intracellular apoptotic events. *Blood* 2000; 95: 2015–2023.
318. Chappell DB, Zaks TZ, Rosenberg SA, Restifo NP. Human melanoma cells do not express Fas (Apo-1/CD95) ligand. *Cancer Res* 1999; 59: 59.
319. Zaks TZ, Chappell DB, Rosenberg SA, Restifo NP. Fas-mediated suicide of tumor-reactive T cells following activation by specific tumor: selective rescue by caspase inhibition. *J Immunol* 1999; 162: 3273.
320. Lee PP, Yee C, Savage PA, et al. Characterization of circulating T cells specific for tumor-associated antigens in melanoma patients. *Nat Med* 1999; 5: 677.

5 Immunotherapy of Advanced Melanoma Directed at Specific Antigens

Stanley P. L. Leong, MD *and Suyu Shu,* PHD

CONTENTS

1. INTRODUCTION

Since the description of melanoma in 1787, its biological behavior has suggested that the immune system may play a significant role in its interaction with melanoma. Several lines of evidence may support this hypothesis: (*i*) in documented cases of children with spontaneous regression of cancer, melanoma has been found to be the cancer second in incidence to neuroblastoma *(1)*; (*ii*) approximately 5% of patients with metastatic melanoma have an unknown primary suggesting that the primary melanoma may have regressed spontaneously *(2,3)*; (*iii*) although widespread vitiligo-like leukoderma is an uncommon clinical entity, its clinical manifestation suggests that an immune mechanism may be the cause of destruction of both normal melanocytes and malignant melanoma *(4)*; (*iv*) in superficial spreading melanoma, it is not infrequent to appreciate areas of regression with tumor-infiltrating lymphocytes (TILs). Lymphocytic infiltration of the primary tumor has been associated with a better prognosis than when the primary tumor is not infiltrated with lymphocytes *(5–7)*; (*v*) although it is not a

From: *Current Clinical Oncology, Melanoma: Biologically Targeted Therapeutics*
Edited by: E. C. Borden

common finding, there are patients whose melanoma may remain dormant for over 20 yr after the diagnosis of the primary melanoma, who subsequently recur and die from melanoma *(8)*. This may suggest tumor escape following a long period of host tumor interaction; and (*vi*) finally, the significantly increased incidence and poorer prognosis for melanoma developed in immunosuppressed renal transplant recipients *(9)* provides additional clinical evidence for the role of immune surveillance in the evolution of melanoma.

The results of laboratory studies also support the notion that melanoma cells are immunogenic in their autochthonous hosts *(10,11)*. In the mid 1970s, Shiku et al. demonstrated the presence of antibodies in the sera of melanoma patients reactive to autologous melanoma cell surface antigens but not fibroblasts derived from the same patients *(12,13)*. Monoclonal antibodies (mAb) have subsequently identified two glycoproteins (p97/gp95, mCSP) and two glycolipids (GD_2, GD_3) on the melanoma cell surface *(14)*. While these tumor-associated antigens are also present on normal cells in low concentrations, their relatively higher levels of expression by melanoma cells serve as potential targets for an immune response.

Over the past decade or so, both immunologic and molecular studies indicate that melanoma is capable of stimulating both humoral *(14)* and cellular immune responses *(15–18)*. This cellular immune response is mainly mediated by T lymphocytes generated from peripheral blood *(19,20)*, TILs *(21–23)*, and lymph nodes (LNs) either draining the metastatic melanoma or LNs containing metastatic tumor *(24–26)*. Despite the presence of immune suppression associated with progressive disease *(27–30)*, there is evidence for the existence of a cellular antitumor response even in patients with metastatic melanoma *(19–26)*.

More effective therapy is needed, as the incidence of melanoma is doubling every 10 yr *(31)*. Melanoma has been found to be most applicable as a model for immunotherapy, because it is resistant to chemotherapy and radiation therapy and yet appears to be antigenic. Antigen-specific immunotherapy may be either active (vaccines) or passive (sensitized cells or mAb).

2. ACTIVE SPECIFIC IMMUNOTHERAPY

Active specific immunotherapy to mediate tumor regression is an important approach. Active specific immunotherapy attempts to elicit immunity in the tumor bearing host with the use of vaccines, which may be cellular or cellular products. The former includes autologous *(32,33)* and allogenic melanoma cells *(34,35)*. The latter includes extracts of melanoma cells such as purified gangliosides *(36,37)*, shed antigens *(38)*, mechanical melanoma cell lysates *(39)*, and viral melanoma cell lysates *(40,41)*. Another approach is the use of anti-idiotypic antibodies mimicking high molecular weight melanoma-associated antigens (MAA) *(42)*. Although occasional responses have been observed, the overall results have been marginal *(32–34,36,38–54)*.

Table 1
MAAs Recognized by Human Tumor-Reactive T Cells[a] *(103)*

Gene	*Expression pattern*	*Restriction element*	*Epitope*
Gp100	Melanoma, melanocyte	HLA-A2	KTWGQYWQV
			ITDQVPFSV
			YLEPGPVTA
			LLDGTATLRL
			VLYRYGSFSV
			RLMKQDFSV
			RLPRIFCSC
		HLA-A3	ALLAVGATV
		HLA-A24	VYFFLPDHL
		HLA-Cw8	ANDPIFVVL
MART-1/ Melan A	Melanoma, melanocyte	HLA-A2	AAGIGILTV
Tyrosinase	Melanoma, melanocyte	HLA-A1	KCCPICTDEY
		HLA-A2	MLLAVLYCL
			YMDGTMSQV
		HLA-A24	AFLPWHRLF
		HLA-B44	SEIWRDIDF
		HLA-DR0401	SYLQDSDPDSFQD
			QNILLSNAPLGPQFP
TRP-1	Melanoma, melanocyte	HLA-A31	MSLQRQFLR
TRP-2	Melanoma, melanocyte	HLA-A2	SVYDFFDWL
		HLA-A31,33	LLPGGRPYR
		HLA-Cw8	KVSNDGPTLI
MAGE-1	Melanoma, breast, head and neck, lung, colorectal, prostate, bladder cancer, normal testis	HLA-A1	EADPTGHSY
		HLA-Cw-16	SAYGEPRKL
MAGE-3	Similar to MAGE-1	HLA-A1	EVDPIGLHY
		HLA-A2	FLWGPRALV
		HLA-B44	MEVDPIGHLY
BAGE	Similar to MAGE-1	HLA-Cw16	AAARAVFLAL
GAGE-1,2	Similar to MAGE-1	HLACw6	YRPRPRRY

[a]Prepared by Dr. Michael Nishimura, Surgery Branch, National Cancer Institute (NCI).

Recent advances in molecular and cellular immunology have identified numerous melanoma-associated peptide antigens (Tables 1 and 2) and made it possible to conduct clinical trials on immunotherapy of cancer using these peptides. In a recent study with melanoma peptide immunization, interleukin (IL)-2

Table 2
Mutated Melanoma Antigens Recognized by Human Tumor-Reactive T Cells[a]

Gene	*Expression pattern*	*Restriction element*	*Epitope*
MUM-1	Melanoma	HLA-B44	EEKLIVVFL
CDK4	Melanoma	HLA-A2	ACDPHSGHFV
β-Catenin	Melanoma	HLA-24	SYLDSGIHF
p15	Melanoma	HLA-A24	AYGLDFYIL
GnT-V	Melanoma	HLA-A2	BLPDVFIRC
TPI *(104)*	Melanoma	HLA-DR	GELIGILNAAKVPAD

[a]Prepared by Dr. Michael Nishimura, Surgery Branch, NCI

seems to play a key role in tumor regression *(55)*. In this study, immunodominant peptides from a synthetic gp100 MAA with increased binding affinity for human leukocyte antigen (HLA)-A2 molecules was used as a cancer vaccine to treat patients with metastatic melanoma. Ninety-one percent of patients were successfully immunized using the synthetic peptide, and 13 of 31 patients (42%) treated with peptide vaccine plus IL-2 had objective cancer responses, and 4 additional patients had mixed or minor responses. However, analysis of the frequencies of specific T cells in peripheral blood revealed that clinical responses did not correlate well with the in vitro assay.

3. ADOPTIVE IMMUNOTHERAPY

Another form of immunotherapy is cellular therapy. It is often referred to as "adoptive immunotherapy" and represents approaches that capitalize on the relatively weak cellular responses observed in the tumor-bearing host, which can be amplified by experimental methods for therapeutic benefit. Once the mechanism is worked out, the practice and principles of immunotherapy of human melanoma may be used on other solid tumors, which are resistant to chemotherapy and radiation therapy. The focus of this review is mainly on the use of a variety of activated lymphoid cells for adoptive immunotherapy of melanoma.

A central tenet of this approach is the need for a lymphoid cell population capable of recognizing and interacting with antigenic components on the tumor cell surface. The therapeutic potential and clinical problems associated with such adoptive immunotherapy have largely been defined in animal models *(56)*. The passive administration of immune cells shows attractive potential, because it may react against the tumor, independent of the host's immune competence, thereby avoiding immune suppression in cancer patients. Adoptive immunotherapy requires the establishment of methods for isolating, sensitizing, and expanding tumor-reactive lymphoid cells from patients to large enough numbers that can be utilized for therapeutic purposes. The discovery and subsequent cloning of the human T-cell growth factor, IL-2, in the late 1970s have opened the way to grow large quantities of antitumor autologous lymphocytes for adoptive immunotherapy *(57)*.

Adoptive immunotherapy has evolved through several stages of development: (*i*) lymphokine-activated killer (LAK) cells; (*ii*) TILs; (*iii*) in vitro-sensitized lymphocytes; and (*iv*) in vitro-activated lymphocytes. Both in vitro-sensitized and -activated lymphocytes are derived from draining LN cells from patients being immunized with autologous irradiated tumor cells with appropriate adjuvants. The above-described stages of adoptive immunotherapy are summarized below.

3.1. Lyphokine Activated Killer Cells

Incubation of peripheral blood leukocytes (PBLs) in the presence of high concentrations of IL-2 resulted in the generation of cytotoxic cells, so called LAK cells, capable of lysing neoplastic, but not normal nonmalignant cells. The therapeutic efficacy of LAK cells was first demonstrated in a variety of animal tumor models and was found to be dependant on the concomitant administration of IL-2 *(58)*. The first meaningful clinical trial of adoptive immunotherapy was the use of LAK cells *(59)*. IL-2 is a cytokine recognized as the primary messenger by which $CD4^+$ T cells mediate their helper function. While the technique of in vitro stimulation of (PBL) in IL-2 did not induce a specific antitumor T cell response, it was discovered to activate a population of natural killer (NK) cells with demonstrable cytotoxic effects against malignant cells, while sparing normal cells *(60,61)*. These LAK cells were derived from non-T, non-B (NK) cells. The NK origin of LAK cells most likely explains both their ability to be derived from normal as well as tumor-bearing hosts and their nonspecific tumor reactivity. In these studies, LAK cell precursors were leukaphoresed from patients' peripheral blood following a 5-day course of systemic IL-2, and a subsequent 2-day rest period during which a rebound lymphocytosis was observed. LAK cells were generated by ex vivo culture of the leukaphoresed cells in high concentrations of IL-2 for 3 to 4 d and given back to the patient systemically with the concomitant infusion of IL-2. The initial LAK cell/IL-2 therapy reported by Rosenberg et al. resulted in an overall (complete and partial) response rate of 27% in 26 patients with metastatic melanoma *(59)*. All of the side effects of treatment were primarily attributable to the administration of high doses of IL-2. The most frequently observed IL-2 related toxicities were cardiovascular, renal, and hematologic in origin, and reversed rapidly upon discontinuation of IL-2. Subsequent trials using LAK cells in combination with intermittent or continuous IL-2 infusion for metastatic melanoma by other investigators resulted in overall response rates ranging between 0–56% *(62–65)*. During this time, several reports documented the antitumor efficacy of IL-2 administration alone *(66–68)*. Subsequently, two randomized studies have been conducted to formally compare LAK cell/IL-2 versus IL-2 therapy alone *(69,70)*. The response rates in both of these studies were found to be comparable between the two treatment regimens. However, the study conducted by Rosenberg et al. demonstrated a higher complete response rate and improved survival rate in patients with melanoma who received LAK cell/IL-2 therapy *(70)*. Although LAK/IL-2 trials are no longer available, these early trials established the basis for adoptive immunotherapy being a viable therapeutic modality for the treatment of metastatic melanoma.

3.2. Tumor Infiltrating Lymphocytes

The recognition that LAK cell therapy represented a viable therapy for metastatic melanoma resulted in the search for effector cells with greater tumor specificity. Lymphocytes infiltrating the stroma of primary and metastatic melanomas were considered to be tumor-specific by virtue of their location and cytotoxicity studies demonstrating tumor-specific reactivity. In the mid 1980s, Spiess et al. demonstrated that in vitro culture of tumor cell suspensions in high concentrations of IL-2 resulted in the activation and expansion of TILs *(71)*. Unlike LAK cells, this antitumor effect was tumor-specific, showing poor cross-reactivity between different methylcholanthrene-induced tumor cell lines. These studies also demonstrated that in comparison with LAK, TILs had 50–100 times greater therapeutic efficacy in mediating the regression of established microscopic pulmonary metastases. The increased efficacy of TILs compared to LAK cells in mediating the regression of established pulmonary metastases in animal models correlated with quantifiable antitumor effects in clinical trials. In a pilot study by Rosenberg et al., 20 patients with metastatic melanoma were pretreated with a single dose of cyclophosphamide, followed by the combination of TILs and IL-2. This therapeutic regimen resulted in 11 (55%) patients having tumor responses (complete and partial), with response durations ranging from 2 to greater than 13 months *(23)*. In a follow-up report by this group, 22 of 55 (40%) patients with advanced melanoma treated with TILs and IL-2 demonstrated significant tumor responses *(72)*. Lysis of autologous tumor cells by TILs was significantly higher for responding than nonresponding patients. Although TILs appeared to be more specific and efficient than LAK cells against autologous melanoma, there is a lack of consistency in the harvesting and growing of TILs to become a reliable approach for adoptive immunotherapy.

3.3. In Vitro Sensitization

Since most human tumors arise spontaneously and are postulated to be poorly immunogenic *(73)*, and therapeutic TILs cannot be generated from progressively growing poorly immunogenic murine tumors *(71)*, TILs may not be reliable effector cells against cancer in the clinical setting. Therefore, more potent and reliable effector cells need to be developed from tumor-bearing hosts. In animal studies, another source of tumor-reactive lymphocytes was identified. Freshly harvested LN cells lacked apparent antitumor reactivity, but potent immune effector cells could be generated from these cells by subsequent culture with an in vitro sensitization (IVS) method that Shu et al. have established *(56)*. The IVS of tumor-draining LN lymphocytes involved the in vitro culture with irradiated tumor cells in the presence of low concentrations of IL-2. These activated lymphocytes demonstrated the ability to mediate tumor-specific regression of established pulmonary metastases in murine models *(56,74)*. Normal lymphocytes from nontumor-bearing host were incapable of being activated by the IVS culture method to develop into competent effector cells. Therefore, the process of eliciting tumor-reactive lymphocytes required presensitization of the lymphocytes in the tumor-bearing host. It was observed in several studies that these LN cells were tumor-primed yet functionally deficient, being unable to mediate tumor regression. Thus, these lymphocytes were termed "pre-effector" cells, capable of differentiation into effector cells with antitumor reactivity only after IVS. It is postulated that LN-draining progressive tumors might represent an excellent source of antitumor effector cells.

In addition, effector cells generated by IVS culture also offered therapeutic advantages over TILs in the treatment of poorly immunogenic murine tumors. Using the poorly immunogenic MCA 102 murine sarcoma, Shu et al. have shown that the addition of *Corynebacterium parvum* to the tumor vaccine would lead to the generation of pre-effector cells, which, following IVS activation, were capable of mediating the regression of established pulmonary metastases *(75)*. In contrast, TILs were found to be difficult to generate and, in cases in which sufficient number of TILs were generated, they have not been demonstrated to show consistent antitumor reactivity against poorly immunogenic tumors *(71)*. Thus, the IVS culture system has theoretical advantages compared to TILs in the treatment of poorly immunogenic human cancers.

Based on these animal studies, a human trial was conducted using the IVS culture method to generate lymphocytes for the treatment of metastatic melanoma and renal cell cancer (RCC) *(76)*. Bacille Calmette-Guérin (BCG) was admixed with irradiated tumor cells and given as a vaccine to prime draining LNs. Following a 9- to 10-d sensitization period, the draining LNs were harvested, activated by IVS, and administered to patients in conjunction with low dose bolus IL-2(180,000 IU/kg q 8 h for 5 d). Of the 10 patients (7 melanoma, 3 RCC) treated, one patient with melanoma had a partial clinical response. The mean number of effector cells infused was 7×10^9 with 72% characterized as $CD4^+$ cells by flow cytometry. Interestingly, 7 of 9 patients evaluated after cell infusion developed a delayed-type hypersensitivity (DTH) response to autologous tumor cells. In a cohort of patients who underwent tumor vaccination and IL-2 administration without cell infusion, none of 10 patients developed DTH reactivity to autologous tumor. While this represented only a small number of patients studied, the development of DTH reactivity to autologous tumor suggested that tumor immunity was transferred by the IVS cells. Further clinical studies evaluating the antitumor reactivity of vaccine-primed LN cells with larger numbers of transferred cells were warranted.

3.4. Anti-CD3/IL-2 Activation

The IVS culture system for generating immune effector cells for adoptive immunotherapy required that tumor-primed LN cells be antigenically stimulated by autologous tumor cells in vitro. This requirement for a large number of autologous tumor cells was potentially restrictive for the broad clinical application of IVS cells. In our limited trials performed to date, the failure of IVS-activated cells to mediate significant responses was likely due to a limitation of sufficient numbers of effector cells for treatment. Because tumor-draining LN cells contain immunologically committed tumor reactive T cells as a result of in vivo exposure to autologous tumor or to stimulation by tumor cell-BCG vaccination, their activation is likely via the recognition by the T cell antigen receptor (TCR), which is noncovalently associated with a cluster of low molecular weight proteins commonly referred to as CD3 *(77–79)*. In animal experiments, in vitro stimulation of tumor-draining LN cells with anti-CD3 mAb for 2 d, followed by culture in 10 U/mL of IL-2, resulted in a 15- to 30-fold T cell proliferation, with 75 ± 8% of these activated T cells bearing the CD8 phenotype *(80,81)*. Following adoptive transfer, these anti-CD3/IL-2-activated cells were capable of mediating the regression of primary as well as advanced macroscopic tumors *(81)*. Despite the fact that anti-CD3 activation is polyclonal, these activated effector cells maintained exquisite tumor-specific reactivity reflecting the tumor used for the in vivo stimulation of the draining LN. Thus, this mAb activation technique offered practical advantages over the IVS method in eliminating the requirement for autologous tumor cells for in vitro stimulation.

Similar to observations with the use of IVS cells, progressively growing poorly immunogenic murine tumors such as the B16/BL6 melanoma failed to stimulate a tumor-specific pre-effector cell response, because tumor-draining LN cells activated by anti-CD3 did not demonstrate antitumor effects *(82)*. However, the pre-effector response could be elicited by admixing tumor cells with powerful adjuvants such as *Corynebacterium parvum*. Based on these animal data, Chang et al. have initiated a human trial of adoptive immunotherapy with anti-CD3/IL-2-activated effector cells for the treatment of metastatic melanoma and RCC *(83)*. Twenty-three patients (11 melanoma, 12 RCC) with advanced cancer were treated with irradiated autologous tumor cells with BCG. Seven days later, draining LNs were removed for activation with anti-CD3 mAb, followed by expansion in IL-2. Vaccine-primed LN were expanded ex vivo with a mean of 8.4×10^{10} cells administered per patient. Activated LN cells were administered intravenously with the concomitant administration of IL-2. Among 11 melanoma patients, one had a partial tumor response. Among 12 RCC patients, two had complete responses, and two had partial responses.

In a recent pilot study, 14 patients with stage IV melanoma were treated with adoptive immunotherapy to assess the feasibility and toxicity of adoptive immunotherapy using activated T cells *(84)*. Each patient was immunized with autologous melanoma cells plus BCG or rh granulocyte-macrophage colony-stimulating factor (GM-CSF) at two sites distal to a LN area, such as the groin or axilla. Draining LNs were harvested 8 d later and processed into single-cell suspensions. For this group of patients, the first 3 patients had BCG as vaccine adjuvant, and the other 11 patients had rhGM-CSF. The LN cells of all 14 patients were sequentially activated in two cycles with staphylococcal enterotoxin A (SEA) and anti-CD3. Activated cells were expanded in culture with 60 IU/mL IL-2. The average culture time was 25 d. The expanded T cells were infused into the patient in conjunction with systemic IL-2 (36,000 IU/Kg q 8 h IV bolus for 5 d) with a total of 16 infusions (2 patients had 2 infusions at 2 different times). These 14 patients received infusions of 1×10^{10} to 1.7×10^{11} cells. The method of T cell activation and expansion yielded a proliferation index ranging from 10- to 363-fold. Fresh tumor-primed LN cells showed a mean composition of 53% of CD4 cells and 10% of CD8 cells, whereas activated T cells showed 30% of CD4 and 68% of CD8. Grade III toxicity (40%) was encountered in this group of patients. All patients developed progression of disease. The laboratory and clinical protocols were, therefore, modified to activate vaccine-draining LN cells with one cycle of stimulation by SEA followed by IL-2. The short activation schedule yielded a mean ex vivo expansions interval of 8.5 d for the second 8 patients, all of whom had rhGM-CSF as adjuvant based on a previous study that rhGM-CSF may play an active role in tumor regression *(33)*. These patients received infusions of 1.0×10^{10} to 5.1×10^{10}. The T cell proliferation index ranged from 30- to 57-fold. Fresh tumor-primed LN cells showed a mean composition of 63% of CD4 and 8% of CD8, which were similar to the first group of patients. However, in contrast to 2 cycles of activation, the short-term activated T cells showed 75% of CD4 and 24% CD8. In this group of patients, no grade III or IV toxicities were encountered, as no IL-2 infusion was given. Two partial responses, one mixed response, and one stable disease were noted, while others had developed progression of disease. Thus, the modified short-term activation appears to be a reliable method of ex vivo expansion of tumor vaccine-primed lymphocytes for adoptive immunotherapy with increased rate of clinical responses and decreased toxicity *(84,85)*. Improved tumor vaccine may stimulate more potent effector cells in future trials.

4. FUTURE PROSPECTIVES

The conceptual advancement of adoptive immunotherapy of cancer has evolved around strategies for ex vivo T cell activation and better methods for generating and augmenting the antitumor immune T cell response in cancer patients. In addition to new T cell activation strategies, many investigators are attempting to enhance the primary antitumor immune response by genetic modification of tumor cells in an attempt to increase tumor immunogenicity. Several studies have now reported that the introduction of cytokine genes including IL-2, IL-4, interferon (IFN)-γ, tumor necrosis factor (TNF)-α, and GM-CSF into murine tumors results in enhanced immune responses directed against the transfected as well as the unmodified tumors *(86–90)*. Additionally, in the case of IFN-γ, IL-2, and/or IL-4, transfection of poorly immunogenic tumors have been shown to stimulate tumor-reactive lymphocytes capable of mediating the regression of parental tumor in adoptive immunotherapy *(91,92)*. Based on such animal studies, several investigators are initiating human trials to study the effects of cytokine gene transfection as a means of stimulating antitumor lymphocytes against human tumors. Although some investigators have attempted to genetically modify the tumor-reactive lymphocytes, this approach is difficult to evaluate at present because of the inconsistent levels of protein expression and altered survival characteristics observed in transfected lymphocytes *(93)*. Recent application of dendritic cells pulsed with lysates *(94)*, peptides *(95–99)*, or apoptotic melanoma bodies *(100–102)* may be used as a potent source of tumor vaccine to stimulate immune T cells.

Investigation of the immune system on a cellular and molecular level ushers into a new age in the treatment of cancer using immunotherapeutic modalities. As we understand more about the immune system and its interaction with cancer, we will be able to manipulate the system better in order to achieve therapeutic goals of eradicating cancer as a form of treatment. To date, immunotherapy is still experimental. When a cancer becomes clinically apparent, it has grown to be at least a 1-cm nodule, which contains approximately 10^9 cells. In general, at this stage, the tumor burden is considered to be significantly large, which may not be effectively eradicated by the immune system. It is believed that immunotherapy probably will be most effective when the tumor burden is minimal at the microscopic level, such as following surgical resection or during complete response to either chemotherapy or radiation therapy. Learning the techniques and principles of immunotherapy derived from treatment of advanced cancer, adjuvant therapy may be developed with intention to eradicate microscopic disease.

5. CONCLUSION

In conclusion, the future of immunotherapy, either specific active immunization with appropriate vaccines or adoptive immunotherapy, would be based on well-defined molecules and antigenic systems with appropriate enhancement based on the principles of the mechanisms of immune reactions. Ex vivo expansion of potent effector cells offers the advantage of avoiding such expansion in an immunosuppressed environment of the tumor-bearing host. In sufficient numbers, adoptive immunotherapy should be more effective than active immunotherapy alone. Well-designed clinical trials are critical to test further the validity of immunotherapy against melanoma.

ACKNOWLEDGMENT

This work was supported in part by FDA grant nos. FD-R-001058-01, R03 CA 82066, R01 CA 74919 and Eva B. Buck Charitable Trust.

REFERENCES

1. Everson T, Cole W. *Spontaneous Regression of Cancer*. W.B. Saunders, Philadelphia, 1966.
2. Reintgen DS, McCarty KS, Woodard B, et al. Metastatic malignant melanoma with an unknown primary. *Surg Gynecol Obstet* 1983; 156: 335–340.
3. Nathanson L. Spontaneous regression of malignant melanoma: a review of the literature on incidence, clinical features, and possible mechanisms. *Natl Cancer Inst Monogr* 1989; 44.
4. Koh HK, Sober AJ, Nakagawa H, et al. Malignant melanoma and vitiligo-like leukoderma: an electron microscopic study. *J Am Acad Dermatol* 1983; 9: 696–708.
5. Smith J, Stehlin JS Jr. Spontaneous regression of primary malignant melanoma with regional metastases. *Cancer* 1965; 18: 1399.
6. Clark WH, Elder DE, DuPont G IV, et al. Model predicting survival in stage I melanoma based on tumor progression. *J Natl Cancer Inst* 1989; 81: 1893–1904.
7. Tefany FJ, Barnetson RS, Halliday GM, et al. Immunocytochemical analysis of the cellular infiltrate in primary regressing and non-regressing malignant melanoma. *J Invest Dermatol* 1991; 97: 197–202.
8. Briele HA, Beattie CW, Ronan SG, et al. Late recurrence of cutaneous melanoma. *Arch Surg* 1983; 118: 800–803.
9. Penn I. Immunosuppression and skin cancer. *Clin Plast Surg* 1980; 7: 361–368.
10. Mavligit GM, Hersh EM, McBride CM. Lymphocyte blastogenic responses to autochthonous viable and nonviable human tumor cells. *J Natl Cancer Inst* 1973; 51: 337–343.
11. Rossen RD, Crane MM, Morgan AC, et al. Circulating immune complexes and tumor cell cytotoxins as prognostic indicators in malignant melanoma: a prospective study of 53 patients. *Cancer Res* 1983; 43: 422–429.
12. Shiku H, Takahashi T, Resnick LA, et al. Cell surface antigens of human malignant melanoma. III. Recognition of autoantibodies with unusual characteristics. *J Exp Med* 1977; 145: 784–789.
13. Oettgen HF. Immunotherapy of cancer. *N Engl J Med* 1977; 297: 484–491.
14. Steffans T, Bajorin D, Houghton A. Immunotherapy with monoclonal antibodies in metastatic melanoma. *World J Surg* 1992; 16: 261–269.
15. Anichini A, Fossati G, Parmiani G. Clonal analysis of cytotoxic T-lymphocyte response to autologous human metastatic melanoma. *Int J Cancer* 1985; 35: 683–689.
16. Anichini A, Fossati G, Parmiani G. Heterogeneity of clones from a human metastatic melanoma detected by autologous cytotoxic T lymphocyte clones. *J Exp Med* 1986; 163: 215–220.
17. Anichini A, Mazzocchi A, Fossati G, et al. Cytotoxic T lymphocyte clones from peripheral blood and from tumor site detect intratumor heterogeneity of melanoma cells. Analysis of specificity and mechanisms of interaction. *J Immunol* 1989; 142: 3692–3701.
18. van der Bruggen P, Traversari C, Chomez P, et al. A gene encoding an antigen recognized by cytolytic T lymphocytes on a human melanoma. *Science* 1991; 254: 1643–1647.

19. Hersey P, Bindon C, Edwards A, et al. Induction of cytotoxic activity in human lymphocytes against autologous and allogeneic melanoma cells in vitro by culture with interleukin 2. *Int J Cancer* 1981; 28: 695–703.
20. Knuth A, Danowkis B, Oettgen HF, Old LJ. T-cell-mediated cytotoxicity against autologous malignant melanoma: analysis with interleukin 2-dependent T-cell cultures. *Proc Natl Acad Sci USA* 1984; 81: 3511–3515.
21. Topalian S, Mull L, Rosenberg S. Growth and immunologic characteristics of lymphocytes infiltrating human tumors. *Surg Forum* 1986; 37: 390–391.
22. Muul LM, Spiess PJ, Director EP, et al. Identification of specific cytolytic immune responses against autologous tumor in humans bearing malignant melanoma. *J Immunol* 1987; 138: 989–995.
23. Rosenberg SA, Packard BS, Aebersold PM, et al. Use of tumor-infiltrating lymphocytes and interleukin-2 in the immunotherapy of patients with metastatic melanoma. A preliminary report [see comments]. *N Engl J Med* 1988; 319: 1676–1680.
24. Crowley NJ, Darrow TL, Quinn-Allen MA, et al. MHC-restricted recognition of autologous melanoma by tumor-specific cytotoxic T cells. Evidence for restriction by a dominant HLA-A allele. *J Immunol* 1991; 146: 1692–1699.
25. Leong SPL, Granberry ME, Zhou YM, et al. Selection of cytotoxic T lymphocytes against autologous human melanoma from lymph nodes with metastatic melanoma using repeated in vitro sensitization. *Clin Exp Metastasis* 1991; 9: 301–317.
26. Leong SPL, Zhou YM, Granberry ME, et al. Generation of cytotoxic effector cells against human melanoma. *Cancer Immunol Immunother* 1995; 40: 397–409.
27. Mukherji B, Wilhelm SA, Guha A, et al. Regulation of cellular immune response against autologous human melanoma. I. Evidence for cell-mediated suppression of in vitro cytotoxic immune response. *J Immunol* 1986; 136: 1888–1892.
28. Mukherj B, Nashed AL, Guha A, Ergin MT. Regulation of cellular immune response against autologous human melanoma. II. Mechanism of induction and specificity of suppression. *J Immunol* 1986; 136: 1893–1898.
29. Chakraborty NG, Twardzik DR, Sivanandham M, et al. Autologous melanoma-induced activation of regulatory T cells that suppress cytotoxic response. *J Immunol* 1990; 145: 2359–2364.
30. Hoon DS, Foshag LJ, Nizze AS, et al. Suppressor cell activity in a randomized trial of patients receiving active specific immunotherapy with melanoma cell vaccine and low dosages of cyclophosphamide. *Cancer Res* 1990; 50: 5358–5364.
31. Grin-Jorgensen CM, Rigel DS, Friedman RJ. The worldwide incidence of malignant melanoma. In: Balch C, Houghton A, Milton G, et al., eds., *Cutaneous Melanoma*. J.B. Lippincott, Philadelphia, 1992, p. 27.
32. Berd D, Maguire H Jr, Mastrangelo M. Induction of cell-mediated immunity to autologous melanoma cells and regression of metastases after treatment with a melanoma cell vaccine preceded by cyclophosphamide. *Cancer Res* 1986; 46: 2572–2577.
33. Leong SP, Enders-Zohr P, Zhou YM, et al. Recombinant human granulocyte macrophage-colony stimulating factor (rhGM-CSF) and autologous melanoma vaccine mediate tumor regression in patients with metastatic melanoma. *J Immunother* 1999; 22: 166–174.
34. Livingston PO, Kaelin K, Pinsky CM, et al. The serologic response of patients with stage II melanoma to allogeneic melanoma cell vaccines. Cancer 1985; 56: 2194–2200.
35. Morton DL, Foshag LJ, Hoon DS, et al. Prolongation of survival in metastatic melanoma after active specific immunotherapy with a new polyvalent melanoma vaccine [published erratum appears in *Ann Surg* 1993 Mar; 217(3): 309]. *Ann Surg* 1992; 216: 463–482.
36. Vadhan-Raj S, Cordon-Cardo C, Carswell E, et al. Phase I trial of a mouse monoclonal antibody against GD3 ganglioside in patients with melanoma: induction of inflammatory responses at tumor sites. *J Clin Oncol* 1988; 6: 1636–1648.

37. Livingston PO, Natoli EJ, Calves MJ, et al. Vaccines containing purified GM2 ganglioside elicit GM2 antibodies in melanoma patients. *Proc Natl Acad Sci USA* 1987; 84: 2911–2915.
38. Bystryn JC. Immunogenicity and clinical activity of a polyvalent melanoma antigen vaccine prepared from shed antigens. *Ann NY Acad Sci* 1993; 690: 190–203.
39. Mitchell MS, Harel W, Kempf RA, et al. Active-specific immunotherapy for melanoma. *J Clin Oncol* 1990; 8: 856–869.
40. Hersey P. Evaluation of vaccinia viral lysates as therapeutic vaccines in the treatment of melanoma. *Ann NY Acad Sci* 1993; 690: 167–177.
41. Wallack M, Muthukumaran S, Whooley B, et al. Favorable clinical responses in subsets of patients from a randomized, multi-institutional melanoma vaccine trial. *Ann Surg Oncol* 1995; 3: 110–117.
42. Giacomini P, Veglia F, Cordiali Fei P, et al. Level of a membrane-bound high-molecular-weight melanoma-associated antigen and a cytoplasmic melanoma-associated antigen in surgically removed tissues and in sera from patients with melanoma. *Cancer Res* 1984; 44: 1281–1287.
43. Ahn SS, Irie RF, Weisenburger TH, et al. Humoral immune response to intralymphatic immunotherapy for disseminated melanoma: correlation with clinical response. *Surgery* 1982; 92: 362–367.
44. Berd D, Maguire JR. Potentiation of human cell-mediated and humoral immunity by low-dose cyclophosphamide. *Cancer Res* 1984; 44: 5439–5443.
45. Estin C, Stevenson U, Plowman G, et al. Recombinant vaccinia virus vaccine against the human melanoma antigen p97 for use in immunotherapy. *Proc Natl Acad Sci USA* 1986; 83: 1261–1265.
46. Cheung NK, Lazarus H, Miraldi FD, et al. Ganglioside GD2 specific monoclonal antibody 3F8: a phase I study in patients with neuroblastoma and malignant melanoma [see comments]. *J Clin Oncol* 1987; 5: 1430–1440.
47. Berd D, Maguire H Jr, McCue P, et al. Treatment of metastatic melanoma with an autologous tumor-cell vaccine: clinical and immunologic results in 64 patients. *J Clin Oncol* 1990; 8: 1858–1867.
48. Berd D, Maguire HC Jr, McCue P, et al. Treatment of metastatic melanoma with an autologous tumor-cell vaccine: clinical and immunologic results in 64 patients. *J Clin Oncol* 1990; 8: 1858–1867.
49. Mittelman A, Chen ZJ, Kageshita T, et al. Active specific immunotherapy in patients with melanoma. A clinical trial with mouse antiidiotypic monoclonal antibodies elicited with syngeneic anti-high-molecular-weight-melanoma-associated antigen monoclonal antibodies [published erratum appears in *J Clin Invest* 1991 Feb; 87(2): 757]. *J Clin Invest* 1990; 86: 2136–2144.
50. Mittelman A, Chen ZJ, Yang H, et al. Human high molecular weight melanoma-associated antigen (HMW-MAA) mimicry by mouse anti-idiotypic monoclonal antibody MK2-23: induction of humoral anti-HMW-MAA immunity and prolongation of survival in patients with stage IV melanoma. *Proc Natl Acad Sci USA* 1992; 89: 466–470.
51. Mitchell MS, Harel W, Kan-Mitchell J, et al. Active specific immunotherapy of melanoma with allogeneic cell lysates. Rationale, results, and possible mechanisms of action. *Ann NY Acad Sci* 1993; 690: 153–166.
52. Livingston P, Wong G, Adluri S, et al. A randomized trial of adjuvant vaccination with BCG versus BCG plus the melanoma ganglioside GM2 in patients with AJCC stage III melanoma. *Ann NY Acad Sci* 1993; 690: 204–213.
53. Goodman G, Hellstrom I, Hu S, et al. Phase I trial of a melanoma vaccine expressing the p97 antigen [abstract]. *Proc Natl Acad Sci USA* 1993; 83: 1052–1056.
54. Chapman P, Livinston P, Morrison M, et al. Use of BEC2 anti-idiotypic monoclonal antibody (Mab) to induce antibodies against GD3 ganglioside in melanoma patients [abstract]. *Proc Am Soc Clin Oncol* 1993; 12: 388.

55. Rosenberg SA, Yang JC, Schwartzentruber DJ, et al. Immunologic and therapeutic evaluation of a synthetic peptide vaccine for the treatment of patients with metastatic melanoma [see comments]. *Nat Med* 1998; 4: 321–327.
56. Shu SY, Chou T, Rosenberg SA. Generation from tumor-bearing mice of lymphocytes with in vivo therapeutic efficacy. *J Immunol* 1987; 139: 295–304.
57. Taniguchi T, Matsui H, Fujita T, et al. Structure and expression of a cloned cDNA for human interleukin-2. *Nature* 1983; 302: 305–310.
58. Mule JJ, Shu S, Schwarz SL, et al. Adoptive immunotherapy of established pulmonary metastases with LAK cells and recombinant interleukin-2. *Science* 1984; 225: 1487–1489.
59. Rosenberg SA, Lotze MT, Muul LM, et al. A progress report on the treatment of 157 patients with advanced cancer using lymphokine-activated killer cells and interleukin-2 or high-dose interleukin-2 alone. *N Engl J Med* 1987; 316: 889–897.
60. Grimm EA, Mazumder A, Zhang HZ, et al. Lymphokine-activated killer cell phenomenon. Lysis of natural killer-resistant fresh solid tumor cells by interleukin 2-activated autologous human peripheral blood lymphocytes. *J Exp Med* 1982; 155: 1823–1841.
61. Grimm EA, Robb RJ, Roth JA, et al. Lymphokine-activated killer cell phenomenon. III. Evidence that IL-2 is sufficient for direct activation of peripheral blood lymphocytes into lymphokine-activated killer cells. *J Exp Med* 1983; 158: 1356–1361.
62. Schoof DD, Gramolini BA, Davidson DL, et al. Adoptive immunotherapy of human cancer using low-dose recombinant interleukin 2 and lymphokine-activated killer cells. *Cancer Res* 1988; 48: 5007–5010.
63. Dutcher JP, Creekmore S, Weiss GR, et al. A phase II study of interleukin-2 and lymphokine-activated killer cells in patients with metastatic malignant melanoma. *J Clin Oncol* 1989; 7: 477–485.
64. Bar MH, Sznol M, Atkins MB, et al. Metastatic malignant melanoma treated with combined bolus and continuous infusion interleukin-2 and lymphokine-activated killer cells [see comments]. *J Clin Oncol* 1990; 8: 1138–1147.
65. Dutcher JP, Gaynor ER, Boldt DH, et al. A phase II study of high-dose continuous infusion interleukin-2 with lymphokine-activated killer cells in patients with metastatic melanoma. *J Clin Oncol* 1991; 9: 641–648.
66. Atkins MB, Gould JA, Allegretta M, et al. Phase I evaluation of recombinant interleukin-2 in patients with advanced malignant disease. *J Clin Oncol* 1986; 4: 1380–1391.
67. Lotze MT, Chang AE, Seipp CA, et al. High-dose recombinant interleukin 2 in the treatment of patients with disseminated cancer. Responses, treatment-related morbidity, and histologic findings. *JAMA* 1986; 256: 3117–3124.
68. Mitchell MS, Kempf RA, Harel W, et al. Effectiveness and tolerability of low-dose cyclophosphamide and low-dose intravenous interleukin-2 in disseminated melanoma [corrected]. [published erratum appears in *J Clin Oncol* 1988 Jun; 6(6): 1067]. *J Clin Oncol* 1988; 6: 409–424.
69. McCabe M, Stablein D, Hawkins M. The modified group C experience-phase III randomized trials of IL-2 vs. IL-2/LAK in advanced renal cell carcinoma and advanced melanoma. *Proc Am Soc Clin Oncol* 1991; 10: 213.
70. Rosenberg SA, Lotze MT, Yang JC, et al. Prospective randomized trial of high-dose interleukin-2 alone or in conjunction with lymphokine-activated killer cells for the treatment of patients with advanced cancer. [published erratum appears in *J Natl Cancer Inst* 1993 Jul 7; 85(13): 1091]. *J Natl Cancer Inst* 1993; 85: 622–632.
71. Spiess PJ, Yang JC, Rosenberg SA. In vivo antitumor activity of tumor-infiltrating lymphocytes expanded in recombinant interleukin-2. *J Natl Cancer Inst* 1987; 79: 1067–1075.
72. Aebersold P, Hyatt C, Johnson S, et al. Lysis of autologous melanoma cells by tumor-infiltrating lymphocytes: association with clinical response. *J Natl Cancer Inst* 1991; 83: 932–937.

73. Hewitt HB, Blake ER, Walder AS. A critique of the evidence for active host defence against cancer, based on personal studies of 27 murine tumours of spontaneous origin. *Br J Cancer* 1976; 33: 241–259.
74. Chou T, Chang AE, Shu SY. Generation of therapeutic T lymphocytes from tumor-bearing mice by in vitro sensitization. Culture requirements and characterization of immunologic specificity. *J Immunol* 1988; 140: 2453–2461.
75. Shu SY, Chou T, Sakai K. Lymphocytes generated by in vivo priming and in vitro sensitization demonstrate therapeutic efficacy against a murine tumor that lacks apparent immunogenicity. *J Immunol* 1989; 143: 740–748.
76. Chang A, Yoshizawa H, Sakai K, et al. Clinical observations on adoptive immunotherapy with vaccine-primed T lymphocytes secondarily sensitized to tumor *in vitro*. *Cancer Res* 1993; 53: 1043–1050.
77. Van Wauwe JP, De Mey JR, Goossens JG. OKT3: a monoclonal anti-human T lymphocyte antibody with potent mitogenic properties. *J Immunol* 1980; 124: 2708–2713.
78. Kronenberg M, Siu G, Hood LE, Shastri N. The molecular genetics of the T-cell antigen receptor and T-cell antigen recognition. *Annu Rev Immunol* 1986; 4: 529–591.
79. Clevers H, Alarcon B, Wileman T, Terhorst C. The T cell receptor/CD3 complex: a dynamic protein ensemble. *Annu Rev Immunol* 1988; 6: 629–662.
80. Yoshizawa H, Sakai K, Chang A, et al. Specific adoptive immunotherapy mediated by tumor-draining lymph node cells sequentially activated with anti-CD3 and rIL-2. *J Immunol* 1991; 147: 729–737.
81. Yoshizawa H, Sakai K, Chang A, et al. Activation by anti-CD3 of tumor-draining lymph node cells for specific adoptive immunotherapy. *Cell Immunol* 1991; 134: 473–479.
82. Geiger JD, Wagner PD, Shu S, et al. A novel role for autologous tumour cell vaccination in the immunotherapy of the poorly immunogenic B16-BL6 melanoma. *Surg Oncol* 1992; 1: 199–208.
83. Chang A, Aruga A, Cameron M, et al. Adoptive immunotherapy with vaccine-primed lymph node cells secondarily activated with anti-CD3 and interleukin-2. *J Clin Oncol* 1997; 15: 796–807.
84. Leong SPL, Zhou YM, Peng M, et al. Adoptive immunotherapy of malignant melanoma using activated tumor draining lymph node T cells. Manuscript in preparation; 2001.
85. Shu S, Plautz G, Leong SPL. T-cell immunotherapy of melanoma and glioma. *J Surg Oncol* 2001; in press.
86. Gansbacher B, Zier K, Daniels B, et al. Interleukin 2 gene transfer into tumor cells abrogates tumorigenicity and induces protective immunity. *J Exp Med* 1990; 172: 1217–1224.
87. Gansbacher B, Bannerji R, Daniels B, et al. Retroviral vector-mediated gamma-interferon gene transfer into tumor cells generates potent and long lasting antitumor immunity. *Cancer Res* 1990; 50: 7820–7825.
88. Asher AL, Mulâe JJ, Kasid A, et al. Murine tumor cells transduced with the gene for tumor necrosis factor-alpha. Evidence for paracrine immune effects of tumor necrosis factor against tumors. *J Immunol* 1991; 146: 3227–3234.
89. Tepper RI, Coffman RL, Leder P. An eosinophil-dependent mechanism for the antitumor effect of interleukin-4. *Science* 1992; 257: 548–551.
90. Dranoff G, Jaffee E, Lazenby A, et al. Vaccination with irradiated tumor cells engineered to secrete murine granulocyte-macrophage colony-stimulating factor stimulates potent, specific, and long-lasting anti-tumor immunity. *Proc Natl Acad Sci USA* 1993; 90: 3539–3543.
91. Restifo NP, Spiess PJ, Karp SE, et al. A nonimmunogenic sarcoma transduced with the cDNA for interferon gamma elicits $CD8^+$ T cells against the wild-type tumor: correlation with antigen presentation capability. *J Exp Med* 1992; 175: 1423–1431.
92. Strome S, Chang A, Shu S, et al. Secretion of both IL-2 and IL-4 by tumor cells results in rejection and immunity. *J. Immunother* 1996; 19: 21–32.

93. Rosenberg SA, Aebersold P, Cornetta K, et al. Gene transfer into humans—immunotherapy of patients with advanced melanoma, using tumor-infiltrating lymphocytes modified by retroviral gene transduction [see comments]. *N Engl J Med* 1990; 323: 570–578.
94. Grabbe S, Bruvers S, Gallo RL, et al. Tumor antigen presentation by murine epidermal cells. *J Immunol* 1991; 146: 3656–3661.
95. Shimizu J, Zou JP, Ikegame K, et al. Evidence for the functional binding in vivo of tumor rejection antigens to antigen-presenting cells in tumor-bearing hosts. *J Immunol* 1991; 146: 1708–1714.
96. Storkus WJ, Zeh HJd, Salter RD, et al. Identification of T-cell epitopes: rapid isolation of class I-presented peptides from viable cells by mild acid elution. *J Immunother* 1993; 14: 94–103.
97. Celluzzi CM, Mayordomo JI, Storkus WJ, et al. Peptide-pulsed dendritic cells induce antigen-specific CTL-mediated protective tumor immunity [see comments]. *J Exp Med* 1996; 183: 283–287.
98. Hu X, Chakraborty NG, Sporn JR, et al. Enhancement of cytolytic T lymphocyte precursor frequency in melanoma patients following immunization with the MAGE-1 peptide loaded antigen presenting cell-based vaccine. *Cancer Res* 1996; 56: 2479–2483.
99. Ribas A, Butterfield LH, McBride WH, et al. Genetic immunization for the melanoma antigen MART-1/Melan-A using recombinant adenovirus-transduced murine dendritic cells. *Cancer Res* 1997; 57: 2865–2869.
100. Albert ML, Sauter B, Bhardwaj N. Dendritic cells acquire antigen from apoptotic cells and induce class I-restricted CTLs. *Nature* 1998; 392: 86–89.
101. Nouri-Shirazi M, Palucka KA, Chomarat P, et al. Dendritic cells phagocytose carcinoma-derived apoptotic bodies. *J Leukoc Biol Suppl* 1998; 2: 49.
102. Chang J, Peng M, Vaquerano J, et al. Induction of Th1 response by dendritic cells pulsed with autologous melanoma apoptotic bodies. *Anticancer Res* 2001; 20: 1329–1336.
103. Rosenberg SA, Zhai Y, Yang JC, et al. Immunizing patients with metastatic melanoma using recombinant adenoviruses encoding MART-1 or gp100 melanoma antigens. *J Natl Cancer Inst* 1998; 90: 1894–1900.
104. Pieper R, Christian RE, Gonzales MI, et al. Biochemical identification of a mutated human melanoma antigen recognized by CD4(+) T cells [see comments]. *J Exp Med* 1999; 189: 757–766.

6 Melanoma Antigens

Vaccines and Monoclonal Antibodies

Paul B. Chapman, MD
and Jedd D. Wolchok, MD, PhD

Contents

1. INTRODUCTION

Physicians have been intrigued with the idea of immunizing against cancer well before there was any coherent understanding of immune mechanisms. The most simple approach seemed to be to inject subjects with crude tumor material, and there have been well over a hundred reports from 1902 through 1990 of patients being injected with tumor extracts *(1)*. Few of these reports are interpretable, however. Early studies in the 1950s using inbred strains of mice showed that among chemically induced tumors, there were tumor-specific antigens that could serve as tumor rejection antigens *(2,3)*. However, experiments by Hewitt and colleagues demonstrated that spontaneously arising tumors, such as those seen in patients, are far less immunogenic than chemically induced tumors making it unclear whether these observations could be extended to spontaneously arising tumors *(4)*. This generated a question and controversy, which persists today; namely, do experiments using inbred strains of mice and tumor cell lines from artificially induced tumors have relevance to the clinical setting?

In an attempt to identify antigens that could be recognized by the human immune system, Old and colleagues used autologous serum to identify antibody-defined antigens on melanoma cells *(5)*. Using this technique, it was possible to

From: *Current Clinical Oncology, Melanoma: Biologically Targeted Therapeutics*
Edited by: E. C. Borden © Humana Press Inc., Totowa, NJ

identify both unique antigens, as well as antigens shared by more than one patient's tumor. One of the shared antigens was eventually identified as GD2, a ganglioside. These observations were important for two reasons. First, they demonstrated that the human immune system could recognize shared antigens on tumor cells. Second, by identifying gangliosides as a class of antigens which could be used to target tumors, it suggested that tumor immunologists need not look only to proteins as antigenic targets.

In this chapter, we will review passive immunotherapy strategies using monoclonal antibodies directed against specific antigens expressed on melanoma cells. We will also review attempts to induce active immunity against melanoma cells using either defined antigen constructs or undefined tumor vaccines.

2. PASSIVE IMMUNOTHERAPY USING MONOCLONAL ANTIBODIES

A variety of monoclonal antibodies (MAbs) with specificity against antigens on tumor cells have been shown to have antitumor effects in murine models. Typically, these experiments are conducted by injecting human tumor xenografts in immunodeficient mice and then treating the mice with a MAb that binds to the tumor cell. It is often possible to show that treatment either delays or prevents tumor outgrowth. In some situations it has been possible to conduct these experiments using immunocompetent animals injected with syngeneic tumor cell lines. In one set of experiments, we showed that immunocompetent hamsters injected with a hamster melanoma could be successfully treated with R24 MAb against GD3 ganglioside, even if the treatment was started 6 d after tumor cell injection *(6)*. Despite the fact that these experiments can sometimes be carried out in syngeneic systems, it must be noted that these animal experiments are somewhat artificial and probably do not reflect accurately the clinical setting in which we wish to use MAb.

Most of the experience in melanoma has been with MAb against either GD3 ganglioside such as MAb R24 (Table 1) or against GD2 ganglioside such as MAb 3F8, 14G2a, or the chimeric form of 14G2a designated ch14.18 (Table 2). Experience with anti-GD3 or anti-GD2 MAb used alone has shown an objective response rate of approximately 10%. There has been experience in combining R24 with chemotherapy (Table 3), as well as combining MAb against both GD2 and GD3 (Table 4), neither of which has resulted in an obvious improvement in response rate among the small number of patients treated. MAbs against GD3 and GD2 have also been administered with a variety of cytokines (interleukin [IL]-2, granulocyte-macrophage colony-stimulating factor [GM-CSF], M-CSF, tumor necrosis factor [TNF]-α, interferon [IFN] α) without enhanced clinical effects, in general. However, one trial using R24 and IL-2 carried out at the National Cancer Institute reported 10/32 partial responses (31%) in patients with

Table 1
Clinical Trials Using Anti-GD3 MAb R24 Alone in Patients with Melanoma

Reference	*Institution*	*No. of pts*	*R24 dose*	*Route*	*Objective responses*	*Site of response*
101	MSKCC	21	8–80–240–400 mg/m^2	IV/CIV	4 PR	Skin, lymph nodes.
102	MSKCC	7	800–1200 mg/m^2	CIV	None	
103	Pittsburgh Cancer Inst.	12	8–80 mg/m^2	CIV	1 CR/1PR	Not available.
Houghton (unpublished)	MSKCC	43	6–60 mg/m^2	IV	1 CR/1 PR	CR: soft tissue. PR: soft tissue, endobronchial.
104,105	Mainz Univ, Germany	20	7–210 mg/m^2	IV	None	
Total		103			10 (10%)	

MSKCC, Memorial Sloan-Kettering Cancer Center; IV, intravenous; CIV, continuous intravenous infusion; PR, partial response; CR, complete response.

Table 2
Clinical Trials Using MAb Against GD2 Ganglioside

MAb	*Institution*	*No. of pts*	*MAb dose*	*Objective responses*	*Site of response*
3F8 *(107,108)*	MSKCC	17 (9 melanoma patients)	5–100 mg/m^2	2 PR in melanoma patients.	Lymph nodes, liver.
14G2a *(109,110)*	Univ. Alabama, MD Anderson	30 (23 melanoma patients)	10–200 mg/m^2	2 PR in neuroblastoma.	
ch14.18 *(111)*	Univ. Alabama	13	5–100 mg/m^2	None	
ME36.1 *(112)*	Univ. Penn.	13	25–500 mg/m^2	1 CR	Not reported.
Total		58		5 (9%)	

[a]ME36.1 has specificity for both GD2 and GD3, but has higher avidity for GD2.

Table 3
Clinical Trials Using Anti-GD3 MAb R24 Combined with Chemotherapy Active in Patients with Metastatic Melanoma

Combination	*Institution*	*No. of pts*	*Doses*	*Objective responses*	*Site of response*
R24 + Dacarbazine (unpublished)	MSKCC	24	R24: 18 mg/m^2 Dacarbazine: 200–1000 mg/m^2	4 PR	Skin, soft tissue, lymph nodes.
R24 + Cisplatin *(106)*	Cleveland Clinic	19	R24 80-400 mg/m^2 Cisplatin: 120 mg/m^2 WR-2721: 740 mg/m^2	2 PR	Lung, soft tissue.

Table 4
Clinical Trials Using Combinations of MAb Against Both GD2 and GD3 Ganglioside

MAbs	*Institution*	*No. of pts*	*Doses*	*Objective responses*
R24 + 3F8 *(113)*	MSKCC	6	R24: 5, 20, 50 mg/m^2 3F8: 5, 20, 50 mg/m^2	None
R24 + ch14.18 (+ IL-2) *(114)*	Univ. Wisc.	20	R24: 2–7.5 mg/m^2/d ch14.18: 1–10 mg/m^2/d	1 PR

metastatic melanoma, but has been reported only in abstract form *(7)*. This high response rate was not observed in another trial with R24 and IL-2, in which only 1/20 partial responses were reported *(8)*. Among 8 melanoma patients treated with R24 and TNF-α, one patient developed a massive tumor lysis syndrome, which raised the possibility that MAb with TNF-α could activate a massive and specific immune reaction against tumor cells *(9)*.

Overall, the experience in melanoma to date has shown that MAb can induce objective responses in approximately 10% of cases. It should be noted that the majority of the experience has been with fully murine MAb, which are highly immunogenic in humans. This limits the amount and duration of treatment that can be administered. The only chimeric MAb that has been used in melanoma patients is ch14.18, and this appears to induce anti-ch14.18 antibodies in a proportion of patients. This may be due to the fact that the MAb retains significant murine regions. It seems unlikely that an immunogenic MAb will induce a meaningful clinical effect when the MAb cannot be given for more than 10 d. In order for the potential of antiganglioside MAb to be fully assessed, it will be necessary to develop fully humanized antiganglioside MAb that can be administered chronically without inducing anti-MAb antibodies.

3. ACTIVE IMMUNOTHERAPY IN MELANOMA

3.1. Undefined Antigen Targets

3.1.1. Allogeneic Vaccines

Some of the earliest attempts at vaccination against melanoma have used allogeneic cultured melanoma cells as vaccines. The assumption was that among the thousands of different molecules injected, some were relevant tumor-rejection antigens which could be recognized by the immune system. Multiple variations of allogeneic cell vaccines have been developed using whole irradiated cells *(10–12)*, cell lysates *(13–15)*, and shed antigens isolated from tissue culture supernatants *(16,17)*, with literally thousands of patients having been safely vaccinated. These vaccines have been difficult to develop partly because there was no way to monitor a relevant immune response other than measuring responses against specific known antigens (see below). There is also the potential for batch-to-batch variability since the relevant antigen content cannot be measured. It has been possible to show that these vaccines can generate immune responses against numerous antigens present in melanoma cells such as members of the tyrosinase family of melanosomal antigens (gp75/tyrosinase-related protein [TRP-1] and TRP-2) as well as GM2 ganglioside *(18–20)*. Several trials of allogeneic vaccines have suggested clinical benefit based only upon comparison with historical controls *(21,22)*, but conclusions regarding vaccine efficacy cannot be drawn from such nonrandomized trials. Early results of a randomized trial of Melacine, an allogeneic cellular vaccine, used as adjuvant therapy in patients with resected American Joint Committee on Cancer (AJCC) stage II melanoma have been reported, but not yet published. Interpretation of the results is complicated by the 13% of ineligible patients and by some imbalances in prognostic variables between the two groups. However, in the intent-to-treat analysis, there was initial evidence of a statistically significant disease-free survival benefit for patients in the Melacine group. It is not clear if this difference will hold up with further follow up. There was no difference between the two groups when only eligible patients were considered, adding further complexity to the analysis. The same vaccine was evaluated in a randomized trial versus the Dartmouth chemotherapy regimen (cisplatin, carmustine, dacarbazine, tamoxifen) as therapy for metastatic melanoma. Response rates in both treatment arms were low (13% in the Dartmouth arm vs 9% in the Melacine arm), and there was no difference in median survival *(23)*. Based on these data, Melacine was approved for use in Canada for stage IV melanoma, presumably because treatment with Melacine resulted in far less toxicity than the combination chemotherapy.

In an attempt to increase the immunogenicity of potential yet undefined tumor antigens, investigators have infected tumor cells with cytolytic virus, such as vaccinia, and used the viral lysate to immunize. The hope is that the highly immunogenic vaccinia proteins will function as an immunological adjuvant and boost the immune response against the melanoma antigens. A randomized trial of this type of vaccine in which AJCC stage III melanoma patients received vaccinia alone or vaccinia oncolysate did not demonstrate significant survival benefit *(24)*. Despite the fact that this trial had a disappointing clinical outcome, it remains an important paradigm as the first randomized trial of a vaccine as adjuvant therapy for melanoma. The concept of using viruses as melanoma vaccine delivery systems remains appealing and is described below in the context of defined antigen systems.

3.1.2. Autologous Vaccines

Autologous tumor vaccines have several potential advantages over allogeneic vaccines. They are more likely to contain antigens of specific immunologic importance for the individual patient, including any unique antigens resulting from mutations. Also, the absence of irrelevant allogeneic antigens makes immunological monitoring more straightforward. This approach requires that a relatively large amount of tumor tissue be available from each patient for preparation of the customized vaccines, which restricts the eligible patient population and skews it to include patients who have a relatively higher burden of disease.

A novel approach to enhance the immunogenicity of autologous tumor vaccines has been described by Berd et al. using haptenated autologous vaccines for melanoma as well as other epithelial malignancies. This involves conjugation of the hapten dinitroflourobenzene (DNFB) to proteins on autologous tumor cells. The haptenated tumor cells are injected with bacille Calmette-Guérin (BCG) into patients presensitized to DNFB. Although interpretation of efficacy remains clouded by the absence of randomized trials, the haptenated autologous vaccines are intriguing because of their ability to mediate inflammation at tumor sites distant from the point of injection *(25)*. The haptenated autologous vaccines are currently being analyzed in a randomized controlled trial as adjuvant therapy for resected AJCC stage III melanoma.

Another strategy to try to enhance the immunogenicity of tumor cells is to introduce genes encoding a variety of cytokines or chemokines. In syngeneic animal models, expression of almost any cytokine seems to enhance tumor rejection. Special interest has been focused on GM-CSF, largely due to experiments reported by Dranoff et al., who showed that GM-CSF had the greatest ability to enhance tumor rejection in the B16 mouse melanoma model *(26)*. Initial clinical results using autologous vaccine expressing the gene encoding GM-CSF have demonstrated the ability of the vaccine to induce an inflammatory response at the injection site, as well as in distant metastatic lesions in patients *(27–29)*. The cellular composition of the infiltrate includes T-cells, plasma cells, dendritic cells, and eosinophils. Although clinical responses have been reported, interpretation is difficult because of relatively small numbers of patients. Larger trials and longer follow-up are necessary to determine the clinical impact of these new vaccines.

3.2. Defined Melanoma Antigen Targets

3.2.1. Ganglioside Antigens

Gangliosides are a class of acidic glycolipids that consist of a hydrophobic ceramide moiety which anchors the molecule into the plasma membrane exposing the immunogenic sugars. The diversity of gangliosides is expressed by the composition of the glycosidic portion of the molecule which consists of both neutral sugars and sialic acids. Melanocytic cells express a variety of gangliosides including: GM3, GD3, GD2, GM2, and *O*-acetyl GD3. GM3 and GD3 are the gangliosides expressed most abundantly on melanoma *(30)*, but GM3 is ubiquitously expressed on virtually all cells and so is not an attractive target for immunotherapy. The other gangliosides have much more limited expression on normal tissue and, as a result, efforts to develop ganglioside cancer vaccines have focused on these other gangliosides.

3.2.1.1. GM2. GM2 appears to be one of the most immunogenic gangliosides. Initial observations in melanoma patients with naturally-occurring antibodies to GM2 suggested that the presence of anti-GM2 antibodies correlated with improved survival *(31)*. GM2 mixed with BCG can induce anti-GM2 IgM antibodies in over 85% of patients treated. In a trial involving 122 AJCC stage III melanoma patients who were free of disease after surgery but at high risk of recurrence, patients were randomized to receive either GM2 plus BCG or BCG alone *(32)*. Using an intent to treat analysis, there was not a statistically significant difference in relapse-free survival (RFS) between the two groups. However, the presence of anti-GM2 antibodies was clearly associated with improved RFS, and among the 116 patients who did not have antibodies against GM2 prior to entering the trial, there was a clear survival advantage for patients immunized with GM2/BCG ($p = 0.02$). This was the first randomized data suggesting that antiganglioside antibodies might have an impact on the natural history of melanoma. Newer formulations of the GM2 vaccine have been produced, in which the GM2 is conjugated to keyhole limpet hemocyanin (KLH) and mixed with the adjuvant QS-21 (GMK). Using this formulation, nearly 100% of patients developed antibodies to GM2, and almost all of them developed IgG antibodies *(33,34)*.

GMK vaccine has been tested in a phase III randomized multicenter trial to see if the vaccine is at least 15% better than INF-α2b in prolonging RFS. The data accumulated at a median follow-up of 16 mo allows rejection of the hypothesis that GMK vaccine improves RFS by 15% over INF-α2b. At this median follow-up, the survival rate of the GMK group was worse than the IFN-α2b group *(34a)*. We must await further follow-up to determine if the overall survival rates remain different.

Since the original randomized trial using GM2 plus BCG suggested a benefit in RFS evident after 12 mo, and there is evidence that INF-α2b can have an early impact on RFS which is evident after a month of treatment, it may be beneficial to combine these two forms of adjuvant therapy. However, given the toxicity and neutropenia associated with INF, it is possible that INF treatment could blunt the anti-GM2 antibody response induced by the GM2 vaccine. To answer this question, a clinical trial was designed in which patients were randomized to receive the GMK vaccine with or without high dose INF-α2b *(35)*. The primary endpoint of this trial was the anti-GM2 antibody response and the results showed that INF-α2b did not affect the peak titers or the percent of patients responding to GM2. These results show that INF-α2b and the GMK vaccine can be combined without diminishing the immunogenicity of the vaccine.

These data open the way to combine INF-α2b with other experimental vaccines in randomized trials. A critical and controversial issue is what should constitute the control arm of such trials given that no adjuvant treatment has convincingly or consistently been shown to improve overall survival.

Table 5
Immunogenicity of GD3 and Various Congeners

Immunogen	*Anti-GD3 antibody response*	*Reference*
GD3	0/6 patients	*37*
GD3-amide	0/4 patients	*37*
GD3-lactone	4/6 patients	*38*
O-acetyl GD3	0/42 patients	*115*

3.2.1.2. GD2. Although early vaccine studies made it clear that GD2 was less immunogenic than GM2 *(36)*, immunizing patients with GD2 conjugated to KLH and mixed with QS-21 (GD2-KLH/QS-21) can induce anti-GD2 antibodies in a subset of patients. Dose-response studies showed that in doses of GD2-KLH/QS-21, between 30 and 70 μg of GD2 can induce anti-GD2 IgM in 36% of patients and anti-GD2 IgG in 64% of patients immunized *(36a)* without significant toxicity. It remains to be determined whether vaccination against GD2 can have an impact on the natural history of tumors expressing GD2.

3.2.1.3. GD3. GD3 is one of the most abundantly expressed ganglioside on melanoma cells and is expressed on virtually all melanoma tumors *(30)*. This makes it a particularly attractive immunological target. However, compared to GM2 and GD2, GD3 is far less immunogenic. Immunization of patients with melanoma cells, GD3, or congeners of GD3 mixed with BCG adjuvant failed to induce any antibodies against GD3 (Table 5) *(37)*. Recently, Livingston showed that it was possible to induce antibodies against GD3 in 4/6 patients immunized with GD3-lactone conjugated to KLH and mixed with the adjuvant QS-21 *(38)*. Clinical trials are currently underway to determine more precisely what the immunologic response rate is to GD3-lactone-KLH injected with QS-21.

3.2.1.4. Anti-Idiotypic MAb Mimicking Ganglioside Antigens. Given the limited immunogenicity of GD2 and GD3, other approaches were sought to immunize against these gangliosides. One strategy is to develop anti-idiotypic MAb vaccines (Fig. 1). Mice are immunized with a MAb (designated Ab1) against the antigen of interest, and a MAb specifically against the Ab1 is isolated. This MAb is an anti-idiotypic MAb (also designated Ab2). It is possible to identify an Ab2 antibody that binds to the antigen-binding site of Ab1 and contains a region within the variable domains that functionally mimics the original antigen—in this case either GD2 or GD3. That is, an Ab2 can sometimes be used as a surrogate antigen in place of the original antigen. An anti-idiotypic MAb vaccine may be more immunogenic than the ganglioside it mimics since it is a xenogenic protein rather than a carbohydrate self-antigen. An anti-idiotypic MAb vaccine may also contain helper T cell epitopes capable of inducing class switching to IgG antibody responses.

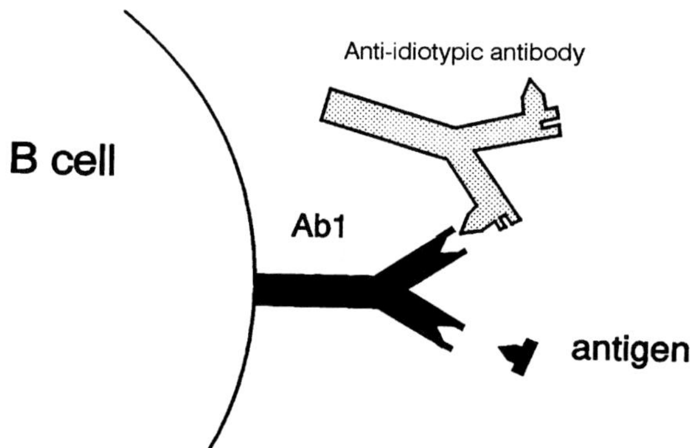

Fig. 1. Anti-idiotypic antibody can mimic antigen. Ab1 is an antibody that recognizes a specific antigen. Some anti-idiotypic antibodies contain regions that bind to the antigen-binding site of the Ab1 in a way that mimics the original antigen. Reproduced with permission from *Biology and Treatment of Melanoma*, edited by Frank G. Haluska, Kluwer Academic Publishers, Norwell, MA, 2000.

Several investigators have developed anti-idiotypic MAb that mimic GD2 ganglioside and that can induce anti-GD2 immune responses in animals *(39–41)*. Immunization of patients with one of these anti-idiotypic MAb vaccines, designated 1A7, can induce detectable antibodies against GD2 if serum is partially purified *(42)*. We have developed an anti-idiotypic MAb (designated BEC2) that mimics GD3, and in approximately 20 to 30% of patients immunized to date, it has been possible to detect circulating antibodies against GD3 without purifying or concentrating the serum *(43,44)*. Clinical trials are on-going with these anti-idiotypic MAb vaccines to optimize the immunogenicity and to determine if further phase III trials are warranted in melanoma.

Whether anti-idiotypic MAb can induce antiganglioside antibodies at high enough titer to influence the course of the disease remains to be seen. It is possible that even low titers of antiganglioside antibodies can have a beneficial effect on relapse-free and overall survival. Experience with antibodies against GM2 suggest that titers as low as 1:40 are associated with improved outcome *(32,45)*. We are also intrigued by our experience using BEC2 to immunize patients with small cell lung carcinoma (SCLC), a GD3$^+$ tumor. In a pilot study *(46)*, 15 SCLC patients (8 patients with extensive disease, 7 patients with limited disease) who had a complete or partial response after chemoradiation therapy were immunized with BEC2 vaccine. The serological results showed that only 33% of the patients developed detectable anti-GD3 antibodies—a proportion similar to that seen previously in melanoma patients. However, after a median follow-up of 4 yr, only one of the 7 patients with limited disease has relapsed with SCLC. This observation may mean that very low levels of anti-GD3 antibodies—even below

Table 6
Types of Antigens on Melanoma Cells

Mutated proteins	Examples: CDK4, b-catenin, MUM-1.
Cancer-testis antigens	Examples: MAGE, BAGE, GAGE, NY-ESO-1.
Differentiation antigens	Examples: Gangliosides, tyrosinase family.

the level of detection by our enzyme-linked immunosorbent assay (ELISA)—can be sufficient to have antitumor effects. An alternative hypothesis is that immune effectors other than antibodies are responsible for this clinical effect. A multicenter randomized European Organization for Research and Treatment of Cancer (EORTC) trial is currently on-going in limited disease SCLC patients to determine if this observation can be confirmed in a larger number of patients.

Once maximally immunogenic formulations have been established for vaccines against GD2 and GD3, it will be possible to test a trivalent ganglioside vaccine. After an initial pilot trial to establish safety and immunogenicity, it will be critical to test the trivalent vaccine in a randomized trial in the adjuvant setting.

3.2.2. Protein Antigens

Significant progress in the area of molecular biology during the last 10–20 yr has led to the identification of protein antigens on melanoma cells recognized by both antibodies and by T cells. Antigen recognition by $CD8^+$ cytotoxic T cells requires that a peptide derived from the full sequence of protein be displayed by cell surface major histocompatibility complex (MHC) class I molecules. Engagement of the T cell receptor, in conjunction with CD8 and co-stimulatory molecules, can lead to killing of the target cell either by release of cytotoxic granules and cytokines or by *fas-fas* ligand interactions. Identification of such peptides bound to MHC class I molecules may, therefore, lead to an understanding of which proteins are capable of being recognized by the immune system (Table 6).

One of the first melanoma antigens recognized by T cells was identified using T cells from patient AV, who had been treated at Memorial Sloan-Kettering Cancer Center for metastatic melanoma with surgery, autologous tumor vaccination, and dacarbazine chemotherapy, and who remains alive today, free of disease. Brisk cytolytic activity was observed when this patient's peripheral blood mononuclear cells were incubated in vitro with autologous tumor cells (SK-MEL-29) in culture. A cDNA library constructed from the SK-MEL-29 cell line was transfected into COS cells, which were subsequently used as targets in lysis assays for cytotoxic T lymphocyte (CTL) clones from patient AV. Based on sequencing of the specific DNA transfected into lysed cell clones, the enzyme tyrosinase was identified as a target for T cells in this patient with melanoma *(47)*.

These findings established a technique for identification of protein antigens recognized by T cells from cancer patients and demonstrated that a normal component of melanocytic cells could serve as an antigen for T cells. Further analysis of this same patient's T cells led to the identification of several other antigens, including the differentiation antigen Melan-A/MART-1 *(48)* and a mutated form of the cyclin-dependent kinase, CDK4 *(49)*.

The identification of tyrosinase as a melanoma antigen established melanosomal differentiation antigens as one category of proteins that could serve as a target for an antimelanoma immune response. Tyrosinase is an enzyme that catalyzes the rate-limiting step in the melanin biosynthetic pathway. It is a member of a family of proteins which includes gp75/TRP-1 and TRP-2, both also enzymes involved in melanin synthesis. In addition, antibodies recognizing gp75/TRP-1 and T cells recognizing TRP-2 have been isolated from melanoma patients *(50,51)*. Other melanosomal differentiation antigens are gp100, a structural component of the melanosome and MART-1/Melan A, a 118-amino acid protein expressed in melanoma cells, which is otherwise poorly characterized. Antibodies and/or T cells directed toward each of these proteins have been found in melanoma patients, supporting the notion that they represent potential targets for active immunization strategies.

The same group which identified tyrosinase as a target for the T cells of patient AV also established a new category of antigens with expression restricted to tumor cells and normal testis. This family, termed the cancer-testis antigens, include the MAGE, BAGE, GAGE, RAGE, and NY-ESO-1 genes *(52)*, and are all encoded on the X chromosome. MAGE-1, the first gene identified, is present on approximately 40% of melanoma tumor samples *(53)*. The attraction of this group of antigens is that they have relatively restricted normal tissue expression, which may lead to less common or less severe autoimmune sequelae when used for vaccination. Undoubtedly, other families of antigens will be identified in the future.

Understanding how peptides bind to human leukocyte antigen (HLA) molecules has led to the observation that amino acids can be substituted to increase the affinity of peptide binding to HLA molecules. This can result in enhanced immunogenicity towards the native peptide *(54)*. One example is the gp100 209–217 peptide, in which substituting a methionine for the threonine at position 210 resulted in a much more immunogenic peptide. These substituted peptides are termed heteroclitic peptides and represent a general strategy of enhancing immunogenicity *(55)*.

Peptides presented by MHC class II molecules are also becoming a source for new vaccine targets. MHC class II epitopes have been identified within melanoma differentiation antigens *(56)* and within tumor-testis antigens *(57)*, and several novel antigens (described below) have recently been described based upon recognition by $CD4^+$ T cells.

Several clinical trials have been reported in which patients were immunized with peptides derived from either cancer-testis antigens *(58,59)* or differentiation antigens *(60–68)*. Some of the gp100 peptide trials used a heteroclitic peptide in which the second amino acid was changed from threonine to methionine in order to increase binding affinity to the HLA-A2.1 molecule. In most of these trials, it was possible to detect a T cell response against the peptide of interest in a proportion of patients, but to detect T cell responses it has been necessary to stimulate the peripheral blood T cells for at least 7 d in vitro in the presence of target peptide before assaying the cells. One concern is that results obtained in this way may not accurately reflect the immunology going on in the patient. This is supported by the observation of Lee and colleagues who noted that the ability to stimulate T cells in vitro did not correlate with clinical responses *(69)*. In fact, several investigators have reported clinical responses in the absence of detectable T cell responses *(58,62,64)*. If these observations hold up, it may indicate that we are not measuring the correct effector cells.

The protein antigens discussed thus far have been normal self proteins. However, another category of antigens are mutated proteins. This category represents the only truly tumor-specific antigens in that expression is limited to the particular cell clones that possess the mutation. Mutations within a normal self protein may result in a new T cell epitope through several mechanisms such as altered processing, enhanced binding to MHC class I or II molecules, or increased affinity for a specific T cell receptor. $CD8^+$ T cells have been identified in patients that recognize mutant forms of cyclin-dependent kinase 4 (CDK4), β-catenin, and MUM-2 present in autologous melanoma cells *(70–73)*. Mutations may also lead to enhanced recognition by MHC class II-restricted T cells. A mutation within the cell cycle control protein CDC27 results in the creation of an MHC class II epitope recognized by $CD4^+$ T cells and a mutated form of the enzyme triosephosphate isomerase also contains an MHC class II-restricted epitope *(74)*. By activating $CD4^+$ T cells, these peptides may mobilize an antimelanoma response through direct cytotoxic effects of $CD4^+$ cells or through generation of T cell help in establishing a more potent $CD8^+$ T cell response.

Aside from the fact that mutated proteins can represent tumor-specific antigens, another appealing characteristic is that the mutated protein can be required for the malignant phenotype of the tumor cell. For example, the mutation in CDK4 renders this cell cycle control protein insensitive to inhibition by p16 and likely contributes to the proliferative capacity of the melanoma. A cell that loses expression of this antigen is also likely to lose the capacity to maintain the transformed phenotype. Thus, antigen-loss variants may also lose the transformed phenotype. No trials using mutated self proteins have been conducted so far because these mutated proteins seem to be present only in sporadic patients.

Simply injecting synthetic peptides is unlikely to stimulate an immune response. Tolerance may result from administration of peptide without an adjuvant capable of eliciting T cell help and any discussion of peptide vaccines must include a description of immunological adjuvants. Some of the most potent adjuvants utilized in animal model systems are thought to be too toxic for routine use in human clinical trials *(75)*. Other adjuvants have been commonly used in vaccine trials such as alum, incomplete Freund's adjuvant, QS-21, and GM-CSF. The latter agent is particularly interesting given its known ability to recruit dendritic cells to the site of administration *(76)*. An important aspect of enhancing the immunogenicity of cancer vaccines in general—and peptide vaccines in particular—is to identify optimal adjuvants. As an initial step, we recently completed a randomized peptide vaccine trial comparing three adjuvants: incomplete Freund's adjuvant, QS-21, and GM-CSF. Immune responses, as assessed using enzyme-linked immunospot (ELISPOT) assays, showed that GM-CSF and QS-21 were superior to incomplete Freund's adjuvant in stimulating a $CD8^+$ T cell responses against tyrosinase and gp100 peptides *(77)*. Further studies comparing adjuvants will be needed to optimize vaccine formulations.

4. FUTURE ISSUES

4.1. Antigen Discovery Using SEREX

As noted in the Introduction of this chapter, some of the early efforts at antigen discovery in melanoma used the technique of autologous typing looking for antibodies that bound to autologous melanoma cells. The SEREX technique represents a vastly upgraded form of autologous tissue typing in which the tumor cell's total cDNA is expressed in viral clones and probed with autologous serum *(78)*. As a method to identify antigens expressed by tumor cells which can be recognized by autologous antibodies, SEREX has several distinct advantages such as allowing the entire cDNA repertoire to be probed and permitting rapid identification of the antigen. At the same time, there are some limitations of the technique. The antigens recognized are all nonglycosylated proteins. This means that antibodies against glycolipids, such as gangliosides, will not be detected. It also raises the possibility that the reactivity identified may not be relevant in vivo against the fully glycosylated protein.

A growing number of antigens have been identified by SEREX on melanoma and other tumor types (http://www.licr.org/SEREX.html), including antigens previously identified using T cell clones, such as MAGE-1 and tyrosinase. One of the surprising observations is that many of the antigens identified appear to be housekeeping proteins, implying that it is common to have circulating antibodies against these normal cellular proteins. The significance of these antibodies is unclear. In addition, novel melanoma antigens have been discovered using SEREX, such as NY-ESO-1 *(79,80)*. Many of the antigens identified by SEREX can also be recognized by T cells demonstrating that SEREX may be able to identify relevant T cell antigens as well. The challenge in the future will be to sort through the growing list of antigens identified by SEREX and identify potential vaccine candidates.

4.2. Antigen Delivery

Once potential protein antigens have been identified, the next important issue is how to immunize patients most efficiently. Several questions immediately arise: (*i*) what form should the antigen take (peptide, protein)? (*ii*) what adjuvant may be required? and (*iii*) how should the vaccine be delivered to the immune system? The use of peptides with adjuvants is described above. Despite the relative simplicity of producing peptide vaccines, their use is restricted to patients who have an MHC haplotype that binds the predefined peptides. Many of the peptides identified to date have been those binding to the HLA-A2.1 molecule. Although this is the most common haplotype among melanoma patients (40–50%), a significant number of patients are ineligible for current vaccine studies because of MHC restriction.

4.2.1. DNA Vaccination

With DNA vaccination, cDNA encoding the antigen of interest is cloned into a bacterial expression plasmid with a constitutively active promoter. The plasmid is introduced into the skin or muscle with an intradermal or intramuscular injection, where it is taken up by professional antigen presenting cells (APCs), particularly dendritic cells. Dendritic cells (DCs) are bone marrow-derived cells of the monocyte lineage which differentiate under the influence of various cytokines to develop the capacity to take up antigens and present them in the context of both MHC class I and II molecules. DCs also express the B7-1 and B7-2 co-stimulatory molecules that are essential as "second signals" for antigen presentation to naive T cells. Precisely how the antigen is introduced into the APC is a topic of recent investigation. One proposed mechanism is direct transfection of DCs by the plasmid DNA *(81)*. Despite the fact that DCs represent a very small percent of the cells in the skin or muscle, the greatly enhanced ability of DCs to present antigen allows this mechanism to be practical. An alternative mechanism of presentation has been termed cross-priming *(82,83)*. This involves transcription and translation of the antigen within non-APCs, such as keratinocytes or myocytes, and release of mature antigen through either secretion or cell death. The antigen is then captured by APCs and presented to naive T cells in local draining lymph nodes. Most likely, both mechanisms (direct transfection of APC and cross-priming) are operative during successful DNA immunization.

DNA immunization offers several potential advantages. The presence of the full-length cDNA provides multiple potential epitopes, thus alleviating the limitations of MHC restriction. Also, the plasmid DNA itself contains immunogenic unmethylated CpG motifs (immunostimulatory sequences), which may act as a

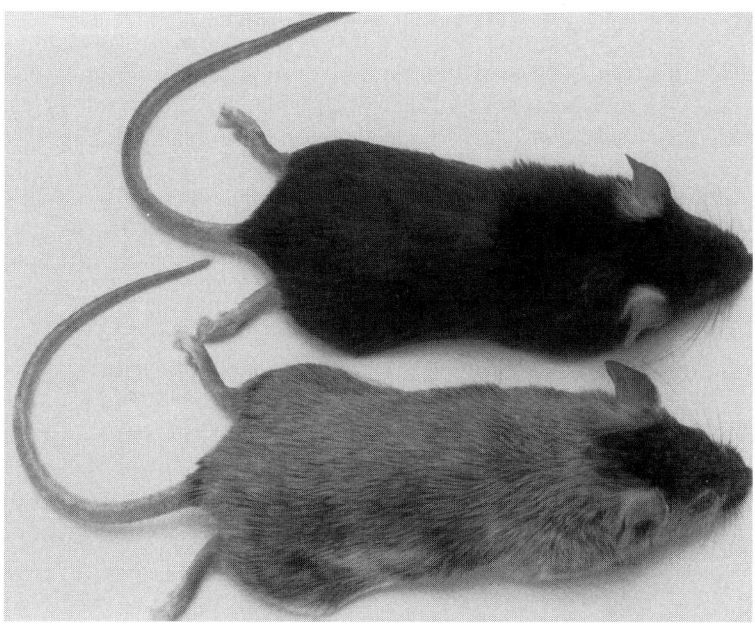

Fig. 2. Autoimmune depigmentation of coat resulting from xenogenic immunization with human TRP-2 DNA. The upper mouse is a nonimmunized C57BL/6 mouse demonstrating normal (black) coat color. The lower mouse has been immunized 5 times with human TRP-2 DNA. Depigmentation began approximately 1 mo after beginning immunization and progressed to involve the entire coat within 3 mo. This animal had no ocular changes and has been healthy for 18 mo since immunization. Depigmentation occurs in the majority of animals immunized with human TRP-2.

potent immunological adjuvant *(84,85)*. A further advantage is that DNA is relatively simple to purify in large quantities.

Our group and others have demonstrated significant activity of DNA vaccines in preclinical animal models of melanoma. Immunization of mice with DNA encoding xenogenic (human) gp100, gp75/TRP-1, or TRP-2 results in protection from syngeneic tumor challenge with B16 mouse melanoma, as well as rapid and extensive depigmentation of coat *(86–88)*. Immunization against self antigens can also induce autoimmune reaction. Black mice immunized against melanosomal proteins develop reproducible depigmentation (Fig. 2) showing the ability of DNA immunization to induce immune recognition of self proteins in mouse melanocytes. In clinical trials for infectious disease, DNA immunization has been shown to be safe and effective in developing immune responses to malaria and human immunodeficiency virus *(89–91)*. Clinical trials are underway in which melanoma patients are being immunized with DNA encoding antigens such as tyrosinase and gp100.

4.2.2. Dendritic Cells

Several different approaches to immunization against antigens present on melanoma cells have been devised to take advantage of the unique properties of DCs. Recently, techniques have been developed to generate large quantities of DCs in vitro using cytokine mixtures, to differentiate peripheral blood mononuclear cells. DCs produced in this fashion can then be "loaded" with peptides of interest and reinfused into patients. Alternatively, several approaches have been used to introduce full-length protein sequences containing multiple potential antigenic epitopes. DCs can be exposed to tumor lysates before injection, as a means of generating a response to numerous antigens, both known and unknown. The loading of DCs with total tumor RNA has also been investigated as a vaccination strategy. Loading with RNA allows for endogenous production and processing of antigens much like the DNA vaccination approach described above. Both the lysate and RNA methods bring forth the possibility of inducing potentially toxic autoimmune responses to unknown antigens in the lysate or RNA pool. Alternative approaches have utilized transduction of DCs with retroviruses, poxviruses, or adenoviruses encoding specific antigens of interest.

The results of two clinical trials using DC-based vaccination in melanoma patients have recently been reported. One trial used immature DCs pulsed with multiple peptides or tumor lysates and showed objective tumor responses in 5/16 patients *(92)*. In the other trial, mature DCs were pulsed with MAGE-3A1 peptide, based on in vitro data suggesting that mature cells were better able to stimulate a Th1 response and were more resistant to the effects of immunosuppressive cytokines, such as tumor-derived IL-10 *(93)*. This trial reported clinical responses in 6/11 patients, including complete resolution of individual metastases in skin, liver, lung, and lymph nodes. This study also demonstrated the ability of peptide-pulsed mature DCs to expand CTL precursors. The number of patients demonstrating an immunologic response was dependent on the specific assay used. Whereas 8/11 patients responded by a semiquantitative recall assay, only 2/11 patients had an increase in IFN-γ-producing cells in an ELISPOT assay. This discrepancy reinforces the importance of developing reproducible immunological assays for quantitative monitoring of T cell responses in vaccine trials that correlate with clinical outcomes. Although these results are encouraging for the further development of immunologic therapies for melanoma, they must be interpreted with caution. Most of the responses were mixed, and the groups of patients were small.

Ex vivo expansion and loading of DCs is a labor-intensive and expensive approach. Several investigators are exploring in vivo strategies to exploit the power of DCs by developing means of DC recruitment to sites of vaccination. One approach is the use of GM-CSF, in either the protein or DNA formulation.

Intradermal or subcutaneous delivery of GM-CSF results in infiltration of DCs to the site of application *(76,94)*. After several days, the same site is used to administer the vaccine (peptide, DNA, virus, etc.), and the hypothesis is that the locally concentrated DCs will present antigen efficiently and induce an immune response to the vaccine. This strategy has been used in a pilot trial of peptide vaccines with GM-CSF protein *(77)*. The use of the GM-CSF gene, however, may offer several advantages over using GM-CSF protein, such as fewer days of GM-CSF injections because of persistent local production of the cytokine and the intrinsic adjuvant effects of the CpG immunostimulatory sequences within the plasmid DNA. Preclinical animal studies have demonstrated that administration of the murine GM-CSF gene results in recruitment of epidermal DCs *(95)*.

4.2.3. Heat-Shock Proteins

Heat-shock proteins (HSPs) are a family of proteins that are highly conserved through evolution and are produced by cells in response to physical, chemical or immunological stress. Largely through the work of Srivastava and colleagues, HSPs have been found to function as intracellular peptide carriers, and there is evidence that the HSP–peptide complexes are readily taken up by DCs for presentation to naive T cells *(96–99)*. HSP–peptide complexes can be purified from individual tumors and theoretically represent the total set of processed peptides from that tumor cell. Pilot trials immunizing patients with autologous HSP–peptide complexes are currently underway for several malignancies, including melanoma. The results of one early study at MD Anderson Cancer Center documented the safety of this approach *(100)*. Future studies will provide more information regarding the ability of HSP-based vaccines to induce both immune and clinical responses against tumor.

4.2.4. Recombinant Viral Vaccines

The use of recombinant viruses encoding melanoma-associated antigens is also an area of active investigation. This approach has its foundation in the inherent immunogenicity of viruses combined with previous experience using viral oncolysate (described above). Currently, investigators are studying recombinant adenovirus and vaccinia viruses encoding melanosomal antigens as potential vaccines. One drawback to the use of vaccinia is the high prevalence of neutralizing antibodies in a large proportion of the adult population that has received vaccinia immunization for prevention of smallpox. To circumvent this problem, the latest generation of recombinant viral vaccines use other members of the poxvirus family (fowlpox, canarypox), which may not be affected by anti-vaccinia immunity.

4.3. Conclusions

A variety of techniques are being used to identify molecules on melanoma that can be recognized by the immune system. At the same time, investigations are underway to learn the optimal ways to present these molecules to the immune system and to measure the immune response generated. The goal is to be able to induce an autoimmune reaction that destroys tumor but causes little damage to normal tissues. It appears that this can be done in mouse models, and our challenge is to translate this into the clinical setting.

REFERENCES

1. Oettgen HF, Old LJ. The history of cancer immunotherapy. In: DeVita VT Jr, Hellman S, Rosenberg SA, eds., *Biologic Therapy of Cancer*. J.B. Lippincott Company, Philadelphia, 1991, pp. 87–120.
2. Foley E. Antigenic properties of methylcholanthrene-induced tumors in mice of the strain of origin. *Cancer Res* 1953; 13: 835–837.
3. Prehn RT, Main JM. Immunity to methylcholanthrene-induced sarcomas. *J Natl Cancer Inst* 1957; 18: 769–778.
4. Hewitt HB, Blake ER, Walder AS. A critique of the evidence for active host defence against cancer, based on personal studies of 27 murine tumours of spontaneous origin. *Br J Cancer* 1976; 33: 241–259.
5. Old LJ. Cancer immunology: the search for specificity—G.H.A. Clowes memorial lecture. *Cancer Res* 1981; 41: 361–375.
6. Nasi M, Meyers M, Livingston P, Houghton A, Chapman P. Anti-melanoma effects of R24, a monoclonal antibody against GD3. *Vaccine Res* 1997; 7(suppl 2): S155–S162.
7. Creekmore S, Urba W, Koop W, et al. Phase IB/II trial of R24 antibody and interleukin-2 (IL2) in melanoma. *Proc Am Soc Clin Oncol* 1992; 11: 345.
8. Bajorin DF, Chapman PB, Dimaggio J, et al. Phase I evaluation of a combination of monoclonal antibody R24 and interleukin 2 in patients with metastatic melanoma. *Cancer Res* 1990; 50: 7490–7495.
9. Minasian LM, Szatrowski TP, Rosenblum M, et al. Hemorrhagic tumor necrosis during a pilot trial of tumor necrosis factor-α and anti-GD3 ganglioside monoclonal antibody in patients with metastatic melanoma. *Blood* 1994; 83: 56–64.
10. Livingston PO, Takeyama H, Pollack MS, et al. Serological responses of melanoma patients to vaccines derived from allogeneic cultured melanoma cells. *Int J Cancer* 1983; 31: 567–575.
11. Gercovich FG, Gutterman JU, Mavligit GM, Hersh EM. Active specific immunization in malignant melanoma. *Med Pediatr Oncol* 1975; 1: 277–287.
12. Slingluff CL Jr, Seigler HF. Immunotherapy for malignant melanoma with a tumor cell vaccine. *Ann Plast Surg* 1992; 28: 104–107.
13. Morton DL, Foshag LJ, Nizze JA, et al. Active specific immunotherapy in malignant melanoma. *Semin Surg Oncol* 1989; 5: 420–425.
14. Haigh PI, Difronzo LA, Gammon G, Morton DL. Vaccine therapy for patients with melanoma. *Oncology (Huntingt)* 1999; 13: 1561–1574.
15. Chan AD, Morton DL. Active immunotherapy with allogeneic tumor cell vaccines: present status. *Semin Oncol* 1998; 25: 611–622.
16. Bystryn JC, Henn M, Li J, Shroba S. Identification of immunogenic human melanoma antigens in a polyvalent melanoma vaccine. *Cancer Res* 1992; 52: 5948–5953.

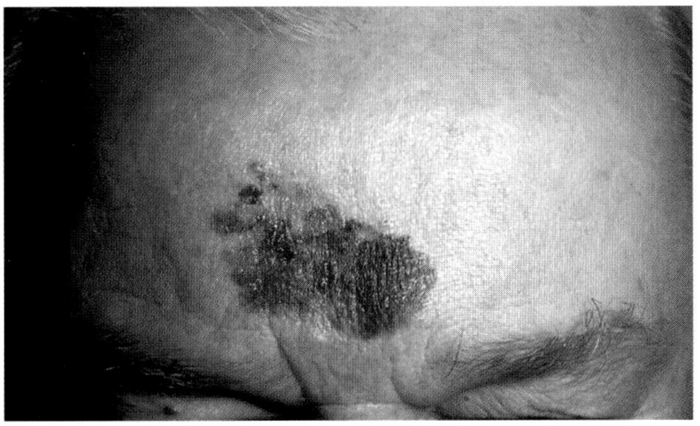

Color Plate 1. Lentigo maligna melanoma (*Fig. 1; see* discussion in Chapter 1 on p. 9).

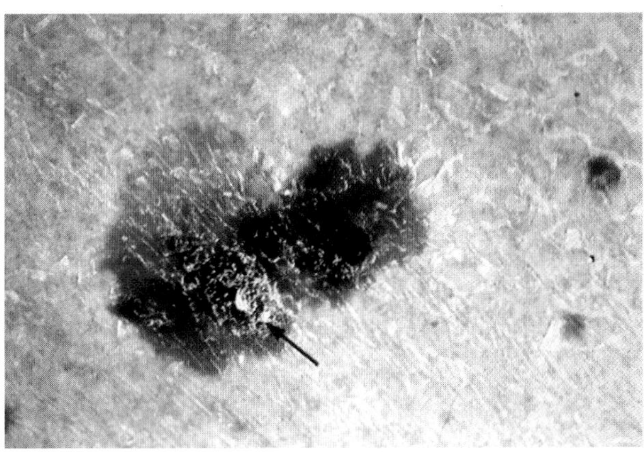

Color Plate 2. Superficial spreading melanoma
(*Fig. 2; see* full caption and discussion in Chapter 1 on pp. 11–12).

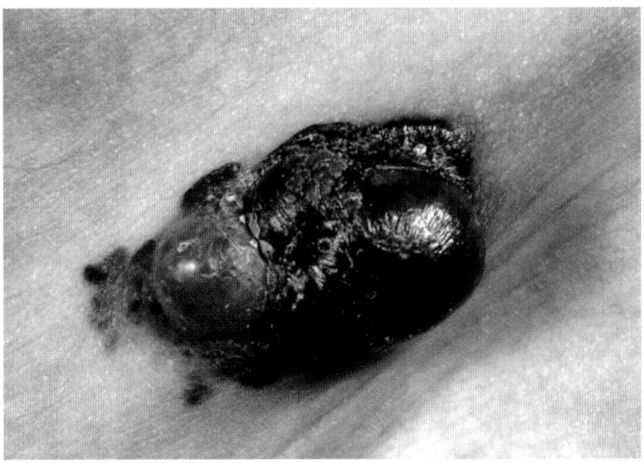

Color Plate 3. Nodular melanoma (*Fig. 3; see* discussion in Chapter 1 on pp. 12–13).

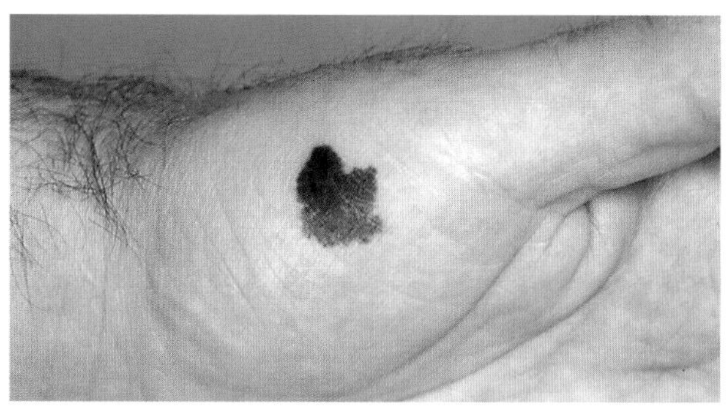

Color Plate 4. Acral lentiginous melanoma (*Fig. 4; see* discussion in Chapter 1 on pp. 13–14).

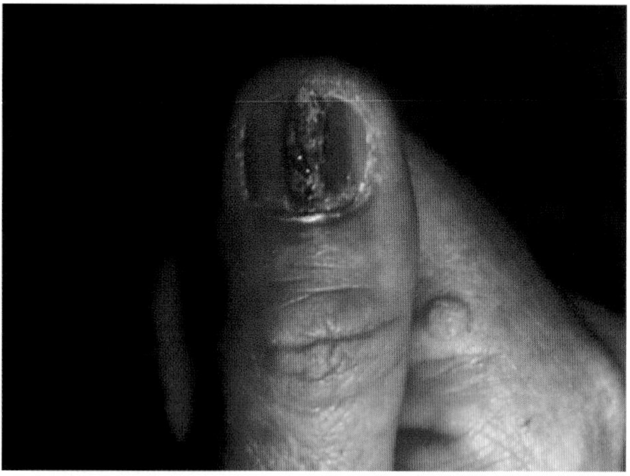

Color Plate 5. Subungual melanoma (*Fig. 5; see* discussion in Chapter 1 on pp. 14–15).

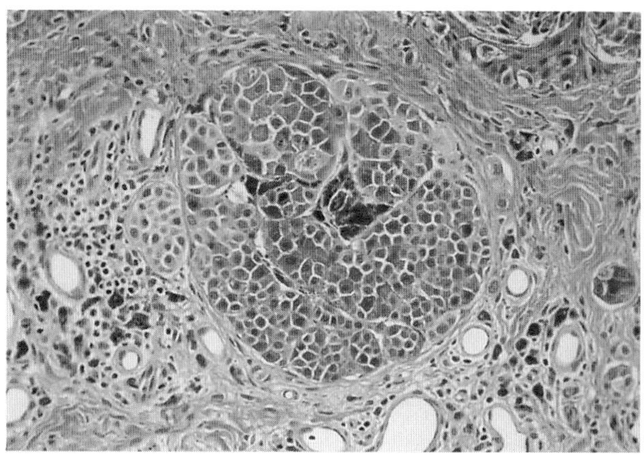

Color Plate 6. Vertical growth (*Fig. 1; see* full caption and discussion in Chapter 2 on pp. 40–41).

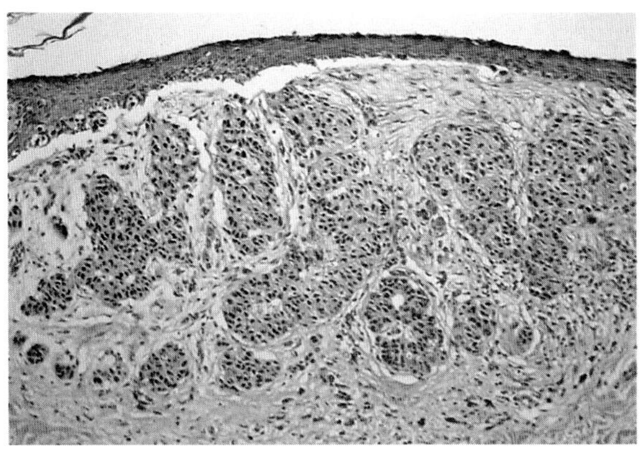

Color Plate 7. Variant vertical growth
(*Fig. 2; see* full caption and discussion in Chapter 2 on pp. 40–41).

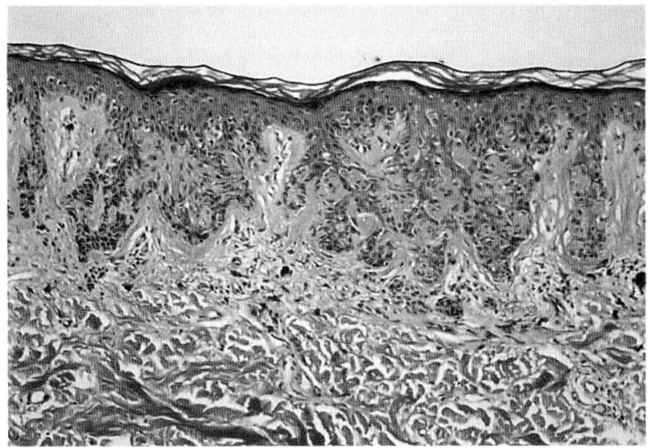

Color Plate 8. Moderate to severe melanocytic dysplasia
(*Fig. 3; see* full caption and discussion in Chapter 2 on p. 43).

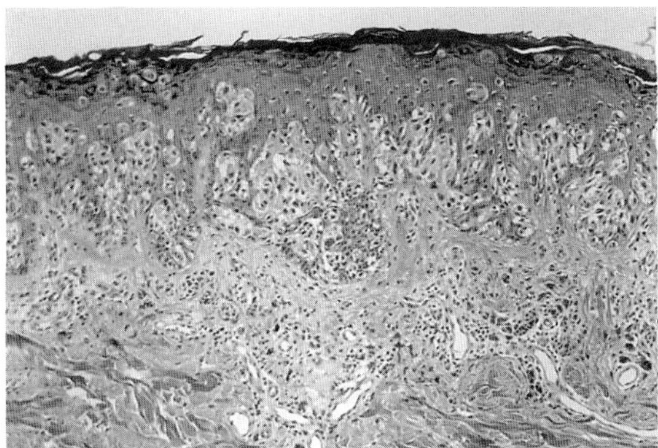

Color Plate 9. Severe melanocytic dysplasia
(*Fig. 4; see* full caption and discussion in Chapter 2 on pp. 43–44).

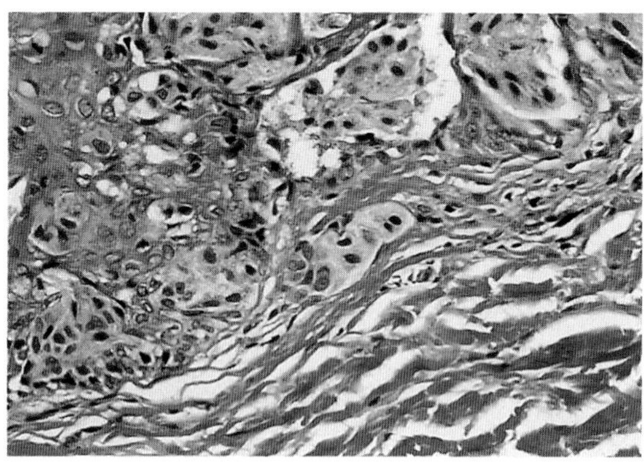

Color Plate 10. Severe compound melanocytic dysplasia.
(*Fig. 5; see* full caption and discussion in Chapter 2 on pp. 43–44).

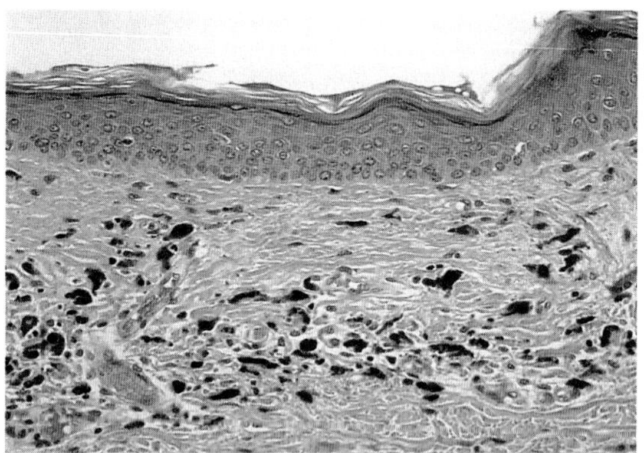

Color Plate 11. Histology of regression
(*Fig. 6; see* full caption and discussion in Chapter 2 on p. 45).

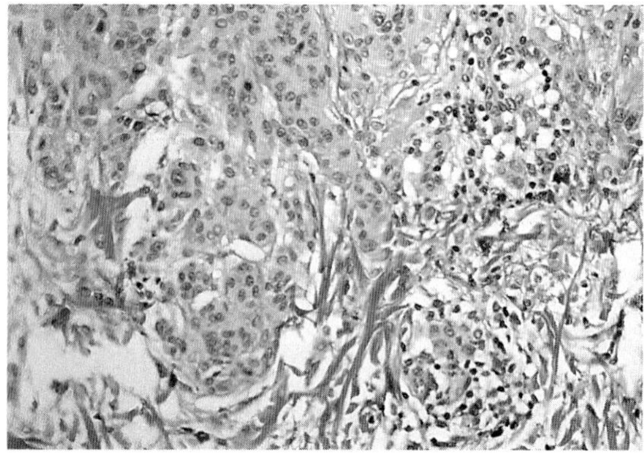

Color Plate 12. Thin (0.76 mm) level IV vertical growth with subsequent metastasis and death (*Fig. 7; see* full caption and discussion in Chapter 2 on p. 46).

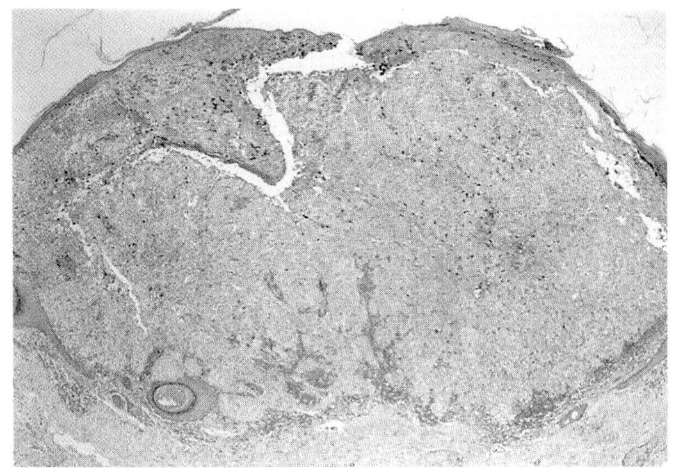

Color Plate 13. Breslow's tumor thickness measurement (*Fig. 8; see* full caption and discussion in Chapter 2 on pp. 47–48).

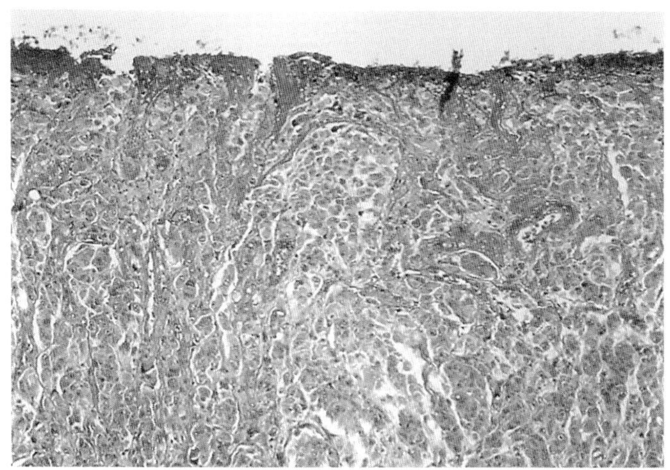

Color Plate 14.
Ulceration (*Fig. 10; see* full caption and discussion in Chapter 2 on p. 49).

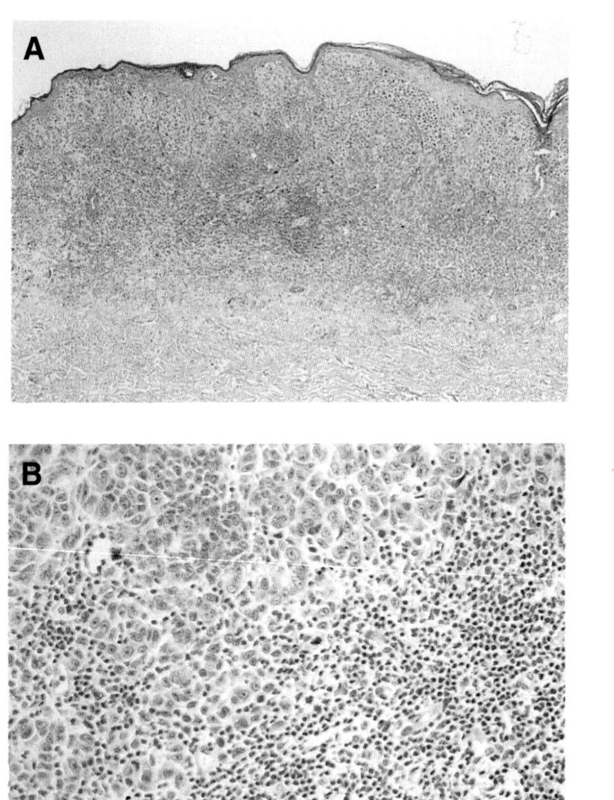

Color Plate 15. Tumor infiltrating lymphocytes (TILs) (*Fig. 11; see* full caption and discussion in Chapter 2 on pp. 50–51).

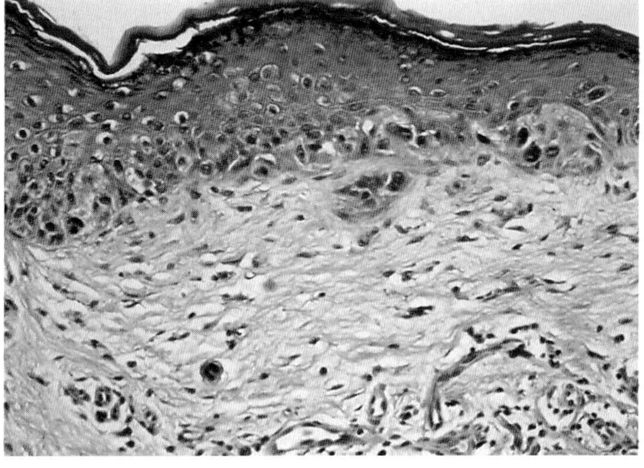

Color Plate 16. Immune-reactive stroma (incomplete regression) (*Fig. 12; see* full caption and discussion in Chapter 2 on p. 53).

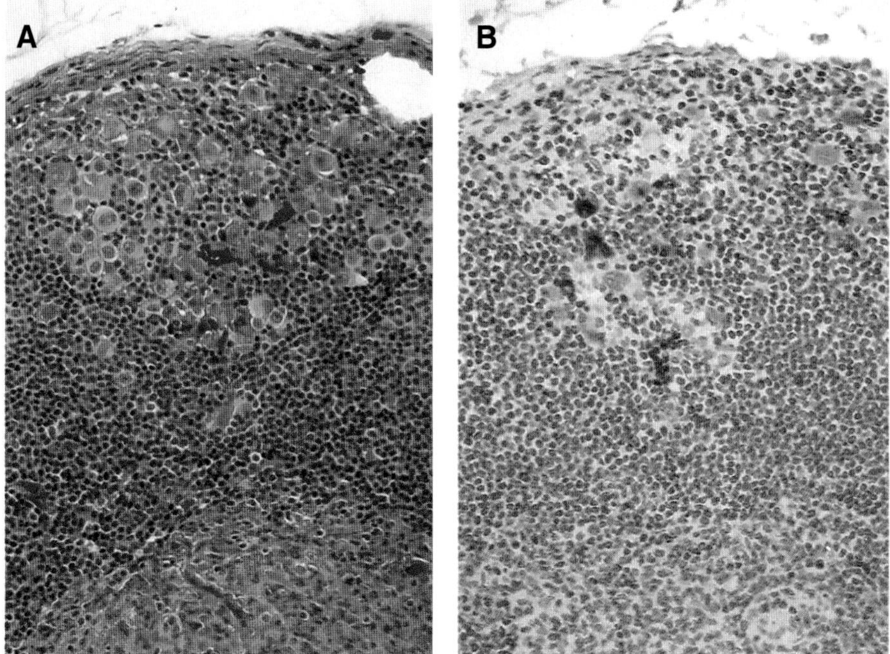

Color Plate 17. Micrometastasis in a sentinel lymph node. H&E stain shows a small group of atypical cells of uncertain nature **(A)** Immunostaining with antibodies to Melan-A (Mart-1) supports the interpretation of micrometastasis of malignant melanoma **(B)**. (*Figs. 13A, 13B; see* discussion in Chapter 2 on pp. 60–63).

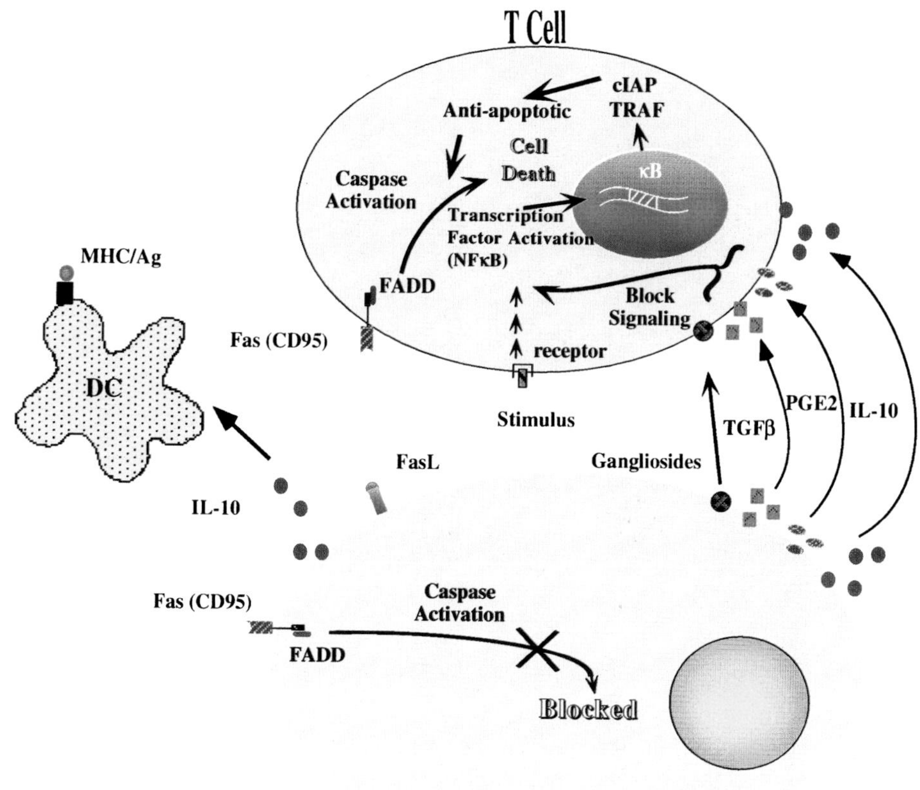

Color Plate 18. Putative mechanisms by which tumor cells can induce immune dysfunction in T cells and dendritic cells. Tumor cells can produce a variety of immunosuppressive products that include IL-10, gangliosides, TGFβ, and PGs. These products can affect T cell signaling and can suppress activation of transcription factors such as NFκB. Blocking NFκB may also reduce expression of certain anti-apoptotic genes that would render T cells more sensitive to apoptosis. IL-10 can also inhibit the Ag-presenting function of DCs. Moreover, some tumors express Fas ligand (Fas-L) that can induce apoptosis in T cells that express Fas receptor. At the same time, some tumor cells that express Fas receptor may themselves be resistant to apoptosis induced by Fas-L expression on the activated T cells. Such resistance, in some cases, appears related to the tumor cells' reduced expression of molecules such as caspase that are essential for activation of apoptotic pathways. (*Fig. 5; see* discussion in Chapter 4 on pp. 121–122).

17. Bystryn JC. Immunogenicity and clinical activity of a polyvalent melanoma antigen vaccine prepared from shed antigens. *Ann NY Acad Sci* 1993; 690: 190–203.
18. Okamoto T, Irie RF, Fujii S, et al. Anti-tyrosinase-related protein-2 immune response in vitiligo patients and melanoma patients receiving active-specific immunotherapy. *J Invest Dermatol* 1998; 111: 1034–1039.
19. Huang SK, Okamoto T, Morton DL, Hoon DS. Antibody responses to melanoma/melanocyte autoantigens in melanoma patients. *J Invest Dermatol* 1998; 111: 662–667.
20. Reynolds SR, Celis E, Sette A, et al. HLA-independent heterogeneity of $CD8^+$ T cell responses to MAGE-3, Melan-A/MART-1, gp100, tyrosinase, MC1R, and TRP-2 in vaccine-treated melanoma patients. *J Immunol* 1998; 161: 6970–6976.
21. Morton DL, Foshag LJ, Hoon DS, et al. Prolongation of survival in metastatic melanoma after active specific immunotherapy with a new polyvalent melanoma vaccine [published erratum appears in *Ann Surg* 1993 Mar; 217(3): 309]. *Ann Surg* 1992; 216: 463–482.
22. Bystryn JC. Clinical activity of a polyvalent melanoma antigen vaccine. *Recent Results Cancer Res* 1995; 139: 337–348.
23. Mitchell MS, Von Eschen KB. Phase III trial of melacine melanoma theraccine versus combination chemotherapy in the treatment of stage IV melanoma. *Proc Am Soc Clin Oncol* 1997; 16: 494a.
24. Wallack MK, Sivanandham M, Balch CM, et al. Surgical adjuvant active specific immunotherapy for patients with stage III melanoma: the final analysis of data from a phase III, randomized, double-blind, multicenter vaccinia melanoma oncolysate trial. *J Am Coll Surg* 1998; 187: 69–77.
25. Berd D, Murphy G, Maguire HC, Mastrangelo MJ. Immunization with haptenized, autologous tumor cells induces inflammation of human melanoma metastases. *Cancer Res* 1991; 51: 2731–2734.
26. Dranoff G, Jaffee E, Lazenby A, et al. Vaccination with irradiated tumor cell engineered to secrete murine granulocyte-macrophage colony-stimulating factor stimulates potent, specific, and long-lasting anti-tumor immunity. *Proc Natl Acad Sci USA* 1993; 90: 35339–33543.
27. Soiffer R, Lynch T, Mihm M, et al. Vaccination with irradiated autologous melanoma cells engineered to secrete human granulocyte-macrophage colony-stimulating factor generates potent antitumor immunity in patients with metastatic melanoma. *Proc Natl Acad Sci USA* 1998; 95: 13141–13146.
28. Ellem KA, O'Rourke MG, Johnson GR, et al. A case report: immune responses and clinical course of the first human use of granulocyte/macrophage-colony-stimulating-factor-transduced autologous melanoma cells for immunotherapy. *Cancer Immunol Immunother* 1997; 44: 10–20.
29. Dranoff G, Soiffer R, Lynch T, et al. A phase I study of vaccination with autologous, irradiated melanoma cells engineered to secrete human granulocyte-macrophage colony stimulating factor. *Hum Gene Ther* 1997; 8: 111–123.
30. Hamilton WB, Helling F, Lloyd KO, Livingston PO. Ganglioside expression on human malignant melanoma assessed by quantitative immune thin-layer chromatography. *Int J Cancer* 1993; 53: 566–573.
31. Jones PC, Lan LS, Liu PY, Morton DL, Irie RF. Prolonged survival for melanoma patients with elevated IgM antibody to oncofetal antigen. *J Natl Cancer Inst* 1981; 66: 249–254.
32. Livingston PO, Wong GYC, Adluri S, et al. Improved survival in stage III melanoma patients with GM2 antibodies: a randomized trial of adjuvant vaccination with GM2 ganglioside. *J Clin Oncol* 1994; 12: 1036–1044.
33. Helling F, Zhang S, Shang A, et al. GM2-KLH conjugate vaccine: increased immunogenicity in melanoma patients after administration with immunological adjuvant QS-21. *Cancer Res* 1995; 55: 2783–2788.

34. Chapman PB, Morrissey DM, Panageas KS, et al. Induction of antibodies against GM2 ganglioside by immunizing melanoma patients using GM2-KLH + QS21 vaccine: a dose-response study. *Clin Cancer Res* 2000; 6: 874–879.
34a. Kirkwood JM, Ibrahim JG, Sosman JA, et al. *J. Clin. Oncol.* High-dose interferon alfa-2b significantly prolongs relapse-free and overall survival compared with the GM2-KLH/QS-21 vaccine in patients with resected stage IIB-III melanoma: results of intergroup trial E1694/S9512/C509801. 2001; 19: 2370–2380.
35. Chapman PB, Morrissey D, Ibrahim J, et al. Eastern Cooperative Oncology Group Phase II randomized adjuvant trial of GM2-KLH + QS21 (GMK) vaccine ± high dose interferon 2b in melanoma. *Proc Am Soc Clin Oncol* 1999; 17: 538a.
36. Tai T, Cahan LD, Tsuchida T, Saxton RE, Irie RF, Morton DL. Immunogenicity of melanoma-associated gangliosides in cancer patients. *Int J Cancer* 1985; 35: 607–612.
36a. Chapman PB, Morrisey D, Panageas KS, et al. Vaccination with a bivalent GM2 and GD2 ganglioside conjugate vaccine: A trial comparing doses of GD2-KLH. *Clin Cancer Res* 2000; 6:4658-4662.
37. Ritter G, Boosfeld E, Adluri R, et al. Antibody response to immunization with ganglioside GD3 and GD3 congeners (lactones, amide and gangliosidol) in patients with malignant melanoma. *Int J Cancer* 1991; 48: 379–385.
38. Ragupathi G, Meyers M, Adluri S, Howard L, Musselli L, Livingston PO. Induction of antibodies against GD3 ganglioside in melanoma patients by vaccination with GD3-lactone-KLH conjugate plus immunological adjuvant QS-21. *Int J Cancer* 2000; 85: 659–666.
39. Cheung N-KV, Canete A, Cheung IY, Ye J-N, Liu C. Disialoganglioside GD2 anti-idiotypic monoclonal antibodies. *Int J Cancer* 1993; 54: 499–505.
40. Saleh MN, Stapleton JD, Khazaeli MB, LoBuglio AF. Generation of a human anti-idiotypic antibody that mimics the GD2 antigen. *J Immunol* 1993; 151: 3390–3398.
41. Sen G, Chakraborty M, Foon KA, Reisfeld RA, Bhattacharya-Chatterjee M. Preclinical evaluation in nonhuman primates of murine monoclonal anti-idiotype antibody that mimics the disialoganglioside GD2. *Clin Cancer Res* 1997; 3: 1969–1976.
42. Foon KA, Lutzky J, Baral RN, et al. Clinical and immune responses in advanced melanoma patients immunized with an anti-idiotype antibody mimicking disialoganglioside GD2. *J Clin Oncol* 2000; 18: 376–384.
43. Yao T-J, Meyers M, Livingston PO, Houghton AN, Chapman PB. Immunization of melanoma patients with BEC2-Keyhole limpet hemocyanin plus BCG intradermally followed by intravenous booster immunizations with BEC2 to induce anti-GD3 ganglioside antibodies. *Clin Cancer Res* 1999; 5: 77–81.
44. McCaffery M, Yao T-J, Williams L, Livingston PO, Houghton AN, Chapman PB. Enhanced immunogenicity of BEC2 anti-idiotypic monoclonal antibody that mimics GD3 ganglioside when combined with adjuvant. *Clin Cancer Res* 1996; 2: 679–686.
45. Tai T, Paulson JC, Cahan LD, Irie RF. Ganglioside GM2 as a human tumor antigen (OFA-I-1). *Proc Natl Acad Sci USA* 1983; 80: 5392–5396.
46. Grant SC, Kris MG, Houghton AN, Chapman PB. Long survival of patients with small cell lung cancer after adjuvant treatment with the anti-idiotypic antibody BEC2 plus BCG. *Clin Cancer Res* 1999; 5: 1319–1324.
47. Brichard V, Van Pel A, Wolfel T, et al. The tyrosinase gene codes for an antigen recognized by autologous cytolytic T lymphocytes on HLA-A2 melanomas. *J Exp Med* 1993; 178: 489–495.
48. Coulie PG, Brichard V, Van Pel A, et al. A new gene coding for a differentiation antigen recognized by autologous cytolytic T lymphocytes on HLA-A2 melanomas. *J Exp Med* 1994; 180: 35–42.
49. Wolfel T, Hauer M, Schneider J, et al. A p16INK4a-insensitive CDK4 mutant targeted by cytolytic T lymphocytes in a human melanoma. *Science* 1995; 269: 1281–1284.

50. Vijayasaradhi S, Bouchard B, Houghton AN. The melanoma antigen gp75 is the human homologue of the mouse *b (brown)* locus gene product. *J Exp Med* 1990; 171: 1375–1380.
51. Wang RF, Appella E, Kawakami Y, Kang X, Rosenberg SA. Identification of TRP-2 as a human tumor antigen recognized by cytotoxic T lymphocytes. *J Exp Med* 1996; 184: 2207–2216.
52. Chen YT, Old LJ. Cancer-testis antigens: targets for cancer immunotherapy [comment]. *Cancer J Sci Am* 1999; 5: 16–17.
53. van der Bruggen P, Traversari C, Chomez P, et al. A gene encoding an antigen recognized by cytolytic T lymphocytes on a human melanoma. *Science* 1991; 254: 1643–1647.
54. Parkhurst MR, Salgaller ML, Southwood S, et al. Improved induction of melanoma-reactive CTL with peptides from the melanoma antigen gp100 modified at HLA-A*0201-binding residues. *J Immunol* 1996; 157: 2539–2548.
55. Dyall R, Bowne WB, Weber LW, et al. Heteroclitic immunization induces tumor immunity. *J Exp Med* 1998; 188: 1553–1561.
56. Topalian SL, Gonzales MI, Parkhurst M, et al. Melanoma-specific $CD4^+$ T cells recognize nonmutated HLA-DR-restricted tyrosinase epitopes. *J Exp Med* 1996; 183: 1965–1971.
57. Jager E, Jager D, Karbach J, et al. Identification of NY-ESO-1 epitopes presented by human histocompatibility antigen (HLA)-DRB4*0101-0103 and recognized by CD4(+) T lymphocytes of patients with NY-ESO-1-expressing melanoma. *J Exp Med* 2000; 191: 625–630.
58. Marchand M, van Baren N, Weynants P, et al. Tumor regressions observed in patients with metastatic melanoma treated with an antigenic peptide encoded by gene MAGE-3 and presented by HLA-A1. *Int J Cancer* 1999; 80: 219–230.
59. Weber JS, Hua FL, Spears L, Marty V, Kuniyoshi C, Celis E. A phase I trial of an HLA-A1 restricted MAGE-3 epitope peptide with incomplete Freund's adjuvant in patients with resected high-risk melanoma. *J Immunother* 1999; 22: 431–440.
60. Lee PP, Yee C, Savage PA, et al. Characterization of circulating T cells specific for tumor-associated antigens in melanoma patients. *Nat Med* 1999; 5: 677–685.
61. Salgaller ML, Marincola FM, Cormier JN, Rosenberg SA. Immunization against epitopes in the human melanoma antigen gp100 following patient immunization with synthetic peptide. *Cancer Res* 1996; 56: 4749–4757.
62. Jaeger E, Bernhard H, Romero P, et al. Generation of cytotoxic T-cell responses with synthetic melanoma-associated peptides in vivo: implications for tumor vaccines with melanoma-associated antigens. *Int J Cancer* 1996; 66: 162–169.
63. Storkus WJ, Kirkwood JM, Mayordomo JI, et al. Melanoma peptide vaccine: a randomized Phase I evaluation of MART-1, gp100, and tyrosinase peptide vaccines in patients with malignant melanoma [meeting abstract]. *Proc Annu Meet Am Soc Clin Oncol* 1996; 15: A1811.
64. Rosenberg SA, Yang JC, Schwartzentruber DJ, et al. Immunologic and therapeutic evaluation of a synthetic peptide vaccine for the treatment of patients with metastatic melanoma [see comments]. *Nat Med* 1998; 4: 321–7.
65. Wang F, Bade E, Kuniyoshi C, et al. Phase I trial of a MART-1 peptide vaccine in incomplete Freund's adjuvant for resected high-risk melanoma. *Clin Cancer Res* 1999; 5: 2756–2765.
66. Jager E, Ringhoffer M, Dienes HP, et al. Granulocyte-macrophage-colony-stimulating factor enhances immune responses to melanoma-associated peptides in vivo. *Int J Cancer* 1996; 67: 54–62.
67. Zarour HM, Kirkwood JM, Kierstead LS, et al. Melan-A/MART-1(51-73) represents an immunogenic HLA-DR4-restricted epitope recognized by melanoma-reactive CD4(+) T cells. *Proc Natl Acad Sci USA* 2000; 97: 400–405.
68. Cormier JN, Salgaller ML, Prevette T, et al. Enhancement of cellular immunity in melanoma patients immunized with a peptide from MART-1/Melan A. *Cancer J* 1997; 3: 37–44.
69. Lee K-H, Wang E, Nielsen MB, et al. Increased vaccine-specific T cell frequency after peptide-based vaccination correlates with increased susceptibility to in vitro stimulation but does not lead to tumor regression. *J Immunol* 1999; 163: 6292–6300.

70. Wolfel T, Hauer M, Schneider J, et al. A p16^{INK4a}-insensitive CDK4 mutant targeted by cytolytic T lymphocytes in a human melanoma. *Science* 1995; 269: 1281–1284.
71. Robbins PF, El-Gamil M, Li YF, et al. A mutated beta-catenin gene encodes a melanoma-specific antigen recognized by tumor infiltrating lymphocytes. *J Exp Med* 1996; 183: 1185–1192.
72. Chiari R, Foury F, De Plaen E, Baurain JF, Thonnard J, Coulie PG. Two antigens recognized by autologous cytolytic T lymphocytes on a melanoma result from a single point mutation in an essential housekeeping gene. *Cancer Res* 1999; 59: 5785–5792.
73. Coulie PG, Lehmann F, Lethe B, et al. A mutated intron sequence codes for an antigenic peptide recognized by cytolytic T lymphocytes on a human melanoma. *Proc Natl Acad Sci USA* 1995; 92: 7976–7980.
74. Wang RF, Wang X, Atwood AC, Topalian SL, Rosenberg SA. Cloning genes encoding MHC class II-restricted antigens: mutated CDC27 as a tumor antigen. *Science* 1999; 284: 1351–1354.
75. Weeratna RD, McCluskie MJ, Xu Y, Davis HL. CpG DNA induces stronger immune responses with less toxicity than other adjuvants. *Vaccine* 2000; 18: 1755–1762.
76. Kaplan G, Walsh G, Guido LS, et al. Novel responses of human skin to intradermal recombinant granulocyte/macrophage-colony-stimulating factor: Langerhans cell recruitment, keratinocyte growth, and enhanced wound healing. *J Exp Med* 1992; 175: 1717–1728.
77. Schaed SG, Houghton AN, Klimek VM, et al. Immunization of melanoma patients with both tyrosinase (370D) and GP100 (210M) peptides: comparison of adjuvants and peptide immunogenicity. *Proc Am Assoc Cancer Res* 1999; 41: 4029.
78. Old LJ, Chen Y-T. New paths in human cancer serology. *J Exp Med* 1998; 187: 1163–1167.
79. Jager E, Chen YT, Drijfhout JW, et al. Simultaneous humoral and cellular immune response against cancer-testis an. *J Exp Med* 1998; 187: 265–270.
80. Jager E, Maeurer M, Hohn H, et al. Clonal expansion of Melan A-specific cytotoxic T lymphocytes in a melanoma patient responding to continued immunization with melanoma-associated peptides. *Int J Cancer* 2000; 86: 538–547.
81. Porgador A, Irvine KR, Iwasaki A, Barber BH, Restifo NP, Germain RN. Predominant role for directly transfected dendritic cells in antigen presentation to CD8$^+$ T cells after gene gun immunization. *J Exp Med* 1998; 188: 1075–1082.
82. Casares S, Inaba K, Brumeanu TD, Steinman RM, Bona CA. Antigen presentation by dendritic cells after immunization with DNA encoding a major histocompatibility complex class II-restricted viral epitope. *J Exp Med* 1997; 186: 1481–1486.
83. Akbari O, Panjwani N, Garcia S, Tascon R, Lowrie D, Stockinger B. DNA vaccination: transfection and activation of dendritic cells as key events for immunity. *J Exp Med* 1999; 189: 169–178.
84. Klinman DM, Yi AK, Beaucage SL, Conover J, Krieg AM. CpG motifs present in bacteria DNA rapidly induce lymphocytes to secrete interleukin 6, interleukin 12, and interferon gamma. *Proc Natl Acad Sci USA* 1996; 93: 2879–2883.
85. Sato Y, Roman M, Tighe H, et al. Immunostimulatory DNA sequences necessary for effective intradermal gene immunization. *Science* 1996; 273: 352–354.
86. Bowne WB, Srinivasan R, Wolchok JD, et al. Coupling and uncoupling of tumor immunity and autoimmunity. *J Exp Med* 1999; 190: 1717–1722.
87. Hawkins WG, Gold JS, Dyall R, et al. Immunization with DNA coding for gp100 results in CD4$^+$ T-cell independent antitumor immunity. *Surgery* 2001; 128: 273–280.
88. Weber LW, Bowne WB, Wolchok JD, et al. Tumor immunity and autoimmunity induced by immunization with homologous DNA. *J Clin Invest* 1998; 102: 1258–1264.
89. Wang R, Doolan DL, Le TP, et al. Induction of antigen-specific cytotoxic T lymphocytes in humans by a malaria DNA vaccine. *Science* 1998; 282: 476–480.
90. Boyer JD, Cohen AD, Vogt S, et al. Vaccination of seronegative volunteers with a human immunodeficiency virus type 1 env/rev DNA vaccine induces antigen-specific proliferation and lymphocyte production of beta-chemokines. *J Infect Dis* 2000; 181: 476–483.

91. Ugen KE, Nyland SB, Boyer JD, et al. DNA vaccination with HIV-1 expressing constructs elicits immune responses in humans. *Vaccine* 1998; 16: 1818–1821.
92. Nestle FO, Alijagic S, Gilliet M, et al. Vaccination of melanoma patients with peptide- or tumor lysate-pulsed dendritic cells [see comments]. *Nat Med* 1998; 4: 328–332.
93. Thurner B, Haendle I, Roder C, et al. Vaccination with mage-3A1 peptide-pulsed mature, monocyte-derived dendritic cells expands specific cytotoxic T cells and induces regression of some metastases in advanced stage IV melanoma. *J Exp Med* 1999; 190: 1669–1678.
94. Nasi ML, Lieberman P, Busam KJ, et al. Intradermal injection of granulocyte-macrophage colony-stimulating factor (GM-CSF) in patients with metastatic melanoma recruits dendritic cells. *Cytokines Cell Mol Ther* 1999; 5: 139–144.
95. Bowne WB, Wolchok JD, Hawkins WG, et al. Injection of DNA encoding granulocyte-macrophage colony-stimulating factor recruits dendritic cells for immune adjuvant effects. *Cytokines Cell Mol Ther* 1999; 5: 217–225.
96. Przepiorka D, Srivastava PK. Heat shock protein—peptide complexes as immunotherapy for human cancer. *Mol Med Today* 1998; 4: 478–484.
97. Srivastava PK. Purification of heat shock protein-peptide complexes for use in vaccination against cancers and intracellular pathogens. *Methods* 1997; 12: 165–171.
98. Blachere NE, Srivastava PK. Heat shock protein-based cancer vaccines and related thoughts on immunogenicity of human tumors. *Semin Cancer Biol* 1995; 6: 349–355.
99. Srivastava PK, Udono H. Heat shock protein-peptide complexes in cancer immunotherapy. *Curr Opin Immunol* 1994; 6: 728–732.
100. Eton O, East MJ, Ross MI, et al. Autologous tumor-derived heat-shock protein peptide complex-96 (HSPPC-96) in patients (pts) with metastatic melanoma. *Proc Am Assoc Cancer Res* 2000; 41: 3463.
101. Vadhan-Raj S, Cordon-Cardo C, Carswell EA, et al. Phase I trial of a mouse monoclonal antibody against GD3 ganglioside in patients with melanoma: induction of inflammatory responses at tumor sites. *J Clin Oncol* 1988; 6: 1636–1648.
102. Bajorin DF, Chapman PB, Wong GY, et al. Treatment with high dose mouse monoclonal (anti-GD3) antibody R24 in patients with metastatic melanoma. *Melanoma Res* 1992; 2: 355–362.
103. Raymond J, Kirkwood J, Vlock D, et al. A phase Ib trial of murine monoclonal antibody R24 (anti-GD3) in metastatic melanoma. *Proc Am Soc Clin Oncol* 1991; 10: 298.
104. Dippold WG, Bernhard H, Dienes HP, Meyer zum Buschenfeld K-H. Treatment of patients with malignant melanoma by monoclonal ganglioside antibodies. *Eur J Cancer Clin Oncol* 1988; 24(suppl 2): 865–867.
105. Dippold W, Bernhard H, Meyer zum Buschenfelde KH. Immunological response to intrathecal and systemic treatment with ganglioside antibody R-24 in patients with malignant melanoma. *Eur J Cancer* 1994; 30A: 137–144.
106. Bukowski RM, Murthy SA, Finke J, et al. Phase I trial of cisplatin, WR-2721, and the murine monoclonal antibody R24 in patients with metastatic melanoma: clinical and biologic effects. *J Immunother* 1994; 15: 273–282.
107. Cheung N, Lazarus H, Miraldi F, et al. Ganglioside GD2 specific monoclonal antibody 3F8: a phase I study in patients with neuroblastoma and malignant melanoma [published erratum appears in *J Clin Oncol* 1992 April 10(4): 671]. *J Clin Oncol* 1987; 5: 1430–1440.
108. Cheung N-KV, Lazarus H, Miraldi FD, et al. Reassessment of patient response to monoclonal antibody 3F8. *J Clin Oncol* 1992; 10: 671–672.
109. Saleh MN, Khazaeli MB, Wheeler RH, et al. Phase I trial of murine monoclonal anti-GD2 antibody 14G2a in metastatic melanoma. *Cancer Res* 1992; 52: 4342–4347.
110. Murray JL, Cunningham JE, Brewer H, et al. Phase I trial of mouse monoclonal antibody 14G2a administered by prolonged intravenous infusion in patients with neuroectodermal tumors. *J Clin Oncol* 1994; 12: 184–193.

111. Saleh MN, Khazaeli MD, Wheeler RH, et al. Phase I trial of the chimeric anti-GD2 monoclonal antibody ch14.18 in patients with malignant melanoma. *Hum Antibodies Hybridomas* 1992; 3: 19–23.
112. Lichtin A, Iliopoulos D, Guerry D, Elder D, Herlyn D, Steplewski Z. Therapy of melanoma with an anti-melanoma ganglioside monoclonal antibody: a possible mechanism of a complete response. *Proc Am Soc Clin Oncol* 1988; 7: 247.
113. Lonberg M, Bajorin D, Cheung N-K, et al. Phase I trial of a combination of two mouse monoclonal antibodies anti-GD3 (R24) and anti-GD2 (3F8) in patients with melanoma and soft tissue sarcoma. *Proc Am Soc Clin Oncol* 1988; 7: 173.
114. Albertini M, Hank J, Schiller J, et al. Phase Ib trial of combined treatment with ch14.18 and R24 monoclonal antibodies and interleukin-2 for patients with melanoma or sarcoma. *Proc Am Soc Clin Oncol* 1998; 17: 437a.
115. Ritter G, Ritter-Boosfeld E, Adluri R, et al. Analysis of the antibody response to immunization with purified O-acetyl GD3 gangliosides in patients with malignant melanoma. *Int J Cancer* 1995; 62: 668–672.

7 Interleukin-2

James W. Mier, MD
and Michael B. Atkins, MD

CONTENTS

1. INTRODUCTION

Interleukin-2 (IL-2) is the first agent available for the treatment of metastatic cancer that functions solely through the activation of the immune system. IL-2 enhances several aspects of cellular immune function and induces tumor regression in numerous murine tumor models. Clinical investigations with recombinant IL-2 have demonstrated that it possesses significant antitumor activity, producing durable complete responses in a small percentage of patients with either metastatic melanoma or renal cell carcinoma. The high-dose intravenous bolus IL-2 regimen developed at the National Cancer Institute (NCI) Surgery Branch received Food and Drug Administration (FDA) approval for the treatment of metastatic renal cell carcinoma in 1992 and malignant melanoma in 1998. This chapter will review the in vitro effects of IL-2, the results of pertinent preclinical studies, and subsequent clinical investigations of IL-2-based regimens in patients with malignant melanoma.

From: *Current Clinical Oncology, Melanoma: Biologically Targeted Therapeutics*
Edited by: E. C. Borden © Humana Press Inc., Totowa, NJ

1.1. IL-2 and Its Receptor

In 1976, the conditioned medium of lectin-stimulated human peripheral blood mononuclear cells (PBMCs) was used to propagate indefinitely pre-activated human T cells ex vivo *(1)*. This initial description of what was then termed T cell growth factor (TCGF) was followed by the isolation, biochemical characterization, and ultimately, the cDNA cloning of the responsible lymphokine *(2,3)*. Subsequently designated IL-2, this factor was shown to be a 15-kDa polypeptide made up of 153 amino acids, the first 20 of which are proteolytically cleaved during secretion. Crystallographic analysis indicates that IL-2 is a spherical molecule comprised of 6 α helical regions.

The various effects of IL-2 are mediated through its binding to specific surface receptors (reviewed in ref. *4*). As is the case with IL-2 itself, the expression of high affinity IL-2 receptors (IL-2Rs) is induced in T cells as a result of an encounter with an antigenic peptide/major histocompatibility complex (MHC), which accommodates the clonotypic T cell antigen receptor (TCR). With the exception of a minor population of memory T cells, which presumably were activated in vivo by a prior antigen exposure, freshly isolated peripheral blood T cells do not constitutively express high affinity IL-2Rs *(5)*.

The high affinity IL-2R consists of three distinct subunits designated the α, β, and γ chains (Fig. 1). The α chain *(6)* is a 251 amino acid polypeptide with a large extracellular domain capable of binding IL-2 with low affinity, a transmembrane span, and a short 13 residue cytoplasmic tail, which is not involved in IL-2-induced signaling. The β chain has a 214 amino acid extracellular domain, a transmembrane motif, and a large 286 residue cytoplasmic tail absolutely essential for IL-2 signaling *(7)*. The IL-2R-β chain has paired cysteines at two sites within the extracellular domain and a perimembrane WSXWS motif, both of which are signature motifs of an enlarging cytokine receptor superfamily, which includes the receptors for IL-3, IL-4, IL-6, IL-7, granulocyte-macrophage colony-stimulating factor (GM-CSF), prolactin, erythropoietin, and growth hormone.

The novel 64 kDa γ chain is another member of the cytokine receptor superfamily *(8)*, which, when paired with the β chain, binds IL-2 with intermediate affinity. This receptor chain is shared by the receptors for several lymphokines, including IL-4, IL-7, IL-9, and IL-15, as well as IL-2 *(9)*. Mutations in the gene encoding this receptor chain account for most, if not all, cases of X-linked severe combined immunodeficiency *(10)*. The three chains together yield a high affinity IL-2R, which transduces signals and is internalized in response to IL-2 binding. Resting T cells constitutively express low levels of the IL-2R-γ chain, but not the α or β chains. All three chains are up-regulated as a result of antigenic stimulation. Resting natural killer (NK) cells constitutively express the β chain, and both the α and γ chains are induced in these cells by exposure to IL-2 or IL-12 *(11)*.

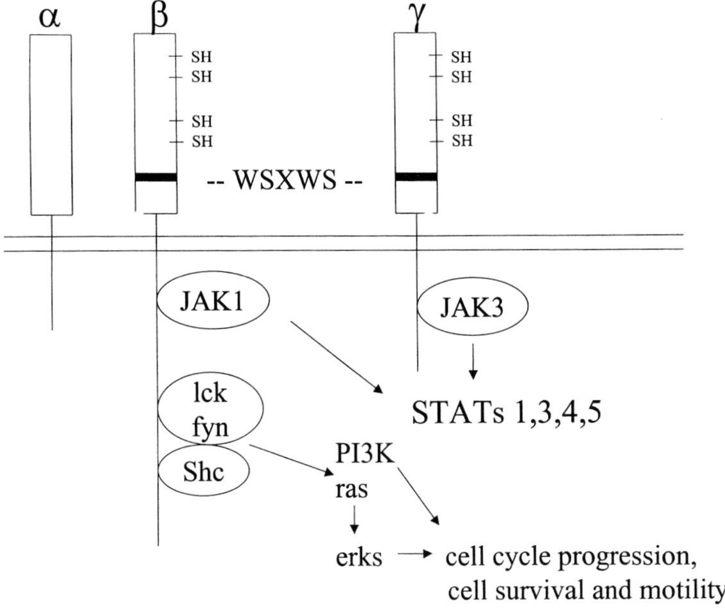

Fig. 1. The high affinity IL-2R and associated signaling pathways. The high affinity IL-2R is a heterotrimer consisting of α, β, and γ chains, the latter two of which are critically involved in the transmission of signals activated by IL-2 binding. Signaling pathways activated include several STATs and src-related protein tyrosine kinases, which are responsible for cell cycle progression, the regulation of motility, and susceptibility to apoptosis.

IL-2 induces the tyrosine phosphorylation of numerous cellular proteins, including the IL-2R-β chain itself. These events are transduced through kinases such as the *src* family member $p56^{lck}$ that physically associate with the cytoplasmic domains of the receptor subunits (Fig. 1) *(12,13)*. IL-2 also induces the recruitment and subsequent tyrosine phosphorylation of the adapter protein *Shc* to the IL-2R-β chain. This particular association is thought to be largely responsible for the activation of $p21^{ras}$ and the downstream microtubule-associated protein (MAP) kinases *erk-1* and *erk-2* in response to IL-2 *(14)*. In addition to the association with *src* family tyrosine kinases, both the β and γ receptor chains associate with members of the Janus kinase (JAK) family of tyrosine kinases *(15)*. JAK3, for example, associates with the IL-2R-γ chain, whereas both JAK1 and JAK2 associate with the β chain. JAKs activate various members of the signal transduction and activators of transcription (STAT) family of transcription factors. The binding of IL-2 to its receptor on antigen-primed T cells results in the phosphorylation and activation of STAT1, STAT3, and STAT5. In NK cells, STAT4 is also activated by IL-2 *(16)*.

1.2. In Vitro Effects of IL-2

In addition to its proliferative effects, IL-2 induces the synthesis of an array of secondary cytokines such as IL-1, tumor necrosis factor (TNF), IL-6, and lymphotoxin *(17)*, several of which are detectable in the circulation of cancer patients receiving IL-2 and thought to contribute to IL-2-induced tumor regression and toxicity *(18)*. The biological effect of IL-2, arguably most pertinent to its use as an antitumor agent, may be its ability to enhance the cytolytic activity of antigen-specific cytotoxic T lymphocyte (CTL) cells and NK cells *(19,20)*. In addition to increasing the cytolytic activity of these cells for their respective targets, IL-2 markedly diversifies the range of target cells these effectors are able to kill *(21,22)*. Indeed, human peripheral blood lymphocytes exposed only to high concentrations of IL-2 without prior exposure to tumor cells are able to kill virtually all tumor cell lines and most freshly isolated tumor cells in vitro regardless of the particular human leukocyte antigen (HLA) class I alleles expressed by the target cell. The cells responsible for this HLA-unrestricted killing in response to IL-2 have been termed "lymphokine-activated killer" or LAK cells *(21,22)* and appear to be a mixture of activated NK cells and $CD3^+/CD8^+$ cytotoxic T cells. As described below, these ex vivo-activated LAK cells featured prominently in the early clinical trials carried out with IL-2 in cancer patients.

1.3. Preclinical Studies with IL-2 in Tumor-Bearing Mice

IL-2 has been extensively evaluated as an antitumor agent in a variety of murine tumor models. The lymphokine has been used alone, in combination with other cytokines, and in conjunction with various adoptively transferred, ex vivo-activated lymphoid preparations to eradicate a wide range of local and metastatic tumors. Early studies demonstrated that IL-2 used alone could reduce or eliminate pulmonary metastases from melanoma and methylcholanthrene-induced sarcoma cell lines and that this antitumor effect was strictly dependent on the dose of IL-2 administered *(23)*. In more recent studies, in which mice were immunized with dendritic cells pulsed with tumor lysates, the concurrent systemic administration of IL-2 was shown to enhance the efficacy of the vaccine *(24)*. In several studies, the effects of IL-2 could be enhanced by the concurrent administration of LAK cells generated by culturing splenocytes ex vivo in IL-2-containing media *(25)*. Mice bearing B16 melanoma pulmonary metastases, for example, are highly responsive to treatment with the combination of IL-2 and LAK cells *(26)*. Lymphocytes present within tumor infiltrates are enriched for effector cells capable of killing tumor cells *(27,28)*, and, when isolated and tested in vitro for cytolytic activity against autologous tumor cells, these tumor-infiltrating lymphocytes (TILs) are 50- to 100-fold more potent than IL-2-activated splenocytes (LAK cells). Several studies have demonstrated the efficacy of TIL/IL-2 in the eradication of disseminated malignancy *(27,28)*.

2. CLINICAL APPLICATIONS OF IL-2

2.1. High-Dose IL-2 Administered as Intravenous Bolus Injections

The encouraging results of studies with tumor-bearing mice prompted the rapid movement of IL-2 into the clinical setting. Early clinical trials were initiated prior to the availability of recombinant material and involved modest doses of highly purified T cell-derived IL-2, the administration of which produced transient fever and lymphopenia, but no sustained ill effects or tumor responses *(29,30)*. The advent of recombinant IL-2 allowed much higher doses to be administered. In order to facilitate comparisons between the various studies reviewed in this and subsequent sections, we have listed all IL-2 doses in International Units (IU) using the following conversion ratios: 1 Cetus Unit = 6 IU; 1 Hoffman-LaRoche Unit = 1 Biologics Response Modifier Program (BRMP) Unit = 2.6 IU *(31)*.

The high dose intravenous bolus IL-2 therapy currently in use at many institutions was initially pioneered by the NCI Surgery Branch in the mid-1980s. This regimen was based on data from previously cited murine studies demonstrating that tumor responses to IL-2 were dose-dependent and enhanced when the daily dosage of IL-2 was divided over 3 daily doses or when IL-2 was combined with LAK cells. The early clinical trials performed at the NCI Surgery Branch established the toxicity, management guidelines, and maximum tolerated dose for the high-dose bolus regimen when administered either alone or in combination with autologous LAK cells *(32,33)*. In the regimen developed at the NCI, IL-2 (Cetus/Chiron) was administered at 600,000–720,000 IU/kg intravenously every 8 h for d 1–5 and 11–15 of a treatment course. In those cases in which LAK cells were given, the cells were prepared from leukapheresis-derived PBMCs obtained on d 8,9, and 11 and administered with IL-2 on d 12,13, and 15. A maximum of 28–30 IL-2 doses per course was administered; however, doses were frequently withheld for excessive toxicity. Treatment courses were repeated at 8- to 12-wk intervals in responding patients. This IL-2 regimen administered either alone or in combination with LAK cells produced overall tumor responses in 15 to 20% of patients with metastatic melanoma in clinical trials conducted at either the NCI Surgery Branch or within the Cytokine Working Group (formerly Extramural IL-2 and LAK Working Group). Complete responses were noted in 4–6% of patients and were frequently durable *(30,34–37)*.

Long-term follow-up data are now available on metastatic melanoma patients that participated in these early high-dose bolus IL-2 trials. These data confirm the efficacy of IL-2 in at least a minority of patients. We recently analyzed data on 270 patients that were treated on the 8 high-dose IL-2 trials conducted between 1985 and 1993 *(37,38)*. Data were initially analyzed through the fall of 1996 *(37)* and then updated through December, 1998 *(38)*. Although this study population was highly selected for excellent organ function and the absence of central nervous system (CNS) metastases or significant cardiovascular disease, it included

Table 1
High-Dose Intravenous Bolus IL-2 Alone Therapy

Author (reference)	*Dose*	*Patients no: evaluable*	*Response*		*Total (%)*	*Comments*
			CR	*PR*		
Atkins et al. *(67)*	600,000–720,000 IU/kg IL-2 (Chiron) IV every 8 h d 1–5 and 15–19.	305	19 (6%)	28 (9%)	47/305 (15%)	5 patients received 360–540,000 IU/kg of IL-2.

IL-2, Interleukin-2; IV, intravenous; IU, International Units.
Adapted from Atkins, Shet, and Sosman *(67)*.

a large percentage of individuals with other poor prognostic features such as visceral metastases, multiple metastatic sites, and/or prior systemic therapy. Objective responses were seen in 43 (16%) patients (95% confidence interval [CI]: 12 to 21%) including 17 (6%) complete responses and 26 (10%) partial responses (Table 1). Responses were noted in all disease sites, including lung, liver, lymph nodes, soft tissue, adrenal, bone, and subcutaneous tissue, and were observed in some patients with large tumor burdens or bulky individual lesions. Ten of 17 complete responses (59%) and two of 26 partial responses (8%) were ongoing at >42 to >122 mo. Progression-free survival for these 12 patients ranged from >70 to >150 mo. The median duration of response for all responders was 8.9 mo (range 1.5 – >122 mo), and 28% of these responding patients remained free of disease progression (Fig. 2). The median duration of complete responses had yet to be reached and exceeded 59 mo. No patient responding for longer than 30 mo exhibited disease recurrence or progression, suggesting that some patients may actually have been "cured" of their disease.

Responses were less frequent in patients with baseline Eastern Cooperative Oncology Group (ECOG) performance status of 1 or greater or in those who had received prior systemic therapy. Involvement of multiple organ sites or visceral metastases did not reduce the likelihood of treatment benefit. Five additional responding patients (1 complete response [CR] and 4 partial response [PR]), who developed an isolated site of progression that was amenable to local therapy, were alive and free of disease at >79 and >104 mo following IL-2 therapy, suggesting a role for regional salvage treatment in patients who develop isolated site relapse after a response to IL-2 therapy. Overall, 31 (11%) were alive at last contact. The median survival (Kaplan-Meyer) for the entire treated population was 12 mo (Fig. 3). Nineteen (44%) of the responding patients remained alive, all having survived more than 5 yr. The six deaths (2.2%) that occurred during these trials were all related to infections and occurred prior to 1991 *(39)*, after which prophylactic antibiotics were routinely incorporated into the treatment protocol.

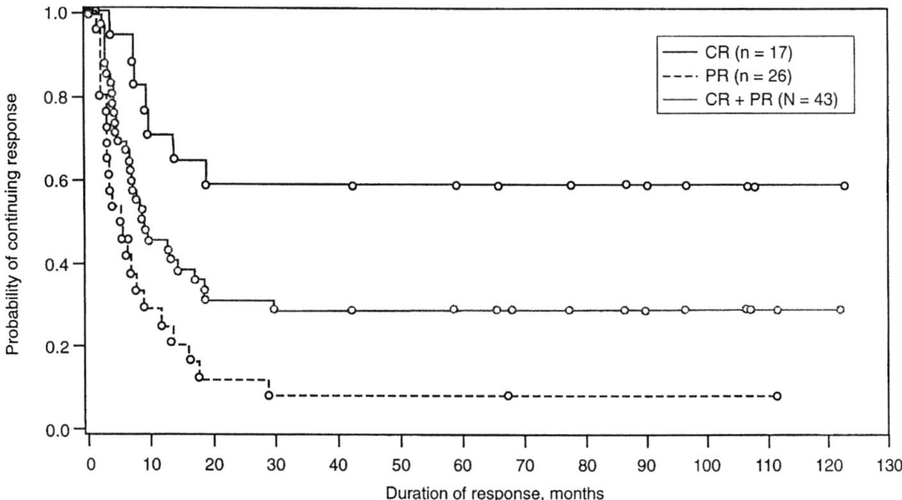

Fig. 2. Kaplan-Meier estimate of response durations for patients with metastatic melanoma exhibiting a complete or partial response to high-dose intravenous bolus IL-2. Adapted with permission from ref. *38*.

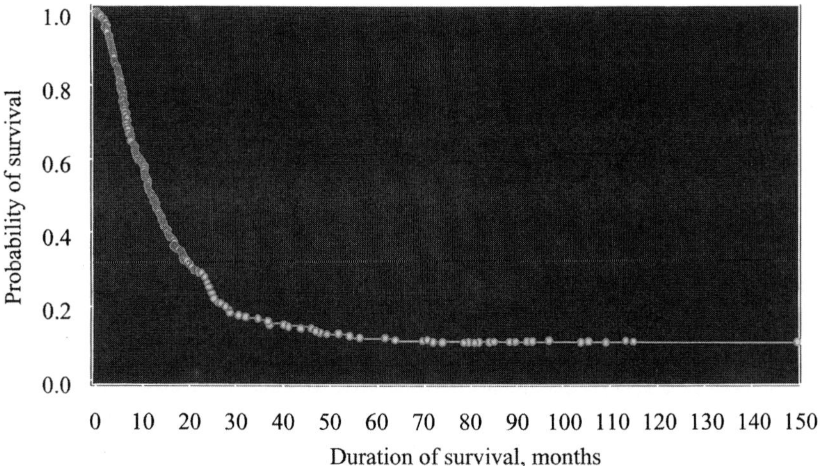

Fig. 3. Kaplan-Meier estimate of overall survival for patients with metastatic melanoma treated with high-dose intravenous bolus IL-2 ($N = 270$). Adapted with permission from ref. *37*.

Rosenberg et al. has reported long-term follow-up data on 409 patients (182 with metastatic melanoma, 217 with renal cell carcinoma) treated with high-dose intravenous bolus IL-2 alone at the NCI Surgery Branch *(40)* between September, 1985 and November, 1996. All patients received 720,000 IU of IL-2 (Cetus/Chiron) every 8 h for a maximum of 15 doses per cycle as clinically tolerated. Some of these patients received a polyethylene glycol (PEG)-conjugated form of IL-2 during the second treatment cycle. These patients fared no differently than those receiving conventional high-dose bolus IL-2 *(41)*. All but 35 of these patients were included in the data set described above (*see* Table 1). Complete regression was observed in 12 (6.6%) of the 182 patients with metastatic melanoma; partial regression occurred in 15 (8.2%) patients. Ten (6%) patients with melanoma exhibited ongoing continuous CR from 83 to 161 + mo from the onset of treatment. In this population, CR was significantly more frequent in patients who had not received prior immunotherapy. Only 2% of previously treated patients achieved a CR. The CRs tended to occur in patients that received a relatively large fraction of the scheduled doses and whose lymphocyte counts had the highest rebound at the completion of the first cycle of IL-2.

2.2. IL-2 Administered at Lower Doses or by Alternative Schedules

The toxicity of high-dose intravenous bolus IL-2 and the expense associated with the obligatory hospitalization of patients receiving this form of therapy have provided impetus for the development of alternative regimens using lower doses of IL-2. Several such regimens involving IL-2 administered either by lower dose intravenous bolus, continuous infusion, or subcutaneous injection have since been evaluated. Generally, treatment schedules using lower doses of IL-2 allow more prolonged treatment. IL-2 administered this way expands the number and enhances the function of circulating NK cells *(42,43)*. Antibody-dependent cellular cytotoxicity (ADCC) and NK/LAK cell activity are increased by relatively low and less toxic doses of IL-2 *(42–45)*. Unfortunately, these immunologic parameters do not correlate with the antitumor effect observed, which in the case of melanoma are often inferior to those achieved with high doses. The results of these various high dose and intermediate dose continuous infusion IL-2 alone regimens, in patients with metastatic melanoma, are summarized in Table 2 and described in detail below.

The alternative IL-2 regimen is currently the most widely used. This treatment consisted of IL-2 administered at 18 MIU/m^2/d by continuous infusion on d 1–5 and 11–15 with or without LAK cells *(46)*. The IL-2/LAK cell regimen produced tumor responses in 5 of 10 (50%) of evaluable patients with melanoma *(46)*. Toxicity was still significant, but generally felt to be more predictable and manageable than with the high-dose intravenous bolus IL-2 schedule developed by the NCI Surgery Branch. The National Biotherapy Study Group (NBSG) studied this continuous infusion IL-2 regimen omitting the LAK cells. Objective responses were seen in 33 of 188 (18%) patients with melanoma *(47)*. An alternative sched ule, which combined bolus and continuous infusion IL-2, was subsequently explored. In this schedule, a total of 90 MIU/m^2 of IL-2 was administered over

Table 2
Continuous Infusion and Low-Dose IL-2 Alone Regimens

IL-2 Administration route/dose level	N	*CR plus PR*	*Response rate (%)*
High-dose continuous infusion	219	40	18
Hybrid (bolus plus continuous infusion)	18	4	22
Low-dose IV or subcutaneous	95	1	1

Adapted from Atkins, Shet, and Sosman *(67)*.

3 instead of 5 d *(48)*. Treatment was administered every 2 wk for 2 mo. Twenty-two patients with melanoma were enrolled, of which 18 had measurable disease. Two patients achieved a CR and another two were PRs (22% overall response rate [RR]; 95% CI of 6–48%). Additional studies of this regimen and long-term follow-up data on the first patients to receive this form of immunotherapy have yet to be reported.

A slightly lower dose of IL-2 (12 MIU/m^2/d) administered by continuous infusion for 4 d on 4 consecutive wk *(49)*. Out of 31 patients, 1 CR and 6 PR for a 22% overall RR (10–41%; 95% CI) resulted. Toxicity was sufficiently mild to allow these patients to be managed on a general hospital ward. Responses lasted from 4–18+ mo. Finally, a regimen using IL-2 at 20 MIU/m^2 for d 1–5, 15–18, and 29–31 was investigated. While toxicity was significant, 8 responses were reported among 24 patients with metastatic melanoma *(50)*. However, 4 of the responses were very transient, lasting less than 1 mo. In summary, the available data suggest that continuous infusion regimens may be comparable to high-dose bolus IL-2 in terms of response rates. However, the long-term follow-up experience with these regimens raises concerns about the durability of these responses. In one study, only 10 of 175 patients (6%) with melanoma and only 25% of the complete responders survived for greater than 3 yr *(51)*.

Several investigators have evaluated still lower dose regimens, which could be safely administered in an outpatient setting. The results achieved with various low dose IL-2 treatment regimens are summarized in Table 2. For example, a low-dose outpatient regimen in which IL-2 was administered at 1.8 MIU/m^2/d by continuous infusion, 24 h/d for 3 consecutive wk (21 d) *(52)*. While toxicity was quite manageable, no responses were observed in the 15 melanoma patients included in their phase II study *(53)*. The Southwest Oncology Group (SWOG) recently explored a regimen in which low doses of IL-2 were administered weekly by bolus injection to patients with metastatic melanoma *(54)*. This regimen produced significant short-term side effects but virtually no antitumor activity. Together, these results suggest that the minimum dose of IL-2 capable of inducing disease regression in even a minority of melanoma patients may exceed that which could be safely administered in an outpatient setting. Very low dose, outpatient IL-2 regimens appear to be completely inactive in metastatic melanoma. Although conventional high-dose bolus IL-2 has not been formally compared with less intensive regimens in randomized trials, the frequency, durability, and quality of the responses noted in melanoma patients treated as outpatients are sufficiently discouraging so as to eliminate any incentive to carry out such large-scale phase III trials.

2.3. Toxicity of IL-2 Therapy

The utility of high-dose IL-2 has been limited by its toxicity, many features of which resemble bacterial sepsis. IL-2 side effects are dose-dependent and, fortunately, predictable and reversible. Common side effects include fever, chills, lethargy, diarrhea, nausea, anemia, thrombocytopenia, eosinophilia, diffuse erythroderma, hepatic dysfunction, and confusion *(55,56)*. Myocarditis also occurs in approximately 5% of patients. IL-2 therapy routinely causes a "capillary leak syndrome" characterized by peripheral edema, hypotension, adult respiratory distress syndrome (ARDS), and pre-renal azotemia. As a consequence of these side effects, few patients are able to receive all of the therapy scheduled in high dose regimens. IL-2 produces a neutrophil chemotactic defect that predisposes patients to infection with gram positive and occasionally gram negative bacteria *(39,55,56)*. Prior to the discovery of this defect, high-dose IL-2 treatment was associated with 2–4% mortality, largely related to infection or cardiac toxicity *(37,42,55,56)*. The routine use of antibiotic prophylaxis, more extensive cardiac screening, and the more judicious IL-2 administration have greatly enhanced the safety of this therapy. Since 1990, the mortality rates at experienced treatment centers have been less than 1% *(57)*. Nonetheless, the considerable toxicity of the high-dose IL-2 regimen has continued to limit its application to highly selected patients with excellent performance status and adequate organ function treated at medical centers with considerable experience with this approach.

As expected, lower dose IL-2 regimens have been generally better tolerated. Side effects have consisted of flu-like symptoms, erythroderma, and fluid retention. The more worrisome pulmonary, renal, cardiac, and hepatic side effects are usually not seen in patients receiving low-dose regimens. Unfortunately, this reduction in toxicity may be associated with an even more dramatic fall off in clinical efficacy, limiting the use of such lower dose regimens.

2.4. IL-2 Toxicity Reduction Strategies

IL-2 is a potent inducer of pro-inflammatory cytokines such as IL-1, TNFα, and interferon gamma (IFNγ) *(17,18,32,58)*. These substances and others, including nitric oxide (NO) *(59)*, may play a role in IL-2 toxicity. To the extent that this is the case, one would expect that suppression of the synthesis of these mediators or selective neutralization of their biological activities might enhance the therapeutic index of IL-2 by dissociating its toxic effects from its antitumor effects.

A number of such toxicity dissociation approaches have been tried with limited success. Most of these approaches have utilized the high-dose intravenous bolus IL-2 schedule described previously. The addition of dexamethasone to this regimen, for example, prevented the induction of circulating TNF and significantly reduced treatment-related fever and hypotension, allowing for a threefold increase in the maximum tolerated dose *(60)*. However, potential interference with the antitumor efficacy of IL-2 by glucocorticoids limited this approach *(60,61)* and highlighted the need for more selective ways of inhibiting the effects of secondary cytokines released in response to IL-2.

More recent investigations have involved the concomitant administration of IL-2 with soluble neutralizing receptors to TNF (sTNFR:IgG) or IL-1 (sIL-1R) or TNF or IL-1 signal transduction inhibitors of the methylxanthine class (e.g., pentoxifylline or CT1501R) *(62–65)*. Several of these approaches showed significant promise in animal models and were able to inhibit some of the biologic effects associated with high-dose IL-2 in patients without interfering with antitumor effects. In fact, responses were seen in 9 (5 CR and 4 PR) of 45 patients (20%) with metastatic melanoma treated as part of these clinical trials *(66,67)*. Unfortunately, none of these agents was able to significantly block IL-2 toxicity as measured by the incidence of hypotension, the use of pressors, or the number of IL-2 doses that could be administered. These results indicate that multiple factors, including a variety of pro-inflammatory cytokines or possibly direct interactions of activated lymphocytes with the vascular endothelium may be responsible for the dose-limiting side effects of IL-2. If such were the case, the neutralization of individual cytokines such as TNF or IL-1 with soluble cytokine receptors would be unlikely to abrogate toxicity.

The tetravalent guanylhydrazone compound CNI-1493 blocks the synthesis of numerous pro-inflammatory cytokines such as TNF and IL-1 through the inhibition of the P38 MAP kinase signaling pathway. At high concentrations, it inhibits lipopolysaccharide- and IFNγ-induced NO production by blocking L-arginine uptake *(68,69)*. This compound is selectively taken up by monocytes and, therefore, has no effect on lymphocyte function or activation. Preclinical experiments suggested that CNI-1493 can broadly block by-products of macrophage activation that may contribute significantly to the toxicity of IL-2 without interfering directly with lymphocyte activation by IL-2. In fact, in a rat hepatoma model, the use of CNI-1493 allowed the administration of IL-2 at doses 10-fold higher than the maximum tolerated dose and protected the animals from toxicity while enhancing the antitumor effects of IL-2 *(70)*. Unfortunately, early clinical trials with this compound have failed to reproduce these preclinical findings. Although a reduction in IL-2-induced hepatic enzyme abnormalities was observed, other IL-2 related toxicities were unaffected by CNI-1493 (Atkins et al., manuscript in preparation).

Another potentially promising approach involves the use of agents that block NO production. NO produced by endothelial cells is one of the major regulators of vascular tone and blood pressure. Kilbourn and colleagues have shown that the NO synthase inhibitor N-methyl arginine was able to rapidly reverse the hypotension induced by high-dose IL-2 in patients with metastatic renal cell carcinoma *(71)*. Additional clinical trials of this agent in combination with IL-2 are in progress.

2.5. Potential Correlates of Response and Resistance

Because of the toxicity of high-dose IL-2 and the fact that only a small minority of patients respond to IL-2-based immunotherapy, several investigators have attempted to identify factors predicting responsiveness to IL-2. As mentioned previously, in the 270 patient database presented to the FDA, tumor response was significantly associated with a baseline ECOG performance status of 0 and the absence of prior systemic therapy *(37)*. There was no association of response with the number of metastatic sites or the amount of therapy administered. Likewise, in the NCI Surgery Branch database, achievement of complete response correlated with the absence of prior immunotherapy. In this analysis, the total dose of IL-2 administered and the degree of rebound lymphocytosis after cessation of IL-2 also correlated with response *(40)*.

In a recent French multicenter study involving patients treated with either IL-2 alone (19 patients), IL-2 plus IFNα (29 patients) or cisplatin (CDDP)/IL-2/IFNα (33 patients), tumor response was shown to correlate inversely with pretreatment levels of IL-6, cAMP-receptor protein (CRP), and lactate dehydrogenase (LDH) *(72)*. In a multivariate analysis, a low baseline serum CRP level and disease confined to skin, subcutaneous tissue, or lymph nodes (Mla) were most predictive of response and survival. In another analysis of 65 patients treated with IL-2 and IFNα, high serum LDH, poor performance status, and large tumor burdens were associated with poor response to treatment and poor overall survival *(73)*.

Several studies have documented correlations between tumor response and the development of vitiligo *(74)* and other autoimmune phenomenon such as thyroid dysfunction *(75)*. Vitiligo has been the most extensively studied and, in one recent study, was observed in 11 of 74 patients with melanoma who were followed for greater than 1 yr after receiving high-dose IL-2 *(74)*. Of note was the fact that it was noted only in patients exhibiting an objective tumor response. None of 27 nonresponding patients with melanoma followed for 1 yr developed vitiligo ($p = 0.0002$). Vitligo did not develop in patients receiving IL-2 for metastatic renal cell cancer, suggesting that a relative abundance of melanocyte derived antigens might be a critical factor in the induction of specific T cell immunity to pigmented cells during IL-2 treatment.

Many groups have attempted to correlate responses to IL-2 treatment with HLA phenotype. The NCI Surgery Branch, for example, reported an association between tumor response and the HLA-A11 and A19 alleles, especially in patients receiving IL-2 with TIL *(76,77)*. HLA-DR4 expression was associated with increased IL-2 toxicity *(77)*. However, these associations were not as strong or convincing in subsequent analyses that included larger numbers of patients *(78)*. Another study correlated HLA-DQI expression with tumor response ($p = 0.0017$) and survival ($p = 0.026$) *(79)*. Finally, Scheibenbogen et al. noted that HLA-CW7 and HLA-A1 phenotypes were more frequent in patients who responded to IL-2 and IFN *(80)*. In general, it has been difficult to confirm the correlations between these various HLA phenotypes and either antitumor response or the severity of side effects. As a consequence, the use of HLA phenotype as an eligibility criterion for access to IL-2-based immunotherapy does not appear justified.

Resistance to IL-2 therapy has been postulated to be due to a number of factors including the induction of apoptosis in activated tumor-infiltrating T cells as a result of tumor cell expression of Fas ligand *(81)* or T cell dysfunction due to diminished expression of the T cell antigen receptor ζ chain and other signaling components *(82)*. Of note, Rabinowich et al. have shown that these T cell receptor abnormalities can be reversed by IL-2 immunotherapy and that such reversal may correlate with tumor response *(83)*. Additional, correlative laboratory studies performed in conjunction with current and future clinical trials will be necessary to sort out the importance of these various molecular phenomena to the antitumor effects of IL-2.

3. IL-2 IN COMBINATION WITH OTHER BIOLOGIC RESPONSE MODIFIERS

3.1. IL-2 in Combination with IFNα

The decision to investigate the antitumor effects of IL-2/IFNα combinations is based on an abundance of persuasive preclinical laboratory and animal studies *(84–87)*. Investigations involving various combinations of IL-2 and IFNα are summarized in Table 3. In one of the first dose escalation phase I/II clinical trials assessing the combination intravenous bolus IL-2 at 2.6–12 MIU/m^2 per dose and intravenous IFNα at 3–6 MU/m^2 per dose (Hoffmann-LaRoche) every 8 h on d 1–5 and 15–19 was administered to 91 patients, 39 of whom had metastatic melanoma *(88)*. Tumor responses were seen in 25 patients (7 CR, 18 PR) including in 13 patients with metastatic melanoma (3 CR, 10 PR). The response rate was as high as 41% among the 27 patients treated at the highest doses of IL-2 (12 MIU/m^2) and IFNα (6 MU). Toxicity was similar to that seen with high-dose IL-2 alone regimens, except for a higher than expected incidence of cardiac and neurologic toxicity. In 1995, Marincola and colleagues published long-term fol-

Table 3
IL-2 and IFNα Containing Treatment Regimens

IL-2 Administration route/dose level	N	*CR/PR*	*Response rate (%)*
High-dose bolus	217	12/36	22
Continuous infusion	259	6/33	15
Subcutaneous injection	51	0/3	6

Adapted from Atkins, Shet, and Sosman *(67)*.

low-up data of the NCI Surgery Branch experience using the combination of IL-2 and IFNα. This update included data from 189 patients, of which 82 had melanoma *(89)*. The response rate was 24% (20/82) in the patients with melanoma. However, of the 20 patients with melanoma that responded to the IL-2/IFN combination, only one was a long-term progression-free survivor. The investigators concluded that this combined regimen provided no obvious benefit relative to high-dose bolus IL-2 alone.

The Cytokine Working Group (CWG) performed a randomized phase III comparison of intravenous bolus IL-2 with or without IFNα. In this study, IL-2 was administered 3 times daily for 5 d, either alone at 6 MU/m^2/dose (16 MIU/m^2) or at 4.5 MU/m^2/dose (12.6 MIU/m^2) in combination with IFNα at 3 MU/m^2/dose *(90)*. As with the NCI Surgery Branch study, both the IL-2 and IFNα were supplied by Hoffmann-LaRoche. The toxicities of these regimens were equivalent. Eighty-five patients were enrolled, with 44 being randomized to IL-2 alone and 41 to IL-2 plus IFNα, respectively. Responses were seen in only 6 patients—2 of 44 (5%) patients receiving IL-2 alone and 4 of 41 (10%) patients receiving both IL-2 and IFNα. There were no complete responses on either arm. The study was terminated early due to the disappointing results on both arms. However, as with the other trials, it was clear that the addition of IFNα failed to result in a meaningful improvement over standard regimens involving high-dose IL-2 alone.

Two alternative IL-2/IFN regimens have also been explored. Patients received IFNα 10 MU/m^2/d subcutaneously for 5 d, followed by IL-2 administered either by a 5-d continuous infusion at 18 MIU/m^2/d or in accordance with a "decrescendo" schedule, in which IL-2 was administered at 18 MIU/m^2 over 6 h, followed by 18 MIU/m^2 over 12 h, 18 MIU/m^2 over 24 h, and finally a maintenance dose of 4.5 MIU/m^2/d for 72 h *(91)*. This decrescendo regimen was designed both to induce optimal IL-2 receptor expression and to minimize toxicity by avoiding the induction of high circulating levels of secondary cytokines. The 18 MIU/m^2/d IL-2 schedule produced 5 responses in 27 patients (1 CR and 4 PR; 18% RR; 6–36%; 95% CI), while the decrescendo IL-2 schedule yielded 11 responses in 27 patients (3 CR, 8 PR; 41% RR; 22–61%; 95% CI) and an impressive 17-mo median survival. Twenty-two percent of patients whose disease had progressed following dacarbazine (DTIC) chemotherapy responded to the decrescendo IL-2/IFN regimen. In addition to this encouraging antitumor activity, this regimen had a more favorable toxicity profile than the more conventional continuous infusion schedule. The European Organization for Research and Treatment of Cancer (EORTC) Melanoma Cooperative Group recently conducted a large-scale phase III randomized trial assessing the effect of adding cisplatin to the aforementioned decrescendo IL-2/IFNα regimen *(92)*. Of the 66 patients assigned to the IL-2/IFNα alone arm, 18% responded (4 CR and 8 PR). Although this response rate was less than that of the cisplatin/IL-2/IFNα combination arm, overall and progression-free survival were equivalent for both limbs of the study.

Investigators at M.D. Anderson recently evaluated the effects of adding IFNα to their previously described continuous infusion IL-2 regimen. They observed only 2 PR out of 23 patients (8% RR; 1–28%; 95% CI) *(93)*. In a large phase II multicenter Netherlands-based trial, 57 patients with melanoma were treated with IL-2 at 7.8 MIU/m^2/d (Hoffmann-LaRoche) by continuous infusion and IFNα at 6 MU administered subcutaneously on d 1–4 every 2 wk. Responses were seen in 16% of the 51 evaluable patients (8 responses; 1 CR, 7 PR) *(94)*. A similar regimen utilizing IL-2 (Hoffmann-LaRoche) at 5.2 MIU/m^2/d plus IFNα was explored with no responses noted in 14 melanoma patients *(95)*. Likewise, no responses occurred among 15 patients with melanoma treated with a similar regimen, in which IL-2 was administered by subcutaneous injection *(96)*.

Finally, 3 times weekly, IFNα with low-dose IL-2 (60,000 IU/kg) was administered as an intravenous bolus injection every 8 h for up to 14 doses on d 1–5 and 15–19 *(97)*. Among 38 evaluable patients, 6 responses were observed with 1 CR and 5 PR (15% RR; 4–27%; 95% CI). Three of the 6 responses were over 12 mo in duration, with 2 ongoing at 26+ and 40+ mo.

Despite promising preclinical data, there is presently no convincing evidence suggesting that IL-2 and IFNα combinations are inherently superior to high-dose IL-2 alone. Nonetheless, because some IL-2 and IFNα combinations have demonstrated an improved therapeutic index relative to high-dose IL-2, this combination has provided a more suitable building block for clinical trials using IL-2 in combination with other biologic agents or cytotoxic chemotherapy.

3.2. IL-2 in Combination with Other Immune Activating Agents

A variety of clinical trials evaluating IL-2 in combination with immune modulators other than IFNα have been performed, and the results of these studies are described in Table 4. A few trials have examined combinations of IFNγ and IL-2. IFNγ activates macrophages and granulocytes and enhances MHC class I and II and tumor antigen expression. The NCI Surgery Branch evaluated the antitumor effects of IFNγ administered prior to standard high-dose intravenous bolus IL-2 *(98)*. Some of the study patients also received TIL. Only 2 of the 20 patients enrolled in this study (and none of the 5 receiving TIL) responded.

Table 4
IL-2 with Other Immune Activating Agents

		Interleukin-2			Results			
						Response		
Author date	*Reference*	*Dose*	*Route*	*Other agent*	*Melanoma*	*CR*	*PR*	*RR (%)*
Viens et al. 1992	*99*	8 MIU/m^2	IVBQ8H	IFNγ 1 × 10^6 IU/m^2 escalating doses	11	1	1	8%
Thatcher et al. 1990	*109*	11 MIU/m^2	IVQOD[a]	FAA 4.8 gm/m^2	34	1	4	15%
O'Reilly et al. 1993	*110*	6–18 MIU/m^2/d	IV CI	FAA 4.8 gm/m^2	21	1	2	14%
Kim et al. 1995	*98*	720,000 IU/kg	IVBQ8H	IFNγ	20	1	1	10%
				IFNγ plus TIL	5	0	0	
Ahmed et al. 1996	*107*	3 MIU/m^2/d	SQ	Levamisole 50 mg tid	18		1	12%
		5.4 MIU/m^2/d escalating doses	SQ	Levamisole 50 mg tid with or without	21		1	12%
Olencki et al. 1996	*101*	3, 12, 48 MIU/m^2	IV 3 times/wk	IL-4 40, 120, 400 μg/m^2	39	0	2	5%
Creagan et al. 1997	*104*	3 MIU/m^2/d	SQ	Levamisole 50 mg/m^2 tid PO	19	0	0	0

[a]Adapted from Atkins, Shet, and Sosman *(67)*. IU, international units; MIU, million international units; IVBQ8H, intravenous bolus every 8 h; IVQOD, intravenous every other day; SQ, subcutaneous; CR, complete response; PR, partial response; RR, response rate.

Other phase I trials assessing IFNγ combined with lower dose, more protracted, IL-2 schedules in patients with melanoma were equally disappointing *(99,100)*.

Several investigators have explored IL-2 in combination with IL-4 *(101,102)*. The rationale for this combination is the known ability of IL-4 to enhance tumor-specific T cell responses and nonspecific NK/LAK cell-mediated cytotoxicity. Thus far, studies with this cytokine combination have been disappointing, in that only a few tumor responses and minimal enhancement of the immunomodulatory effects of IL-2 have been noted. While IL-4 continues to be of interest as a growth factor to be used in combination with GM-CSF to propagate ex vivo dendritic cells for use in vitro or in vaccine development *(103)*, studies involving IL-4/IL-2 combinations as treatment for overt metastatic malignancy have not been further pursued.

The Mayo Clinic has investigated a combination of IL-2 with levamisole, an antiparasitic agent purported to have immunostimulatory properties *(104)*. Levamisole has shown potential benefit as an adjuvant to surgical resection in patients with high-risk melanoma *(105,106)*. Unfortunately, a phase II trial of subcutaneous IL-2 and levamisole demonstrated no objective responses in 19 melanoma patients treated with this combination *(104)*. In a similar study carried out at the Royal Marsden Hospital by Ahmed et al. using subcutaneous IL-2 at 3 and 5.4 MIU/m^2/d with or without levamisole, responses were seen only in those patients receiving IL-2 without levamisole *(107)*, suggesting that the combination offers little advantage over IL-2 alone.

Flavone-8-acetic acid (FAA) activates NK cell activity and, when given with IL-2, exerts synergistic antitumor effects in animal tumor models *(108)*. Based on these preclinical data, Thatcher and colleagues performed a phase II trial of IL-2 in combination with FAA in patients with metastatic melanoma *(109)*. In this study, IL-2 was first administered via a femoral catheter intrasplenically and then by intravenous bolus on alternate days while FAA was administered intravenously as a 6-h infusion prior to the IL-2. Five responses, including 1 CR, were observed among the 34 study patients. Responses occurred mainly in nonvisceral sites. The authors felt that this response rate was not significantly better than IL-2 alone. O'Reilly explored the use of FAA in combination with continuous infusion IL-2 and observed 3 responses (1 CR, 2 PR) in the 21 study patients (overall response rate of 14%), again suggesting no advantage over IL-2 alone *(110)*.

Several investigators have recently become interested in the combination of IL-2 with histamine *(111)*. This biogenic amine can inhibit monocyte-derived oxygen free radical formation. Some investigators believe that monocyte free radical formation inhibits T cell and NK cell tumoricidal activity, hence the rationale for the combination. A randomized trial of IL-2 plus histamine versus IL-2 alone, in patients with metastatic melanoma, has recently been completed and is pending analysis.

IL-2 has been shown to enhance IL-12 receptor expression and IL-12-induced IFNγ production, suggesting that these two cytokines might act synergistically to eradicate tumor cells *(112,113)*. Indeed, Wiggington et al. have shown that the combination of IL-2 with IL-12 has synergistic antitumor activity in a murine renal cell carcinoma model *(114)*. Phase I trials to evaluate this combination in humans have recently opened at the NCI and Beth Israel Deaconess Medical Center in Boston.

Although some of these approaches with combinations of immune modulating agents appear promising, one must conclude that at the moment, no convincing evidence exists that any immunologic agent can add to the antitumor activity of IL-2 alone in metastatic melanoma.

3.3. IL-2 and Adoptive Immunotherapy

The initial reports of effective IL-2 treatment demonstrated that the combination of high-dose IL-2 with ex vivo IL-2-activated PBMCs (LAK cells) had activity against various cancers *(115,116)*. PBMCs were obtained via lymphocytopheresis performed during the rebound lymphocytosis following a 5-d cycle of high-dose IL-2. PBMCs were subsequently activated to create LAK cells by exposure to IL-2 in bags or flasks and reinfused with another cycle of high-dose IL-2. Eleven out of the first 25 patients had objective tumor responses, with most responses occurring in patients with either kidney cancer or melanoma *(115)*. These results were expanded upon in a multiple subsequent reports *(116)*.

The promising results from the initial NCI Surgery Branch studies led other groups to explore the combination of IL-2 and LAK cells (Table 5). In the phase II experience of the 6-member IL-2 Extramural Working Group (IL2-EWG) with high-dose bolus or continuous infusion IL-2 plus LAK cells *(35,117)*, there were 6 responses among 32 patients (19%) in the bolus IL-2/LAK cell trial, while only 1 response among 33 patients (3%) was observed with the continuous infusion IL-2/LAK regimen. The IL2-EWG experience with a combined regimen utilizing bolus IL-2 on d 1–3 and continuous infusion IL-2 with periodic LAK cell infusions on d 10–14 produced 7 responses (1 CR, 6 PR) for a 14% RR in 50 evaluable patients *(118)*. The NBSG reported a long-term follow-up on patients receiving continuous infusion IL-2 together with LAK cells. They observed only 4 responses among 33 melanoma patients (12%) with a median survival of only 6.1 mo *(119)*. Other lower dose IL-2 plus LAK cell regimens have been uniformly disappointing with very few objective responses in melanoma patients *(120)*. In a randomized trial using weekly continuous infusion IL-2 versus IL-2 plus LAK, Koretz et al. observed no objective responses in 18 patients with melanoma despite significant in vivo stimulation of LAK and NK cells *(121)*.

The NCI Surgery Branch performed a phase III trial of high-dose intravenous bolus IL-2 with or without LAK cells *(122)*. Fifty-four of the 181 patients entered into the trial had melanoma. Overall, the survival and response rate was not significantly improved for patients receiving IL-2/LAK treatment; however, survival in melanoma patients was slightly prolonged. Survival rates of 32% vs 15% and 18% vs 4% were observed at 24 and 48 mo for patients treated with IL-2/LAK cells and IL-2 alone, respectively. Nonetheless, because of the general impracticality of the LAK cell generation procedure and the absence of a compelling therapeutic benefit, LAK cell therapy has been abandoned as an adjunct to IL-2.

Subsequently, Rosenberg and his colleagues explored the use of more specific CTLs generated from TILs *(123)*. Animal studies had demonstrated TILs to be greater than fiftyfold more effective in their antitumor activity than LAK cells *(28)*. The initial report of autologous TILs plus IL-2 was very promising, with over a 40% RR in patients with melanoma *(124)*. A larger cumulative experience, including 86 patients with metastatic melanoma treated with TILs and high-dose IL-2, showed a 34% RR *(125)*. Responses were observed as frequently in patients who had failed high-dose IL-2 as those who were previously untreated with IL-2. Most of these responses were partial, however, and of short duration. Considering that this treatment was primarily limited to patients with relatively slow growing disease and biopsy-accessible tumor, which contained expandable TILs, it was uncertain to what extent these apparently improved results relative to high-dose IL-2 alone were a consequence of selection bias.

Numerous other smaller studies have explored the application of TILs plus IL-2 with varying results. Tumor responses have been observed, and at times, these clinical responses have correlated with in vitro cytotoxicity against autologous tumor cells. Thirty-seven consecutive patients (28 with measurable disease after excisional biopsy for TIL isolation) were treated with TIL infusions ($>10^{10}$ cells) and low-dose IL-2 (4.5 MIU subcutaneously 3 times daily for 3 d) *(126)*. Eight of 28 patients had tumor regression (3CR, 2 PR, 3 minor response [MR]). Further analysis revealed that there was a significant correlation between the level of $CD8^+$ cells after IL-2-TIL therapy and both tumor response and overall survival. Median overall survival was 12 mo (range 1–54 mo). After freshly isolating TIL from stage IV melanoma patients, Arienti and colleagues cultured these cells in low-dose IL-2 and then high-dose IL-2 *(127)*. Sixteen patients subsequently received TIL (mean 6.8×10^9 cells) and IL-2 (mean dose 130 MIU; range 28.8–231 MIU). There was 1 CR and 3 PR in 12 evaluable patients. Infused TIL showed an preferential lysis of autologous tumor cells in vitro in all the responding patients. Finally, TIL and IL-2 combinations have been examined in the adjuvant setting with some encouraging results *(128)*.

Other investigators have attempted to activate specific lymphoid effector cell populations using strategies that did not require the harvesting and activation of TIL *(129,130)*. Chang and his colleagues obtained lymphocytes from draining lymph nodes of patients vaccinated with an autologous tumor plus Bacille

Table 5
IL-2 Combined with Adoptive Cellular Therapy

Author year (ref.)	*IL-2 Dose*	*Route*	*Additional treatment*	*Patients (total)*	*Response CR*	*Response PR*	*Total %*	*Comments*
High-dose bolus IL-2								
Dutcher et al. 1989 *(35)*	600,000 IU/kg	IV	LAK cell infusion, on d 12, 13, and 15.	32	1	5	19	Priming dose for 5 d. 8th day leukapheresis, followed by another 5 d IL-2 course.
Bar et al. 1990 *(118)*	600,000 IU/kg 3 MIU/m^2	IV bolus IV CI for 148 h	LAK cell infusion, on d 9, 10, and 12.	50	1	6	14	Priming dose for first 3 d, followed by CI for 148 h on d 9–15. Total 15-d cycle.
Rosenberg et al. 1993 *(122)*	720,000 IU/kg	IV Q8H	LAK cell infusion, on d 11, 12, and 14.	(54)	0	6	22	Randomized control trial: IL-2 vs IL-2 plus LAK.
				22	3	3	27	
Rosenberg et al. 1994 *(124)*	720,000 IU/kg	IV Q8H	TIL plus CTX 25 mg/kg × 1 dose	86	5	24	34	No. of pts reported reflects the no. in whom TILs were successfully harvested.
High-dose continuous IV infusion IL-2								
Dillman et al. 1991 *(119)*	18 MIU/m^2/d	IV CI × 5d IV CI × 5d	LAK cell infusion, on 11, 12, and 13.	53	CR + PR = 12		23	Combined results of studies by NBSG.
Dutcher et al. 1991 *(117)*	18 MIU/m^2/d 22.5 MIU/d	IV CI × 5d IV CI × 5d	LAK cell infusion, on d 11, 12, and 14	33	0	1	3	CWG results using IL-2 CIV.
Arienti et al. 1993 *(127)*	28.8–231 MIU/d	IV CI	TIL infusion no. of cells = 6.8×10^9	16	1	3	33	Mean dose of IL-2 = 130×10^6 IU/d Mean no. of TIL = 6.8×10^9 cells.

			Moderate-dose IL-2					
Chang et al. 1997 *(130)*	3.6 MIU/kg	IVBQ8HR	OKT3 and IL-2-activated TIL	23	0	1	6	TIL harvested from draining lymph nodes after vaccination and activated with IL-2 and OKT3 in vitro.
Calvo et al. 1997 *(126)*	4.5 MIU	SC	TIL	28	3	2	22	3 minor responses not included in results.
Reali et al. 1977 *(128)*	$3–9 \times 10^6$ IU	SC	TIL plus IFNα	24	—	—	—	Escalating dose of IL-2 1.5×10^6 IU/d. Day 0–5
Curti et al. 1998 *(129)*	9 MIU/d	IV CI	CD4 cell infusion CTX 1000 mg/m^2	14	0	1	8	
Koretz et al. 1989 *(121)*	3 MU/m^2/d	IV CI	LAK infusion	18	0	0	0	Randomized trial of IL-2 vs IL-2 plus LAK therapy.

CR, complete response; PR, partial response; IU, international units; MIU, million international units; IV CI, intravenous continuous infusion; IVQ8H, intravenous every 8 h; TIL plus CTX, tumor infiltrating lymphocytes; OKT3, anti-CD3 antibody; SC, subcutaneous.

Calmette-Guérin (BCG) vaccine *(130)*. These lymphocytes were activated in vitro with anti-CD3 and IL-2 and reinfused along with additional IL-2. The T cells expanded this way had minimal cytotoxicity for autologous tumor, but exhibited highly specific cytokine release (IFNγ and GM-CSF). There was one PR observed in 11 patients with melanoma. Curti et al. at the NCI-Biologic Response Modifiers Program (BRMP) explored the merits of CD4-selected T cells activated ex vivo with anti-CD3 and IL-2 *(129)*. These $CD4^+$ T cells were then infused with additional systemic IL-2. $CD4^+$ cells were expanded in vivo following infusion, and cells appeared to traffic to sites of subcutaneous melanoma deposits. Tumor responses were observed in 3 of 31 patients (1 CR, 2 PR). The responses were seen in patients receiving larger numbers of $CD4^+$ T cells. Despite all of the above efforts, and some encouraging results, the true value of TIL and other adoptive immunotherapy approaches in combination with IL-2 relative to IL-2 alone remains to be determined. Nonetheless, the tremendous labor and cell preparation costs involved with this treatment approach have limited or even abrogated its use in future clinical investigations.

3.4. IL-2 and Monoclonal Antibodies

The prospect of combining IL-2 with monoclonal antibodies (MAbs) in the treatment of melanoma is based on several studies that suggest that the two agents may interact in a synergistic fashion to eradicate tumor cells. Antibodies reactive with tumor cells can bind to unique tumor antigens, rendering the tumor cells susceptible to clearance by activated Fc receptor-positive phagocytes and NK cells. Indeed, IL-2 has been repeatedly shown to enhance ADCC *(44,45,131–134)*. Alternatively, antibodies directed at molecules on the surface of the host effector cells (e.g., CD3, CD2, CD16) activate these cells and might render them more receptive to IL-2-mediated expansion *(135–138)*. Recent advances in biotechnology have made possible the creation of bispecific MAbs capable of simultaneously binding to both effector cells and tumor cells, thereby facilitating the formation of effector:target conjugates and the lysis of the tumor target cell. Similar techniques have led to the production of antibody:cytokine conjugates, which bind to tumor cells and activate proximal immune effector cells, expressing receptors for the particular cytokine *(139,140)*.

Much of this research focused on ganglioside-specific MAbs. Gangliosides are glycolipid molecules composed of a sialylated oligosaccharide chain linked to a ceramide fatty acid core. Melanoma cells are rich in gangliosides, two of which (GD2 and GD3) appear to be up-regulated by transformation of melanocytes *(141,142)*. Gangliosides are also present on the surface of certain T cells, where they are able to trigger activation signals when engaged by a specific antibody *(135)*. Phase I clinical trials of unconjugated ganglioside-specific MAbs have shown that they can reach tumor sites after systemic administration. Some tumor responses have been observed with R24, (anti-GD3), 3F8 (anti-GD2), and other murine MAbs *(142–147)*.

The anti-GD3 antibody R24 has been the MAb most actively investigated in combination with IL-2. In the initial study with this antibody at the Memorial Sloan Kettering Cancer Center, IL-2 was administered at 6 MIU/m^2 intravenously over 6 h on d 1–5 and 8–12, while R24 was given at one of 4 dose levels ranging between 1 and 12 mg/m^2 daily on d 8–12 *(148)*. The extent of T cell activation and the magnitude of the rebound lymphocytosis at the completion of the IL-2 treatment correlated with the R24 dose. Of the 20 treated patients, 1 PR and 2 MR were noted. The R24 MAb was combined with very low-dose continuous infusion IL-2 administered over a course of 8 wk with the antibody given during wk 5 and 6 *(149)*. Of the 28 patients with metastatic melanoma enrolled, only 1 PR (regression of liver metastases from a primary ocular melanoma) was observed. Alpaugh et al. recently reported the results of a phase IB trial that utilized a 5-d continuous infusion of R24 followed by 3 wk of subcutaneous IL-2 and IFNα *(150)*. Twenty melanoma patients were enrolled. Tumor biopsies obtained prior to treatment, on d 8 (prior to the initiation of IL-2 and IFNα) and on d 29 revealed progressively increasing chronic inflammation; however, it was difficult to determine to what extent the R24 may have contributed to this inflammatory reaction. In any event, there were no objective responses seen in the 18 evaluable patients.

The administration of murine antibodies to humans inevitably leads to the production of neutralizing human antimouse antibody (HAMA). This limitation, as well as the relatively poor interaction between murine antibodies and human Fc receptor positive immune effectors, has led to the generation of "humanized" antibodies with longer half-lives and better ADCC activation. In a phase I clinical trial evaluating one such antibody, IL-2 was continuously infused along with a chimeric anti-GD2 ganglioside antibody (14.18) *(151)* constructed by ligating DNA sequences encoding the Fab fragment of the mouse 3F8 MAb into sequences specifying a human immunoglobulin molecule. The 14.18 antibody/IL-2 combination enhanced ADCC and LAK activity and reduced human anti-chimera antibody (HACA) formation. Antitumor activity was observed in 2 of the 24 study patients (1 CR, 1 PR). One case of dose-limiting peripheral neuropathy was observed. Concomitant laboratory studies suggested that the addition of IL-2 might have suppressed anti-idiotypic antibody formation induced by the 14.18 chimera *(152)*.

Although some tumor responses have been noted in trials assessing combinations of IL-2 with antiganglioside antibodies, they are sufficiently rare so as to dissuade further clinical investigation in patients with metastatic melanoma at the present time. More potent MAbs and additional data on how to optimally combine MAbs with IL-2 are prerequisites for further investigation of this approach to immunotherapy.

The use of IL-2 in combination with MAbs directed against T cell antigens has also been explored. Preclinical studies support the concept that anti-CD3 MAb administered at low doses can activate T cells to release cytokines and proliferate and mediate antitumor effects *(136–138,153)*. Anti-CD3 MAb OKT3 in doses ranging from 10–600 μg was used in conjunction with IL-2 administered either by continuous low-dose intravenous infusion, subcutaneous injection, or high-dose intravenous bolus *(154–157)*. These trials failed to demonstrate the induction of CD25, a component of the high-affinity IL-2R on circulating T cells despite the fact that this activation antigen is readily induced by OKT3 in vitro. Furthermore, only one objective response was observed among 16 patients with melanoma treated with OKT3 and IL-2 *(157)*. However, it is possible that this strategy of combining IL-2 with T cell-specific MAb might be more effective if bispecific MAbs or fusion antibodies, which are able to activate effector cells directly at the tumor cell surface, were to be used.

In an effort to enhance ADCC at the tumor site, IL-2 was linked to the carboxy-terminus of the aforementioned chimeric 14.18 molecule *(158)*. This fusion protein binds to GD2-expressing tumor cells in vitro as avidly as the unmodified 14.18 antibody and mediates ADCC against GD2-expressing melanoma cells by stimulating both cytotoxic T cells and NK cells expressing IL-2Rs, regardless of whether they express Fc receptors. Animal models using this fusion protein have shown it to be superior to either IL-2 or 14.18 alone or both in combination at comparable stoichiometry *(139,159,160)*. Phase I trials of this fusion protein in melanoma patients have recently been initiated.

3.5. IL-2 and Tumor Vaccines

Melanomas possess tumor antigens that can be recognized by the host immune system *(161)*. Over the past several decades, numerous investigators have attempted to exploit this attribute to develop specific vaccines capable of inducing T cell-mediated tumor rejection. Most of these early attempts made use of crude melanoma cell preparations. While some of these approaches showed initial promise, beneficial effects have yet to be confirmed in phase III trials *(161–167)*. Efforts to develop an effective vaccine have been hindered by poor immunogenicity of certain antigens, tumor-induced tolerance, antigen shedding, and heterogeneity with respect to tumor cell antigen expression. Since IL-2 is able to induce the clonal expansion of antigen-primed T cells, it follows that IL-2 would be a useful adjunct to any vaccine regimen under development. As a consequence, several investigators have included IL-2 as a key component in their various tumor vaccine protocols. A summary of recent trials, pairing IL-2 with some sort of tumor vaccine, is displayed in Table 6.

An allogenic liposomal melanoma vaccine has been administered with or without systemic or regional low-dose IL-2 *(168)*. Nine of the 24 vaccinated patients had objective responses, including 6 responses (3 CR, 3 PR) in the 10 patients

Table 6
IL-2 Combined with Vaccines

	Interleukin-2						*Response*		*Total response*
Author year (ref.)	*Dose*	*Route*	*Schedule*	*Type of vaccine*	*Schedule*	*N*	*CR*	*PR*	*%*
1. Adler et al. 1995 *(168)*	Variable bolus	Intravenous or regional	Q8H	Allogenic liposomal melanoma vaccine	SQ injection at 2 sites every week × 10 wk	24[a]	3	6	50%[a]
2. Oratz et al. 1996 *(169)*	$0–5 \times 10^5$ IU	Liposome encapsulated d IL-2		Polyvalent melanoma vaccine encapsulated in liposomal IL-2	ID Q2 wk × 4 and monthly × 3	8[b]	1	1	25%
3. Rosenberg et al. 1998 *(180)*	720,000 IU/kg	IVB	Q8 H × 5 d for 2 cycles	Modified gp100 peptide vaccine (G209–2M)	1.0 mg SQ into thigh. 2–6 Immunizations at 3-wk intervals	31	1	12	42%

[a]Study included 4 arms of which responses were seen in the IL-2 plus vaccine arm and the regionally administered IL-2 arm only.
[b]Only 8 patients had measurable disease of the 36 in the group studied.
CR, complete response; PR, partial response; SQ, subcutaneous; ID, intradermal; IVB, intravenous bolus; IU, international units.

who received the vaccine plus low-dose regional IL-2. Unfortunately, neither follow-up reports on these patients nor additional trials confirming these remarkable results have been forthcoming. Oratz and colleagues have evaluated a polyvalent vaccine, in which shed melanoma antigens and IL-2 were both encapsulated into liposomes in an effort to increase vaccine immunogenicity *(169)*. Thirty-six patients with stage IV melanoma received this vaccine, followed by daily low-dose IL-2 injections (2–5 × 10^5 IU) for 2 wk. This regimen was felt to induce a higher frequency and duration of vaccine-induced delayed-type hypersensitivity (DTH) responses relative to historical controls receiving vaccine alone, an effect attributed to the addition of IL-2 *(169)*. Of 28 patients whose metastatic disease had been completely resected at entry, 9 of 12 that had been followed for 2 yr and remained alive compared with only 15–30% of "matched" historical controls. There were 2 tumor responses (1 CR, 1 PR) observed in the 8 patients with measurable disease. Longer follow-up and randomized controlled studies are clearly necessary in order to determine the true value of this combination.

The recent identification and characterization of melanoma antigens specifically recognized by cytotoxic T cells has led to a shift in vaccine development towards the use of defined peptides rather than crude tumor cell lysates as a source of antigen *(170–172)*. These antigens include embryonic proteins (MAGE family), as well as tissue-restricted (melanocyte differentiation) proteins such as tyrosinase, MART-1, and gp100 *(173–179)*. Rosenberg and colleagues have investigated the immunogenicity of an 8-amino acid peptide derived from the gp100 protein (residues 209–217) and a mutated version of this peptide (gp100 peptide 209-2M) which binds HLA-A2.1 more effectively than the wild-type peptide *(180)*. While the mutated peptide (gp100:209-2M) administered in incomplete Freund's adjuvant alone was quite effective in inducing specific T cell immune responses (10/11 patients), few antitumor effects were observed. However, 13 (42%) of 31 patients who received the peptide together with high-dose IL-2 had an objective tumor response. A confirmatory trial of this combination is currently underway within the CWG and a phase III trial randomizing patients to either high-dose IL-2 alone or in combination with the gp100:209-2M peptide is being contemplated.

4. IL-2 GENE THERAPY

As previously discussed, IL-2 administered systemically enhances the immunogenicity of dendritic cell-based vaccines *(24)*. In an effort to develop melanoma vaccine protocols that take advantage of the proliferative effects of IL-2 on activated T cells, but avoid the toxicity associated with the systemic administration of the cytokine, several investigators have pioneered vaccine regimens utilizing tumor cells genetically engineered to secrete IL-2 or mixtures of tumor cells with IL-2-secreting fibroblasts. For example, murine melanoma cells engineered to secrete IL-2 elicited a greater degree of T cell activation in the lymph nodes draining the vaccination site than could be achieved with the parental untransfected tumor cells *(181)*. In a small clinical trial in which 12 melanoma patients were vaccinated with one of two IL-2-transduced human melanoma cell lines, the investigators observed disease stabilization in 4 of the 12 patients treated *(182)*. Likewise, in a clinical trial using autologous melanoma cells co-suspended with an allogenic immortalized fibroblast line engineered to secrete IL-2, vaccinated patients developed inflammatory reactions at the vaccination site, but little systemic toxicity. The DTH reactions at the vaccination site were characterized histologically by dense infiltrates of both $CD4^+$ and $CD8^+$ T cells. $CD8^+$ T cells isolated from the vaccine sites and propagated ex vivo were cytolytic for autologous tumor cells *(183)*. These results suggest that the high local concentrations of IL-2 achieved at the vaccine site by the aforementioned genetic manipulations might prove superior to the high circulating levels achieved by systemic administration as a means of enhancing the T cell response to tumor cell-based vaccines.

5. IL-2-BASED BIOCHEMOTHERAPY

Many investigators have studied combinations of IL-2-based immunotherapy and cytotoxic chemotherapy in this disease. Combinations including cisplatin and IL-2 have been the most promising, producing response rates consistently higher than those observed with either IL-2 or chemotherapy alone *(184,185)*. It is, however, unclear if these combinations increase the number of patients surviving long-term disease-free. Multiple phase III trials comparing biochemotherapy to either chemotherapy alone or IL-2-based immunotherapy in patients with metastatic melanoma have been initiated. These trials should definitively address the value of biochemotherapy in this disease. This information is discussed in more detail in Chapter 10.

6. CONCLUSIONS

Modest progress has been made in the treatment of metastatic melanoma over the past decade. With the advent of high-dose IL-2, it is now possible to talk about "cure", albeit in a small minority of patients. Abundant preclinical data support the use of IL-2 in combination with other cytokines, toxicity blocking agents, monoclonal antibodies, adoptive immunotherapy, or vaccines, and many of these approaches have yet to fully tested clinically. The wealth of promising new treatment strategies offers hope that "cure" for more than the rare patient with metastatic melanoma will be achieved within the coming generation. It is likely that IL-2 will be a critical component of whichever new approach gains ascendancy in the future.

ACKNOWLEDGMENT

The authors are indebted to Susan Graham-McLaughlin for her assistance in the preparation of this manuscript.

REFERENCES

1. Morgan D, Ruscetti FW, Gallo R. Selective in vitro growth of T-lymphocytes from normal bone marrows. *Science* 1976; 193: 1007–1008.
2. Mier J, Gallo R. Purification and some characteristics of human T cell growth factor (TCGF) from PHA-stimulated lymphocyte conditioned media. *Proc Natl Acad Sci USA* 1980; 77: 6134–6138.
3. Taniguchi T, Matsui H, Fujita T, et al. Structure and expression of a cloned cDNA for human interleukin-2. *Nature* 1983; 302: 305–310.
4. Taniguchi T, Minami Y. The IL-2/IL-2 receptor system: a current overview. *Cell* 1993; 73: 5–8.
5. Gootenberg J, Ruscetti F, Mier J, Gazdar A, Gallo R. Human cutaneous T-cell lymphoma and leukemia cell lines produce and respond to T-cell growth factor. *J Exp Med* 1981; 154: 1403–1413.
6. Leonard WJ, Depper J, Uchiyama T, Smith KA, Waldmann TA, Greene WC. A monoclonal antibody that appears to recognize the receptor for T cell growth factor: partial purification of the receptor. *Nature* 1982; 300: 267–270.
7. Hatakeyama M, Tsudo M, Minamoto S, et al. Interleukin-2 receptor beta chain gene: generation of three receptor forms by cloned human alpha and beta chain cDNAs. *Science* 1989; 244: 551–556.
8. Takeshita T, Asao H, Ohtani K, et al. Cloning of the gamma-chain of the human IL-2 receptor. *Science* 1992; 257: 379–381.
9. Lodolce JP, Boone DL, Chai S, et al. IL-15 receptor maintains lymphoid homeostasis by supporting lymphocyte homing and proliferation. *Immunity* 1998; 9: 669–676.
10. Noguchi M, Yi H, Rosenblatt HM, et al. Interleukin-2 receptor gamma chain mutation results in X-linked severe combined immunodeficiency in humans. *Cell* 1983; 73: 147–155.
11. Nakarai T, Robertson MJ, Streuli M, et al. Interleukin-2 receptor gamma chain expression on resting and activated lymphoid cells. *J Exp Med* 1994; 180: 241–251.
12. Hatakeyama M, Kono T, Kobayashi N, et al. Interaction of the IL-2 receptor with the *src*-family kinase p56^{lck}: Identification of novel intermolecular association. *Science* 1991; 252: 1523–1528.
13. Friedmann MC, Migone T-S, Russell SM, Leonard WJ. Different interleukin-2 receptor beta chain tyrosines couple to at least two signaling pathways and synergistically mediate interleukin-2-induced proliferation. *Proc Natl Acad Sci USA* 1996; 93: 2077–2082.
14. Asao H, Takeshita T, Ishii N, Kumaki S, Nakamura M, Sugamura K. Reconstitution of functional interleukin 2 receptor complexes on fibroblastoid cells: involvement of the cytoplasmic domain of the gamma chain in two distinct signaling pathways. *Proc Natl Acad Sci USA* 1993; 90: 4127–4131.
15. Russell SM, Johnston JA, Noguchi M, et al. Interaction of IL-2 receptor beta and gamma c chains with JAK1 and JAK3: implications for XSCID and XCID. *Science* 1994; 266: 1042–1045.
16. Wang KS, Ritz J, Frank DA. IL-2 induces STAT4 activation in primary NK cells and NK cell lines, but not in T cells. *J Immunol* 1999; 162: 299–304.
17. Numerof R, Aronson F, Mier J. Interleukin-2 stimulates the production of interleukin-1 alpha and interleukin-1 beta by human peripheral blood mononuclear cells. *J Immunol* 1988; 141: 4250–4256.

18. Gemlo BT, Palladino MA, Jaffe HS, Espevik TP, Rayner AA. Circulating cytokines in patients with metastatic cancer treated with recombinant interleukin-2 and lymphokine-activated killer cells. *Cancer Res* 1988; 48: 5864–5869.
19. Strasser JL, Rosenberg SA. In vitro growth of cytotoxic human lymphocytes. I. Growth of cells sensitized in vitro to alloantigens. *J Immunol* 1978; 121: 1951–1955.
20. Lotze MT, Grimm EA, Mazumder A, Strausser JL, Rosenberg SA. Lysis of fresh and cultured autologous tumor by human lymphocytes cultured in T-cell growth factor. *Cancer Res* 1981; 41: 4420–4425.
21. Grimm EA, Mazumder A, Zhang HZ, Rosenberg SA. Lymphokine-activated killing phenomenon: lysis of natural killer resistant fresh solid tumor cells by interleukin-2 activated autologous human peripheral blood lymphocytes. *J Exp Med* 1982; 155: 1823–1841.
22. Grimm EA, Robb RJ, Roth JA, et al. The lymphokine activated killer cell phenomenon. III. Evidence that IL-2 alone is sufficient for direct activation of PBL into lymphokine-activated killer cells. *J Exp Med* 1983; 158: 1356–1361.
23. Rosenberg SA, Mule JJ, Spiess PJ, Reichert CM, Schwarz SL. Regression of established pulmonary metastases and subcutaneous tumors mediated by the systemic administration of high-dose recombinant interleukin-2. *J Exp Med* 1985; 161: 1169–1181.
24. Shimizu K, Fields RC, Giedlin M, Mule JJ. Systemic administration of interleukin-2 enhances the therapeutic efficacy of dendritic cell-based tumor vaccines. *Proc Natl Acad Sci USA* 1999; 96: 2268–2273.
25. Lafreniere R, Rosenberg SA. Adoptive immunotherapy of murine hepatic metastases with lymphokine activated killer (LAK) cells and recombinant interleukin-2 (RIL-2) can mediate the regression of both immunogenic and nonimmunogenic sarcomas and an adenocarcinoma. *J Immunol* 1985; 135: 4273–4278.
26. Mule JJ, Shu S, Rosenberg SA. The anti-tumor efficacy of lymphokine-activated killer cells and recombinant interleukin 2 in vivo. *J Immunol* 1985; 135: 646–652.
27. Belldegrun A, Muul LM, Rosenberg SA. Interleukin-2 expanded tumor infiltrating lymphocytes in human cancer: isolation, characterization and antitumor activity. *Cancer Res* 1988; 48: 206–210.
28. Spiess PJ, Yang JC, Rosenberg SA. In vivo antitumor activity of tumor-infiltrating lymphocytes expanded in recombinant interleukin-2. *J Natl Cancer Inst* 1987; 79: 1067–1071.
29. Lotze MT, Frana LW, Sharrow SO, et al. In vivo administration of purified human interleukin 2. I. Half-life and immunologic effects of the Jurkat cell line-derived interleukin 2. *J Immunol* 1985; 134: 157–166.
30. Sznol M, Dutcher JP, Atkins MB, et al. Review of interleukin-2 alone and interleukin-2/LAK clinical trials in metastatic malignant melanoma. *Cancer Treat Rev* 1989; 16(suppl A): 29–38.
31. Marincola FM, Rosenberg SA. Interleukin 2—clinical applications: melanoma. In: Devita VT, Hellman S, Rosenberg SA, eds. *Biologic Therapy of Cancer, 2nd ed.* JB Lippincott, Philadelphia, 1995, p. 250.
32. Lotze MT, Matory YL, Ettinghausen SE, et al. In vivo administration of purified human interleukin 2. II. Half-life, immunologic effects and expansion of peripheral lymphoid cells in vivo with recombinant IL 2. *J Immunol* 1985; 135: 2865–2875.
33. Rosenberg SA, Lotze MT, Muul LM, et al. Observations on the systemic administration of autologous lymphokine-activated killer cells and recombinant interleukin-2 to patients with metastatic cancer. *N Engl J Med* 1985; 313: 1485–1492.
34. Rosenberg SA, Yang JC, Topalian SL, et al. Treatment of 283 consecutive patients with metastatic melanoma or renal cell cancer using high-dose bolus interleukin-2. *JAMA* 1994; 271: 907–913.
35. Dutcher JP, Creekmore S, Weiss GR, et al. A phase II study of interleukin-2 and lymphokine activated killer (LAK) cells in patients with metastatic malignant melanoma. *J Clin Oncol* 1989; 7: 477–485.

36. Parkinson D, Abrams J, Wiernik P, et al. Interleukin-2 therapy in patients with metastatic malignant melanoma: a phase II study. *J Clin Oncol* 1990; 8: 1650–1656.
37. Atkins MB, Lotze M, Dutcher JP, et al. High-dose recombinant interleukin-2 therapy for patients with metastatic melanoma: analysis of 270 patients treated from 1985-1993. *J Clin Oncol* 1999; 17: 2105–2116.
38. Atkins MB, Kunkel L, Sznol M, Rosenberg SA. High-dose recombinant interleukin-2 therapy in patients with metastatic melanoma: long-term survival update. *Cancer J Sci Am* 2000; 6(suppl 1): S11–S14.
39. Klempner MS, Snydman DR. Infectious complications associated with interleukin-2. In: Atkins MB, Mier JW, eds. *Therapeutic Application of Interleukin-2, ed. 1*. Marcel Dekker, New York, 1993, pp. 409–424.
40. Rosenberg SA, Yang JC, White DE, Steinberg SM. Durability of complete responses in patients with metastatic cancer treated with high-dose interleukin-2: identification of the antigens mediating response. *Ann Surg* 1998; 228: 307–319.
41. Yang JC, Topalian SL, Schwartzentruber DJ, et al. The use of polyethylene glycol-modified interleukin-s (PEG-IL-2) in the treatment of patients with metastatic renal cell carcinoma and melanoma. A phase I study and a randomized prospective study comparing IL-2 alone versus IL-2 combined with PEG-IL-2. *Cancer* 1995; 76: 687–694.
42. Sondel PM, Kohler PC, Hank JA, et al. Clinical and immunological effects of recombinant interleukin 2 given by repetitive weekly cycles to patients with cancer. *Cancer Res* 1988; 48: 2561–2567.
43. Thompson JA, Lee DJ, Lindgren CG, et al. Influence of dose and duration of infusion of interleukin-2 on toxicity and immunomodulation. *J Clin Oncol* 1988; 6: 669–678.
44. Hank JA, Robinson RR, Surfus J, et al. Augmentation of antibody dependent cell mediated cytotoxicity following in vivo therapy with interleukin-2. *Cancer Res* 1990; 50: 5234–5239.
45. Munn DH, Cheung NK. Interleukin-2 enhancement of monoclonal antibody-mediated cellular cytotoxicity against human melanoma. *Cancer Res* 1987; 47: 6600–6605.
46. West WH, Tauer KW, Yannelli JR, et al. Constant-infusion recombinant interleukin-2 in adoptive immunotherapy of advanced cancer. *N Engl J Med* 987; 16: 898–905.
47. Dillman RO, Church C, Oldham RK, et al. In patient continuous infusion IL-2 in 788 patients with cancer. The national biotherapy study group experience. *Cancer* 1993; 71: 2358–2370.
48. Dillman RO, Wiemann MC, VanderMolen LA, et al. Hybrid high-dose bolus/continuous infusion interleukin-2 in patients with metastatic melanoma: a phase II trial of the cancer biotherapy research group (formerly the National Biotherapy Study Group). *Cancer Biother Radiopharm* 1997; 12: 249–255.
49. Legha SS, Gianan MA, Plager C, et al. Evaluation of interleukin-2 administered by continuous infusion in patients with metastatic melanoma. *Cancer* 1996; 77: 89–96.
50. Dorval T, Mathiot C, Chosidow O, et al. IL-2 phase II trial in metastatic melanoma: analysis of clinical and immunological parameters. *Biotechnol Ther* 1992; 3: 63–79.
51. Dillman RO, Church C, Barth NM, et al. Long-term survival after continuous infusion interleukin-2. *Cancer Biother Radiopharm* 1997; 12: 243–248.
52. Vlasveld LT, Rankin EM, Heckman A, et al. A phase I study of prolonged continuous infusion of low dose recombinant IL-2 in melanoma and renal cell cancer. Part I clinical aspect. *Br J Cancer* 1992; 65: 744–750.
53. Vlasveld LT, Horenblas S, Hekman A, et al. Phase II study of intermittent continuous infusion of low-dose recombinant interleukin-2 in advanced melanoma and renal cell cancer. *Ann Oncol* 1994; 5: 179–181.
54. Whitehead RP, Kopecky KJ, Samson MK, et al. Phase II study of intravenous bolus recombinant interleukin-2 in advanced malignant melanoma: Southwest Oncology Group study. *J Natl Cancer Inst* 1991; 83: 1250–1252.

55. Margolin K. The clinical toxicities of high-dose interleukin-2. In: Atkins MB, Mier JW, eds. *Therapeutic Applications of Interleukin-2*. Marcel Dekker, New York, 1993, pp. 331–362.
56. Schwartzentruber DJ. Biologic therapy with interleukin-2: clinical applications: principles of administration and management of side effects. In: DeVita V, Hellman S, Rosenberg SA, eds. *Biologic Therapy of Cancer, ed. 2*. Lippincott, Philadelphia, 1995, pp. 235–249.
57. Kammula US, White DE, Rosenberg SA. Trends in the safety of high dose bolus interleukin-2 administration in patients with metastatic cancer. *Cancer* 1998; 83: 797–805.
58. Mier J, Vachino G, Van der Meer J, et al. Induction of circulating tumor necrosis factor (TNF) as the mechanism for the febrile response to interleukin-2 (IL-2) in cancer patients. *J Clin Immunol* 1988; 8: 426–436.
59. Hibbs JB, Westenfelder C, Taintor R, et al. Evidence for cytokine inducible nitric oxide synthesis from L-arginine in patients receiving interleukin-2 therapy. *J Clin Invest* 1992; 89: 867–877.
60. Mier JW, Vachino G, Klempner MS, et al. Inhibition of interleukin-2 induced tumor necrosis factor release by dexamethasone: prevention of an acquired neutrophil chemotactic defect and differential suppression of interleukin-2 associated side effects. *Blood* 1990; 76: 1933–1940.
61. Vetto JT, Papa MZ, Lotze MT, Chang AE, Rosenberg SA. Reduction of toxicity of interleukin-2 and lymphokine-activated killer cells in humans by the administration of corticosteroids. *J Clin Oncol* 1987; 5: 496–503.
62. Trehu EG, Mier JW, Shapiro L, et al. A phase I trial of interleukin-2 in combination with the soluble tumor necrosis factor receptor p75 IgG Chimera (TNFR: Fc). *Clin Cancer Res* 1996; 2: 1341–1351.
63. DuBois J, Trehu EG, Mier JW, et al. Randomized placebo-controlled clinical trial of high-dose interleukin-2 (IL-2) in combination with the soluble TNF receptor IgG Chimera (TNFR: Fc). *J Clin Oncol* 1997; 15: 1052–1062.
64. Margolin K, Weiss G, Dutcher J, et al. Prospective randomized trial of lisophylline (CT1501R) for the modulation of interleukin-2 (IL-2) toxicity. *Clin Cancer Res* 1997; 3: 565–579.
65. McDermott D, Trehu E, DuBois J, et al. Phase I clinical trial of the soluble IL-1 receptor either alone or in combination with high-dose IL-2 in patients with advanced malignancies. *Clin Cancer Res* 1998; 5: 1203–1213.
66. Atkins MB. Immunotherapy and experimental approaches for metastatic melanoma. *Hematol Oncol Clin North Am* 1998; 12: 877–902.
67. Atkins MB, Shet A, Sosman J. IL-2: clinical applications—melanoma. In: Devita V, Hellman S, Roseberg S, eds. *Principles and Practice of the Biologic Therapy of Cancer, 3rd ed.* 2000; JB Lippincott, Philadelphia, PA, pp. 50–73.
68. Bianchi M, Bloom O, Raabe T, et al. Suppression of proinflammatory cytokines in monocytes by a tetravalent guanylhydrazone. *J Exp Med* 1996; 183: 927–936.
69. Bianchi M, Ulrich P, Bloom O. An inhibitor of macrophage arginine transport and nitric oxide production (CNI-1493) prevents acute inflammation and endotoxin lethality. *Mol Med* 1995; 1: 254–266.
70. Kemeny MM, Botchkina GI, Ochani M, Bianchi M, Urmacher C, Tracey KJ. The tetravalent guanylhydrazone CNI-1493 blocks the toxic effects of interleukin-2 without diminishing antitumor activity. *Proc Natl Acad Sci USA* 1998; 95: 4561–4566.
71. Kilbourn RG, Fonseca GA, Griffith OW, et al. NG-methyl-L-arginine, an inhibitor of nitric oxide synthase, reverses interleukin-2-induced hypotension. *Crit Care Med* 1995; 23: 1018–1024.
72. Tartour E, Blay JY, Dorval T, et al. Predictors of clinical response to interleukin-2 based immunotherapy in melanoma patients: a French multiinstitutional study. *J Clin Oncol* 1996; 14: 1697–1703.

73. Keilholz U, Scheibogen C, Sommer M, Pritsch M, Geuke AM. Prognostic factors for response and survival in patients with metastatic melanoma receiving immunotherapy. *Melanoma Res* 1996; 6: 173–178.
74. Rosenberg SA, White DE. Vitiligo in patients with melanoma: normal tissue antigens can be targets for cancer immunotherapy. *J Immunother Emphasis Tumor Immunol* 1996; 19: 81–84.
75. Atkins MB. Autoimmune disorders induced by interleukin-2 therapy. In: Atkins MB, Mier JW, eds. *Therapeutic Applications of Interleukin-2*. Marcel Dekker, New York, 1993, pp. 389–408.
76. Schwartzentruber DJ, Hom SS, Dadmarz R, et al. In vitro predictors of therapeutic response in melanoma patients receiving tumor-infiltrating lymphocytes and interleukin-2. *J Clin Oncol* 1994; 12: 1475–1483.
77. Marincola FM, Venzon D, White D, et al. HLA association with response and toxicity in melanoma patients treated with interleukin-2-based immunotherapy. *Cancer Res* 1992; 52: 6561–6566.
78. Marincola FM, Shamamian P, Rivoltini L, et al. HLA associations in the anti-tumor response against malignant melanoma. *J Immunol* 1996; 18: 242–252.
79. Rubin JT, Day R, Duquesnoy R, et al. HLA-DQ1 is associated with clinical response and survival of patients with melanoma who are treated with interleukin-2. *Ther Immunol* 1995; 2: 1–6.
80. Scheibenbogen C, Keilholz U, Mytilineos J, et al. HLA class I alleles and responsiveness of melanoma to immunotherapy with interferon-alpha (INF-alpha) and interleukin-2 (IL-2). *Melanoma Res* 1994; 4: 191–194.
81. Hahne M, Rimoldi D, Schroter M, et al. Melanoma cell expression of Fas (Apo 1/CD95) ligand: implications for tumor immune escape. *Science* 1996; 274: 1363–1366.
82. Zea AH, Cutri BD, Longo, et al. Alterations in T cell receptor and signal transduction molecules in melanoma patients. *Clin Cancer Res* 1995; 1: 1327–1335.
83. Rabinowich H, Banks M, Reichert TE, et al. Expression and activity of signaling molecules in T lymphocytes obtained from patients with metastatic melanoma before and after interleukin 2 therapy. *Clin Cancer Res* 1996; 2: 1263–1274.
84. Iigo M, Sakurai M, Tamura T, Saijo N, Hoshi A. In vivo anti-tumor activity of multiple injections of recombinant interleukin-2, alone and in combination with three different types of recombinant interferon, on various syngeneic murine tumors. *Cancer Res* 1988; 48: 260–264.
85. Rosenberg SA, Schwartz SL, Spiess PJ. Combination immunotherapy for cancer: synergistic antitumor interactions of interleukin-2, alfa interferon, and tumor-infiltrating lymphocytes. *J Natl Cancer Inst* 1988; 80: 1393–1397.
86. Brunda MJ, Bellantoni D, Sulich V. In vivo antitumor activity of combinations of interferon alpha and interleukin-2 in murine model. Correlation of efficacy with the induction of cytotoxic cells resembling natural killer cells. *Int J Cancer* 1987; 40: 365–371.
87. Cameron RB, McIntosh JK, Rosenberg SA. Synergistic anti-tumor effects of combination immunotherapy with recombinant interleukin-2 and a recombinant hybrid alpha-interferon in the treatment of established murine hepatic metastases. *Cancer Res* 1988; 48: 5810–5817.
88. Rosenberg SA, Lotze MT, Yang JC, et al. Combination therapy with interleukin-2 and alpha-interferon for the treatment of patients with advanced cancer. *J Clin Oncol* 1989; 7: 1863–1874.
89. Marincola FM, White DE, Wise AP, Rosenberg SA. Combination therapy with interferon alfa-2a and interleukin-2 for the treatment of metastatic cancer. *J Clin Oncol* 1995; 13: 1110–1122.
90. Sparano JA, Fishcr RI, Sunderland M, et al. Randomized phase III trial of treatment with high dose interleukin-2 either alone or in combination with alfa-2A in patients with advanced melanoma. *J Clin Oncol* 1993; 11: 1969–1977.

91. Keilholz U, Scheibenbogen C, Tilgen W, et al. Interferon-α and interleukin-2 in the treatment of metastatic melanoma: comparison of two phase II trials. *Cancer* 1993; 72: 607–614.
92. Keilholz U, Goey SH, Punt CJ, et al. Interferon alfa-2a and interleukin-2 with or without cisplatin in metastatic melanoma: a randomized trial of the European organization for research and treatment of cancer melanoma cooperative group. *J Clin Oncol* 1997; 15: 2579–2588.
93. Eton O, Talpaz M, Lee KH, et al. Phase II trial of recombinant human interleukin-2 and interferon-alpha 2a. Cancer 1996; 77: 893–899.
94. Kruit WHJ, Goey SH, Calabresi F, et al. Final report of a phase II study of interleukin-2 and interferon-alpha in patients with metastatic melanoma. *Br J Cancer* 1995; 71: 1319–1321.
95. Whitehead RP, Figlin R, Citron ML, et al. A phase II trial of concomitant human interleukin-2 and interferon-alpha-2a in patients with disseminated malignant melanoma. *J Immunother* 1993; 13: 117–121.
96. Castello G, Comella P, Manzo T, et al. Immunological and clinical effects of intramuscular rIFNα-2a and low-dose subcutaneous rIL-2 in patients with advanced malignant melanoma. *Melanoma Res* 1993; 3: 43–49.
97. Karp SE. Low-dose intravenous bolus interleukin-2 with interferon-alpha therapy for metastatic melanoma and renal cell carcinoma. *J Immunother* 1998; 21: 56–61.
98. Kim CJ, Taubenberger JK, Simonis TB, et al. Combination therapy with interferon-γ and interleukin-2 for the treatment of metastatic melanoma. *J Immunol* 1996; 19: 50–58.
99. Viens P, Blaise D, Stoppa AM, et al. Interleukin-2 in association with increasing doses of interferon-gamma in patients with advanced cancer. *J Immunother* 1992; 11: 218–224.
100. Reddy SP, Harwood RM, Moore DF, et al. Recombinant interleukin-2 in combination with recombinant interferon-gamma in patients with advance malignancy: a phase I study. *J Immunother* 1997; 20: 79–87.
101. Olencki T, Finke J, Tubbs R, et al. Immunomodulatory effects on interleukin-2 and interleukin-4 in patients with malignancy. *J Immunother* 1996; 19: 69–80.
102. Sosman JA, Fisher SG, Kefer C, et al. A phase I trial of continuous infusion interleukin-4 (IL-4) alone and following interleukin-2 (IL-2) in cancer patients. *Ann Oncol* 1994; 5: 447–452.
103. Shimizu K, Fields RC, Giedlin M, Mule JJ. Systemic administration of interleukin 2 enhances the therapeutic efficacy of dendritic cell-based tumor vaccines. *Proc Natl Acad Sci USA* 1999; 96: 2268–2273.
104. Creagan ET, Rowlan KM Jr, Suman VJ, et al. Phase II study of combined levamisole with recombinant interleukin-2 in patients with advanced malignant melanoma. *Am J Clin Oncol* 1997; 20: 490–492.
105. Quirt IC, Shelley WE, Pater JL, et al. Improved survival in patients with poor-prognosis malignant melanoma treated with adjuvant levamisole: a phase III study by the National Cancer Institute of Canada clinical trials group. *J Clin Oncol* 1991; 9: 729–735.
106. Spitler LE. A randomized trial of levamisole versus placebo as adjuvant therapy in malignant melanoma. *J Clin Oncol* 1991; 9: 736–740.
107. Ahmed FY, Leonard GA, A'Hern R, et al. A randomized dose escalation study of subcutaneous interleukin-2 with and without levamisole in patients with metastatic renal cell carcinoma or malignant melanoma. *Br J Cancer* 1996; 74: 1109–1113.
108. Salup RR, Sicker DC, Wolmark N, et al. Chemoimmunotherapy of metastatic murine renal cell carcinoma using flavone acetic acid and interleukin 2. *J Urol* 1992; 147: 1120–1123.
109. Thatcher N, Dazzi H, Mellor M, et al. Recombinant IL-2 with flavone acetic acid in advanced malignant melanoma: a phase II study. *Br J Cancer* 1990; 61: 618–621.
110. O'Reilly SM, Rustin GJ, Farmer K, et al. Flavone acetic acid (FAA) with recombinant interleukin-2 (rIL-2) in advanced malignant melanoma I. Clinical and vascular studies. *Br J Cancer* 1993; 67: 1342–1345.

111. Hellstrand K, Hermodsson S, Noredi P, et al. Histamine and cytokine therapy. *Acta Oncol* 1998; 37: 347–353.
112. Gollob JA, Schnipper CP, Orsini E, et al. Characterization of a novel subset of $CD8^+$ T cells that expands in patients receiving interleukin-12. *J Clin Invest* 1998; 102: 561–575.
113. Gollob JA, Mier JW, Veenstra K, et al. Phase I trial of twice weekly intravenous interleukin-12 in patients with metastatic renal cell cancer of malignant melanoma: ability to maintain IFN-γ induction is associated with clinical response. *Clin Cancer Res* 2000; 6: 1678–1692.
114. Wiggington JM, Komschlies KL, Back TC, Franco JL, Brunda MJ, Wiltrout RH. Administration of interleukin-12 with pulse interleukin-2 and the rapid and complete eradication of murine renal cell carcinoma. *J Natl Cancer Inst* 1996; 88: 38–43.
115. Rosenberg SA, Lotze MT, Muul LM, et al. Observations on the systemic administration of autologous lymphokine-activated killer cells and recombinant interleukin-2 to patients with metastatic cancer. *N Engl J Med* 1985; 313: 1485–1492.
116. Rosenberg SA, Lotze MT, Muul LM, et al. A progress report on the treatment of 157 patients with advanced cancer using lymphokine-activated killer cells and interleukin-2 or high-dose interleukin-2 alone. *N Engl J Med* 1987; 316: 889–897.
117. Dutcher JP, Gaynor ER, Boldt DH, et al. A phase II study of high-dose continuous infusion interleukin-2 with lymphokine-activated killer cells in patients with metastatic melanoma. *J Clin Oncol* 1991; 9: 641–648.
118. Bar MH, Sznol M, Atkins MB, et al. Metastatic malignant melanoma treated with combined bolus and continuous infusion interleukin-2 and lymphokine-activated killer cells. *J Clin Oncol* 1990; 8: 1138–1147.
119. Dillman RO, Oldham RK, Tauer KW, et al. Continuous interleukin-2 and lymphokine-activated killer cells for advanced cancer: a National Biotherapy Group trial. *J Clin Oncol* 1991; 9: 1233–1240.
120. Clark JW, Smith W 2nd, Steis RG, et al. Interleukin-2 and lymphokine-activated killer cell therapy: analysis of a bolus interleukin-2 and a continuous infusion interleukin-2 regimen. *Cancer Res* 1990; 50: 7343–7350.
121. Koretz MJ, Lawson DH, York RM, et al. Randomized study of interleukin-2 (IL-2) alone vs. IL-2 plus lymphokine-activated killer cells for treatment of melanoma and renal cell cancer. *J Clin Oncol* 1989; 7: 869–878.
122. Rosenberg SA, Lotze MT, Yang JC, et al. Prospective randomized trial of high-dose interleukin-2 alone or in conjunction with lymphokine-activated killer cells for the treatment of patients with advanced cancer. *J Natl Cancer Inst* 1993; 85: 622–632.
123. Rosenberg SA, Speiss P, Lafreniere R. A new approach to the adoptive immunotherapy of cancer with tumor-infiltrating lymphocytes. *Science* 1986; 233: 1318–1321.
124. Rosenberg SA, Yannelli JR, Yang JC, et al. Treatment of patients with metastatic melanoma with autologous tumor-infiltration lymphocytes and interleukin-2. *J Natl Cancer Inst* 1994; 8: 1159–1166.
125. Rosenberg SA. Treatment of patients with metastatic melanoma with autologous tumor-infiltrating lymphocytes and interleukin-2. *J Natl Cancer Inst* 1995; 87: 319.
126. Calvo E, Garcia-Foncillas J, Aramendia JM, et al. Increase of peripheral blood CD8+ T cells after therapy with tumor infiltrating lymphocytes and IL-2 correlates with response and survival in metastatic melanoma patients. *Proc Annu Meet Am Assoc Cancer Res* 1997; 38: A3270.
127. Arienti F, Belli F, Rivoltini L, et al. Adoptive immunotherapy of advanced melanoma patients with interleukin-2 (IL-2) and tumor-infiltrating lymphocytes selected in vitro with low doses of IL-2. *Cancer Immunol Immunother* 1993; 36: 315–322.
128. Reali UM, Martini L, Borgognoni L, et al. Infusion of in vitro expanded tumour-infiltrating lymphocytes and recombinant interleukin-2 in patients with surgically resected lymph node metastases of malignant melanoma: a pilot study. *Melanoma Res* 1977; 8: 77–82.

129. Curti BD, Ochoa AC, Powers GC, et al. Phase I trial of anti-CD3-stimulated CD4+ T cells, infusional interleukin-2, and cyclophosphamide in patients with advance cancer. *J Clin Oncol* 1998; 16: 2752–2760.
130. Chang AE, Aruga A, Cameron MJ, et al. Adoptive immunotherapy with vaccine-primed lymph node cells secondarily activated with anti-CD3 and interleukin-2. *J Clin Oncol* 1997; 15: 796–807.
131. Vuist WM, v Buitenen F, de Rie MA, Hekman A, Rumke P, Melief CJ. Potentiation by interleukin-2 of Burkitt's lymphoma therapy with anti-pan B (anti-CD19) monoclonal antibodies in a mouse xenotransplantation model. *Cancer Res* 1989; 49: 3783–3788.
132. Gill I, Agab R, Hu E, Mazumder A. Synergistic anti-tumor effects of interleukin-2 and the monoclonal Lym-1 against human Burkitt lymphoma cells in vivo and in vitro. *Cancer Res* 1989; 49: 5377–5379.
133. Schultz KR, Klarnet JP, Peace DJ, et al. Monoclonal antibody therapy of murine lymphoma: enhanced efficacy by concurrent administration of interleukin-2 or lymphokine-activated killer cells. *Cancer Res* 1990; 50: 5421–5425.
134. Eisenthal A, Lafreniere R, Lefor AT, Rosenberg SA. Effect of anti-B16 melanoma monoclonal antibody on established murine B16 melanoma liver metastases. *Cancer Res* 1987; 47: 2771–2776.
135. Welte K, Miller G, Chapman, et al. Stimulation of T lymphocyte proliferation by monoclonal antibodies against GD3 ganglioside. *J Immunol* 1987; 139: 1763–1771.
136. Hirsh R, Gress RE, Pluznile DH, et al. Effects of in vivo administration of anti CD3 monoclonal antibody on T cell function in mice. II. In vivo activation of T cells. *J Immunol* 1989; 142: 737–742.
137. Hirsh R, Eckhans M, Auchincloss H, et al. Effects of in vivo administration of anti CD3 monoclonal antibodies on T cell function in mice I. Immunosuppression or transplantation response. *J Immunol* 1988; 140: 3766–3772.
138. Ellenhorn JD, Hirsh R., Schreiber H, Bluestone JA. In vivo administration of anti-CD3 prevents progressor tumor growth. *Science* 1988; 242: 569–571.
139. Reisfeld RA, Gillies SD. Antibody-interleukin 2 fusion proteins: a new approach to cancer therapy. *J Clin Lab Anal* 1996; 10: 160–166.
140. Sondel PM, Hank JA. Combination therapy with interleukin-2 and antitumor monoclonal antibodies. *Cancer J Sci Am* 1997; 3: S121–S127.
141. Albino AP, Houghton AN, Eisinger M, et al. Class II histocompatibility antigen expression in human melanocytes transformed by Harvery murine sarcoma virus (Ha-MSV) and Kirsten MSV retroviruses. *J Exp Med* 1986; 164: 1710–1722.
142. Thurin J, Thurin M, Elder DE, et al. GD2 ganglioside biosynthesis is a distinct biochemical event in human melanoma tumor progression. *FEBS Lett* 1982; 107: 357–361.
143. Bajorin DF, Chapman PB, Wong GY, et al. Treatment with high dose mouse monoclonal (anti-GD3) antibody R24 in patients with metastatic melanoma. *Melanoma Res* 1992; 2: 355–362.
144. Cheung NV, Lazarus H, Miraldi FD, et al. Ganglioside GD2 specific monoclonal antibody 3F8: a phase I study in patients with neuroblastoma and malignant melanoma (published erratum appears in *J Clin Oncol* 1992; 10: 671). *J Clin Oncol* 1987; 5: 1430–1440.
145. Saleh MN, Khazaeli MB, Wheeler RH, et al. Phase I trial of mouse monoclonal anti-GD2 antibody 14G2a in metastatic melanoma. *Cancer Res* 1992; 52: 4342–4347.
146. Coit D, Houghton AN, Cordon-Cardo C, et al. Isolated limb perfusion with monoclonal antibody R24 in patients with malignant melanoma. *Proc Am Soc Clin Oncol* 1988; 7: 248.
147. Dippold WG, Bernhard H, Meyer zum Bushenfelde K-H. Immunological response to intrathecal GD3-ganglioside antibody treatment in cerebrospinal fluid melanosis. In: Oettgen HF, ed. *Gangliosides and Cancer*. VCH, Weinheim, 1989, pp. 241–247.

148. Bajorin DF, Chapman PB, Dimaggio J, et al. Phase I evaluation of a combination of monoclonal antibody R24 and interleukin 2 in patients with metastatic melanoma. *Cancer Res* 1990; 50: 7490–7495.
149. Soiffer RJ, Chapman PB, Murray C, et al. Administration of R24 monoclonal antibody and low-dose interleukin-2 for malignant melanoma. *Clin Cancer Res* 1997; 3: 17–24.
150. Alpaugh RK, von Mehren M, Palazzo I, et al. Phase IB trial for malignant melanoma using R24 monoclonal antibody, interleukin-2/alpha-interferon. *Med Oncol* 1998; 15: 191–198.
151. Albertini MR, Hank JA, Schuller JH, et al. Phase IB trial of chimeric antidisialoganglioside antibody interleukin-2 for melanoma patients. *Clin Cancer Res* 1997; 3: 1277–1288.
152. Albertini MR, Gan J, Jaeger P, et al. Systemic interleukin-2 modulates the anti-idiotypic response to chimeric anti-GD2 antibody in patients with melanoma. 1996; 19: 278–295.
153. Hoskins DW, Stankova J, Anderson SK, et al. Amelioration of experimental lung metastases in mice by therapy with anti CD3 monoclonal antibodies. *Cancer Immunol Immunother* 1989; 29: 226–230.
154. Sosman JA, Weiss GR, Margolin KA, et al. Phase IB clinical trial of anti-CD3 followed by high-dose bolus interleukin-2 in patients with metastatic melanoma and advanced renal cell carcinoma: clinical and immunologic effects. *J Clin Oncol* 1993; 11: 1496–1505.
155. Hank JA, Albertini M, Wesley OH, et al. Clinical and immunological effects of treatment with murine anti-CD3 monoclonal antibody along with interleukin-2 in patients with cancer. *Clin Cancer Res* 1995; 1: 481–491.
156. Buter J, Janssen RA, Martens A, et al. Phase I/II study of low-dose intravenous OKT3 and subcutaneous interleukin-2 in metastatic cancer. *Eur J Cancer* 1993; 29A: 2108–2113.
157. Sosman JA, Kefer C, Fisher RI, et al. A phase IA/IB trial of anti-CD3 murine monoclonal antibody plus low-dose continuous-infusion interleukin-2 in advanced cancer patients. *J Immunother* 1995; 17: 171–180.
158. Gillies SD, Reilly EB, Lo KM, et al. Antibody targeted interleukin 2 stimulates T cell killing of autologous tumor cells. *Proc Natl Acad Sci USA* 1992; 89: 1428–1432.
159. Becker JC, Pancook JD, Gillies SD, et al. T cell mediated eradication of murine metastatic melanoma induced by targeted interleukin 2 therapy. *J Exp Med* 1996; 183: 2361–2366.
160. Becker JC, Pancook JD, Gillies SD, et al. Eradication of human hepatic and pulmonary melanoma metastases in SCID mice by antibody-interleukin fusion proteins. *Proc Natl Acad Sci USA* 1996; 93: 2702–2707.
161. Livingston P, Sznol M. In: Balch CM, Houghton AN, Sober AJ, Soong S, eds. *Cutaneous Melanoma, ed. 3.* Quality Medical Publishing, St. Louis, 1998, pp. 437–450.
162. Morton DL, Foshag LJ, Hoon DS, et al. Prolongation of survival in metastatic melanoma after active specific immunotherapy with a new polyvalent melanoma vaccine (published erratum appears in *Ann Surg* 1993; 217: 3091). *Ann Surg* 1992; 216: 463–482.
163. Bystryn JC. Clinical activity of a polyvalent melanoma antigen vaccine. *Recent Results Cancer Res* 1995; 139: 337–348.
164. Berd D, Maguire HC Jr, McCue P, Mastrangelo MJ. Treatment of metastatic melanoma with an autologous tumor-cell vaccine: clinical and immunologic results in 64 patients. *J Clin Oncol* 1990; 8: 1858–1867.
165. Mitchell MS, Harel W, Kempf RA, et al. Active-specific immunotherapy for melanoma. *J Clin Oncol* 1990; 8: 856–869.
166. Jones PC, Sze LL, Liu PY, et al. Prolonged survival for melanoma patients with elevated IgM antibody to oncofetal antigen. *J Natl Cancer Inst* 1981; 66: 249–254.
167. Livingston PO, Wong GY, Adhuri S, et al. Improved survival in stage II melanoma patients with GM2 antibodies: a randomized trial of adjuvant vaccination with GM2 antibodies: a randomized trial of adjuvant vaccination with GM2 ganglioside. *J Clin Oncol* 1994; 12: 1036–1044.

168. Adler A, Schachter J, Barenholz Y, et al. Allogeneic human liposomal melanoma vaccine with or without IL-2 in metastatic melanoma patients: clinical and immunobiological effects. *Cancer Biother* 1995; 10: 293–306.
169. Oratz R, Shapiro R, Johnson D, et al. IL-2 liposomes markedly enhance the activity of a polyvalent melanoma vaccine. *Proc Annu Meet Am Soc Clin Oncol* 1996; 15: A1356.
170. van Pel A, van der Bruggen P, Coulie PG, et al. Genes coding for tumor antigens recognized by cytolytic T lymphocytes. *Immunol Rev* 1995; 145: 229–250.
171. Rosenberg SA. The immunotherapy of solid cancers based on cloning the genes encoding tumor-rejection antigens. *Annu Rev Med* 1996; 47: 481–491.
172. Cole DJ, Weil DP, Shilyansky J, et al. Characterization of the functional specificity of a cloned T-cell receptor heterodimer recognizing the MART-1 melanoma antigen. *Cancer Res* 1995; 55: 748–752.
173. Zhai Y, Yang JC, Kawakami Y, et al. Antigen-specific tumor vaccines. Development and characterization or recombinant adenovirus encoding MART-1 or gp100 for cancer therapy. *J Immunol* 1996; 156: 700–710.
174. Parkhurst MR, Salgaller ML, Southwood S, et al. Improved induction of melanoma-reactive CTL with peptides from the melanoma antigen gp100 modified at HLA-A*0201-binding residues. *J Immunol* 1996; 157: 2539–2548.
175. Rivoltini L, Kawakami Y, Sakaguchi K, et al. Induction of tumor-reactive CTLs from peripheral blood and tumor-infiltrating lymphocytes of melanoma patients by in vitro stimulation with and immunodominant peptide of the human melanoma antigen MART-1. *J Immunol* 1995; 54: 2257–2265.
176. Salgaller ML, Afshar A, Marencola FM, et al. Recognition of multiple epitopes in the human melanoma antigen gp100 by peripheral blood lymphocytes stimulated in vitro with synthetic peptides. *Cancer Res* 1995; 55: 4972–4979.
177. Marincola FM, Rivoltini L, Salgaller ML, et al. Differential anti-MART-1/Melan A CTL activity in peripheral blood of HLA-A2 melanoma patients in comparison to healthy donors: evidence for in vivo priming by tumor cells. *J Immunother* 1996; 19: 266–277.
178. Cormier JN, Salgaller ML, Prevette T, et al. Enhancement of cellular immunity in melanoma patients immunized with a peptide from MART-1/Melan A. *Cancer J Sci Am* 1997; 3: 37–44.
179. Salgaller ML, Marincola FM, Comier JN, Rosenberg SA. Immunization against epitopes in the human melanoma antigen gp100 following patient immunization with synthetic peptides. *Cancer Res* 1996; 56: 4749–4757.
180. Rosenberg SA, Yang JC, Schwartzentruber DJ, et al. Immunologic and therapeutic evaluation of a synthetic peptide vaccine for the treatment of patients with metastatic melanoma. *Nat Med* 1998; 4: 321–327.
181. Maass G, Schmidt W, Berger M, et al. Priming of tumor-specific T cells in the draining lymph nodes after immunization with interleukin-2-secreting tumor cells: three consecutive stages may be required for successful tumor vaccination. *Proc Natl Acad Sci USA* 1995; 92: 5540–5544.
182. Belli F, Arienti F, Sule-Suso J, et al. Active immunization of metastatic melanoma patients with interleukin-2-transduced allogeneic melanoma cells: evaluation of efficacy and tolerability. *Cancer Immunol Immunother* 1997; 44: 197–203.
183. Veelken H, Mackensen A, Lahn M, et al. A Phase I clinical study of autologous tumor cells plus interleukin-2-gene-transfected allogeneic fibroblasts as a vaccine in patients with cancer. *Int J Cancer* 1997; 70: 269–277.
184. Legha SA, Ring S, Eton O, et al. Development of a biochemotherapy regimen with concurrent administration of cisplatin, vinblastine, dacarbazine, interferon alfa and interleukin-2 for patients with metastatic melanoma. *J Clin Oncol* 1998; 16: 1752–1759.
185. McDermott D, Mier J, Lawrence D, et al. Phase I pilot trial of concurrent biochemotherapy with cisplatin, vinblastine, dacarbazine, interleukin-2, and interferon-alpha-2B in patients with metastatic melanoma. *Clin Cancer Res* 2000; 6: 2201–2208.

8 Interleukin-12

Immunologic and Antitumor Effects in Human Malignant Melanoma

Ronald M. Bukowski, MD
and Charles Tannenbaum, PhD

Contents

1. INTRODUCTION

Interleukin-12 (IL-12) is a pleotrophic cytokine originally referred to as a natural killer (NK) cell stimulatory factor or a cytotoxic lymphocyte maturation factor *(1,2)*. It was identified as a factor secreted by Epstein Barr virus-transformed B cell lines. Its production can be induced by bacteria, intracellular parasites, viruses, or their products in T cell-dependent and -independent pathways. IL-12 has proinflammatory and immunoregulatory activities, with major effects on T and NK cells. It is an inducer of a type 1 (Th-1) immune response and appears to have critical roles in resistance to both infections and tumors *(3–5)*. These observations stimulated clinical trials with this cytokine in patients with viral infections, e.g., hepatitis, and with neoplasms such as malignant melanoma.

2. STRUCTURE

Following its purification, IL-12 was found to be a 70-kDa disulfide-linked heterodimeric protein composed of two polypeptides with approximate molecular weights of 35 and 40 kDa *(1,6,7)*. Further characterization revealed that the

From: *Current Clinical Oncology, Melanoma: Biologically Targeted Therapeutics*
Edited by: E. C. Borden © Humana Press Inc., Totowa, NJ

p35 component is a 219-amino acid polypeptide with 7 cysteine residues, and the p40 subunit is a 328-amino acid polypeptide, 10 of which are cysteines *(8,9)*. The protein encoded by the p35 cDNA has a molecular weight of 27,500, but appears larger because of extensive glycosylation. The p40 protein has a molecular weight of 34,700 and is comparatively less glycosylated than the p35 molecule *(8–10)*. The p35 gene transcripts are distributed widely, but the p40 transcripts are found only in cells producing biologically active IL-12, such as, monocytes, macrophages, dendritic cells, and B cells *(11)*.

The genes encoding the p40 and p35 subunits are unrelated and are located on different chromosomes *(12)*. The p35 gene maps to human chromosome 3p12-3q13.2 *(12)*. IL-5 and granulocyte-macrophage colony-stimulating factor (GM-CSF) share many amino acid positions with this subunit *(13)*. The p40 gene maps to human chromosome 5q31-33. It resembles members of the hematopoietic cytokine receptor family *(12)*, regions of the IL-6 ciliary neurotropic factor *(14)*, and monocyte colony stimulating factor receptors *(12)*. The p70 heterodimer, thus, has the characteristics of a complex formed between a cytokine and a receptor *(15)*.

3. MECHANISMS OF ACTION

3.1. Cellular Responses

A variety of cell types secret of IL-12. Among peripheral blood mononuclear cells (PBMCs), monocytes and monocyte-derived macrophages are perhaps the most significant producers of this cytokine *(16,17)*. Production of IL-12 by dendritic cells during antigen presentation, however, is a crucial signal for induction of a Th-1 response pattern and effective cell-mediated immunity *(12,17)*. Recent studies also suggest that IL-12 is the "third signal", which can participate with Class I major histocompatibility complex (MHC)/antigen complexes and B7 to induce the proliferation and activation of $CD8^+$ T cells *(18)*. Neutrophils have also been reported to produce IL-12 *(19)*. Finally, production by B lymphocytes has also been noted, although this is considered controversial *(19,20)*.

The most potent inducers of this cytokine are bacteria, lipopolysaccharide (LPS), and intracellular parasites *(16,21,22)*. In addition, IL-12 synthesis is regulated by a variety of cytokines. Interferon (IFN)γ and GM-CSF can stimulate production by phagocytic cells *(23)*. Cytokines that inhibit IL-12 production include IL-10, IL-4, and transformation growth factor β (TGFβ) *(24,25)*. These effects are mediated both at the level of RNA and protein, by inhibiting secretion of the p70 heterodimeric protein, and the accumulation of mRNAs encoding the two subunits *(24,25)*. IL-10-mediated inhibition of IFNγ production by T and NK cells occurs indirectly secondary to prevention phagocytic cell *(11,24)* synthesis of IL-12.

Membrane-bound proteins present on activated T lymphocytes also stimulate mononuclear phagocytes to synthesize and secrete IL-12 *(26,27)*. While not yet fully defined, at least several receptor–ligand interactions have been characterized, which mediate this induction. IL-12 production by antigen-presenting cells is augmented upon engagement of CD40R by CD40 ligand expressed on antigen phytohemagglutinin (PHA)-stimulated T cells *(26,28)*. The importance of this CD40/CD40L binding in mediating IL-12 induction has been demonstrated for both murine and human cells. In human PBMCs, CD40/CD40L interactions stimulated IFNγ production via an IL-12-dependent mechanism when the PBMCs are prestimulated with PHA *(28)*.

IL-12 was originally described as a cytokine that induced proliferation and cytolytic activity of NK cells, lymphokine activated killer (LAK) cells, and cytolytic T lymphocytes (CTLs). This stimulatory activity is now known to be specific for T cells and NK cells pre-activated with either antireceptor antibody *(29)*, mitogens, or IL-2 *(4)*. Freshly isolated T lymphocytes are minimally responsive to IL-12 *(29)*. The requirement for activation is related to the absence of IL-12 receptors on resting cells *(29)* and their induction upon mitogenic stimulation *(29–31)*. Studies have demonstrated that both $CD4^+$ and $CD8^+$ T cell subsets can be stimulated by IL-12 *(2,3,7,32)*.

This cytokine has a pivotal role in promoting the Th-1 vs Th-2 balance of a developing immune response *(33,34)*. Dendritic cell secretion of IL-12 during antigen processing can synergize with IFNγ to promote a Th-1 cellular immune response in T cells *(19)* and with IL-2 to further augment IFNγ production and cytotoxic lymphocyte responses *(1,4,7)*.

3.2. Signaling Pathways–Receptor

Recent studies have demonstrated that the functional IL-12 receptor is a heterodimer composed of a β1 and β2 polypeptide. Each mediates a specific activity required for IL-12 responsiveness *(35,36)*. The IL-12 receptor (IL-12R) β1 chain binds IL-12 *(37)*. The β2 chain is the component that transduces the IL-12 signal *(36,38,39)*. Th-1 cells express both chains and respond to IL-12. Th-2 cells express only the IL-12Rβ1 chain. Though binding occurs, no reactivity is exhibited in the absence of signal transduction capacity *(36,40)*. The loss of IL-12Rβ2 expression is a correlate of Th-2 cell differentiation *(35)*. IFNγ and IFNα have been shown to induce IL-12Rβ2 expression in the mouse and human, respectively *(38)*. Other reports have noted the expression of both IL-12Rβ1 and β2 mRNA is increased in the lymph nodes of naive mice following systemic administration of recombinant IL-12 *(35)*. The possibility that IL-12 induces IL-12Rβ2 mRNA indirectly via IFNγ was suggested by the finding that in IFNγ receptor (IFNγR)-/- mice, β2 mRNA levels are significantly lower than in wild-type mice following IL-12 treatment *(41)*. Conditions in which a Th-2 cell response is dominant have lymphocytes that do not display IL-12Rβ2 chains as a result of high levels of IL-4, IL-5, IL-10, and/or TGFβ *(36,42)*. The immunostimulatory effects of IL-12 are, therefore, regulated at both the agonist and receptor levels.

IL-12 binding to its receptor induces dimerization of the IL-12Rβ1 and IL-12Rβ2 chains, leading to the interaction of their receptor-associated tyrosine kinases *(43)*. These kinases allow functional enzymes to phosphorylate the IL-12Rβ2 chain *(39)*. Signal transducer and activator of transcription (STAT)4 has specificity for the resulting unique phosphorylated peptide sequence on IL-12Rβ2 *(39,44)* and is itself phosphorylated *(44)*. Phosphorylated STAT4 molecules dimerize and migrate to the nucleus, where they bind specific DNA sequences and activate transcription of genes resulting in the activities of IL-12 *(45,46)*.

3.3. Preclinical Antitumor Effects

IL-12 is an effective antitumor agent in a number of murine models, including the renal cell carcinoma Renca *(47,48)*, CT-26 colon adenocarcinoma *(48)*, MCA-105 sarcoma *(49)*, MT5076 reticulum cell sarcoma, B16F10 melanoma *(47)*, MC38/colon *(49)*, KA 31 sarcoma *(50)*, OV-HM ovarian carcinoma *(51)*, HTH-K breast carcinoma *(52)*, MBT-2 bladder carcinoma *(53)*, and MB-48 transitional cell carcinoma *(53)*. Numerous studies have demonstrated that IL-12 administration inhibits tumor growth, reduces the number of metastatic lesions, and increases survival time. In selected models, regression and resistance to secondary tumor challenge are seen *(47,53)*. The antineoplastic effects of this cytokine are found even when therapy is initiated in the presence of a significant tumor burden *(47,48,53)*.

IL-12 has no effects on cultured tumor cells, suggesting the antitumor effect is mediated indirectly through IL-12-inducible cellular and molecular intermediates *(47)*. The molecule induced by IL-12 and central to this activity is IFNγ. IFNγ antibodies essentially abrogate IL-12 mediated antitumor effects *(49,54)*. Although IFNγ is required for IL-12 activity, it does not have the potent antitumor effects characteristic of IL-12 *(55)* when it is administered in vivo. Several factors have been proposed to explain this, including the differential half lives of the two cytokines and lower concentrations of IFNγ at the tumor site.

It has been demonstrated that IL-12 can enhance NK and CTL activity, stimulate antigen primed T cells to proliferate, promote differentiation into Th-1 cells, and induce NK and T cells to secrete IFNγ. A recent report demonstrated that a preexisting CD8 and NK cell tumor infiltrates are required for maximal IL-12 antitumor *(55)*. It was suggested that these IL-12-responsive cells synthesize IFNγ within the tumor bed, which induces the local molecular events required for tumor eradication *(55)*.

Three distinct mechanisms of IL-12 mediated antitumor activity have been identified. Tannenbaum et al. *(56)* demonstrated that a molecular correlate of effective IL-12 antitumor activity in the Renca model is expression of the chemokines monokine induced by IFNγ (MIG) and IFNγ inducible protein (IP-10) within the regressing tumor. These molecules are chemotactic for NK and activated T cells, correlating with immunohistological data demonstrating an influx of $CD8^+$ and $CD4^+$ cells into the treated tumors *(56)* expressing elevated levels of perforin and granzyme. A role for the IFNγ-inducible chemokines in the antitumor effects of IL-12 was demonstrated in studies where antibodies to MIG and IP-10 abrogated the IL-12-mediated tumor regression. Additionally, synthesis of IFNγ and IP-10 mRNA was reported when explants of human renal cancer were treated in vitro with IL-12 *(57)*.

Other studies also support the role of enhanced cellular immunity in IL-12 antitumor effects. These effects of are essentially abrogated in nude mice and in mice depleted of $CD8^+$ T cells *(47)*. Multiple investigators have also reported a significant infiltration of macrophages *(56,58)* in treated tumors of IL-12-treated animals. Finally, the tumors in perforin knock-out mice are unresponsive to IL-12 administration *(59)*.

A comparison of local immune responses during tumor regression produced by either intratumor or systemically administered IL-12, demonstrates the latter is more efficacious. IFNγ expression, chemokine expression, and inflammatory cell infiltration into the tumor bed during systemic therapy appear to be enhanced *(60)*.

A second mechanism by which IL-12-induced IFNγ mediates antitumor activity is through its stimulation of other cytotoxic molecules, such as nitric oxide synthase (iNOS). iNOS is produced by endothelial cells, epithelial cells, macrophages, and tumor cells and can catalyze the production of nitric oxide (NO) *(61)*. NO is an important contributor to macrophage antitumor activity, and it has a central role as demonstrated by the ability of the NO inhibitors L-NMMA to abrogate the antitumor activity of IL-12 *(61)*.

The third possible mechanism involved in antitumor effects of IL-12 is the IFNγ-dependent induction of various anti-angiogenic factors *(62–64)*. Growing tumors require ongoing neovascularization for nourishment, expansion, and metastatic spread *(65)*. The IFN-inducible chemokines MIG, IP-10, and platelet factor 4, have been demonstrated to inhibit IL-8-stimulated angiogenic activity *(63,66)* and in vitro correlates *(62,67)* of blood vessel formation. The mechanisms by which chemokines mediate anti-angiogenic function is uncertain, but in vitro studies show that nanogram concentrations of IP-10 can inhibit endothelial cell chemotaxis *(67)*, proliferation *(68)*, and/or differentiation into tubelike structures *(62)*. The actual contribution of anti-angiogenic molecules to IL-12 antitumor activity is uncertain, but reports indicate a significant role for MIG and IP-10 in tumor necrosis and damage to tumor vasculature following of tumors in nude mice *(69,70)*.

Table 1
IL-12 Clinical Toxicity:
Subcutaneous Administration

Fever and chills
Fatigue
Leukopenia
Nausea and vomiting
Cough and shortness of breath
Elevated transaminase
Mucositis

4. CLINICAL TRIALS

4.1. Pharmacokinetics

Recombinant human IL-12 is manufactured by Genetics Institute and is currently in clinical trials. It is a lyophilized product, which is reconstituted with sterile water. Phase I trials utilizing either intravenous or subcutaneous cytokine have been performed to characterize the effects of this cytokine in patients. Initially, a weekly schedule was chosen in view of the prolonged half-life found in preclinical studies. Motzer et al. *(71)* performed a phase I trial in which IL-12 was administered subcutaneously at a fixed dose (0.1, 0.5, and 1.0 µg/kg) weekly for 3 wk. A maximal tolerated dose (MTD) of 0.5 µg/kg/wk was identified, with hepatic, hematopoietic, and pulmonary toxicity being dose limiting. The toxicity reported secondary to IL-12 is described in Table 1. A second portion of this study involved gradual dose escalation (0.5, 0.75, 1.0, 1.25, and 1.50 µg/kg) of IL-12 following administration of 0.1 µg/kg. In this portion, the MTD was 1.25 µg/kg.

Intravenous IL-12 has also been investigated in a phase I trial. Forty patients (20 with renal cancer, 12 with melanoma, 5 with colon cancer) were enrolled *(72)*. Two weeks after a single injection of IL-12 (3–1000 ng/kg), patients received an additional 6-wk course of intravenous IL-12 therapy, administered for 5 consecutive days every 3 wk. The MTD was 0.5 µg/kg/day, and toxicities include fever and chills, fatigue, nausea, and headaches. Laboratory findings included anemia, neutropenia, lymphopenia, hyperglycemia, thrombocytopenia, and hypoalbuminemia.

A phase II trial of intravenous IL-12 in renal cell carcinoma patients was then initiated utilizing 0.5 µg/kg/day for 5 d *(73)*. Seventeen patients were entered, and due to unexpected severe toxicity, the study was abandoned. The data from both the subcutaneous and intravenous phase I trials suggest a single predose of IL-12 may be associated with a decrease in toxicity and permits escalation to high doses.

The pharmacokinetic parameters reported in this study are outlined in Table 2. Serum IL-12 levels were also examined during continued administration of this

Table 2
Pharmacokinetics of Subcutaneous IL-12 *(71)*

	Fixed dose schedule[a]		*Escalating dose schedule*[a]		
	0.5 µg/kg	*1.0 µg/kg*	*0.5 µg/kg*	*1.0 µg/kg*	*1.5 µg/kg*
No. patients	*15*	*6*	*3*	*3*	*12*
C_{max} (pg/mL)[b]	320 ± 70	1092 ± 275	70 ± 35	353 ± 79	706 ± 159
T_{max} (h)[b]	13	16	16	14	15
$T_{1/2}$ (h)[b]	13 ± 2	10 ± 2	9	15 ± 7	12 ± 1

[a]For fixed schedule, cycle 1, d 1; and for escalation schedule, cycle 1, d 15.
[b]Mean values + standard error.

cytokine (wk 7) *(71)*. A significant decrease in C_{max} levels was noted. This has been referred to as an adoptive response and attributed to antibody formation or a regulatory feedback response. In the report by Motzer et al. *(71)*, antibody formation versus recombinant IL-12 was not detected. Rakhit et al. *(74)* studied this down-regulation of serum IL-12 levels in a murine model and noted this correlated with up-regulation of IL-12R expression and was not seen in IL-12Rβ -/- mice. These observations are consistent with receptor-mediated clearance of IL-12.

4.2. Pharmacodynamics

The pharmacodynamics of IL-12 administration have also been examined. In preclinical studies, the secondary production of IFNγ by peripheral blood lymphocytes is one of the major findings following IL-12 stimulation of lymphocytes. Increases in serum IFNγ have been reported with either subcutaneous *(72)* or intravenous *(73)* administration of IL-12. Peak serum IFNγ levels were noted approximately 24 h following IL-12 administration and returned to baseline within 3 to 6 d *(75)*. With continued administration, or during subsequent cycles of IL-12, serum levels are considerably lower. Other cytokine levels including IL-10, tumor necrosis factor (TNF)α, vascular endothelial growth factor (VEGF), and basic fibroblast growth factor (bFGF) have also been examined *(75)*. Consistent increases in IL-10 are seen, which normalize in 3 to 6 d. Unlike IFNγ levels, increased levels of IL-10 have been seen in later cycles of IL-12 therapy *(75)*. No consistent alterations in TNFα or VEGF levels have been noted, but, Bajetta et al. *(75)* reported a reduction of urinary bFGF levels in several responding melanoma patients.

Alterations in peripheral blood lymphocyte subsets has also been reported. Following IL-12 administration, profound lymphopenia neutropenia and reduction in monocyte numbers is observed *(71,72,75)*. These values return to baseline in 5 to 7 d. Examination of lymphocyte subsets indicates a shift in the CD4:CD8

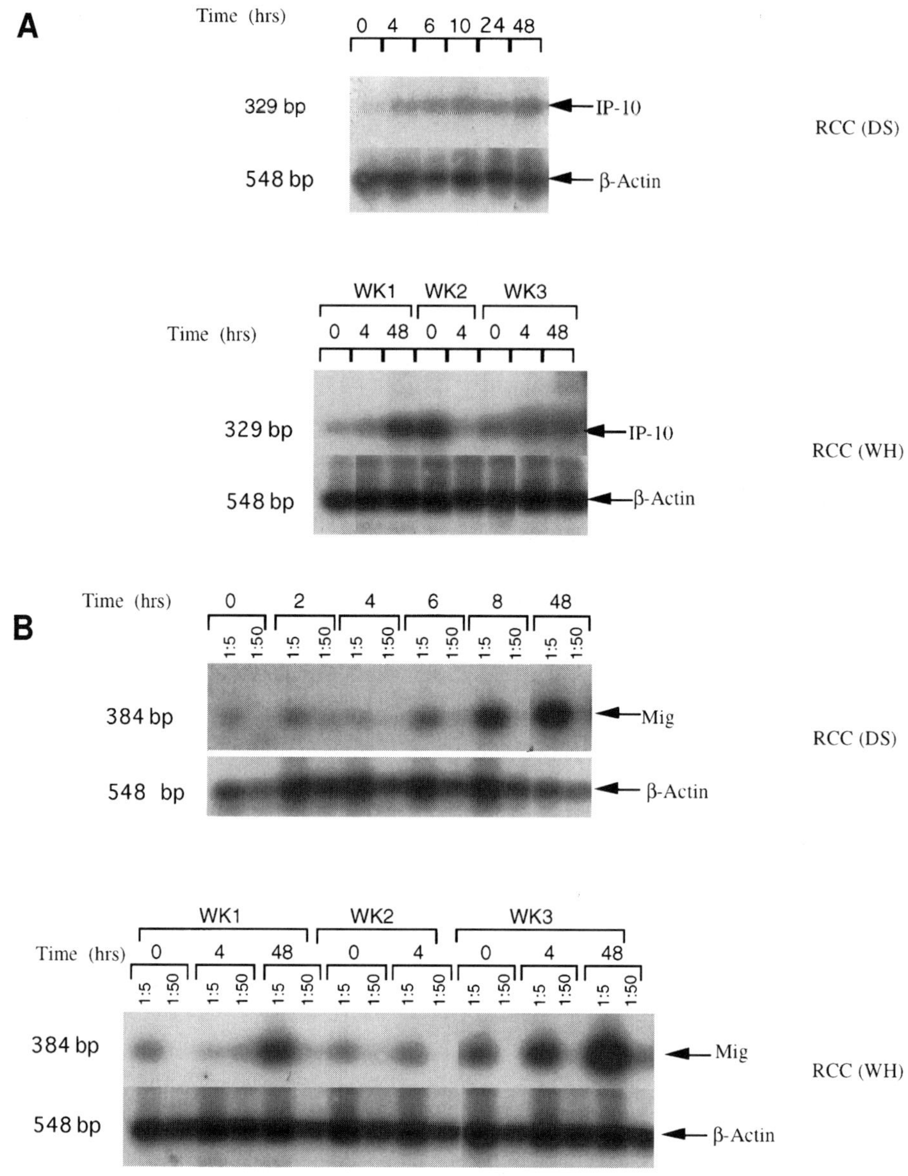

Fig. 1. A series of patients (DS, RH) with renal cell cancer (RCC) receiving subcutaneous IL-12 once weekly are illustrated. PBMCs were isolated at the time points specified, RNA isolated, and amplified utilizing reverse transcription polymerase chain reaction (RT-PCR). The induction of IP-10 and MIG mRNA are illustrated, with β-actin serving as the control. For MIG, dilutions of 1:5 and 1:50 were used. Reproduced with permission from Bukowski et al. *(57)*.

ratio 24 h after the injection of IL-12 *(75)*. There is a marked reduction in CD8$^+$ cells, and an increase in CD4$^+$, and a decrease in CD16$^+$ cells. These alterations were noted 24 h after the first dose of subcutaneous IL-12 and, with the exception of CD16$^+$ cells, had returned to normal by d 44. Augmented NK cytolytic activity and T cell proliferative responses are also seen *(76)*. Other surrogate markers such as neopterin also increase *(71)*. Peak concentrations are noted between 72 to 96 h following a single IL-12 dose.

Bukowski et al. *(57)* have investigated changes in the expression of a variety of genes in PBMCs following subcutaneous IL-12. Rapid induction of IFNγ mRNA was found and was accompanied by subsequent induction mRNA for IP-10 and MIG (*see* Fig. 1). These chemokines are IFNγ inducible and mediate chemotaxis of T-lymphocytes *(56)*. As noted previously, IP-10 appears to have antiangiogenic effects and decreases proliferation of endothelial cells *(68)*.

Pharmacodynamic studies in patients and preclinical models suggest that IL-12 has complex immunoregulatory effects on cytokine networks and lymphoid cell populations. Attempts to associate these changes with clinical responses have been unsuccessful, however.

4.3. Clinical Trials in Melanoma

The notion that selected human melanomas may be immunogenic provided a rationale for investigation of a cytokine such as IL-12, which can impact the activation, proliferation, and function of T lymphocytes. The significant preclinical activity in murine tumor models has also been of interest. Additionally, the production of angiogenic factors, such as VEGF, by human melanomas *(77)* suggests a cytokine such as IL-12 that can induce IP-10, an anti-angiogenic chemokine, may have activity in this neoplasm.

Atkins et al. *(72)* included 12 patients with metastatic melanoma in a phase I trial with intravenous IL-12. One patient with pleural nodules and lymphadenopathy experienced a brief complete response (duration 4 wk). Bajetta et al. *(75)* performed a pilot study of subcutaneous IL-12 (0.5 μg/kg/d 1, 8, 15). Ten previously treated patients were included, and three demonstrated some clinical tumor regression (subcutaneous nodules, lymph nodes, hepatic metastases), which however did not qualify as partial responses.

5. CONCLUSION

Studies to date suggest only minimal activity for IL-12 in this patient population. In experimental models, therapeutic effects of this cytokine are dose-dependent *(47,55)*, and it has been suggested that increasing the intensity of IL-12 therapy may, therefore, be desirable. The adaptive response to IL-12 may be significant in this regard, since serum IL-12 levels decrease in response to repetitive administration. Strategies to decrease the intensity of this response may, therefore, be of interest. Additionally, secondary induction of cytokines, such as IFNγ or IL-10, may play a role in the antitumor response associated with IL-12 administration or its abrogation. Methods to diminish the production of IL-10 may be relevant. Studies *(55)* suggest paracrine production of cytokines and chemokines may be the most important components producing antitumor effects of IL-12. Methods to augment local delivery and/or paracrine production of cytokines may, therefore, be useful. Finally, preclinical studies suggest combinations of IL-12 with other cytokines, such as IFNα or IL-2, may enhance its efficacy. Clinical studies with these approaches are underway.

REFERENCES

1. Kobayashi M, Fitz L, Ryan M, et al. Identification and purification of natural killer cell stimulatory factor (NKSF), a cytokine with multiple biologic effects on human lymphocytes. *J Exp Med* 1989; 170: 827–845.
2. Gately MK, Wilson DE, Wong HL. Synergy between recombinant interleukin 2 (rIL 2) and IL 2-depleted lymphokine-containing supernatants in facilitating allogeneic human cytolytic T lymphocyte responses in vitro. *J Immunol* 1986; 136: 1274–1282.
3. Gately MK, Wolitzky AG, Quinn PM, Chizzonite R. Regulation of human cytolytic lymphocyte responses by interleukin-12. *Cell Immunol* 1992; 143: 127–142.
4. Gately MK, Desai BB, Wolitzky AG, et al. Regulation of human lymphocyte proliferation by a heterodimeric cytokine IL-12 (cytotoxic lymphocyte maturation factor). *J Immunol* 1992; 147: 874–882.
5. Chan SH, Perussai B, Gupta JW, et al. Induction of interferon gamma production by natural killer cell stimulatory factor: characterization of the responder cells and synergy with other inducers. *J Exp Med* 1991; 173: 869–879.
6. Podlaski FJ, Nanduri VB, Hulmes JD, et al. Molecular characterization of interleukin 12. *Arch Biochem Biophys* 1992; 294: 230–237.
7. Stern AS, Podlaski FJ, Hulmes JD, et al. Purification to homogeneity and partial characterization of cytotoxic lymphocyte maturation factor from human B-lymphoblastoid cells. *Proc Natl Acad Sci USA* 1990; 87: 6808–6812.
8. Wolf SF, Temple PA, Kobayashi M, et al. Cloning of cDNA for natural killer cell stimulatory factor, a heterodimeric cytokine with multiple biologic effects on T and natural killer cells. *J Immunol* 1991; 146: 3074–3081.
9. Gubler U, Chua AO, Schoenhaut DS, et al. Coexpression of two distinct genes is required to generate secreted bioactive cytotoxic lymphocyte maturation factor. *Proc Natl Acad Sci USA* 1991; 88: 4143–4147.
10. Schoenhaut DS, Chua AO, Wolitzky AG, et al. Cloning and expression of murine IL-12. *J Immunol* 1992; 148: 3433–3440.
11. Trinchieri G. Interleukin-12: a cytokine produced by antigen-presenting cells with immunoregulatory functions in the generation of T-helper cells type I and cytotoxic lymphocytes. *Blood* 1994; 84: 4008–4027.
12. Murphy EE, Terres G, Macatonia SE, et al. B7 and interleukin 12 cooperate for proliferation and interferon gamma production by mouse T helper clones that are unresponsive to B7 costimulation. *J Exp Med* 1994; 180: 223–231.
13. Mergerg DM, Wolf SF, Clark SC. Sequence similarity between NKSF and the IL-6/G-CSF family (letter). *Immunol Today* 1992; 13: 77–78.
14. Gearing DP, Cosman D. Homology of the p40 subunit of natural killer cell stimulatory factor (NKSF) with the extracellular domain of the interleukin-6 receptor (letter). *Cell* 1991; 66: 9–10.

15. Sieburth D, Jabs EW, Warrington JA, et al. Assignment of genes encoding a unique cytokine (IL12) composed of two unrelated subunits to chromosomes 3 and 5. *Genomics* 1992; 14: 59–62.
16. D'Andrea A, Rengaraju M, Valiante NM, et al. Production of natural killer cell stimulatory factor (interleukin 12) by peripheral blood mononuclear cells. *J Exp Med* 1992; 176: 1387–1398.
17. Macatonia SE, Hsieh CS, Murphy KM, O'Garra A. Dendritic cells and macrophages are required for Th1 development of CD4+ T cells from alpha beta TCR transgenic mice: IL-12 substitution for macrophages to stimulate IFN-gamma production is FIN-gamma-dependent. *Int Immunol* 1993; 5: 1119–1128.
18. Curtsinger JM, Schmidt CS, Mondino A, et al. Inflammatory cytokines provide a third signal for activation of naive $CD4^+$ and $CD8^+$ cells. *J Immunol* 1991; 162: 3256–3262.
19. Hall SS. IL-12 at the crossroads (news) [see comments]. *Science* 1995; 268: 1432–1434.
20. Guery JC, Ria F, Galgiati F, Adorini L. Normal B cells fail to secrete interleukin-12. *Eur J Immunol* 1997; 27: 1632–1639.
21. Macatonia SE, Hosken NA, Litton M, et al. Dendritic cells produce IL-12 and direct the development of Th1 cells from naive $CD4^+$ T cells. *J Immunol* 1995; 154: 5071–5079.
22. Cassatella MA, Meda L, Gasperini S, D'Andrea A, Ma X, Trinchieri G. Interleukin-12 production by human polymorphonuclear leukocytes. *Eur J Immunol* 1995; 25: 1–5.
23. Kubin M, Chow JM, Trinchieri G. Differential regulation of interleukin-12 (IL-12) tumor necrosis factor alpha, and IL-1 beta production in human myeloid leukemia cell lines and peripheral blood mononuclear cells. *Blood* 1994; 83: 1847–1855.
24. D'Andrea A, Aste-Amezaga M, Valiante NM, Ma X, Kubin M, Trinchieri G. Interleukin 10 (IL-10) inhibits human lymphocyte interferon gamma- production by suppressive natural killer cell stimulatory factor/IL-12 synthesis in accessory cells. *J Exp Med* 1993; 178: 1041–1048.
25. D'Andrea A, Ma X, Ate-Amezaga M, Paganin C, Tinchieri G. Stimulatory and inhibitory effects of interleukin (IL)-4 and IL-13 on the production of cytokines by human peripheral blood mononuclear cells: priming for IL-12 and tumor necrosis factor alpha production. *J Exp Med* 1995; 181: 537–546.
26. Shu U, Kiniwa M, Wu CY, et al. Activated T cells induce interleukin-12 production by monocytes via CD40-CD40 ligand interaction. *Eur J Immunol* 1995; 25: 1125–1128.
27. Hunter CA, Ellis-Neyer L, Gabriel KE, et al. The role of the CD28/B7 interaction in the regulation of NK cell responses during infection with Toxoplasma gondii. *J Immunol* 1997; 158: 2285–2293.
28. McDyer JF, Goletz TJ, Thomas E, June CH, Seder RA. CD40 ligand/CD40 stimulation regulates the production of IFN-gamma from human peripheral blood mononuclear cells in an IL-12- and/or CD27-dependent manner. *J Immunol* 1998; 160: 1701–1707.
29. Gollob JA, Schnipper CP, Orsini E, et al. Characterization of a novel subset of CD8(+) T cells that expands in patients receiving interleukin-12. *J Clin Invest* 1998; 102: 561–575.
30. Gately MK, Renzetti LM, Magram J, et al. The interleukin-12/interleukin-12-receptor system: role in normal and pathologic immune responses. *Annu Rev Immunol* 1998; 16: 495–521.
31. Adorini L. Interleukin-12, a key cytokine in Th1-mediated autoimmune diseases. *Cell Mol Life Sci* 1999; 55: 1610–1625.
32. Aste-Amezaga M, Ma X, Sartori A, Trinchieri G. Molecular mechanisms of the induction of IL-12 and its inhibition by IL-10. *J Immunol* 1998; 160: 5936–5940.
33. Mosmann TR, Coffman RL. Heterogeneity of cytokine secretion patterns and functions of helper T cells. *Adv Immunol* 1989; 46: 111–147.
34. Mosmann TR, Coffman RL. Th1 and Th2 cells: different patterns of lymphokine secretion lead to different functional properties. *Annu Rev Immunol* 1989; 7: 145–173.
35. Thibodeaux DK, Hunter SE, Waldburger KE, et al. Autocrine regulation of IL-12 receptor expression is independent of secondary IFN-gamma secretion and not restricted to T and Nκ cells. *J Immunol* 1999; 163: 5257–5264.

36. Showe LC, Fox FE, Williams D, Au K, Niu Z, Rook AH. Depressed IL-12-mediated signal transduction in T cells from patients with Sézary syndrome is associated with the absence of IL-12 receptor beta 2 mRNA and high reduced levels of STAT4. *J Immunol* 1999; 163: 4073–4079.
37. Wang X, Wilkinson VL, Podlaski FJ, et al. Characterization of mouse interleukin-12 p40 homodimer binding to the interleukin-12 rector subunits. *Eur J Immunol* 1999; 29: 2007–2013.
38. Murphy KM, Ouyang W, Szabo SJ, et al. T helper differentiation proceeds through Stat1-dependent, Stat4-dependent and Stat4-independent phases. *Curr Top Microbiol Immunol* 1999; 238: 13–26.
39. Naeger LK, McKinney J, Salvekar A, Hoey T. Identification of a STAT4 binding site in the interleukin-12 receptor required for signaling. *J Biol Chem* 1999; 273: 1875–1878.
40. Rogge L, Papi A, Presky DH, et al. Antibodies to the IL-12 receptor beta 2 chain mark human Th1 but not Th2 cells in vitro and in vivo. *J Immunol* 1999; 162: 3926–3932.
41. Mountford AP, Coulson PS, Cheever AW, Sher A, Wilson RA, Wynn TA. Interleukin-12 can directly induce T-helper 1 responses in interferon-gamma (IFN-gamma) receptor-deficient mice, but requires IFN-gamma signaling to downregulate T-helper 2 responses. *Immunology* 1999; 97: 588–594.
42. Zhang F, Nakamura T, Aune TM. TCR and IL-12 receptor signals cooperative to activate an individual response element in the IFN-gamma promoter in effector Th cells. *J Immunol* 1999; 163: 728–735.
43. Yamamoto K, Shibata F, Miura O, Kamiyama R, Hirosawa S, Miyasaka N. Physical interaction between interleukin-12 receptor beta 2 subunit and Jak2 tyrosine kinase: Jak2 associates with cytoplasmic membrane-proximal region of interleukin-12 and receptor beta 2 via aminoterminus. *Biochem Biophys Res Commun* 1999: 275: 400–404.
44. Yao BB, Niu P, Surowy CS, Faltynek CR. Direct interaction of STAT4 with the IL-12 receptor. *Arch Biochem Biophys* 1999; 368: 147: 155.
45. Akira S. Functional roles of STAT family proteins: lessons from knockout mice. *Stem Cells* 1999; 17: 138–146.
46. Ouyang W. Jacobson NG, Bhattacharya D, et al. The Ets transcription factor ERM is Th1-specific and induced by IL-12 through a Stat4-dependent pathway. *Proc Natl Acad Sci USA* 1999; 96: 3888–3893.
47. Brunda MJ, Luistro L, Warrier RR, et al. Antitumor and antimetastatic activity of interleukin 12 against murine tumors. *J Exp Med* 1993; 178: 1223–1230.
48. Tannenbaum CS, Tubbs R, Armstrong D, Finke JH, Bukowski RM, Hamilton TA. The CXC chemokines IP-10 and Mig are necessary for IL-12-mediated regression of the mouse RENCA tumor. *J Immunol* 1998; 161: 927–932.
49. Nastala CL, Edington HD, McKinney TG, et al. Recombinant IL-12 administration induces tumor regression in association with IFN-gamma production. *J Immunol* 1994; 153: 1697–1706.
50. Gately MK, Gubler U, Brunda MJ, et al. Interleukin-12: a cytokine with therapeutic potential in oncology and infectious diseases. *Ther Immunol* 1994; 1: 187–196.
51. Mu Z, Zou JP, Yamamoto N, et al. Administration of recombinant interleukin 12 prevents outgrowth of tumor cells metastasizing spontaneously to lung and lymph nodes. *Cancer Res* 1995; 55: 4404–4408.
52. Dias S, Thomas H, Balkwill F. Multiple molecular and cellular changes associated with tumour statis and regression during IL-12 therapy of a murine breast cancer model. *Int J Cancer* 1998; 75: 151–157.
53. Brunda MJ, Luistro L, Rumennik L, et al. Antitumor activity of interleukin 12 in preclinical models. *Cancer Chemother Pharmacol* 1996; 38(Suppl): S16–S21.
54. Brunda MJ, Luistro L, Hendrzak JA, Fountoulakis M, Garotta G, Gately MK. Role of interferon-gamma in mediating the antitumor efficacy of interleukin-12. *J Immunother Emphasis Tumor Immunol* 1995; 17: 71–77.

55. Colombo MP, Vagliani M. Spreafico F, et al. Amount of interleukin 12 available at the tumor site is critical for tumor regression. *Cancer Res* 1996; 56: 2531–2534.
56. Tannenbaum CS, Wicker N, Armstrong D, et al. Cytokine and chemokine expression in tumors of mice receiving systemic therapy with IL-12. *J Immunol* 1996; 156: 693–699.
57. Bukowski RM, Rayman P, Molto L, et al. Interferon-gamma and CXC chemokine induction by interleukin 12 in renal cell carcinoma *Clin Cancer Res* 1999; 5; 2780–2789.
58. Ha SJ, Lee SB, Kim CM, Shin HS, Sung YC. Rapid recruitment of macrophages in interleukin-12 mediated tumour regression. *Immunology* 1998; 95: 156–153.
59. Hashimoto W, Osaki T, Okamura H, et al. Differential antitumor effects of administration of recombinant IL-18 or recombinant IL-12 are mediated primarily by Fas-Fas ligand and perforin-induced tumor apoptosis, respectively. *J Immunol* 1999; 163: 583–589.
60. Cavallo F, Di Carolo E, Butera M, et al. Immune events associated with the cure of established tumors and spontaneous metastases by local and systemic interleukin 12. *Cancer Res* 1999; 59: 414–421.
61. Wiggington JM, Kuhns DB, Back TC, Brunda MJ, Wiltroug RH, Cox GW. Interleukin 12 primes macrophages for nitric oxide production in vivo and restores depressed nitric oxide production by macrophages from tumor-bearing mice: implications for the antitumor activity of interleukin 12 and/or interleukin 2. *Cancer Res* 1996; 56: 1131–1136.
62. Angiolillo AL, Sgadari C, Tosato G. A role for interferon-inducible protein 10 in inhibition of angiogenesis by interleukin-12. *Ann NY Acad Sci* 1996; 795: 158–167.
63. Kerbel RS, Hawley RG. Interleukin 12: newest member of the antiangiogenesis club [editorial; comment]. *J Natl Cancer Inst* 1995; 87: 557–559.
64. Sgadari C, Angiolillo AL, Tosato G. Inhibition of angiogenesis by interleukin-12 is mediated by the interferon-inducible protein 10. *Blood* 1996; 87: 3877–3882.
65. O'Reilly MS, Boehm T, Shing Y, et al. Endostatin: an endogenous inhibitor of angiogenesis and tumor growth. *Cell* 1997; 88: 277–285.
66. Voest EE, Kenyon BM, O'Reilly MS, Truitt G, D'Amato RJ, Folkman J. Inhibition of angiogenesis in vivo by interleukin 12 [see comments]. *J Natl Cancer Inst* 1995; 87: 581–586.
67. Strieter RM, Kunkel SL, Arenberg DA, Burdick MD, Polverini PJ. Interferon gamma-inducible protein 10 (IP-10), a member of the C-X-C chemokine family, is an inhibitor of angiogenesis. *Biochem Biophys Res Commun* 1995; 210: 51–57.
68. Luster AD, Greenberg SM, Leder P. The IP-10 chemokine binds to a specific cell surface heparan sulfate site shared with platelet factor 4 and inhibits endothelial cell proliferation. *J Exp Med* 1995; 182: 219–231.
69. Sgadari C, Farber JM, Angiolillo AL, et al. Mig, the monokine induced by interferon-gamma, promotes tumor necrosis in vivo. *Blood* 1997; 89: 2635–2643.
70. Kanegane C, Sgadari C, Kanagane H, et al. Contribution of the CXC chemokines IP-10 and Mig to the antitumor effects of IL-12. *J Leukoc Biol* 1998; 64: 384–392.
71. Motzer RJ, Rakhit A, Schwartz LH, et al. Phase I trial of subcutaneous recombinant human interleukin-12 in patients with advanced renal cell carcinoma. *Clin Cancer Res* 1998; 4: 1183–1191.
72. Atkins MB, Robertson MJ, Gordon M, et al. Phase I evaluation of intravenous recombinant human interleukin 12 in patients with advanced malignancies. *Clin Cancer Res* 1997; 3: 409–417.
73. Mier J, Dollob JA, Atkins M. Interleukin 12, a new antitumor cytokine. *Int J Immunopath Pharm* 1998; 11: 109–115.
74. Rakhit A, Yeon MM, Ferrante J, et al. Down-regulation of the pharmacokinetic-pharmacodynamic response to interleukin-12 during long-term administration to patients with renal cell carcinoma and evaluation of the mechanism of this "adaptive response" in mice. *Clin Pharmacol Ther* 1999; 65: 615–629.

75. Bajetta E, Del Vecchio M, Mortarini R, et al. Pilot study of subcutaneous recombinant human interleukin 12 in metastatic melanoma. *Clin Cancer Res* 1998; 4: 75–85.
76. Robertson MJ, Camerin C, Atkins MB, et al. Immunological effects of interleukin 12 administered by bolus intravenous injection to patients with cancer. *Clin Cancer Res* 1999; 5: 9–16.
77. Arenberg DA, Kunkel SL, Polverini PJ, et al. Interferon-gamma-inducible protein 10 (IP-10) is an angiostatic factor that inhibits human non-small cell lung cancer (NSCLC) tumorigenesis and spontaneous metastases. *J Exp Med* 1996; 184: 981–992.

9 Interferons

Preclinical and Clinical Studies in Melanoma

Ernest C. Borden, MD

Contents

1. INTRODUCTION

Interferons (IFNs) were the first therapeutic protein effective in melanoma in humans. IFNs brought to clinical fruition years of research on the potential role of biological strategies for melanoma. IFN-α2 is now licensed in more than 50 countries for more than a dozen clinical indications including melanoma. The clinical effectiveness of IFN-α2 has been established both in the adjuvant and metastatic clinical settings. IFNs were the first previously unavailable therapeutic proteins resulting from recombinant DNA technology. Thus in 1980, *Time* magazine had published a cover story, "*Interferons: the IF Drug for Cancer*". IFNs are no longer an "IF?" for either melanoma or cancer.

However, there is much to be learned. The full therapeutic potential of the IFN system for melanoma has yet to be realized. Major research challenges for full understanding and application are the following: (*i*) role of endogenous production; (*ii*) actions of the diverse IFN family of proteins; (*iii*) molecular mechanism of action; (*iv*) cellular modulatory effects; (*v*) augmenting therapeutic effects and overcoming resistance; and (*vi*) advantages of combinations. To provide additional insights to begin to answer these challenges, preclinical findings with

From: *Current Clinical Oncology, Melanoma: Biologically Targeted Therapeutics*
Edited by: E. C. Borden

particular reference to melanoma will be reviewed. In addition, clinical results to date with IFN-α2 as an adjuvant for the high risk patient after surgery and for metastatic disease will be reviewed. These data provide the basis on which future progress will occur.

2. IFNs AS PART OF THE HOST RESPONSE TO CANCER

Molecules which are chemically-defined inducers could have several therapeutic advantages. They may possess differing and advantageous pharmacokinetics of IFN effects, induce additional cytokines, activate immune effector cells, and if administered orally, be more convenient. They might prove more effective as therapeutic agents. They could also be effective as chemopreventive agents in individuals such as those with familial dysplastic nevi or a prior melanoma. The first identified, chemically-defined inducers of IFNs were double-stranded polyribonucleotides. Although potent IFN inducers and immunomodulators in mice, polyriboinosinic-polyribocytidilic acid (poly I:poly C) or various modifications do not consistently induce IFN or have any antitumor activity in humans at clinically tolerable doses *(1)*. Subsequently, low molecular weight organic compounds such as tilorone, halopyrimidinones, acridines, substituted quinolines, and flavone acetic acid were identified as inducers of IFNs in different animal species. Several of these IFN inducers have been in human clinical trials. Some induced substantial amounts of IFN and induce IFN-stimulated genes, but all were associated with various unacceptable side effects. The induction of IFN itself is associated with the cytokine symptomatology of chills, fever, and fatigue. These symptoms both confirm the in vivo physiological activity of the inducers and also demonstrate the need to better define both biologically and clinically effective molecules *(2–6)*.

In addition to being therapeutic when exogenously administered, loss of endogenous IFNs may contribute to melanoma development. One chromosomal locus, often lost in melanoma, at 9p21 codes for at least two protein products which influence cell cycle progression *(7–9)*. The genes for production of IFN-α and IFN-β lie at 9p22, another locus commonly lost in melanoma *(10,11)*. In melanoma patients, a loss of IFNs may lead to a lessened host response to the transformed cells. It may also result in additional perturbations of melanocyte proliferation resulting from lack of induction of such IFN-regulated genes as protein kinase R, RNase L, interferon regulatory factor (IRF)-2, and the p202-related family—all genes whose products may influence the cell cycle. Acting in concert with the loss of the cell cycle regulatory proteins at 9p21, p16 and p19 (ARF [alternate reading frame]), the IFN system may be a critical element in controlling progression of transformed melanocytes to malignant tumor masses.

3. FIRST AND SECOND GENERATION IFNs

Human IFNs are a family of more than 20 cytokines defined by inhibition of replication of both RNA and DNA viruses. The family diversity has been retained through evolution and also occurs among vertebrate species. This suggests that unique biological effects may exist for each IFN in modulating cell response and, potentially, in therapeutic roles. IFNs are related by similarities in primary amino acid sequence, although for IFN-γ, only slightly *(12–15)*. As would be predicted by differences in primary sequence, each protein is distinct antigenically in both homologous and heterologous vertebrates. Biologically, IFNs are very species-restricted in biological activity.

IFNs-α, IFN-β, and IFN-ω all bind to a common 2-component receptor. Despite the binding of these three IFN families to a common receptor, differing cellular and clinical effects result. This has been most clearly shown by the differing patterns of gene expression induced in a single cell type *(16,17)*. The biological and clinical effects of IFN-ω remain largely unexplored *(18)*. IFN-τ, identified only in ruminants, is critical for trophoblastic implantation into the endometrium *(19)*.

Each IFN resides at a specific genetic locus. The three most studied classes of IFNs (α, β, γ) were initially defined on the basis of chemical, antigenic, and biologic differences *(12–15)*. Human IFNs-α, IFN-β, and IFN-ω are structurally similar and located on chromosome 9p21. Both IFN-α and IFN-β are 166 amino acids in length with an additional 20-amino acid secretory peptide, which is cleaved from the amino terminus. Comparison of the sequences of IFN-α and IFN-β has defined approximately 45% homology of nucleotides and 29% homology of amino acids. Each of the nonallelic human IFN-α genes differ by approximately 10% in nucleotide sequence, and 15 to 25% in amino acid sequence. IFN-γ, 143 amino acids in length, is located on chromosome 12q14 and also contains a 20-amino acid secretory peptide. IFN-γ has only minimal sequence homology with IFN-α or IFN-β. Although IFN-β and IFN-γ, when produced by eukaryotic cells, are glycosylated, biologic differences from the unglycosylated IFNs produced in prokaryotic cells have not yet been identified.

Studies of natural killer (NK) cell cytotoxicity have defined differences in potency of IFNs-α *(20,21)*. Different IFNs-α also result in varying effects on augmentation of tumor-associated antigen (TAA) expression *(22)*. Quantitative differences in vitro in the various IFNs-α, found in eukaryotic cell-produced IFNs-α preparations, have also been reported *(15)*. Only one of the individual IFN-α types, IFN-α2, has yet been broadly assessed clinically. Limited phase I trials of IFN-α1 have been conducted in the United States. Significantly few side effects resulted *(23)*. For example, in this randomized clinical comparison, maximum peak temperature was significantly less from IFN-α1 than resulting from IFN-α2. Yet IFN-α1 was as effective in inducing 2-5A synthetase and NK cell cytotoxicity as was IFN-α2 *(23,24)*. IFN-α1 has been more widely assessed in China. Reported side effects have been fewer and less severe. IFN-α1 has been used in China mostly for chronic hepatitis B and hepatitis C infections with good effectiveness. In China, it has had only limited trial in malignancies, although it has clinical activity in chronic myelogeneous leukemia and hairy cell leukemia.

In both cancer and multiple sclerosis, IFN-β has proven better tolerated than anticipated based upon expected side effects observed with IFN-α2. For example, in studies in cancer, little or no weight loss has resulted *(25,26)*. In multiple sclerosis, frequency of cumulative side effects over the first 3 mo between placebo and control have been difficult to discern *(27)*.

IFNs were assessed against 40 freshly derived melanomas in human tumor stem cell assay. A dose response relationship was identified and, in comparison to other IFNs, IFN-β had greater antiproliferative effects *(28)*. This study has been extended, subsequently, by others to both freshly derived and continuous melanoma cell lines with consistent findings of greater activity of IFN-β *(29–33)*. To further probe potential mechanisms of antitumor effects, we have assessed apoptosis in response to IFN-α2 and IFN-β in cell lines of varied histologies with focus on melanomas *(34)*. In general, IFN-β had greater antiproliferative and pro-apoptotic effects than IFN-α2 on all cell lines. Evidence of induction of apoptosis by IFNs generally required more than 48 h of treatment. IFN-β-induced apoptosis for the WM-9 melanoma cell lines was dependent on activation of the caspase cascade. Changes in phospholipid symmetry on plasma membrane, movement of cytochrome c from mitochondria to cytoplasm, and DNA fragmentation were also observed. In conjunction with caspase activation, IFN-β, but not IFN-α2, resulted in cleavage of the anti-apoptotic protein Bcl-2. An interferon-stimulated gene (ISG), Apo2L ligand (TRAIL) was one of the genes induced by IFN-β. Conversely, in melanoma cells resistant to the apoptotic effects of IFN-β, there was no induction of TRAIL/Apo2L in response to IFN-β. Induction of TRAIL by IFNs in melanoma may initiate the apoptotic cascade *(34)*.

In vivo studies have suggested antitumor effectiveness of IFN-β. In the nude mouse, human IFN-β inhibited growth of three different melanoma xenografts and resulted in greater antitumor effects than IFN-α2 *(29,35)*. Antitumor effects occurred despite the absence of immune response in the immunodeficient mice. In humans, a deficiency in IFN-β production has been identified in the epidermis overlying melanomas with a concomitant increase in angiogenesis *(36)*. Since IFN-β has antiangiogenic effects in the nude mouse *(37)*, these antitumor effects could be resulting from vascular inhibition in addition to direct effects on tumor. A high dose daily infusion of IFN-β (60 million U) for 4 d resulted in partial responses in 3/15 patients with metastatic melanoma *(38)*. A lower dose (up to 20 million U intravenously) 2 times weekly was ineffective *(39)*.

Table 1
Cellular Effects of IFNs Potentially Important for Antitumor Effects in Melanoma

Protein induction
Adhesion proteins
Enzyme induction
Chemokines–cytokines
Cell modulation
Oncogene depression
Slow mitotic cycle
Differentiation induction
Apoptosis
Immune augmentation
Dendritic cell
T cell
NK/LAK cell
Monocytes
Antigen processing
Antibody-dependent cytotoxicity
Vascular
Angiogenesis inhibition

Clinical effectiveness for melanoma may thus be further enhanced by the introduction of second generation IFNs, whether different IFNs-α, IFN-β, or chemically-modified IFNs, with either different biological effects and/or pharmacokinetic–pharmacodynamic profiles. Pegylated IFNs-α have polyethylene glycol (PEG) linked with a single covalent bond. Multi-institutional trials, including at the Taussig Cancer Center, have identified a prolonged plasma half-life. Pegylated IFN-α2 has proven to be safe and tolerated and may allow once weekly dosing. Tumor regressions have resulted in renal carcinomas and chronic myelogenous leukemia and in the phase I trials in 2/6 patients with metastatic melanoma *(40)*. IFN-β has also been complexed with various molecules, including PEG and the soluble portion of its receptor. Will therapeutically important differences be identified in clinical trials in melanoma with second generation IFNs? We already know from phase I and limited phase II trials, discussed above, that objective responses can occur with IFNs other than IFN-α2 in patients with melanoma.

4. MECHANISMS OF ANTITUMOR ACTION IN MELANOMA

IFNs are cellular modulators with pleiotropic actions (Table 1). IFNs regulate gene expression, modulate expression of proteins on the cell surface, and induce synthesis of new enzymes. Alterations in gene expression result in modulation

Table 2
Modulation of Gene Expression by IFNs

Induced proteins
Antigen processing
MHC
Class I (A, B, C)[a]
Class II (DR, DP, DQ)[a]
β_2-Microglobulin[a]
Invariant chain
Cell surface proteins
ICAM-1
Leu-13
Depressed functional activities
Ornithine decarboxylase
Oncogenes
p450 Microsomal enzymes
Fibroblast growth factor β
Enzymes and other proteins
2-5A synthetase[a]
Protein/kinase R
Indoleamine dioxygenase[a]
Guanylate-binding proteins[a]
GTP cyclohydrolase[a]
Metallothionein II
Mn^{2+} superoxide dismutase
ISG 15[a]
Phospholipid scramblase
p56
Transcription factors
IRF-1 (ISGF-2)
IRF2
Stat 1
Stat 2
ICSBP/PML

[a]Modulation demonstrated after IFN-α in patients in vitro and in vivo.

MHC, major histocompatibility complex; ICAM, intercellular adhesion molecule; GTP, guanylate binding protein; ISG, interferon stimulated gene; ICSBP, interferon consensus sequence binding protein; PML, promyelocytic leukemia.

of levels of receptors for other cytokines, concentration of regulatory proteins on the surface of immune effector cells, and activities of enzymes that modulate cellular growth and function. Antitumor effects may result from either a direct effect on tumor cells such as proliferative capacity, apoptosis, or antigenic composition. Complementing this, indirect effects may occur through modulation of immune effector cell function or through inhibition of angiogenesis.

IFNs induce expression of hundreds of new proteins, mostly on a transcriptional level (Table 2). This diversity in alterations in gene expression has been a problem in attributing the effects of IFNs to any specific gene product(s). The extent of stimulation of genes of diverse function has been mostly clearly demonstrated by determining mRNA profiles from IFN-α, IFN-β, or IFN-γ treatments of a human fibrosarcoma and melanoma using oligonucleotide arrays with probe sets corresponding to more than 5600 human genes *(16,17)*. Until overexpression or deletion can manipulate these genes, delineation of their specific role in cellular response to IFNs can only be speculative. However, a number of genes induced by type I IFNs are involved in apoptosis including protein kinase (PKR), promyelocytic leukemia (PML), RAP46/Bag-1, phospholipid scramblase, TRAIL, and hypoxia inducible factor-1α *(16)*.

4.1. Enzyme Induction

Among the enzymes induced are 2-5 oligoadenylate synthetase (2-5A synthetase), PKR, indoleamine 2,3-dioxygenase (IDO), GTPases, and phospholipid scramblases (Table 2). 2-5A synthetase has been shown to transfer a nucleoside 5' monophosphate to the 2' position of an accepting chain. 2-5A synthetases are multiple isoform products of a 3-gene family *(41)* and are relatively specific markers of IFN system activation. A latent ribonuclease is activated by 2-5A. Expression of an enzymatically inactive RNase L in cells resulted in inhibition of the antiviral and antiproliferative effects of IFNs *(42)*. Apoptosis is suppressed in Rnase L null mice treated with different apoptotic agents *(43)*. Elevated levels of RNase L mRNA and enzymatic activity have been detected in human colorectal carcinomas when compared to corresponding normal mucosa *(44)*. This suggests RNA turnover may be an important step in tumor progression.

A constitutive serine–threonine kinase, PKR, with a unique requirement for double-stranded RNA (dsRNA) undergoes induction and activation by IFNs and dsRNAs *(45)*. The activated PKR phosphorylates several cellular proteins including protein synthesis initiation factor 2a *(45)* and IκB, resulting in activation of nuclear factor (NF)κB *(46)*. A major function of this kinase is growth control; it can also induce apoptosis *(47)*. Cells expressing PKR mutants form colonies in soft agar, and upon injection into nude mice produce large tumors *(48)*. PKR levels correlate inversely with proliferative activity in different human tumors and tumor cell lines with clinical correlations to invasive breast carcinomas *(49,50)*. PKR expression may be partially controlled by an IFN-induced transcription factor, IRF-1. Since IRF-1 increased rapidly in growth-arrested cells, it may influence expression of genes involved in negative control of cell growth and may mediate antiproliferative effects of IFNs. A second transcription factor, IRF-2, identified in murine cells, has sequence hematology to IRF-1 and is a functional antagonist of IRF-1. Upon constitutive expression, IRF-2 can result in cell transformation, which is inhibited by IRF-1 *(51)*. Degradation of tryptophan to kynurenine by IDO has been implicated in protein synthesis inhibition and antiproliferative effects as a result of depletion of tryptophan *(52)*.

There are at least three families of GTPases that are induced by IFNs. The best characterized is the Mx family. The Mx proteins belong to the dynamin superfamily of large GTPases, which are proteins involved in endocytosis and vesicle transport *(53)*. Other GTPases are some of the most abundant proteins in IFN-treated human cells *(54)*.

Phospholipid scramblase flips phosphatidylserine from the inner layer of the plasma membrane to the outer layer *(55)*. The appearancc of phosphatidylserine on the outer layer of the cell membrane has been observed in apoptotic cells. IFNs also down-regulate expression of the multidrug resistance gene (mdr1) in human colon carcinoma cells *(56)*.

Several IFN-induced proteins have been localized to small domains having a speckled appearance in the nucleus, called nuclear bodies (NBs). The best studied of these NB proteins is the PML *(57)*. PML knock-out mice were used to demonstrate that PML is necessary for programmed cell death induced by IFNs-α and IFN-β *(58)*.

Induced proteins and their products can be identified on cells and in serum of treated patients. Their measurement or the quantitation of immune effector cell function can be used to define biologically active molecules, doses, schedules, and routes of administration. Most biologic response modulatory effects peak at 24 to 48 h, which contrasts with maximal serum levels in pharmacokinetic studies *(59,60)*. After intravenous bolus administration, the t1/2*a* of IFN-α2 is short (<60 min); mean terminal half-life is 4 to 5 h with no serum levels measurable at 12 h. After intramuscular or subcutaneous administration, peak levels are 6 to 10 h *(61)*. The pharmacologic hallmark of IFN-β has been virtual absence of serum levels with subcutaneous or intramuscular administration; yet, biologic response modulatory and therapeutic effects occur *(62)*.

4.2. Antiproliferative, Apoptotic, and Differentiative Effects

Proliferation of normal cells is regulated by proteins that serve as checkpoints for the control of cell cycle progression. Melanomas develop defects in one or more proteins in these pathways. Proto-oncogenes regulated by IFNs in different cell types include c-myc *(63,64)*, bcl-2 *(65)*, and c-Ha-ras *(66)*. Melanoma cells were differentiated by IFN-β, an effect that did not correlate directly with an antiproliferative effect *(67)*. Mouse 3T3 cells transformed with the human HA-*ras*-1 gene and cultured continuously, in the presence of murine IFN-α/β, produced revertant colonies in which transcription of the *ras* gene was inhibited. Most cells retained the revertant phenotype during many cell generations despite renewed high levels of transcription of the *ras* gene and of p21 Ras protein *(68)*. A checkpoint protein mutated in many cancers is the retinoblastoma protein (Rb). Underphosphorylated Rb (the active form) specifically binds and inhibits the transcription factor E2F, thus inhibiting cell cycle progression. The primary influence of IFN-α on Rb is inhibition of its hyperphosphorylation by IFN treatment *(69,70)*. Inhibition of Rb hyperphosphorylation by IFN-α may result from rapid reduction of the expression of cyclin D3, which in turn, results in a reduction in the formation of cyclin D-cdk4 and cyclin D-cdk6 kinase complexes *(71)*. E2F controls a number of cell cycle-related genes such as c-myc and cdc2. IFN-α cells results in the reduction of one of the E2F proteins, E2F-1 *(72)*. Downstream of Rb and E2F, IFN-α reduces the amount of the cdc25 tyrosine phosphatase, resulting in the loss of activation of cyclin E-cdk2 and cyclin A-cdk2 kinase complexes *(72)*. Also, the cdk-inhibitor $p21^{WAF1}$ is induced by IFN-γ *(73)*, which negatively regulates cyclinE:cdk2. Although these mechanisms have been examined little in melanoma, some likely contribute to antiproliferative effects.

IFN-β, but not IFN-α, induced apoptosis in a number of melanoma cell lines *(74)*. To understand the mechanism by which this process occurred, proteins associated with apoptosis were examined for inducibility. An oligonucleotide-based analysis in WM9 cells revealed preferential induction of TRAIL/APO2L by IFN-β as compared to IFN-α2 *(17)*. To confirm these results, RNase protection assays were performed with probes for various apoptotic pathways. Caspase8, FasL, DR5, DR4, TNFRp55, and tumor necrosis factor receptor associated death domain protein (TRADD) mRNA were expressed constitutively but not upregulated in melanomas. In contrast, TRAIL was induced in response to IFN-β and IFN-α as early as 8 h, but persisted after IFN-β, but not IFN-α. No basal level of TRAIL mRNA was observed in untreated cells These results suggest TRAIL is an ISG, which may be activated directly or indirectly by IFN-β or IFN-α2 *(34)*.

Another pathway for the induction of apoptosis involves binding of Fas to FasL, which results in recruitment of the death domain containing protein, FADD, and the subsequent activation of caspases, such as caspase-8. IFN-γ up-regulated expression of both Fas and FasL on the human colon adenocarcinoma cell line, HT29 *(74)*. IFNs up-regulate FasL and FasR expression and, therefore, may work through the Fas-mediated apoptotic pathway in other cells but, as noted above, not apparently with IFN-α and IFN-β in melanomas *(34,75–77)*. For example, in chronic myelogenous leukemia, fas expression in vitro has been correlated with clinical response *(78,79)*.

4.3. Immune Effector Cells

IFNs augment the effectiveness of all immune effector cell types that have the potential to kill tumor target cells (see Chapter 4). These include dendritic cells, cytotoxic T cells, NK/lymphokine-activated killer (LAK) cells, and monocytes. Antibody-dependent, cell-mediated cytotoxicity, mediated by subpopulations of these effectors, can also be boosted by IFNs. In addition to augmenting expression of human leukocyte antigen (HLA) molecules (see below), IFNs directly augment T cell functions relevant to tumor cell cytotoxicity *(80,81)*. The ability of IFNs to augment NK cell activity and monocyte function has been demonstrated both in vitro and in vivo *(24,82,83)*. The addition of IFNs to NK cells, even those of depressed lytic activity, can result in augmented tumor cell cytotoxicity. Patients given IFNs demonstrate augmented NK cell and monocyte activity 24 to 72 h after IFN administration.

Equivalent antitumor effectiveness of IFNs in mice has been identified for tumor cells sensitive or resistant to antiproliferative effects of IFNs in vitro *(84,85)*. Additional evidence, supporting a role for host immune effector cell response to IFNs, comes from studies in which mice with Friend leukemia, syngeneic tumor, or human prostate and HeLa tumor xenografts received antibody to murine IFN *(86)*. These mice, in the absence of exogenous IFN, experienced enhanced tumor growth and transplantability, suggesting that neutralization of endogenous IFN removes aspects of host defense to tumor *(87)*. As mentioned above, studies in nude mice with human melanoma xenografts have also demonstrated antitumor effects of human IFNs *(29,35, 88,89)*. This demonstrates, in view of the strict species specificity of IFNs, that the direct effects can also limit tumor growth.

Host modulatory effects of IFNs are part of the network of cytokine and cellular interactions. Induced expression of gene products must underlie immune regulatory effects of IFNs. IFNs enhance cell surface expression of major histocompatibility complex (MHC) antigens, TAA, and Fc receptors. All IFNs augment MHC class I expression, and IFN-γ enhances MHC class II expression on tumor cells as well *(90,91)*. IFN-β and IFN-γ also increase MHC class I and II expression on monocytes *(92)*. Increase in MHC expression may contribute to enhancement of dendritic cell antigen-presenting functions *(93,94)*. Following IFN-γ, respiratory activity in macrophages has increased with production of toxic oxygen intermediates, such as hydrogen peroxide and superoxide anion *(95)*. Monocytes stimulated by IFNs secrete monokines including colony-stimulating factor (CSF), tumor necrosis factor (TNF), and IL-1 as well as plasminogen activator, complement, and a variety of enzymes and other cytotoxic mediators *(96)*.

4.4. Angiogenesis Inhibition

Another component of IFN-mediated antitumor effects is inhibition of angiogenesis. Following IFN, tumor endothelial cells exhibits microvascular injury and a pattern of coagulation necrosis *(97)*. Systemic administration of IFN-α reduces tumor cell growth in IFN-sensitive cells by directly regulating the expression of the angiogenic protein, basic fibroblast growth factor (bFGF) *(98)*. IFN-α and IFN-β down-regulate bFGF in human carcinomas *(99,100)*. Interruption of the angiogenic signal by IFNs precedes the antiproliferative effect and is detectable between 24 to 48 h after tumor inoculation *(37)*. Down-regulation of bFGF correlates with reduced vascularization and reduced growth of the tumors in nude mice *(98)*. IFN-γ may also inhibit angiogenesis by inhibiting collagen synthesis by blocking proliferation of endothelial cells *(101,102)*. Interleukin-8 (IL-8) has also been shown to be a potent mediator of angiogenesis and consequently tumorigenesis *(103–105)*. IL-8 production was inhibited by IFN-α *(106)*. In addition to inhibiting angiogenic proteins, IFN-γ up-regulates the expression of an angiostatic protein, IP-10 *(107)*. IP-10 is an IFN-γ induced C-X-C chemokine with the ability to repress the angiogenic activities of both bFGF and IL-8 *(107)*. Clinically, IFN-α treatment has been successful in inducing regression of bulky hemangiomas, which are tumors consisting of abnormal endothelial cells *(108)*. Kaposi's sarcoma, a neoplastic disease of endothelial origin, also responds to treatment with IFN-α *(109)*.

5. CLINICAL RESULTS

Melanoma trials with IFN-α from leukocytes of blood donor units began under American Cancer Society auspices in 1979. Because the amounts of naturally produced IFNs were limited, in these initial trials, it was difficult either to determine maximally tolerated doses or to treat patients who had metastatic melanoma for extended periods. In the initial trials with buffy-coat IFN-α administered intramuscularly *(110)*, enough evidence of antitumor activity was observed to warrant extension using pure IFN-α produced by recombinant technology. Production of bulk quantities of pure IFNs from prokaryotic cells by recombinant DNA technology made possible rational systematic evaluation of the various IFNs as therapeutic agents. Over this period, both an extensive experience in the clinical use of the IFNs and a marked expansion in our understanding of the effects of IFNs on cellular function have been obtained. Results from phase II and phase III trials of IFN-α2 in patients with measurable metastatic melanoma indicate that these molecules, given as single agents to patients with measurable disease and to the patient at high risk for recurrence following surgery, have clinical activity.

As predicted by the experience with nonrecombinant IFN, both IFN-α2a and IFN-α2b had therapeutic activity against metastatic melanoma *(111–113)*. In a trial at the Mayo Clinic *(111)*, 31 patients were treated with IFN-α2a at a dose of 50 million U/m^2 given intramuscularly 3×/wk for 12 wk. Seven of these patients had regression of their disease (4 partial and 3 complete responses);

these responses lasted from 3 to 11 mo. However, treatments with this dose and schedule resulted in the development of severe fatigue and deterioration in performance status in more than 80% of patients. A lower dose (12 million U/m^2) delivered on the same schedule was utilized in a subsequent trial *(113)*. Although fewer complete responses occurred, the results were statistically indistinguishable (6 responses in 30 patients) from those of the higher dose trial. Forty patients with metastatic melanoma were assessed in a trial using IFN-α2b at a dose of 10 million U/m^2 given subcutaneously 3×/wk. Ten patients had objective responses; 4 of these were complete responses *(114)*. IFN-α produced 4 responses (2 complete) in 23 evaluable patients treated intravenously or intramuscularly 5 d/wk for 4 wk at daily doses of 10, 20, 50, or 100 million U *(115)*. A cyclic schedule was used in 29 patients treated intravenously at doses of 30 million U/m^2 daily for 5 d; 2 patients responded, including 1 patient who had a complete response that was sustained through more than 5 yr of observation. In a study using IFN-α2a on a daily dose schedule escalating to 36 million U daily or on a fixed schedule of 18 million U 3×/wk, 5 patients of 62 treated responded *(116)*. In a trial using IFN-α2b given as an induction regimen of 20 million U intravenously for 5 d for 4 wk, followed by 10 million U subcutaneously 3×/wk, 3 of 26 patients with good performance status, approximately one-third of whom had had prior chemotherapy, responded; 2 of these responses were complete *(117)*. IFN-γ has been evaluated in phases I and II trials and has little activity against melanoma (between 6% and 11% response rate) *(113,118–120)*. Even low doses resulted in occasional objective response.

Overall, trials of recombinant IFN-α2a or IFN-α2b have resulted in an overall objective response rate of 18% (37 of 241 patients) (Table 3). All trials have reported complete responses, and the durable nature of some complete responses has been emphasized *(121)*. For metastatic melanoma, the overall level of activity of IFN-α is in the range of active single agents, including dacarbazine and the nitrosoureas.

Combinations of IFNs with hormones, chemotherapy, and/or IL-2 may increase response rates and potentially survival in metastatic melanoma. Integration of these modalities of therapy into effective biochemotherapy has been limited by significant toxicities requiring careful identification of tolerable sequences and doses (see Chapter 10). However, several investigators have reported high complete response and overall response rates *(122–126)*. But, like other efforts to improve on results in metastatic melanoma, results have not been replicated by all investigators *(127,128)*. Thus prospective, randomized trials have been initiated.

Based upon potentiated antitumor effects in preclinical studies, tamoxifen has been proposed to add to effectiveness of IFNs *(129)*. Completed trials have not utilized the higher doses of tamoxifen, which will be required to reach effective concentrations in preclinical studies *(130)*.

Table 3
Phase II Trials Using IFN-α in Metastatic Melanoma

No.	IFN			Response				
of patients	*Type*	*Dose*	*Schedule*	*PR*	*CR*	*Total (%)*	*TTF*[a]	*References*
30	IFN-α-2a	12.0×10^6 U/m^2	IM 3×/wk for 3 mo	5	1	6(20)	1.9–12.9+	*143*
31	IFN-α-2a	50.0×10^6 U/m^2	IM 3×/wk for 3 mo	4	3	7(23)	3–11.2+	*144*
15	IFN-α-2a	50.0×10^6 U/m^2[b]	IM 3×/wk[c]	0	2	2(13)	6.5–12.0	*145*
24	IFN-α-2b	10.0×10^6 U/m^2	IM 3×/wk[c]	5	2	7(29)	NR[d]	*146*
31	IFN-α-2b	36.0×10^6 U/m^2	IM daily for 61 d	3	0	3(9.7)	7.25–22.0+	*147*
31	IFN-α-2a	18.0×10^6 U/m^2	IM 3×/wk[c]	2	0	2(6.5)	7.25–22.0+	*147*
45	IFN-α-2b	10.0×10^6 U/m^2	IM 3×/wk for 12 mo	6	4	10(22)	1.0–28.0+	*148*
23	IFN-α-2b	$10.0–50.0 \times 10^6$ U/m^2	IV daily	2	2	4(16)	NR	*149*
53	IFN-α-2b	20.0×10^6 U/m^2	IV daily[d]	3	3	6(13)	NR	*150*
283				30	17	47(18)		

[a]TTF, time to treatment failure (range in months).
[b]Escalating doses were used to initiate treatment, i.e., 15.0×10^6 U/m^2 3×/wk for 2 doses, then 15.0×10^6 U/m^2 3×/wk for 2 doses.
[c]Until disease progression or intolerable toxicity occurred.
[d]Dose was given daily 5 d/wk for 4 wk followed by 10×10^6 U/m^2 subcutaneously 3×/wk.
PR, partial response; CR, complete response; IM, intramuscularly; NR, not reported; IV, intravenous.

Findings in metastatic disease stimulated evaluation of the potential benefit of IFN-α2 as an adjuvant for the patient with high risk primary melanoma. For this purpose, multi-institutional trials have been conducted in the United States and Europe. Intergroup trials, Eastern Cooperative Oncology Group (ECOG) 1684, ECOG 1690, and ECOG 1694 have had greatest prominence in North America. Eligible for these trials have been patients with deeply invasive primary melanomas or those with node metastasis, but no evidence of distant metastatic disease.

ECOG 1684 enrolled 287 patients from 1985 until 1990 *(131)*. Patients were randomized to either observation of 1 yr of IFN-α2b. With a median follow-up of patients of 6.9 yr with a range of 0.6 to 9.6 yr, a significant impact on disease-free survival (DFS) from IFN-α2b was identified; 1.72 vs 0.98 yr, ($p < 0.01$). This translated to a 42% improvement in relapse-free survival for patients treated with IFN-α2b compared to those randomized to observation. Overall survival (OS) was also positively impacted ($p = 0.04$). Benefit of IFN appeared in the first year of treatment, the period during which the patients were receiving therapy. Ten-year follow-up data has now confirmed impact on DFS, but not OS in this trial.

To extend the results of ECOG 1684, another trial—ECOG 1690—was initiated. This latter trial has now reached a median follow-up of 4.9 yr. Intent to treat analysis of 642 patients has identified an almost identical survival curve for patients receiving high dose IFN-α2b compared to those receiving it on ECOG 1684. However, the patients randomized to observation alone had a better outcome than occurred in ECOG 1684 *(11)*. Median overall survival for the observation patients in ECOG 1684 was 2.8 yr, with a 5-yr survival of 37%, compared to a median OS of the observation patients in ECOG 1690 of 5.9 yr, with a 5-yr survival of 55%. Thus, survival of patients randomized to observation on ECOG 1690 had a 3.1-yr improvement in median survival compared to ECOG 1684, begun 6 yr earlier *(132)*. With recurrence, a significant number of the patients on the observation arm received IFN, which may have confounded interpretation of the effect of IFN-α2b. No other major difference in study eligibility criteria or patient management could be identified that would account for this marked improvement in survival on the observation arm of IFN-α2b on ECOG 1690.

A subsequent trial of high dose IFN-α2b (ECOG 1694) has identified superiority in survival to patients randomized to a vaccine program *(133)*. This latter trial entered 774 eligible patients. With a median follow-up of 16 mo, a highly significant effect on both DFS and OS emerged in favor of IFN-α2b (DFS, $p = 0.0015$; OS, $p = 0.009$). Survival of patients randomized to vaccine was similar to that observed on ECOG 1690, suggesting that the positive difference resulted from IFN-α2b rather than a detrimental effect of the vaccine. Other large trials have also randomized patients to IFN-α2 or observation following surgery for high risk primary melanoma. In one, 262 patients with stage IIA or stage III disease were prospectively randomized to 12 wk of high-dose IFN-α2a *(134)*. This contrasted with the 52 wk utilized in ECOG 1684 and ECOG 1690. A trend

Table 4
Dose Intensity and Therapeutic Effects of IFN-α2 for Adjuvant Melanoma

International cooperative studies[a]				
Stage	*Study*	*Dose × 10^6 sq*	*DFS*	*OS*
II (T_3NO)	Austria	3×/wk × 1 yr[b]	+	–
	French	3×/wk × 1.5 yr	+	0.06
III ($T_{3\text{-}4}N_1$)	WHO	3×/wk × 3 yr	–	–
	NCCTG	20/m^2 (IM) 3×/wk × 3 mo	–	–
	ECOG 1680	10/m^2 3×/wk × 1 yr[b]	+	0.04
	ECOG 1690	10/m^2 3×/wk × 1 yr[b]	+	–
	ECOG 1694	10/m^2 3×/wk × 1 yr[b]	+	+

[a]All studies >250 patients with median follow-up >3 yr except EST 1694.
[b]Included for 1 mo either daily (Austria) or 20/m^2 intravenously × 20 d (ECOG).

toward a delay in recurrence, particularly in the node-positive patients ($p = 0.04$), was identified. However, no impact on survival was apparent for either stage IIA or stage III patients. A trial undertaken by a cooperative group of French investigators randomized 499 patients with melanoma >1.5 mm in depth who had no clinical evidence of lymph node metastases *(135)*. Patients were treated with 3 million U of IFN-α2a for 18 mo. Significant progression-free survival difference favoring IFN-α2a ($p = 0.04$) was identified. This corresponded to a 25% reduction in the risk of relapse. There was a borderline impact on survival ($p = 0.06$). Another study has used IFN-α2a subcutaneously at a dose of 3 million U 3×/wk subcutaneously for 1 yr in patients with >1.5 mm primary melanomas *(135)*. With a median follow-up of 3.5 yr, DFS was prolonged significantly ($p = 0.02$). Thus, all trials in high-risk primary patients have established effectiveness in increasing DFS (Table 4). The data suggest higher doses may improve survival.

Data suggest dose intensity and duration may be most important in higher risk patients. ECOG 1684 and ECOG 1690 both included patients receiving high-dose IFN-α2b (10×10^6 U/m^2 3×/wk) after a month of even higher dose intravenous induction. ECOG 1690 also evaluated a low-dose IFN-α2b given at 3×10^6 U. This latter lower dose regimen resulted in no significant impact on therapeutic outcome. Thus, the weight of evidence in the adjuvant setting points to greater effectiveness of higher doses (Table 4). The data for patients with metastatic disease is less clear. However, in phase I trials of PEG-IFN-α2b, 2/6 patients with metastatic melanoma responded *(40)*. Thus, PEG-IFN-α2 is active in melanoma and as a result of greater effectiveness of high doses for adjuvant treatment and for treatment of metastatic disease, will certainly be evaluated in phase II and phase III trials. More difficult, however, in the chronic and gradually cumulative anorexia and fatigue, sometimes with depression and decrease in performance

Table 5
Melanoma and IFNs: *Unanswered Questions*

Role of different IFN types.	Dose intensity.
Mechanism of antitumor action.	Cause of side effects.
Prediction of therapeutic response.	Duration of therapy.
Role in suppression of transformation.	Effectiveness of combinations.

high dose IFN as an adjuvant has been associated with the constellation of acute and chronic side effects associated with cytokines. The acute fever and chills of the first few days of administration, while unpleasant, are usually tolerated. More difficult however is the chronic and gradually cumulative anorexia and fatigue, sometimes with depression and decrease in performance. Although an anti-depressive may provide some benefit, neither the cause nor effective treatment for this syndrome have been identified *(136–139)*. Thus, it has been difficult, not only for patients, but also for nurses and physicians involved in their management—particularly since these patients, in contrast to many of those with metastatic disease, are otherwise well.

Fortunately however in younger individuals, who may be receiving adjuvant therapy for melanoma, it is less severe than in older. And despite side effects, 80% of protocol-defined doses were received by patients treated on ECOG 1684 *(131)*. Dose modifications in this study were mandated not only for weight loss and fatigue, but also for the expected leukopenia and hepatic transaminase elevations identified from other studies. Despite the fatigue and anorexia associated with 1 yr of IFN administration, quality of life analysis of ECOG 1684 identified a significant advantage in favor of treatment *(140)*. This quality adjusted time without symptoms and toxicity (Q-TWiST) analysis identified more quality adjusted survival time for the patient receiving treatment, even considering side effects of IFN-α2b. And since a survival advantage accrued to patients treated on this study, results could be demonstrated to have a magnitude of economic benefit associated with advantageous medical interventions *(141)*. In patients with metastatic disease, benefit is most likely to accrue to those with the best prognostic factors *(142)*.

6. CONCLUSION

During the final decade of the 20th century, the effectiveness of IFNs as part of multi-modality regimens for melanoma was clearly established. IFNs remain the most active adjuvant therapy for melanoma for patients staged as at highest risk for recurrence *(12)*. Yet, IFNs have yet to reach their full potential for therapy of this disease. Of several outstanding questions (Table 5), understanding the mechanism of antitumor action will be particularly key. Answers to many, perhaps even most, of these questions in the next decade will likely provide a basis for substantial broadening of clinical use of IFNs for melanoma.

REFERENCES

1. Hawkins MJ, Levin M, Borden EC. An ECOG phase I-II pilot study of polyriboinosinic-polyribocytidylic acid poly-L-Lysine complex (Poly ICLC) in patients with metastatic malignant melanoma. *J Biol Response Mod* 1985; 4: 664–668.
2. Litton G, Hong R, Grossberg SE, Echlekar D, Goodavish CN, Borden EC. Biological and clinical effects of the oral immunomodulator 3,6-bis (2-piperidinoethoxy) acridine trihydrochloride in patients with advanced malignancy. *J Biol Response Mod* 1990; 9: 61–70.
3. Rios A, Stringfellow DA, Fitzpatrick FA, et al. Phase I study of 2-amino-5bromo-6-phenyl-4 (eH)-pyrimidinone (ABPP), an oral interferon inducer, in cancer patients. *J Biol Response Mod* 1986; 5: 330–338.
4. Urba WJ, Longo DL, Weiss RB. Enhancement of natural killer activity in human peripheral blood by flavone acetic acid. *J Natl Cancer Inst* 1988; 80: 521–525.
5. Goldstein D, Hertzod P, Tomkinson E, et al. Administration of imiquimod, an interferon inducer, in asymptomatic human immunodeficiency virus-infected persons to determine safety and biologic response modification. *J Infect Dis* 1998; 178: 858–861.
6. Witt Pl, Ritch PS, Reding D, et al. Phase I trials of an oral immunomodulator and interferon inducer in cancer patients. *Cancer Res* 1993; 53: 5176–5180.
7. Greene MH. The genetics of hereditary melanoma and nevi. *Cancer* 1999; 86: 2464–2477.
8. Cowan JM, Halaban R, Francke U. Cytogenetic analysis of melanocytes from premalignant nevi and melanomas. *J Natl Cancer Inst* 1988; 80: 1159–1164.
9. Kamb A, Gruis NA, Weaver-Feldhaus J, et al. A cell cycle regulator potentially involved in genesis of many tumor types. *Science* 1994; 264: 436–550.
10. Borden EC. Interferon. In: Holland JF, et al., eds. *Cancer Medicine, 3rd ed.*, Lea & Febiger, Philadelphia, 1997, pp. 1199–1212; 1993, pp. 927–936.
11. Pfeffer LM, Dinarello CA, Herberman RB, et al. Biologic properties of recombinant alfa interferons: 40th anniversary of the discovery of interferons. *Cancer Res* 1998; 58: 2489–2499.
12. Nagata S, Mantei N, Weissmann C. The structure of one of the eight or more distinct chromosomal genes for human interferon-α. *Nature* 1980; 287: 401–408.
13. Goeddel DV, Leung DW, Dull TJ, et al. The structure of eight distinct cloned human leukocyte interferon cDNAs. *Nature* 1981; 290: 20–26.
14. Gray PW, Goeddel DV. Structure of the human immune interferon gene. *Nature* 1982; 298: 859–863.
15. Pestka S. The human interferon-alpha species and hybrid proteins. *Semin Oncol* 1997; 24: S9-4–S9-17.
16. Der SD, Zhou A, Williams BR, Silverman RH. Identification of genes differentially regulated by interferon alpha, beta, or gamma using oligonucleotide arrays. *Proc Natl Acad Sci USA* 1998; 95: 15623–15628.
17. Borden EC, Leaman DW, Chawla-Sarkar M, Ozdemir A, Williams BR, Silverman RH. Novel ISGs potently induced by IFN-α in WM9 melanoma cells. *Eur Cytokine Network* 2000; 11: 101.
18. Flores I, Mariano TM, Pestka S. Human interferon omega binds to the alpha/beta receptor. *J Biol Chem* 1991; 266: 19875–19877.
19. Roberts RM, Cross JC, Leaman DW. Unique features of the trophoblast interferons. *Pharmacol Ther* 1991; 51: 329–345.
20. Ozes ON, Reiter Z, Klein S, Blatt LM, Taylor MW. A comparison of interferon-Con1 with natural recombinant interferons-alpha: antiviral, antiproliferative, and natural killer-inducing activities. *J Interferon Cytokine Res* 1992; 12: 55–59.
21. Ortaldo J, Mantovani A, Hobbs D, Rubinstein M, Pestka S, Herberman RB. Effects of several species of human leukocyte interferon on cytotoxic activity of NK cells and monocytes. *Int J Cancer* 1983; 31: 285–289.

22. Greiner JW, Fisher PB, Pestka S, Schlom J. Differential effects of recombinant human leukocyte interferons on cell surface antigen expression. *Cancer Res* 1986; 46: 4984–4990.
23. Hawkins MJ, Borden EC, Merritt JA, et al. Comparison of the biologic effects of two recombinant human interferons alpha (rAand rD) in humans. *J Clin Oncol* 1984; 2: 221–226.
24. Edwards BS, Hawkins MJ, Borden EC. Comparative in vivo and in vitro activation of human natural killer cells by two recombinant alpha interferons differing in antiviral activity. *Cancer Res* 1984; 44: 3135–3139.
25. Borden EC, Rinehart J, Storer BM, Trump DL, Paulnock DM, Teitelbaum AP. Biological and clinical effects of interferon $beta_{ser}$ at two doses. *J Interferon Cytokine Res* 1990; 10: 559–570.
26. Hawkins M, Horning S, Konrad M, et al. Phase I evaluation of a synthetic mutant of interferon b. *Cancer Res* 1985; 45: 5914–5920.
27. PRISMS Study Group. Randomised double-blind placebo-controlled study of interferon beta-1a in relapsing/remitting multiple sclerosis. *Lancet* 1998; 352: 1498–1504.
28. Schiller JH, Willson JKV, Bittner G, Wolberg WH, Hawkins MJ, Borden EC. Antiproliferative effects of interferons on human melanoma cells in the human tumor colony forming assay. *J Interferon Cytokine Res* 1986; 6: 615–625.
29. Johns TG, Mackay IR, Callister KA, Hertzog PJ, Devenish RJ, Linnane AW. Antiproliferative potencies of interferons on melanoma cell lines and xenografts: higher efficacy of interferon beta. *J Natl Cancer Inst* 1992; 84: 1185–1190.
30. Kopf, J, Hanson C, Delle U, et al. Action of interferon alpha and beta on four human melanoma cell lines in vitro. *Anticancer Res* 1996; 2: 791–798.
31. Krasagakis K, Garbe C, Kruger S, Orfanos CE. Effects of interferons on cultured human melanocytes in vitro: interferons-beta but not-alpha or -gamma inhibit proliferation and all interferons significantly modulate the cell phenotype. *J Invest Dermatol* 1991; 2: 364–372.
32. Nagatani T, Okazawa H, Kambara T, et al. Effect of natural interferon-beta on the growth of melanoma cell lines. *Melanoma Res* 1998; 8: 295–299.
33. von Hoff DD, Huong AM. Effect of recombinant interferon-beta ser on primary human tumor colony forming units. *J Interferon Cytokine Res* 1988; 6: 813–820.
34. Chawla-Sarkar M, Leaman DW, Borden EC. Preferential induction of apoptosis by IFN-β compared to interferon-α 2: correlation with TRAIL/Apo 2L induction in melanoma cell lines. *Clin Cancer Res* 2001; 7: 1821–1831.
35. Gomi K, Morimoto M, Nakamizo N. Antitumor effect of recombinant interferon-beta against human melanomas transplanted into nude mice. *J Pharmacobiodyn* 1984; 12: 951–961.
36. McCarthy MG, Bucan CD, Fidler IJ. Melanoma-induced epidermal hyperplasia and increased angiogenesis is mediated by TGF-α through down-regulation of IFN-β. *Cancer Res* 2000; 41: 5155–5161.
37. Sidky Y, Borden EC. Inhibition of angiogenesis by interferons: effects on tumor- and lymphocyte-induced vascular responses. *Cancer Res* 1987; 47: 5155–5161.
38. Abdi EA, Tan YH, McPherson TA. Natural human interferon-beta in metastatic melanoma. A phase II study. *Acta Oncol* 1988; 6: 815–817.
39. Sarna G, Figlin RA, Pertcheck M. Phase II study of betaseron (beta ser17-interferon) as treatment of advanced malignant melanoma. *J Biol Response Mod* 1987; 4: 375–378.
40. Bukowski R, Ernstoff M, Gore M, et al. Phase I study of polyethylene glycol (PEG) interferon alpha-2b (PEG intron) in patients with solid tumors. *Proc ASCO* 1999; 18: 446a.
41. Rebouillat D, Hovanessin A. The human 2', 5' oligoadenylate synthetase family: activation by 2-5A. *J Interferon Cytokine Res* 1999; 19: 295–308.
42. Hassel BA, Zhou A, Sotomayor C, Maran A, Silverman RH. A dominant negative mutant of 2-5 A-dependent RNase suppresses antiproliferative and antiviral effects of interferon. *EMBO J* 1993; 12: 3297–3304.

43. Zhou A, Paranjape J, Brown TL, et al. Interferon action and apoptosis are defective in mice devoid of 2',5'-oligoadenylate-dependent RNase L. *EMBO J* 1997; 16: 6355–6363.
44. Wang LZA, Vasavada S, Dong B, et al. Elevated levels of 2', 5'-linked oligoadenylate-dependent ribonuclease L occur as an early event in colorectal tumorigenesis. *Clin Cancer Res* 1995; 1: 1421–1428.
45. Hovanessian AG. Interferon-induced dsRNA-activated protein kinase (PKR): antiproliferative, antiviral and antitumoral functions. *Semin Virol* 1993; 4: 237–245.
46. Kumar AHJ, Locaste J, Hiscott J, Williams BRG. The dsRNA-dependent protein kinase, PKR, activates transcription factor NF-κB by phosphorylating IκB. *Proc Natl Acad Sci USA* 1994; 91: 6288–6292.
47. Balachandran S, Kim CN, Yeh W-C, Mak TW, Bhalla K, Barber GN. Activation of the dsRNA-dependent protein kinase PKR, induces apoptosis through FADD-mediated death signaling. *EMBO J* 1998; 17: 6888–6902.
48. Koromilas AE, Roy S, Barber GN, Katze MG, Sonenberg N. Malignant transformation by a mutant of the IFN-inducible dsRNA-dependent protein kinase. *Science* 1992; 257: 1685–1689.
49. Haines GK, Cajulis R, Hayden R, Duda R, Talamonti M, Radosevich JA. Expression of the double-stranded RNA-dependent protein kinase (p68) in human breast tissues. *Tumour Biol* 1996; 17: 5–12.
50. Savinova O, Joshi B, Jagus R. Abnormal levels and minimal activity of the dsRNA-activated protein kinase, PKR, in breast carcinoma cells. *Int J Biochem Cell Biol* 1999; 31: 175–189.
51. Harada H, Fujita T, Miyamoto M, et al. Structurally similar but functionally distinct factors, IRF-1 and IRF-2, bind to the same regulatory elements of IFN and IFN-inducible genes. *Cell* 1989; 58: 729–739.
52. Byrne G, Lehmann LK, Kirschbaum JG, Borden EC, Lee CM, Brown RR. Induction of tryptophan degradation in vitro and in vivo: a gamma-interferon stimulated activity. *J Interferon Cytokine Res* 1986; 6: 389–396.
53. Obar RA, Collins CA, Hammerback JA, Shpetner HS, Valee RB. Molecular cloning of the microtubule-associated mechanochemical enzyme dynamin reveals homology with a new family of GTP-binding protein. *Nature* 1990; 347: 256–261.
54. Cheng YSE, Colonno RJ, Yin FY. Interferon induction of fibroblast proteins with guanylate binding activity. *J Biol Chem* 1983; 258: 7746–7750.
55. Zhao J, Zhou Q, Wiedmer T, Sims PJ. Level of expression of phospholipid scramblase regulates induced movement of phosphatidylserine to the cell surface. *J Biol Chem* 1998; 273: 6603–6606.
56. Stein U, Walther W, Shoemaker RH. Modulation of mdr1 expression by cytokines in human colon carcinoma cells: an approach for reversal of multidrug resistance. *Br J Cancer* 1996; 74: 1384–1391.
57. Kakizuka A, Miller WH, Umesono K, et al. Chromosomal translocation t(15; 17) in human acute promyelocytic leukemia fuses RARalpha with a novel putative transcription factor, PML. *Cell* 1991; 66: 663–674.
58. Wang Z-G, Ruggero D, Ronchetti S, et al. PML is essential for multiple apoptotic pathways. *Nat Genet* 1998; 20: 266–272.
59. Goldstein D, Sielaff KM, Storer BE, et al. Human biologic response modification by interferon in the absence of measurable serum concentrations: a comparative trial of subcutaneous and intravenous interferon betaserine. *J Natl Cancer Inst* 1989; 81: 1061–1068.
60. Merritt JA, Ball LA, Sielaff KM, Meltzer DM, Borden EC. Modulation of 2',5'-oligoadenylate synthetase in patients treated with alpha-interferon: effects of dose, schedule, and route of administration. *J Interferon Cytokine Res* 1986; 6: 189–198.
61. Gutterman JU, Fine S, Quesada J, et al. Recombinant leukocyte A interferon: pharmacokinetics, single-dose tolerance, and biologic effects in cancer patients. *Ann Intern Med* 1982; 96: 549–555.

62. Goldstein D, Sielaff KM, Storer BE, et al. Human biologic response modification by interferon in the absence of measurable serum concentrations: a comparative trial of subcutaneous and intravenous interferon beta serine. *J Natl Cancer Inst* 1989; 81: 1061–1068.
63. Ramana CV, Grammatikakis N, Chernov M, et al. Regulation of c-myc expression by IFN-γ through Stat1-dependent and Stat1-independent pathways. *EMBO J* 2000; 19: 263–272.
64. Raveh T, Hovanessian AG, Meurs EF, Sonenberg N, Kimchi A. Double-stranded RNA-dependent protein kinase mediates c-Myc suppression induced by type I interferons. *J Biol Chem* 1996; 271: 25479–25484.
65. Koshiji M, Adachi Y, Sogo S, et al. Apoptosis of colorectal adenocarcinoma (COLO 201) by tumour necrosis factor-alpha (INF-α) and/or interferon-gamma (IFN-γ), resulting from down-regulation of Bcl-2 expression. *Clin Exp Immunol* 1998; 111: 211–218.
66. Samid D, Chang EH, Friedman RM. Biochemical correlates of phenotypic reversion in interferon-treated mouse cells transformed by a human oncogene. *Biochem Biophys Res Commun* 1984; 119: 21–28.
67. Fisher P, Prignoli DR, Hermo H Jr, Weinstein IB, Pestka S. Effects of combined treatment with interferon and mezerein on melanogenesis and growth in human melanoma cells. *J Interferon Res* 1985; 5: 11–22.
68. Samid D, Flessate DM, Greene JJ, Chang EH, Friedman RM. Persisting revertant after interferon treatment of oncogene-transformed cells. In: Stewart WI, Schellekens, H, eds. *The Biology of the Interferon System*. Elsevier, Amsterdam, 1986, p. 327.
69. Kumar R, Atlad I. Interferon-α induces the expression of retinoblastoma gene product in human Burkitt lymphoma Daudi cells: role in growth regulation. *Proc Natl Acad Sci USA* 1992; 89: 6599–6603.
70. Resnitzky D, Tiefenbrun N, Berissi H, Kimchi A. Interferons and interleukin 6 suppress phosphorylation of the retinoblastoma protein in growth-sensitive hematopoietic cells. *Proc Natl Acad Sci USA* 1992; 89: 402–406.
71. Tiefenbrun N, Melamed D, Levy N, et al. Alpha interferon suppresses the cyclin D3 and cdc25A genes, leading to a reversible G0-like arrest. *Mol Cell Biol* 1996; 16: 3934–3944.
72. Melamed D, Tiefenbrun N, Yarden A, Kimchi A. Interferons and interleukin-6 suppress the DNA-binding activity of E2F in growth-sensitive hematopoietic cells. *Mol Cell Biol* 1993; 13: 5255–5265.
73. Subramaniam PS, Cruz PE, Hobeika AC, Johnson HM. Type I interferon induction of the Cdk-inhibitor p21WAF1 is accompanied by order G1 arrest, differentiation and apoptosis of the Daudi B-cell line. *Oncogene* 1998; 16: 1885–1890.
74. Xu X, Fu X-Y, Plate J, Chong AS-F. IFN-γ induces cells growth inhibition by Fas-mediated apoptosis: requirement of STAT1 protein for up-regulation of Fas and FasL expression. *Cancer Res* 1998; 58: 2832–2837.
75. Weller M, Frei K, Groscurth P, Krammer PH, Yonekawa Y, Fontana A. Anti-Fas/APO-1 antibody-mediated apoptosis of cultured human glioma cells. Induction and modulation of sensitivity by cytokines. *J Clin Invest* 1994; 94: 954–964.
76. Spets H, Georgii-Hemming P, Siljason J, Nilsson K, Jernberg-Wiklund H. Fas/APO-1 (CD95)-mediated apoptosis is activated by interferon-γ and interferon-β in interleukin-6 (IL-6)-dependent and IL-6-independent multiple myeloma cell lines. *Blood* 1998; 92: 2914–2923.
77. Cornelissen J, Ploemacher RE, Wognum BW, et al. An in vitro model for cytogenetic conversion in CML: Interferon-alpha preferentially inhibits the outgrowth of malignant stem cells preserved in long-term culture. *J Clin Invest* 1998; 102: 976–983.
78. Gordon M, Marley SB, Lewis JL, et al. Treatment with interferon-alpha preferentially reduces the capacity for amplification of granulocyte-macrophage progenitors (CFU-GM) from patients with chronic myeloid leukemia but spares normal CFU-GM. *J Clin Invest* 1998; 102: 710–715.

79. Selleri C, Maciejewski JP, Pane F, et al. Fas-mediated modulation of Bcr/Abl in chronic myelogenous leukemia results in differential effects on apoptosis. *Blood* 1998; 92: 981–989.
80. Kayagaki N, Yamaguchi N, Nakayama M, Eto H, Okumura K, Yagita H. Type I interferons regulate tumor necrosis factor-related apoptosis-inducing ligand (TRAIL) expression on human T cells: a novel mechanism for the antitumor effects of type I IFNs. *J Exp Med* 1999; 189: 1451–1460.
81. Bellardelli F, Gresser I. The neglected role of type I interferon in the T-cell response. *Immunol Today* 1996; 17: 369–372.
82. Herberman R, Djeu JY, Ortaldo JR, Holden HT, West WH, Bonnard GD. Role of interferon in augmentation of natural and antibody-dependent cytotoxicity. *Cancer Treat Rep* 1978; 62: 1893–1896.
83. Kleinerman ES, Kurzrock R, Wyatt D, Quesada JR, Gutterman JU, Fidler IJ. Activation or suppression of the tumoricidal properties of monocytes from cancer patients following treatment with human recombinant gamma-interferon. *Cancer Res* 1986; 46: 5401–5405.
84. Belardelli F, Gresser I, Maury C, Maunoury MT. Antitumor effects of interferon in mice injected with interferon-sensitive and interferon-resistant Friend leukemia cells. II. Role of host mechanisms. *Int J Cancer* 1982; 30: 821–825.
85. Reid TR, Race ER, Wolff BH, Friedman RM, Merigan TC, Basham TY. Enhanced in vivo therapeutic response to IFN in mice with an in vitro interferon-resistant B-cell lymphoma. *Cancer Res* 1989; 49: 4163–4169.
86. Reid LM, Minato N, Gresser I, Holland J, Kadish A, Bloom BR. Influence of anti-mouse interferon serum on the growth and metastasis of tumor cells persistently infected with virus and of human prostatic tumors in athymic nude mice. *Proc Natl Acad Sci USA* 1981; 78: 1171–1175.
87. Balkwill FR, Moodie EM, Freedman V, Fantes KH. Human interferon inhibits the growth of established human breast tumours in the nude mouse. *Int J Cancer* 1982; 30: 231–235.
88. Sakurai M. Iigo M, Tamura T, et al. Comparative study of the antitumor effect of two types of murine recombinant interferons, (beta) and (gamma), against B16-F10 melanoma. *Cancer Immunol Immunother* 1988; 26: 109–113.
89. Horton HM, Hernandez P, Parker SE, Barnhart KM. Antitumor effects of interferon-omega: in vivo therapy of human tumor xenografts in nude mice. *Cancer Res* 1999; 59: 4064–4068.
90. Basham TY, Bourgeade MF, Creasey AA, Merigan TC. Interferon increases HLA synthesis in melanoma cells: interferon-resistant and -sensitive cell lines. *Proc Natl Acad Sci USA* 1982; 79: 3265–3269.
91. Fellous M, Nir U, Wallach D, Merlin G, Rubinstein M, Revel M. Interferon-dependent induction of mRNA for the major histocompatibility antigens in human fibroblasts and lymphoblastoid cells. *Proc Natl Acad Sci USA* 1982; 76: 3082–3086.
92. Paulnock DM, Havlin KA, Storer BM, Spear GT, Sielaff KM, Borden EC. Induced proteins in human peripheral mononuclear cells over a range of clinically tolerable doses of interferon gamma. *J Interferon Cytokine Res* 1989; 9: 457–473.
93. Kadowaki N, Antonenko S, Lau JY, Liu YJ. Natural interferon alpha/beta-producing cells link innate and adaptive immunity. *J Exp Med* 2000; 192: 219–226.
94. Santini SM, Lapenta C, Logozzi M, et al. Type I interferon as a powerful adjuvant for monocyte-derived dendritic cell development and activity in vitro and in Hu-PBL-SCID mice. *J Exp Med* 2000; 191: 1777–1788.
95. Nathan C. Secretory products of macrophages. *J Clin Invest* 1987; 79: 319–326.
96. Arenzana-Seisdedos F, Virelizier JL, Fiers W. Interferons as macrophage-activating factors. III. Preferential effects of interferon-gamma on the interleukin 1 secretory potential of fresh or aged human monocytes. *J Immunol* 1985; 134: 2444–2448.
97. Dvorak HF, Gresser I. Microvascular injury in pathogenesis of interferon-induced necrosis of subcutaneous tumors in mice. *J Natl Cancer Inst* 1989; 81: 497–502.

98. Dinney CP, Bielenberg DR, Perrotte P, et al. Inhibition of basic fibroblast growth factor expression, angiogenesis, and growth of human bladder carcinoma in mice by systemic interferon- alpha administration. *Cancer Res* 1998; 58: 808–814.
99. Singh RK, Gutman M, Bucana CD, Sanchez R, Llansa N, Fidler IJ. Interferons alpha and beta down-regulate the expression of basic fibroblast growth factor in human carcinomas. *Proc Natl Acad Sci USA* 1995; 92: 4562–4566.
100. Slaton J, Perrote P, Inoue K, Dinney CPN, Fidler IJ. Interferon-α-mediated down-regulation of angiogenesis-related genes and therapy of bladder cancer are dependent on optimization of biological dose and schedule. *Clin Cancer Res* 1999; 5: 2726–2734.
101. Albini A, Marchisone C, Del Grosso F, et al. Inhibition of angiogenesis and vascular tumor growth by interferon-producing cells: a gene therapy approach. *Am J Pathol* 2000; 156: 1381–1393.
102. Wang W, Chen HJ, Schwartz A, Cannon PJ, Rabbani LE. T cell lymphokines modulate bFGF-induced smooth muscle cell fibrinolysis and migration. *Am J Physiol* 1997; 272: C392–C398.
103. Koch AE, Polverini PJ, Kunkel SL, et al. Interleukin-8 as a macrophage-derived mediator of angiogenesis. *Science* 1992; 258: 1798–1801.
104. Yoshida S, Ono M, Shono T, et al. Involvement of interleukin-8, vascular endothelial growth factor, and basic fibroblast growth factor in tumor necrosis factor alpha-dependent angiogenesis. *Mol Cell Biol* 1997; 17: 4015–4023.
105. Arenberg DA, Kunkel SL, Polverini PJ, Glass M, Burdick MD, Strieter RM. Inhibition of interleukin-8 reduces tumorigenesis of human non-small cell lung cancer in SCID mice. *J Clin Invest* 1996; 97: 2792–2802.
106. Reznikov LL, Puren AJ, Fantuzzi G, et al. Spontaneous and inducible cytokine responses in healthy humans receiving a single dose of IFN-α2b: increased production of interleukin-1 receptor antagonist and suppression of IL-1-induced IL-8. *J Interferon Cytokine Res* 1998; 18: 897–903.
107. Strieter RM, Kunkel SL, Arenberg DA, Burdick MD, Polverini PJ. Interferon gamma-inducible protein 10 (IP-10), a member of the C-X-C chemokine family, is an inhibitor of angiogenesis. *Biochem Biophys Res Commun* 1995; 210: 51–57.
108. Ezekowitz RAB, Milliken JB, Folkman J. Interferon alfa-2a therapy for life-threatening hemangiomas of infancy. *N Engl J Med* 1992; 326: 1456–1463.
109. Krown SE. Interferon-α: evolving therapy for AIDS-associated Kaposi's sarcoma. *J Interferon Cytokine Res* 1998; 18: 209–214.
110. Krown SE, Burk MW, Kirkwood JM, Kerr D, Morton DL, Oettgen HF. Human leukocyte (alpha) interferon in metastatic malignant melanoma: the American Cancer Society phase II trial. *Cancer Treat Rep* 1984; 68: 723–726.
111. Creagan ET, Ahmann DL, Green SJ, et al. Phase II study of recombinant leukocyte A interferon (rIFN-alpha A) in disseminated malignant melanoma. *Cancer* 1984; 54: 2844–2849.
112. Creagan ET, Ahmann DL, Green SJ, et al. Phase II study of low-dose recombinant leukocyte A interferon in disseminated malignant melanoma. *J Clin Oncol* 1984; 2: 1002–1005.
113. Creagan ET, Ahmann DL, Long HJ, Frytak S, Sherwin SA, Chang MN. Phase II study of recombinant interferon-gamma in patients with disseminated malignant melanoma. *Cancer Treat Rep* 1987; 71: 843–844.
114. Robinson WA, Mughal TI, Thomas MR, Johnson M, Spiegel RJ. Treatment of metastatic malignant melanoma with recombinant interferon alpha-2. *Immunobiology* 1986; 172: 275–282.
115. Kirkwood JM, Ernstoff MS, Davis CA, Reiss M, Ferraresi R, Rudnick SA. Comparison of intramuscular and intravenous recombinant interferon in melanoma and other cancer. *Ann Intern Med* 1985; 103: 32–36.

116. Legha SS, Papadopoulos NEJ, Plager C, et al. Clinical evaluation of recombinant interferon alfa-2A (Roferon-A) in metastatic melanoma using two different schedules. *J Clin Oncol* 1987; 5: 1240–1246.
117. Miller LL, Spitler LE, Allen RE, Minor DR. A randomized, double-bind, placebo-controlled trial of transfer factor as adjuvant therapy for melanoma. *Cancer* 1988; 61: 1543–1549.
118. Ernstoff MS, Trautman T, Davis CA, et al. A randomized phase I/II study of cutaneous versus intermittent intravenous interferon gamma inpatients with metastatic malignant melanoma. *J Clin Oncol* 1987; 5: 1804–1810.
119. Gutterman JU, Rosenblum MG, Rios A, Fritsche HA, Quesada JR. Pharmacokinetic study of partially pure gamma-interferon in cancer patients. *Cancer Res* 1984; 44: 4164–4171.
120. Kurzrock R, Quesada JR, Talpaz M, et al. Phase I study of multiple dose intramuscularly administered recombinant gamma interferon. *J Clin Oncol* 1986; 4: 1101–1109.
121. Creagan ET, Ahmann DL, Frytak S, Long HJ, Chang MN, Itri LM. Phase II trials of recombinant leukocyte A interferon in disseminated malignant melanoma: results in 96 patients. *Cancer Treat Rep* 1986; 70: 619–624.
122. Legha SS, Ring S, Eton O, Bedikian A, Plager C, Papadopoulos N. Development and results of biochemotherapy in metastatic melanoma: the University of Texas M.D. Anderson Cancer Center Experience. *Cancer J Sci Am* 1997; 3: S3–S15.
123. Legha SS, Ring S, Eton O, Bedikian A, Buzaid AC, Plager C, Papadopoulos N. Development of a biochemotherapy regimen with concurrent administration of cisplatin, vinblastine, dacarbazine, interferon alfa and interleukin-2 for patients with metastatic melanoma. *J Clin Oncol* 1998; 16: 1752–1759.
124. Richards J, Gale D, Mehta N, Lestingi T. Combination of chemotherapy with interleukin-2 and interferon alfa for the treatment of metastatic melanoma. *J Clin Oncol* 1999; 17: 651–657.
125. Thompson JA, Gold PT, Markowitz DR, Byrd DR, Lindgren CG, Fefer A. Updated analysis of an outpatient chemoimmunotherapy regimen for treating metastatic melanoma. *Cancer J Sci Am* 1997; 3: S29–S34.
126. Antoine E, Benhammouda A, Bernard A, et al. Salpetriere Hospital experience with biochemotherapy in metastatic melanoma. *Cancer J Sci Am* 1997; 3: S16–S21.
127. Johnston S, Constenla DO, Moore J, et al. Randomized phase II trial of BCDT [carmustine (BCNU), cisplatin, dacarbazine (DTIC) and tamoxifen] with or without interferon alpha (IFN-alpha) and interleukin (IL-2) in patients with metastatic melanoma. *Br J Cancer* 1998; 77: 1280–1286.
128. Margolin K, Liu PY, Unger JM, et al. Phase II trial of biochemotherapy with interferon alpha, dacarbazine, cisplatin and tamoxifen in metastatic melanoma: a Southwest Oncology Group trial. *J Cancer Res Clin Oncol* 1999; 125: 292–296.
129. Falkson CI, Ibrahim J, Kirkwood JM, Coates AS, Atkins MB, Blum RH. Phase III trial of dacarbazine versus dacarbazine with interferon alpha-2b versus dacarbazine with tamoxifen versus dacarbazine with interferon alpha-2b and tamoxifen in patients with metastatic malignant melanoma: an Eastern Cooperative Oncology Group study. *J Clin Oncol* 1998; 16: 1743–1751.
130. Lindner DJ, Borden EC, Kalvakolanu D. Increasing effectiveness of interferon alpha for malignancies. *Semin Oncol* 1998; 25: 3–8.
131. Kirkwood JM, Strawderman MH, Ernstoff MS, et al. Interferon alfa-2b adjuvant therapy of high-risk resected cutaneous melanoma: the Eastern Cooperative Oncology Group trial EST 1684. *J Clin Oncol* 1996; 14: 7–17.
132. Kirkwood JM, Ibrahim JG, Sondak VK, et al. High- and low-dose interferon alfa-2b in high-risk melanoma: first analysis intergroup trial E1690/S9111/C9190. *J Clin Oncol* 2000; 18: 2444–2458.
133. Kirkwood JM, Ibrahim JG, Sosman JA, et al. High-dose interferon alfa-2b significantly prolongs relapse-free and overall survival compared with the GM2-KLH/QS-21 vaccine in

patients with resected stage IIB-III melanoma: results of intergroup trial E1694/S9512/C509801. *J Clin Oncol* 2001; 19: 2370–2380.

134. Creagan ET, Dalton RJ, Ahman DL, et al. Randomized, surgical adjuvant clinical trial of recombinant interferon alfa-2a in selected patients with malignant melanoma. *J Clin Oncol* 1995; 13: 2776–2783.
135. Pehamerger H, Soyer HP, Steiner A, et al. Adjuvant interferon alfa-2a treatment in resected primary stage II cutaneous melanoma. *J Clin Oncol* 1998; 16: 1425–1429.
136. Musselman DL, Lawson DH, Gumnick JF, Manatunga AK, Penna S, Goodkin RS, Greiner K, Nemeroff CB, Miller AH. Paroxetine for the prevention of depression induced by high-dose interferon alfa. *N Engl J Med* 2001; 344: 961–966.
137. Borden EC, Parkinson D. A perspective on the clinical effectiveness and tolerance of interferon-α. *Semin Oncol* 1998; 25(Suppl 1): 3–8.
138. Licinio J, Kling MA, Hauser P. Cytokines and Brain Function: Relevance to Interferon-α-induced mood and cognitive changes. *Semin Oncol* 1998; 25(Suppl 1): 30–38.
139. Plata-Salama'n, CR. Cytokines and anorexia: a brief overview. *Semin Oncol* 1998; 25(Suppl 1): 64–72.
140. Cole BF, Gelber RD, Kirkwood JM, et al. A quality-of-life-adjusted survival analysis of interferon alfa-2b adjuvant treatment for high-risk resected cutaneous melanoma: an Eastern Cooperative Oncology Group study (E1684). *J Clin Oncol* 1996; 14: 2666–2673.
141. Hillner BE, Kirkwood JM, Atkins MB, et al. Economic analysis of adjuvant interferon alfa-2b in high-risk melanoma based on projections from Eastern Cooperative Oncology Group 1684. *J Clin Oncol* 1997; 15: 2351–2358.
142. Barth A, Wanek LA, Morton DL. Prognostic factors in 1,521 melanoma patients with distant metastases. *J Am Coll Surg* 1995; 181: 193–201.
143. Creagan ET, Ahmann DL, Green SJ, et al. Phase II study of low-dose recombinant leukocyte A interferon in disseminated malignant melanoma. *J Clin Oncol* 1984; 2: 1002–1005.
144. Creagan ET, Ahmann DL, Green SJ, et al. Phase II study of recombinant leukocyte A interferon (rIFN-αA) in disseminated malignant melanoma. *Cancer* 1984; 54: 2844–2949.
145. Hersey P, Hasic E, MacDonald M, et al. Effects of recombinant leukocyte interferon (rIFN-αA) on tumour growth and immune responses in patients with metastatic melanoma. *Br J Cancer* 1985; 51: 815–826.
146. Dorval T, Palangie T, Jouve M, et al. Treatment of metastatic malignant melanoma with recombinant interferon alfa-2b. *Invest New Drugs* 1987; 5: 61–64.
147. Legha SS, Papadopoulos NEJ, Plager C, et al. Clinical evaluation of recombinant interferon alfa-2A (Roferon-A) in metastatic melanoma using two different schedules. *J Clin Oncol* 1987; 5: 1240–1246.
148. Robinson WA, Mughal TI, Thomas MR, Johnson M, Spiegel RJ. Treatment of metastatic malignant melanoma with recombinant interferon alpha 2. *Immunobiology* 1986; 172: 275–282.
149. Kirkwood JM, Ernstoff MS, Davis CA, Reiss M, Ferraresi R, Rudnick SA. Comparison of intramuscular and intravenous recombinant alpha-2 interferon in melanoma and other cancers. *Ann Intern Med* 1985; 103: 32–36.
150. Miller RL, Steis RG, Clark JW, et al. Randomized trial of recombinant α2b-interferon with or without indomethacin in patients with metastatic malignant melanoma. *Cancer Res* 1989; 49: 1871–1876.

10 Biochemotherapy of Melanoma

Lawrence E. Flaherty, MD
and Philip Agop Philip, MD, PhD, MRCP

Contents

1. INTRODUCTION

Malignant melanoma poses an increasingly important health problem. The incidence of this disease has increased 4% per year from 5.7 per 100,000 individuals per year in 1973 to 13.3 in 1995. It is estimated that by the end of 1999, the lifetime risk of developing melanoma in the United States will have reached one in 75 *(1)*. Over 47,000 individuals are diagnosed with melanoma annually, and melanoma accounts for in excess of 7500 deaths each year *(2)*. Melanoma ranks second only to testicular tumors in "years of life lost" when death occurs, because the majority of patients with advanced melanoma are young at the time of diagnosis. Stage IV melanoma is associated with a mortality rate of more than 95% within the first 5 yr of diagnosis. In several large series, survival has correlated inversely with the sites of tumor involvement, the number of involved organ sites, the absence or presence of visceral involvement, disease-free interval, performance status, and whether there was an elevated serum lactate dehydrogenase (LDH) level *(3)*.

The lack of curative therapies for metastatic melanoma, coupled with the modest antitumor activity of chemotherapy and biologic agents available to date, has prompted many investigators to explore various combinations of drugs to

From: *Current Clinical Oncology, Melanoma: Biologically Targeted Therapeutics*
Edited by: E. C. Borden

Table 1
Single Agent Therapies

Agent	*Evaluable patients*	*CR plus PR*	*95% CI (%)*
Chemotherapy			
Dacarbazine	1936	20%	18–22
Carmustine	122	18%	11–25
Cisplatin	188	23%	17–29
Vincristine	52	12%	3–20
Vinblastine	62	13%	5–21
Paclitaxel	65	18%	9–28
Biologic agents			
Interferon α	380	16%	N/A
Interleukin-2	270	16%	12–21

improve the outcome for this group of patients. One of the most promising areas of clinical investigation in this field has been the development of treatment regimens that have combined both chemotherapy and biologic agents. These combinations have generally been referred to as biochemotherapy, particularly when they include the use of interleukin-2 (IL-2). Understanding the rationale for the development of this approach requires an understanding of the development and evaluation of many of the single and multi-agent treatment regimens that have occurred within the past few decades. The results of many single and multi-agent chemotherapy treatment regimens, which have led to our present understanding of treatment for melanoma, are outlined below. These results were evolving at the time that many of the biochemotherapy regimens were under development and explain, in part, the rationale for inclusion of many of the drugs, doses, and schedules chosen.

2. CYTOTOXIC THERAPY

2.1. Single Agent Therapy

There is extensive experience with cytotoxic therapy administered as single agents in patients with metastatic melanoma. Table 1 outlines some of the most commonly used drugs in this setting and their efficacy. Taken as a group, single agent therapies have had modest responses, which have usually been of short duration *(1)*. Dacarbazine (DTIC) remains the most commonly used single agent in melanoma and the standard for many comparisons. It produces response rates of approximately 10–20%, with a median response duration of 4 to 6 mo, and a 5 yr survival rate of 2%, with a median survival time of 6–9 mo. The major toxicities associated with its use are hematological and gastrointestinal. Cisplatin (DDP), as a single agent, has activity that is similar to DTIC and many other

Table 2
DTIC Combination Chemotherapy Single Institution Phase II Trials

Regimen	*Response rate*
DTIC plus cisplatin	20–53%
DTIC plus cisplatin plus velban (CVD)	20–40%
Bleomycin plus vincristine plus CCNU plus DTIC (BOLD)	22–44%
DTIC plus cisplatin plus BCNU plus tamoxifen (CDBT or Dartmouth)	15–55%

CCNU, lomustine.

single agents. Cisplatin, however, has a different toxicity profile than most other chemotherapeutic agents used for melanoma. Cisplatin's major dose-limiting toxicity is its nephrotoxicity, gastrointestinal toxicity, and ototoxicity. Cisplatin has been associated with considerably less hematologic toxicity than other agents. Cisplatin may also possess some unique immunomodulatory effects (*see* Subheading 4.2.) not seen with other cytotoxic agents. This unique feature, along with its toxicity profile, has frequently made cisplatin an obvious choice for use in combination with other chemotherapy agents for melanoma.

2.2. Chemotherapy Combinations

Several drug combinations using cytotoxic agents with different mechanisms of action have been evaluated in metastatic melanoma. By choosing drugs that have had little to no overlapping toxicities, it has been possible to create combination regimens that have minimal additive toxicity (Table 2). Several of these combinations have utilized DTIC and/or cisplatin and have demonstrated response rates in the range of 20–50%, in single institution phase II trials *(4–12)*. The "Dartmouth" regimen, which combines DTIC, cisplatin, carmustine (BCNU), and tamoxifen, has been one of the more commonly used regimens in recent years. Response rates to this regimen have been in the 40–50% range in several single institution phase II studies *(5,6)*. However, lower response rates for all these combinations were identified in multi-institutional and in the cooperative group setting *(12–14)*. For example, the Southwest Oncology Group (SWOG) recently completed and reported a trial of 79 eligible patients treated with the Dartmouth regimen and reported a 15% response rate with a median survival of 9.0 mo *(13)*.

Phase III trials to compare DTIC alone with several of the more promising combinations have been reported in the past *(15,16)*. Most have been small trials performed within single institutions. Improvement in the response rate for combination therapy has occasionally been demonstrated, but without statistical significance. No improvement in median or overall survival has been seen. Recently, a large cooperative group phase III trials has compared DTIC alone with the

Dartmouth regimen in over 240 advanced stage melanoma patients *(17)*. There was no survival advantage for the combination chemotherapy group ($p = 0.52$). The response rate trend was higher for the combination chemotherapy (16.8%) than for DTIC alone (9.9%), however, this was not statistically significant ($p = 0.13$). Toxicity, particularly neutropenia and thrombocytopenia, was significantly more common and severe with the combination chemotherapy.

Based on the available data at the present time, though there may be a trend toward higher response rates, there does not appear to be an advantage associated with the use of multi-agent chemotherapy regimens in the management of metastatic melanoma when compared to DTIC alone.

2.3. Tamoxifen

Early studies suggested that melanoma cells expressed estrogen receptors and, therefore, might be candidates for treatment trials with the anti-estrogen drug, tamoxifen *(18,19)*. A large number of phase II treatment trials in patients with metastatic melanoma were reported in the early 1980s *(20–24)* and identified a response rate of 5%, few of which were durable. Women appeared to benefit more often than men, with most responses confined to soft tissue and lymph node sites. Renewed interest in tamoxifen emerged in 1992, following a small phase III trial reported by Cocconi et al., which compared DTIC alone to DTIC combined with tamoxifen *(25)*. There was a significant difference in the response rates (28% vs 12%, $p = 0.03$) and survival (median, 48 vs 29 wk, $p = 0.02$) in favor of patients who received the combination. Interestingly, the greatest benefit occurred in women. Subsequently, several large phase III trials have investigated the contribution of tamoxifen to the chemotherapy of metastatic melanoma. A National Cancer Institute of Canada (NCIC) trial compared cisplatin, BCNU, and DTIC with or without high-dose tamoxifen. No progression-free or overall survival advantage was demonstrated for those patients who received tamoxifen *(26)*. Although the response rate for the group receiving tamoxifen with chemotherapy was slightly higher (30% vs 21%), the difference was not statistically significant ($p = 0.187$). More recently, the Eastern Cooperative Oncology Group (ECOG) reported a study of tamoxifen added to either DTIC alone or DTIC plus interferon (IFN)α in over 250 patients with metastatic melanoma. There was no difference in overall survival ($p = 0.91$) or time to treatment failure ($p = 0.74$) for the addition of tamoxifen *(17)* with equivalent response rates in the two groups *(27)*.

In conclusion, it does not appear that tamoxifen adds significantly to the benefit of either single agent or multi-agent chemotherapy regimens for patients with metastatic melanoma.

2.4. Interferon Alone and Combined with DTIC

IFN has pleiotropic actions at a cellular level, including direct and indirect antiproliferative and immunomodulatory effects, which appear responsible for its mechanism of action *(28)*. Early studies with IFN demonstrated responsiveness in patients with metastatic melanoma *(29)*.

Most studies have demonstrated a response rate to IFN, particularly IFN-α, in the 15% range in patients with metastatic melanoma with a small but consistent number of durable remissions *(30)*.

Several investigators have combined IFN with DTIC in an effort to improve response rates and survival *(31–33)*. Bajetta et al. *(31)* randomized 266 patients with metastatic melanoma to either DTIC alone (800 mg/m^2 intravenously [IV] d 1 every 21 d) or DTIC plus IFN. Two different low-dose IFN regimens were chosen, either 9 million international units (MIU) intramuscularly (IM) daily or 3 MIU IM 3×/wk (t.i.w). Although there was no difference in response rates noted between the groups (20, 28, and 23%), the IFN arms were associated with a prolongation of response duration (2.6 vs 8.4 vs 5.5 mo, respectively), which, unfortunately, did not translate into overall survival advantage.

Thomson et al. *(32)*, randomized 170 patients on a two arm phase III trial in metastatic melanoma, which compared an escalating dose of DTIC, which reached 800 mg/m^2 every 3 wk alone or combined with IFN. The IFN was administered subcutaneously (s.c.) at 3 MU daily for d 1–3, then 9 MU daily on d 4–70, then 9 MU t.i.w. Treatment was continued for 6 mo or disease progression. The combination produced response rates of 21% for the combination and 17% for DTIC alone. There was no significant difference in response duration or overall survival.

A third but smaller randomized phase III trial that evaluated the addition of IFN to DTIC was reported by Kirkwood et al. *(33)*. Patients with metastatic melanoma were randomized to either: (group A) DTIC 250 mg/m^2/d × 5 d every 3 wk; (group B) IFN 30 MIU/d, Monday through Friday for 3 wk, then 10 MIU/m^2 s.c. 3×/wk; or (group C) DTIC plus IFN. Of the 68 evaluable patients, there were 5 responses (21%) among the 24 patients in group A, 1 response (4%) among the 23 patients in group B, and 4 responses (19%) among the 21 patients receiving DTIC plus IFN in group C.

In 1991, Falkson et al. *(34)* reported the results of a small randomized phase III trial in metastatic melanoma, in which single agent DTIC was compared with DTIC combined with IFN. The response rate in the 30 patients who received DTIC alone was 20%, with a response duration of 2.5 mo, compared to a response rate of 53% and a response duration of 9.0 mo for the 30 patients receiving DTIC combined with IFN. This trial was unique in its schedule and dose of IFN compared with previous trials. The IFN was administered IV in high dose and preceded the administration of DTIC by 4 wk. This schedule and route of IFN was similar to that which had been successfully employed in the adjuvant setting in the ECOG trial E-1684 reported by Kirkwood et al. *(35)*. To test this further, a large phase III trial in metastatic melanoma was conducted by the ECOG (E-3690) and has recently been reported *(27)*. In that 2 × 2 factorial design trial, IFNα was added to DTIC alone or DTIC plus tamoxifen. The IFNα schedule used in this important trial was the high-dose IV IFNα administration originally reported by Falkson et al. *(34)*. This trial, with over 120 patients in each arm, demonstrated a response rate for the IFNα-containing arm of 20% compared to 16% for the non-IFNα-containing arms. There was, however, no overall survival advantage ($p = 0.85$) and no improvement in time to treatment failure ($p = 0.74$). The IFNα arms were associated with greater toxicity.

At least one investigation has evaluated the addition of high-dose IFN to multi-agent chemotherapy. This phase II trial combined high-dose IFN with DTIC, cisplatin, and tamoxifen in 25 patients with metastatic melanoma in the Southwest Oncology Group (SWOG). The response rate was 4% with moderate hematologic and constitutional side effects for the patients enrolled in this study *(36)*. The investigators concluded that there was no benefit to pursuing this strategy further given the toxicity and lack of clinical activity.

Based on the above experience, it does not appear that adding IFNα alone, either in high-dose or low-dose regimens, to single or multi-agent chemotherapy regimens is beneficial, and, in all circumstances, it has been associated with greater toxicity.

3. INTERLEUKIN-2

IL-2 is a pleiotropic immunostimulatory cytokine whose antitumor effect is not entirely clear and may be multi-factorial. IL-2's action is thought to be mediated indirectly through its activation of natural killer (NK) and specific cytotoxic T cells. The recommended dose when used as a single agent is 600,000 IU/kg given IV, every 8 h for up to 14 doses. Treatment is repeated once after a 1-wk rest period. A review of 270 patients from 8 clinical trials treated with this dose and schedule, conducted between 1985 and 1993, revealed an objective tumor response rate of 16% with complete responses (CR) in 6% *(37)*. Of particular importance was the number of durable CR. IL-2 has been approved by the FDA for treatment in patients with metastatic melanoma in the dose and schedule above. Because of the protean nature of IL-2 stimulation however, systemic toxicity is a major potential drawback of therapy. Due to the toxicity associated with its administration in this schedule, treatment with this dose and schedule has been confined to a relatively small number of tertiary referral centers throughout the United States. Early trials evaluated different schedules of IL-2 dose in an attempt to overcome this problem. In 1987, West et al. *(38)* administered IL-2, 18.0 MIU/m^2/d by continuous infusion over 5 d in 48 cancer patients, including 10 with metastatic melanoma. Less toxicity was associated with this dose and schedule, and responses were seen in 5 of the 10 patients with melanoma in this small trial. This experience prompted many investigators to adopt this approach to IL-2 administration in subsequent melanoma trials, often in combination with other biologics and single and multi-agent chemotherapy. The clinical activity of IL-2 as a single agent has established the principal that this immunologic manipulation can mediate the regression of established tumor deposits. It is likely that IL-2 will continue to play a pivotal role in the immunotherapy of melanoma.

4. BIOCHEMOTHERAPY WITH IL-2

4.1. Rationale for Biochemotherapy

The antitumor activity of IL-2 and its unique mechanism of action have suggested to many investigators that IL-2 could be combined with cytotoxic chemotherapy to produce additive or synergistic antitumor effects. To rationally combine IL-2 and chemotherapy however, the mechanisms of action of each component, as well as any potential interactions, must be taken into account. IL-2 is a pleiotropic immunostimulatory protein whose antineoplastic activity is probably mediated indirectly through its ability to activate NK and specific cytotoxic T lymphocyte (CTL) cells and to induce the generation of lymphokine-activated killer (LAK) cells. In contrast, most chemotherapeutic agents mediate their effects through either direct cytotoxic action on tumor cells or their interference with mechanisms of cellular growth and division leading to apoptosis.

Many chemotherapeutic agents have demonstrated immune-modulating effects ranging from immune suppression, probably mediated through direct lymphocytotoxicity, to immune augmentation, possibly mediated through interference with immune regulatory mechanisms *(39)*. Mitchell *(40)* has reviewed and classified some common chemotherapeutic drugs according to their general effects on the immune system. Despite this information, the lack of a standard quantifiable definition of immunocompetence and the lack of understanding of the biologic effects of IL-2 that correlate with tumor regression, make it difficult to predict or assess the outcome of a particular chemotherapy and IL-2 combination on either the immune system or the tumor.

The sequence and timing of IL-2 and chemotherapy administration may potentially have a major influence on the activity and the toxicity of a particular combination. Theoretical arguments can be made to support administering the chemotherapy before, after, or concurrently with the IL-2. Reasons for administering the chemotherapy first include: (*i*) priming the immune system (if the chemotherapeutic agent itself is immunoaugmentive) for later response to IL-2; and (*ii*) reducing the tumor burden, thereby optimizing the chance that IL-2 might produce additional benefit. The principal reason for administering chemotherapy concurrently with IL-2 is to provide maximal opportunity for additive or synergistic interactions. Potential favorable interactions could include: (*i*) chemotherapy altering the tumor cell membrane, rendering the tumor more susceptible to immunologic attack; or (*ii*) IL-2 creating a selective intratumoral capillary leak, allowing chemotherapy better access to the tumor. The reason for administering chemotherapy after the IL-2 include: (*i*) allowing IL-2 to mediate its effect unencumbered by any immunosuppressive effect of cytotoxic chemotherapy; and (*ii*) potential modification of tumor cells by IL-2 or secondary cytokines, making them more susceptible to the cytotoxic effects of chemotherapy (e.g., decreased multidrug resistance [MDR] protein expression). Despite these theoretical considerations, most combinations tested to date have been empirical in nature and are based primarily on observations that both treatments possess activity against melanoma.

4.2. Preclinical Investigations

The primary focus of preclinical investigations of IL-2 and chemotherapy combinations were to determine whether chemotherapy would block host immunologic response to IL-2 and to confirm non-cross-resistance between these two classes of drugs. However, in vitro studies have been difficult to perform with IL-2 and chemotherapy drugs because IL-2's primary biologic effect is on effector cells and, therefore, requires an intact host to demonstrate its antineoplastic effect. In addition, only a few cytotoxic agents are viewed as having immunomodulatory effects that would be beneficial. These have generally included cyclophosphamide *(41,42)*, cisplatin *(43)*, and 5-FU *(44)*. Of these agents, only cisplatin has been considered to be a clinically active agent in the management of melanoma, and, therefore, many of the following studies have focused on its effects and potential mechanism of interaction.

Allavena et al. *(45)* demonstrated that cisplatin exposure rendered peripheral blood lymphocytes (PBL) resistant to recombinant IL-2 activation in vitro, with spontaneous recovery within 24–48 h. In contrast however, in clinical studies, no inhibition of PBL-derived LAK activity was detected in ovarian cancer patients after receiving 50 mg/m^2 of cisplatin. In vitro studies of PBL exposed to cisplatin by other investigators failed to demonstrate an alteration of LAK cell generation or activity at cisplatin concentrations achievable in humans *(46)*. Other in vitro and in vivo studies have suggested that cisplatin enhances NK cells, LAK cells, and T cell function *(47–49)*. The clinical impact of these findings has been more difficult to identify. A number of in-vitro studies *(47,50,51)* have also suggested that cisplatin may have a beneficial effect on host monocyte and macrophage function. Clinical studies seem to support this possibility when comparing monocyte cytotoxicity of untreated cancer patients to controls and the effects of cisplatin compared to non-cisplatin-containing regimens on a patient's monocyte function *(52,53)*.

Several investigators have assessed the sensitivity of chemotherapy-resistant cell lines to NK and LAK cell-mediated killing. Samlowski et al. *(54)* showed that the parent and drug-resistant variants of the human leukemia (HL)-60 leukemia, squamous cell carcinoma (SCC)-25, and MES-SA sarcoma cell lines exhibited similar patterns of NK and LAK cell susceptibility in vitro. Additional studies *(55)* suggested that resistant cell lines might be more sensitive to LAK cell-mediated lysis than their chemotherapy-sensitive parent cell lines. Finally, prior cisplatin administration actually enhanced the cytolytic activity of LAK cells against the chemotherapy-resistant human lung adenocarcinoma cell lines PC-9 and PC-14 *(56)*.

In addition to the immunomodulatory effects, it has also been proposed that nitric oxide (NO) generation contributes to IL-2-induced antitumor activity and systemic toxicity. The production of NO in tumor cells may also be a potential mechanism of interaction between IL-2 and cisplatin. IL-2 has been identified to enhance NO production in tumor cells, and studies have demonstrated a synergy between NO production and cisplatin in melanoma cell lines *(57,58)*. Therefore, NO produced by tumor cells stimulated by IL-2 or other cytokine production may enhance the toxicity of cytotoxic agents and potentiate directly cisplatin DNA damage.

Sequence issues have been addressed in vivo in a number of murine models. Rhinehart et al. demonstrated that the combination of cytoxan, etoposide, and cisplatin chemotherapy and IL-2 improved survival in C57BL/6 mice injected with B16 melanoma if the IL-2 was administered first, but not if the order were reversed *(59)*. Furthermore, BCNU and doxorubicin did not appear to enhance survival when given before IL-2 in mice bearing MCA-105 sarcoma *(60)*. Guany et al., working with mice implanted either with MethA sarcoma or B16 melanoma *(61,62)*, found highly variable results, further supporting the view that antitumor efficacy was dependent on sequence and schedule. In the MethA model, greater efficacy was seen if bleomycin, cisplatin, or doxorubicin was administered either before or concurrently with IL-2. Synergy was reported with cisplatin when it was given before IL-2 administration, but was only seen with etoposide and DTIC when they were given concurrently with IL-2. In contrast to prior models, synergy was not seen when the chemotherapy was administered after IL-2. Bernsen et al. *(63)* identified different sensitivities to cisplatin and IL-2 in sequence in two murine models that were equally sensitive to these agents individually. These conflicting results highlighted the potential complexity involved with combining these two modalities.

Many possible mechanisms of action and interaction may exist between IL-2 and the cytotoxic agents evaluated in the investigations above and in the clinical setting. Although our understanding and investigations have become ever more sophisticated, our lack of a biologic correlate for response to these therapies has left this an area of intense speculation and interest. To date, no firm conclusions can be drawn regarding the optimal drug combinations and sequencing in the absence of a nonclinical endpoint that corresponds with clinical outcome.

4.3. Clinical Experience with IL-2-Based Biochemotherapy

The development of clinical studies combining cytotoxic agents with IL-2 was based in part on the preclinical information above, as well as a knowledge of the active cytotoxic agents for melanoma. Investigators have looked to combine these agents in ways that might be additive or synergistic with an eye to avoiding and evaluating possible toxic interactions. Several looked at biologic endpoints as correlates of improved activity or deleterious interaction. Initial efforts began with the combination of DTIC and IL-2, but, as tolerability and activity was identified, rapidly moved to the incorporation of a wider range of cytotoxic drugs and the incorporation of IFN. Over the past 15 yr, efforts to understand the individual contribution of drugs, the sequencing of therapy, efforts to reduce toxicity, and incorporation of outpatient treatment strategies have all evolved. The following highlights some, but not all, of the studies that have led us to our present understanding of IL-2-based biochemotherapy.

4.4. DTIC and IL-2

Several early biochemotherapy investigations combined DTIC and IL-2 in an effort to evaluate dose, schedule, toxicity, and, in some circumstances, immunologic effects (Table 3). DTIC followed by IL-2 was the focus of an investigation by Flaherty et al. *(64)*. A phase I/II trial was performed combining DTIC, 1000 mg/m^2 IV as a 24-h infusion with IL-2 administered in the outpatient setting on d 15–19 and 22–26 of a 28-d cycle. IL-2 was initially administered at 12.0×10^6 IU/m^2 daily with dose escalation of 6.0×10^6 IU/m^2 in subsequent groups of 3 patients to define the maximally tolerated dose (MTD). The last 11 patients on the study began treatment at a dose of 24.0×10^6 IU/m^2 as the MTD dose of IL-2. Plasma and urinary DTIC and 5-aminoimidazole 4-carboximide (AIC) levels were measured in the first 2 cycles in 14 patients. A decrease in DTIC area under the curve (AUC) was observed in cycle 2, possibly as a result of increased volume of distribution related to a vascular leak associated with the prior IL-2 administration. There was no change in the elimination half-lives or urinary excretion of DTIC or AIC, and no change in the AIC AUC *(65)*. Of the 32 patients registered onto the study, there was 1 CR and 6 partial responses (PR) for an overall response rate of 22%. Responses were seen in soft tissue, lymph node, liver, lung, and adrenals. The overall median survival and the median survival for the nonresponders was 8.5 mo. The median survival for the responders was 24 mo, with 3 patients in unmaintained remissions for over 10 yr. In the 120 treatment cycles, 2 patients required overnight hospitalization for hydration. There were 5 grade IV hematologic events during the IL-2 phase of therapy. All patients had complete recovery of their counts despite continued IL-2 therapy suggesting that the DTIC was primarily responsible for the hematologic toxicity. Lymphocyte counts were measured in the last 19 patients after each cycle of

Table 3
DTIC and IL-2 Trials in Melanoma

Author (reference)	*DTIC*	*IL-2*	*N*	*RR%*	*CR*
Flaherty et al. *(64)*	1000 mg/m^2 d 1 every 28 d.	24 MIU IVPB d 15–19, 22–26.	32	22	1
Papadopoulos et al. *(68)*	200 mg/m^2 d 1–5 every 28 d.	24 MIU IVPB d 1–5, 8–12.	30	33	4
Stoter et al. *(66)*	850 mg/m^2 d 26 every 28 d.	18 MIU CVI d 1–5, 12–17.	24	25	2
Dillman et al. *(67)*	1200 mg/m^2 d 29.	18 MIU CVI d 1–5, 11–15.	27	26	2
Totals			113	27	9

DTIC, dacarbazine; N, number of patients; IL-2, interleukin-2; RR, response rate; CR, complete response; d, day; MIU, Million International Units; IVPB, intravenous piggyback; CVI, continuous venous infusion.

treatment, and a repeated lymphocytosis was identified with each cycle, suggesting that the DTIC did not appear to interfere with the ability of IL-2 to generate a lymphocytosis.

The opposite sequence of IL-2 first followed by DTIC was the focus of a trial by Stoter et al. *(66)*. This phase II multicenter European trial consisted of IL-2 as a continuous intravenous infusion (CI) on d 1–5 and d 12–17, followed by DTIC (850 mg/m^2) given as a bolus over 30 min on d 26 of a 35-d cycle. Thrombocytopenia was observed in only 2 patients. Tumor response was seen in 6 (2 CR and 4 PR) of 24 (25%) evaluable patients. The median time to progression was 4 mo, and the median survival time was 13 mo for the patients on the study.

Another trial, which evaluated biotherapy with infusional IL-2 first, followed by DTIC, was reported by Dillman et al. *(67)*. Therapy consisted of IL-2 (18.0 $\times 10^6$ IU/m^2/d) by CI on d 1–5 and 11–15 and DTIC (1200 mg/m^2) administered over 1–3 d beginning on d 29. Platelet counts less than 20,000 mm^{-3} were seen in 5 patients, and 4 patients developed granulocyte counts < 500 mm^{-3}. There were 2 CR and 5 PR in 27 response-evaluable patients, for a 26% response rate. The overall median survival for the group was 10 mo, with a 36% survival at 1 yr. The only durable responses (13$^+$ and 24$^+$ mo) were seen in the 2 patients achieving CR.

The only trial to evaluate concurrent administration of IL-2 and DTIC was reported by Papadoupolous et al. *(68)*. DTIC (200 mg/m^2/d) by CI on d 1–5 was combined with IL-2 (24.0 $\times$ 10^6 IU) IV piggyback (IVPB) over 30 min daily on d 1–5 and 8–12, every 28 d. Treatment was in the outpatient setting. Only 3 patients required hospitalization during the treatment, and in an additional 3 patients, the platelet count fell to <75,000. Of 30 patients treated, there were

4 CR and 6 PR, for an overall response rate of 33%. Responses were noted in all sites, including liver and bone, but the response duration was only 16 wk.

In summary, early investigations combining DTIC and IL-2 demonstrated no unusual or unexpected toxicities. Both agents were generally administered in full doses. Responses were seen in all organ sites, and durable unmaintained remissions were identified. Where measured, neither agent appeared to have a detrimental effect on the pharmacokinetics or immunostimulatory effect of the other. The overall clinical benefit in terms of response rates and median survival did not suggest synergy, but rather at best, additive benefits. No advantage for infusion or IV bolus IL-2 or sequence of administration between chemotherapy and IL-2 could be identified. Encouraged by these initial results, many investigators pursued additional trials using multi-agent chemotherapy and added IFN to the biotherapy in hopes of generating better clinical results.

4.5. IL-2 with Multi-Agent Chemotherapy and IFN

In the late 1980s, a number of investigators were reporting their results from single institution phase II trials with multi-agent chemotherapy in melanoma (see above). These encouraging results, coupled with the emerging data combining DTIC and IL-2 in the schedules above, prompted a series of investigations. These trials are characterized by their frequent incorporation of DTIC and cisplatin with IL-2 in a variety of doses and schedules often in combination with IFN (Table 4). Due to the choice of IL-2 dose and schedule, all of these trials required in-patient management. The several trials listed below are typical of the strategies used to learn new information about combining these therapies.

A trial by Demchak et al. was an important effort to separate and identify the individual contributions of chemotherapy and IL-2 *(69)*. IL-2 was administered at 6×10^5 IU/kg by IV bolus every 8 h on d 1–5 and 15–19, followed by 2 courses of high-dose cisplatin beginning on d 32 and 53 of a 74-d cycle. Cisplatin was administered by 2 different schedules: regimen A, 135–150 mg/m^2 IV bolus over 30 min with the chemoprotectant WR-2721 (910 mg/m^2); or regimen B, 50 mg/m^2 IV over 2 h every day for 3 d. Among 27 evaluable patients, there were 10 (37%) overall responses, including 3 (11%) CR with durations of 9, 15, and 27$^+$ mo. Tumor regression was noted in 7 patients (4 PR and 3 minor response [MR]; 26%) following the first IL-2 treatment phase and 12 patients (12 PR; 44%) in response to the chemotherapy component. These results were similar to what has been reported for each component used independently, implying at least additive effects. Responses to chemotherapy were seen in 3 of 13 patients, whose disease progressed during the IL-2 phase of treatment, indicating some level of non-cross-resistance. Of 7 patients responding to IL-2, 6 achieved an additional PR to chemotherapy, possibly implying some synergy in the subset of patients whose disease was sensitive to IL-2. Durable major responses (>90% PR or CR) were seen only in patients responding to IL-2. The toxicity during the IL-2 phase of

Table 4
Biochemotherapy Inpatient Regimens IL-2-Based

Author (reference)	*Regimen*	*Route*	*N*	*RR*	*CR*
McDermott et al. *(80)*	CVD/IL-2/IFN	CIV	42	45%	6
Antoine et al. *(72)*	C/IL-2/IFN	CIV	127	49%	13
Richards et al. *(71)*	DCBT/IL-2/IFN	IVPB	42	57%	10
Legha et al. *(78)*	CVD/IL-2/IFN	CIV	114	60%	24
Keiholz et al. *(74)*	C/IL-2/IFN	CIV	60	33%	3
Demchak et al. *(69)*	CD/IL-2	IVPB	38	42%	3
O'Day et al. *(75)*	CVDT/IL-2/IFN	CIV	35	57%	7
Totals			458		66(14.4%)

C, cisplatin; D, DTIC (dacarbazine); V, velban; T, tamoxifen; IL-2, interleukin-2; IFN, interferon α; CIV, continuous intravenous infusion; DCBT, cisplatin, BCNU, and tamoxifen; IVPB, intravenous piggyback; N, number of patients; RR, response rate; CR, complete response.

therapy was typical of high-dose protocols and completely reversible. The authors concluded that the individual components of this combination appear to be non-cross-resistant and possess at least additive antitumor activity against melanoma.

Insight on this issue of non-cross-resistance also comes from a report by Richards et al. *(70)* who evaluated the benefit of chemotherapy on melanoma patients after treatment with IL-2 had been completed. Twenty patients with metastatic melanoma, who had previously received IL-2 regimens by CI or IVPB regimens and failed, were treated with DTIC, cisplatin, BCNU, and tamoxifen (Dartmouth regimen). Eleven patients (55%) had an objective PR to treatment. This response rate is similar to that reported in phase II trials for this regimen in untreated patients, leading these investigators to conclude that prior IL-2 does not appear to select for chemoresistant disease. In addition, in the trials of high-dose IV bolus IL-2 *(37)*, responses to IL-2 were seen both in patients that had not received prior systemic therapy, as well as those that had received systemic therapy, though it was higher in the former group. These results suggest that IL-2 and chemotherapy may not be cross-resistant and that strategies to combine them might be beneficial.

A more direct look at the issue of sequencing was also undertaken by Richards et al. *(71)* based on the data above. IL-2 and IFN were combined and given sequentially both after and before chemotherapy in 42 patients with metastatic melanoma. The chemotherapy chosen was the Dartmouth regimen consisting of DTIC 220 mg/m^2 IV and cisplatin 25 mg/m^2 IV on d 1–3 and 23–25, BCNU 150 mg/m^2 IV every 6 wk, and tamoxifen 20 mg daily. IL-2 3.9 MIU/m^2 IV every 8 h × 15 doses and IFN 6 MIU/m^2 s.c. daily were administered on d 4–8 and 17–21. There were 10 complete remissions (24%) and 14 partial remissions (33%) for an overall response rate of 57% and a median survival of 11.5 mo.

The Salpetriere Hospital group has reported an experience, which evaluates sequential treatment, that begins with the administration of chemotherapy, in this case using only cisplatin *(72)*. One hundred twenty-seven response-evaluable patients with metastatic melanoma were treated with cisplatin 100 mg/m^2 IV d 0, IFN 9 MIU s.c. t.i.w., and infusional IL-2 18.0 MIU/m^2/d on d 3–6 and 17–21. Treatment was administered every 28 d in 94 patients and every 21 d in 11 patients. Another 24 patients received in addition, tamoxifen 160 mg/m^2 from d –5 to +5. Among the entire 126 patient group there were 13 CR (10%) and 49 PR for an overall response rate of 49%. The median overall survival was 11.0 mo.

A number of investigators have developed novel regimens to maintain IL-2 benefit but reduce its toxicity. Based on the concept that initial high concentrations of IL-2 may be necessary to saturate, but lower concentrations may be sufficient to stimulate CTL cells, reports have emerged using a "decrescendo" schedule of IL-2. Keilholz et al. *(73)* evaluated this strategy first by combining IL-2 and IFN alone. They performed sequential phase II trials, which sequenced IFN 10 MIU/m^2 s.c. for 5 d followed by IL-2 18.0 MIU/m^2 by CI for 5 d in schedule (A) and in their next trial sequenced the same IFN dose and schedule followed by a decrescendo IL-2 described as 18 MIU/m^2 by CI over 6 h, then 18 MIU/m^2 CI over 12 h, then 18 MIU/m^2 over 24 h, then 4.5 MIU/m^2 over 24 h for 3 d, schedule (B). Among 27 patients in group (A) there was 1 CR and 4 PR for a 20% response rate, and in group (B), there were 3 CR and 8 PR for a 41% response rate. These investigators identified a significant reduction in IL-2 toxicity with this schedule and, encouraged by the activity in schedule (B), initiated a randomized phase III trial *(74)* comparing the decrescendo IL-2 plus IFN schedule with or without cisplatin (*see* Subheading 4.8.). Sixty patients on one arm of the randomized trial received cisplatin 100 mg/m^2 IV on d 1, followed by the IFN and IL-2 schedule (B) above on d 1–10. There were 3 CR and 17 PR for a 33% overall response rate. O'Day and colleagues *(75)* used a similar decrescendo approach to IL-2 administration in order to modify the concurrent biochemotherapy regimen described by Legha et al. (*see* Subheading 4.6.). DTIC 800 mg/m^2 IV d 1, vinblastine 1.5 mg/m^2 IV d 1–4, and cisplatin 20 mg/m^2 IV d 1–4 were administered IV and given concurrently with IFN and IL-2. The IFN was given s.c. at a dose of 5 MIU/m^2 d 1–5, and the IL-2 was given by CI, 18.0 MIU/m^2 on d 1, 9.0 MIU/m^2 on d 2, and 4.5 MIU/m^2 on d 3 and 4 of a 21-d cycle. Tamoxifen was also administered in a dose of 20 mg by mouth (p.o.) daily. Forty-five patients with metastatic melanoma were treated. There were 10 CR (23%) and 15 PR (34%) for a 57% response rate and a median survival duration of 11.4 mo. Hospital stays were 4–5 d in 86% of cycles, and readmission rates were low. Despite granulocyte colony-stimulating factor (G-CSF) support, 20 and 24% of cycles experienced grade III and IV neutropenia respectively, 60% of patients required red blood cell (RBC) transfusions, and 40% required platelet transfusions. This suggests that additional modifications in chemotherapy may be necessary to further reduce the toxicity associated with this regimen.

Two recent large reviews have summarized experience with IL-2 both alone and in combination. Keilholz et al. *(76)* compared the results of IL-2 alone, IL-2 plus IFNα, IL-2 plus chemotherapy, and IL-2 plus IFNα and chemotherapy. The IL-2 was given by CI in all of the 631 patients in their analysis. IL-2 with IFN and chemotherapy was associated with the highest response rates (44.8%, $p < 0.001$) and the longest median survival durations (11.4 mo). The 5-yr survival of patients treated with IL-2, IFN, and chemotherapy was 12%. Allen et al. *(77)* in a meta-analysis compared chemotherapy (with DTIC- or cisplatin-based regimens) with IL-2 alone, IL-2 plus IFNα, and IL-2 combined with IFNα, and chemotherapy. One hundred and fifty-four studies involving over 7000 patients were analyzed. The highest response rates (47%) were found when IL-2 was combined with IFN, cisplatin, and DTIC. Response durations for IL-2, IFN, and chemotherapy (10.0 mo) were statistically superior ($p < 0.05$) to either IL-2 alone or chemotherapy alone (8 and 7 mo, respectively).

The results of this collection of single institution phase II trials above points to an improvement in response rates and survival durations for multi-agent biochemotherapy regimens compared to single agent combinations and historic controls. Durable complete responses continue to be identified. All required management on an inpatient basis. Still to be defined for the field was whether there was an advantage for one sequence over another and whether these strategies were truly an improvement over chemotherapy or biotherapy alone.

4.6. Sequence of Biochemotherapy

The optimum combination and sequence of chemotherapy with biologic therapies remains to be determined. Legha et al. *(78)* in several phase II trials has evaluated various schedules (Fig. 1) of cisplatin, vinblastine, DTIC (CVD), chemotherapy combined with IL-2 and IFN-α. These serial phase II trials with a large number of patients from a single institution have provided some of the most useful clinical data thus far reported to address the issue of sequence. The chemotherapy used in these studies was cisplatin 20 mg/m^2 IV and vinblastine 1.5 mg/m^2 IV on d 1–4 combined with DTIC 800 mg/m^2 IV on d 1 of a 21-d cycle. The biotherapy consisted of IL-2 9.0 MU/m^{2}d/d as a CI on d 1–4 (96-h infusion) combined with IFNα 5.0 MU/m^2 s.c. on d 1–5, 8, 10, and 12, of a 21-d cycle. Their first trial compared alternating chemotherapy with biotherapy. One group of patients received a 6-wk course of chemotherapy (2 cycles) followed by a 6-wk course of biotherapy (2 cycles). The other group received the biotherapy first, followed 6 wk later by chemotherapy. The overall response rate for both groups of patients was 33%, which was not superior to chemotherapy alone. This strategy was not pursued further. A second series of trials evaluated the sequential administration of chemotherapy and biotherapy. The first group

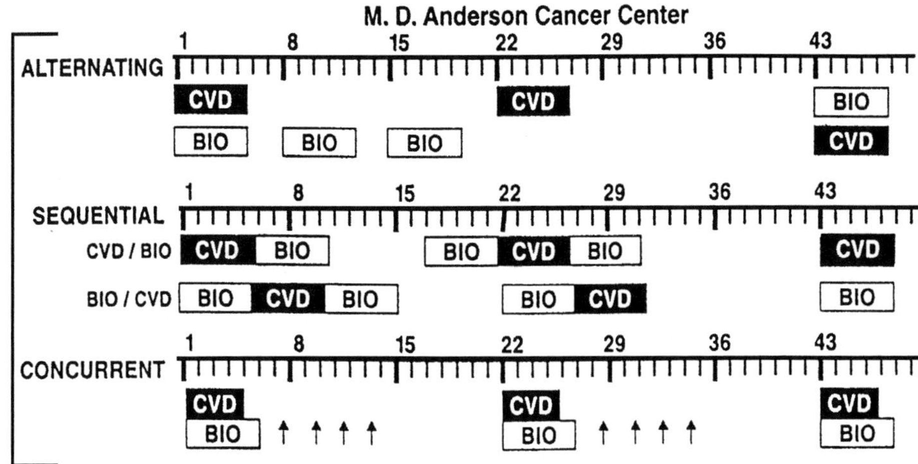

Fig. 1. Treatment schema of select biochemotherapy regimens. C, cisplatin; B, BCNU; D, decarbazine; V, vinblastine; BIO, IL-2 plus IFNα; arrow, IFNα only.

of patients received chemotherapy immediately followed by biotherapy and then, after a week rest, received biotherapy followed by chemotherapy, and then biotherapy again. Cycles were repeated every 6 wk. The second group of patients receiving sequential treatment began their treatment with biotherapy, followed by chemotherapy, followed by biotherapy again. After a 1-wk break, they received biotherapy followed by chemotherapy. The response rate for those beginning with chemotherapy was 66% compared to 50% for those starting with biotherapy, with a progression-free survival of 8 vs 7 mo for those beginning with chemotherapy. No overall survival advantage was seen in either group. There were 10 CR in the chemotherapy first group, compared with 3 CR in the biotherapy first group. All the durable CR received chemotherapy first. Compared with CVD chemotherapy alone from earlier trials within the same institution (historic controls) the sequential trial demonstrated superior response rates (66% vs 40%) and overall survival (12 mo vs 9 mo). The last in these series of investigations evaluated concurrent biochemotherapy by giving the chemotherapy and biotherapy components of treatment on the same days. This reduces the delivery time of treatment to 5 d in a 21-d cycle. Experience with this approach in 53 patients has a reported response rate of 64% with 20% of patients achieving a CR, of which approximately one-half have been durable *(79)*.

The high response rates along with the complete remissions and their durability have made the concurrent and chemotherapy first sequential regimens of interest. The concurrent regimen appears more practical considering it only requires a 5-d hospitalization for treatment. Unfortunately, it is associated with a high incidence of neutropenic fevers (64%) and bacteremia (51%). In addition, two-thirds of patients required transfusion with packed cells, and almost 50% required platelet transfusions. The concurrent regimen as outlined above, has been modified to reduce its toxicity and evaluated again as a phase II trial by McDermott et al. *(80)*. Adjustments have included; the addition of prophylactic antibiotics, the reduction of the vinblastine dose to 4.8 mg/m^2, the addition of G-CSF on days 7–16, the replacement of central lines with each cycle, the aggressive use of antiemetics, and strict conservative dose modifications. Incorporating those changes has significantly lowered the incidence of hematologic toxicity and maintained a response rate of 48%, with 20% of patients achieving a complete remission. Of particular note is that one-half of the patients that were entered onto the trial had received, and subsequently failed, high-dose adjuvant IFN. The modifications above have allowed a phase III randomized intergroup trial to be initiated using biochemotherapy as the experimental arm (*see* Subheading 4.8.).

4.7. Outpatient Biochemotherapy

There has been considerable interest in outpatient regimens of biochemotherapy in recent years. If the present inpatient regimens establish a role for this therapy in the management of melanoma, it would be useful to identify regimens with similar activity that could be administered in an outpatient setting. Potential advantages would be a reduction in toxicity and an elimination of inpatient costs, which would make acceptance of these regimens more attractive to managing patients and physicians alike. Table 5 lists some of the reported trials to date, along with their response rates and the number of complete responders. Results appear generally similar to those reported with the inpatient biochemotherapy regimens. Several of the trials have differed in the dose and schedule of the administered IL-2.

Sequential biochemotherapy using DTIC and cisplatin first, followed by outpatient IV bolus IL-2 was the focus of a trial by Flaherty et al. *(81)*. DTIC (750 mg/m^2) IV bolus and cisplatin (100 mg/m^2) IV bolus were administered on d 1, and IL-2 (24.0 × 10^6 IU/m^2/d) by IV bolus was administered on d 12–16 and 19–23 of a repeating 28-d cycle. Of the first 91 courses, 11 were associated with a creatinine clearance less than 60 mL/min. No unusual toxicities were observed. NK and LAK cell assays performed before and after the IL-2 phase of treatment in the first 2 treatment cycles demonstrated that the chemotherapy did not interfere with the in vitro generation of NK and LAK cell activity *(82)*. Responses were seen in 13 (5 CR and 8 PR) of 32 (41%) registered patients. Complete remissions were observed in soft tissue and lymph node sites. The median response duration was 8.0 mo (3.0–24.0 mo).

Thompson et al. *(83)* has also evaluated sequential biochemotherapy, administering chemotherapy first in a phase II trial in 53 patients with metastatic melanoma. The chemotherapy consisted of BCNU (150 mg/m^2 every other

Table 5
Biochemotherapy Outpatient Regimens IL-2

Author (reference)	*Regimen*	*IL-2 route*	*N*	*RR%*	*CR*
Flaherty et al. *(81)*	CD/IL-2	IVPB	32	41	5
Thompson et al. *(83)*	DCBT/IL-2/IFN	SC	53	42	10
Atzpodien et al. *(89)*	DCBT/IL-2/IFN	SC	27	55	3
Bernengo et al. *(90)*	CT/IL-2/IFN	SC	36	47	5
Guida et al. *(91)*	CD/IL-2	SC	24	42	2
Flaherty et al. *(84)*	CD/IL-2/IFN	IVPB	43	37	5
Flaherty et al. *(84)*	CD/IL-2/IFN	SC	36	17	1
Kamanabrou et al. *(92)*	CDB/IL-2/IFN	SC	109	38	12
Dillman et al. *(93)*	CDBT/IL-2/IFN	SC	26	34	3
Totals			386		46(12.0%)

C, cisplatin; D, DTIC (dacarbazine); V, velban; T, tamoxifen; IL-2, interleukin-2; IFN, interferon α; SC, subcutaneous; IVPB, intravenous piggyback; N, number of patients; RR, response rate; CR, complete response.

cycle), DTIC (660 mg/m^2), and cisplatin (75 mg/m^2) administered on d 1 IV. Treatment was preceded by tamoxifen 40 mg b.i.d. for 3 d, and then given at 20 mg daily for the remainder of the cycle. Patients received IL-2 s.c. at 3 MIU/m^2 on d 3–9 and IFN 3 MIU s.c. on d 3, then 5 MIU/m^2 on d 5, 7, and 9 of a 21- or 28-d cycle. There were 10 CR (19%) and 12 PR (23%) for a 42% overall response rate. The median survival was 12 mo. Grade IV thrombocytopenia or neutropenia occurred in only 9% and 8% of cycles, respectively, suggesting that this type of approach may be less toxic with a potentially equivalent clinical benefit.

Recently, the Cytokine Working Group (CWG) has completed and reported the results of a randomized phase II trial evaluating DTIC and cisplatin chemotherapy combined with IFN and IL-2 *(84)*. These 2 phase II trials used identical doses and schedules of DTIC, cisplatin, and IFN. The 2 regimens differed in the dose of IL-2 and route of administration. In group 1, IL-2 was given in a dose of 18.0 MU/m^2 IV, and in group 2, the IL-2 was given in a dose of 5.0 MU/m^2 s.c. A randomized strategy was used to create comparable treatment groups and provide results in a similar time frame in order to choose a regimen to propose for future phase III trials. The group receiving IV IL-2 had a response rate of 37% with 12% CR, including 13 patients who are alive with a median follow-up exceeding 2.5 yr. The group receiving IL-2 s.c. had a response rate of 17% with 3% CR and 3 patients alive with the same follow-up. No patient in either group required admission for neutropenic fever or infection. There was a 23% incidence of grade III/IV neutropenia in group 1 and an 11% incidence of similar grade neutropenia in group 2. Both regimens were well tolerated.

The results of the trials listed in Table 5 suggest response rates that are comparable, though in some cases slightly lower for the outpatient regimens than for in-patient biochemotherapy. More of these trials are multi-institutional, which have generally been associated with lower response rates. The percentage of complete responses and their durability in these trials however remains encouraging. Should inpatient biochemotherapy regimens prove useful in the management of metastatic melanoma, a logical next step would be a comparison with outpatient regimens. The regimen using IV IL-2 would appear to be a reasonable choice for that type of trial.

4.8. Randomized Phase III Trials of Biochemotherapy

Several randomized phase III trials in metastatic melanoma, comparing either chemotherapy with IL-2 biochemotherapy regimens or IL-2 biotherapy regimens with IL-2 biochemotherapy, have either been completed or are nearing completion. They have varied in size, their choice of the biochemotherapy regimen under investigation, the schedule, route, and dose of IL-2 administered, and their choice of the chemotherapy or biotherapy control arm. In none of these studies has the control arm been DTIC alone. These features have made conclusions difficult at this time.

An effort to isolate the contribution of cisplatin to biotherapy was the focus of a small European Organization for Research and Treatment of Cancer Melanoma Cooperative Group (EORTC) phase III trial that randomized 138 patients to either IL-2 plus IFN alone or cisplatin followed by IL-2 plus IFN *(74)*. Among the 126 evaluable patients, the biochemotherapy regimen produced superior response rates (33% vs 18%, $p = 0.04$) and superior progression-free survival (92 vs 53 d, $p = 0.02$, Wilcoxon; $p = 0.09$, log rank), but no difference in median overall survival (9 mo) *(73)*.

Rosenberg et al. recently published the results of a small prospective randomized single institution trial in metastatic melanoma undertaken to compare the response rate of chemotherapy to biochemotherapy *(85)*. One hundred two patients were randomized to chemotherapy composed of tamoxifen, cisplatin, and DTIC or this same chemotherapy followed by IFN-α-2b and IL-2. There was a 44% response rate in the biochemotherapy arm compared to 27% in chemotherapy alone ($p = 0.071$). There was a trend, however, toward a survival advantage for patients receiving chemotherapy alone (15.8 mo vs 10.7 mo).

A larger phase III trial (EORTC 18951) involving 325 patients is accruing, and an interim analysis of the first 118 patients with 1-yr follow-up has been reported *(86)*. This trial attempts to isolate the potential contribution of IL-2 to biochemotherapy. Patients were randomized to DTIC, cisplatin, and IFN alone or combined with decrescendo IL-2. The response rates between the two arms have not differed significantly ($p = 0.12$), however, the number of patients with-

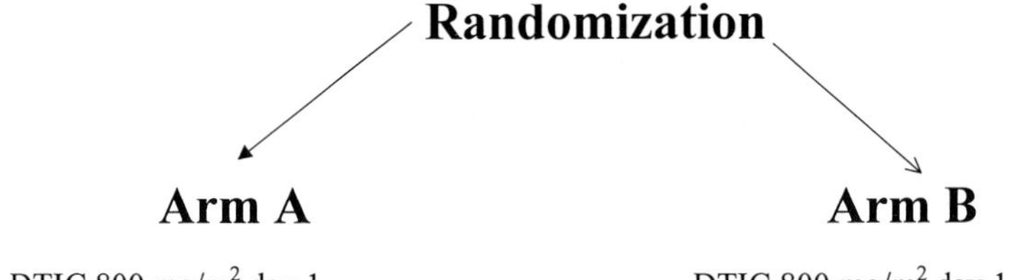

Arm A	Arm B
DTIC 800 mg/m^2 day 1	DTIC 800 mg/m^2 day 1
CDDP 20 mg/m^2 day 1-4	CDDP 20 mg/m^2/d day 1-4
VBL 1.2 mg/m^2/d day 1-4	VBL 1.2 mg/m^2/d day 1-4
	IFN alpha 2b 5 MU/m^2 SC day 1-5,8,10,12
	IL-2 9 MU/m^2/d by CIV x 4 days
	G-CSF 5 mcg/kg SC days 7-16

Fig. 2. Concurrent BCT vs CVD protocol: E3695. Cycle every 21 d; assess response on d 42; for a maximum of 4 cycles.

out relapse (10 for the IL-2 arm vs 2 for the non-IL-2) has been significant to date ($p = 0.028$). Further long-term follow-up and complete accrual will be necessary before any further conclusions can be drawn.

The M.D. Anderson Hospital group has recently reported their single institution randomized phase III trial involving 190 patients, which assesses the contribution of biotherapy to chemotherapy alone *(87)*. Patients were randomized to either CVD or to a biochemotherapy regimen consisting of CVD with IL-2 by CI combined with IFN administered sequentially before and after the chemotherapy regimen. The biochemotherapy arm was associated with a response rate of 48% compared to 25% for the CVD chemotherapy alone ($p = 0.001$). The time to treatment failure for biochemotherapy was 4.9 mo vs 2.4 mo for chemotherapy ($p = 0.007$), and the median survival was 11.9 mo for the biochemotherapy arm compared to 9.2 mo for chemotherapy ($p = 0.055$).

One additional large cooperative group randomized phase III trial is still accruing and should be additionally informative when it is completed. This trial, E-3695, is an intergroup trial performed by ECOG, SWOG, and the Cancer and Leukemia Group B (CALGB). This trial compares CVD chemotherapy with a concurrent biochemotherapy regimen, which has been modified to reduce its toxicity (Fig. 2). It is similar in design to the M.D. Anderson phase III trial reported above and attempts to identify whether biotherapy, when added to chemotherapy, is superior to chemotherapy alone. This trial has accrued 350 of the planned 485 patients. It should be completed in mid-2002 and reported within the next few years.

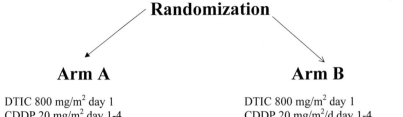

Few definitive conclusions can be drawn from this data to date. Several of these trials have demonstrated improvement for one or more important endpoint, suggesting a potential advantage for biochemotherapy as initial management, but others have not. Unfortunately, none of these trials compares biochemotherapy to DTIC alone. Additional time and the maturing results of trials presently underway, however, will hopefully improve our understanding of the role of biochemotherapy in the management of metastatic melanoma.

4.9. Biochemotherapy in the Adjuvant Setting

Patients with stage III melanoma have a high risk of metastasis and death within 5 yr of diagnosis. Estimates suggest that even in patients who have been treated with adjuvant high-dose IFN, the overall likelihood of further disease progression and death is 50% or more. In the last several intergroup trials, the median age of patients enrolled was 50 yr of age. This high-risk young group of patients makes melanoma one of the leading tumors in "years of life lost" when death occurs. Clearly, more effective therapies are needed for this group of patients. Data from existing experience suggests that biochemotherapy regimens could be more effective in this setting. Biochemotherapy has adequately demonstrated response rates of 40–60% in numerous phase II and phase III trials in stage IV disease. Durable complete responses have been identified in most if not all of these trials. Patients that have received IFN in the adjuvant setting and progressed to stage IV disease have been identified to benefit from these treatment regimens in several studies. A modification of the M.D. Anderson concurrent biochemotherapy regimen is being used in the present stage IV intergroup trial (E-3695) and has been identified to have an acceptable toxicity profile for use in the cooperative group setting. The M.D. Anderson group has treated patients with local regional metastases neoadjuvantly with biochemotherapy regimens and identified response rates of 51% *(88)*. Finally, the ability to receive a treatment that would be complete in 9 wk (three 3-wk cycles) may have considerable appeal to patients when compared with the present standard of treatment with IFN that requires a year of therapy.

Two trials have been initiated in the United States to look at this important question. The first is an M.D. Anderson randomized phase III trial that will enroll 200 or more patients with node-positive melanoma to a 1:1 randomization between IFN for 1 yr and 4 cycles of biochemotherapy. The group randomized to IFN will undergo further randomization between standard high-dose IFN and IFN given in maintenance doses for 1 yr. The second trial is an intergroup trial, S-0008. This trial will accrue 420 patients who will be randomized between standard high-dose IFN and 3 cycles of concurrent biochemotherapy, as administered in E-3695 trial (Fig. 2). Eligibility for this trial will include patients with nodal involvement that are at the highest risk, including those with 2 or more microscopic or 1 or more macroscopic node involved by tumor. It will include patients with in-transit and satellite presentation, those with extranodal extension, those with recurrence in a previously resected nodal basin, and patients with nodal involvement and an ulcerated primary lesion.

5. SUMMARY AND FUTURE DIRECTIONS

Aggregate results from multiple phase II trials indicate that biochemotherapy produces responses in approximate 50% of patients, and approximately 10% of patients achieve an unmaintained durable complete response. Studies of biochemotherapy suggest that both IL-2 and chemotherapy can be administered in combination schedules in approximately the same doses as when used alone. Chemotherapy does not appear to interfere with the immunomodulatory effects of IL-2, nor does IL-2 appear to interfere with the pharmacokinetics of chemotherapy in the few studies in which these issues have been evaluated. Toxicities have generally been nonoverlapping, but there has been an increased incidence of neutropenia and thrombocytopenia when the IL-2 is administered shortly after DTIC chemotherapy, and a possible increased risk of significant renal and gastrointestinal toxicity when cisplatin is administered shortly after IL-2. Responses have been seen in all tumor locations, but durable responses have been more frequent in patients with metastases limited to subcutaneous tissue, lymph nodes, or lung. The overall objective response rate and median survivals for many of the phase II trials appear clearly superior to prior trials of chemotherapy alone. Phase III trials to date have been small and have chosen inconsistent regimens and controls to be able to draw broad conclusions. Despite this, however, several of these trials have demonstrated some response rate advantage for those patients receiving biochemotherapy. The completion of the ongoing phase III trials, their results, and interpretation in the next few years will clearly set the tone for whether this type of therapy becomes more than investigational in nature.

The future directions for biochemotherapy will, of course, depend in part on the results of many of the ongoing phase III trials. Evaluation in well designed randomized trials in the adjuvant setting appears appropriate given the activity demonstrated to date in stage IV disease regardless of the outcome of the present stage IV randomized trials. Efforts to reduce the toxicity and to identify regimens, which can be used in an outpatient setting, would make biochemotherapy more practical and cost-effective for patients and physicians alike. Strategies to prolong the response durations for the many patients who experience partial but not complete responses would also be valuable. These could include additional immunomodulations or the use of antiangiogensis treatment strategies. As new active chemotherapy or immunotherapy agents are identified, their addition or substitution for existing agents in the present combinations provide important opportunities as well.

REFERENCES

1. Balch CM, Reintgen DS, Kirkwood JM, et al. *Cutaneous Melanoma in Cancer: Principles and Practice of Oncology—5th ed.* Devita VT, Hellman S, Rosenberg SA, eds. Lippincott, Philadelphia, 1997.

2. Greenlee RT, Murry T, Bolden S, et al. Cancer statistics 2000. *CA Cancer J Clin* 2000; 50: 7–33.
3. Ryan L, Kramar A, Borden E. Prognostic factors in metastatic melanoma. *Cancer* 1993; 71, 2995–3005.
4. Legha SS, Ring S, Papadopoulos N, et al. A prospective evaluation of a triple-drug regimen containing cisplatin, vinblastine, and dacarbazine (CVD) for metastatic melanoma. *Cancer* 1989; 64: 2024–2029.
5. McClay EF, Mastrangelo MJ, Bellet RE, et al. Combination chemotherapy and hormonal therapy in the treatment of malignant melanoma. *Cancer Treat Rep* 1987; 71: 465–469.
6. DelPrete SA, Maurer LH, O'Donnell J, et al. Combination chemotherapy with cisplatin, carmustine, dacarbazine, and tamoxifen in metastatic melanoma. *Cancer Treat Rep* 1984; 68: 1403–1405.
7. Murren JR, DeRosa W, Durivage HJ, et al. High-dose cisplatin plus dacarbazine in the treatment of metastatic melanoma. *Cancer* 1991; 67: 1514–1517.
8. Fletcher WS, Green S, Fletcher JR, et al. Evaluation of cis-platinum and DTIC combination chemotherapy in disseminated melanoma. A Southwest Oncology Group study. *Am J Clin Oncol* 1988; 11: 589–593.
9. Seigler HF, Lucas VS, Pickelt NJ, et al. DTIC, CCNU, bleomycin and vincristine (BOLD) in metastatic melanoma. *Cancer* 1980; 46: 2346–2348.
10. York RM, Foltz AT. Bleomycin, vincristine, lomustine, and DTIC chemotherapy for metastatic melanoma. *Cancer* 1988; 61: 2183–2186.
11. McClay EF, Mastrangelo MJ, Berd D, et al. Effective combination chemo/hormonal therapy for malignant melanoma: experience with three consecutive trials. *Int J Cancer* 1992; 50: 553–556.
12. Flaherty LE, Liu PY, Mitchell MS, et al. The addition of tamoxifen to dacarbazine and cisplatin in metastatic malignant melanoma. A phase II trial of the Southwest Oncology Group, (SWOG-8921). *Am J Clin Oncol* 1996; 19: 108–113.
13. Margolin KA, Liu PY, Flaherty LE, et al. Phase II study of carmustine, dacarbazine, cisplatin, and tamoxifen in advanced melanoma: a Southwest Oncology Group study. *J Clin Oncol* 1998; 16: 664–669.
14. Fletcher WS, Daniels DS, Sondak VK, et al. Evaluation of cisplatin and DTIC in inoperable stage III and IV melanoma. A Southwest Oncology Group study. *Am J Clin Oncol* 1993; 16: 359–362.
15. Luikart SD, Kennealey GT, Kirkwood JM. Randomized phase III trial of vinblastine, bleomycin, and cis-dichlorodiammine-platinum versus dacarbazine in malignant melanoma. *J Clin Oncol* 1984; 2: 164–168.
16. Buzaid AC, Legha S, Winn R, et al. Cisplatin, vinblastine, and dacarbazine versus dacarbazine alone in metastatic melanoma: preliminary results of a phase III Cancer Community Oncology Program trial. *Proc Am Soc Clin Oncol* 1993; 12: 389.
17. Chapman PB, Einhorn LH, Meyers ML, et al. Phase III multicenter randomized trial of the Dartmouth regimen versus dacarbazine in patients with metastatic melanoma. *J Clin Oncol* 1999; 17: 2745–2751.
18. Walker MJ, Beattie CW, Patel MK, et al. Estrogen receptor in malignant melanoma. *J Clin Oncol* 1987; 5: 1256–1261.
19. Fisher RI, Neifeld JP, Lippman ME. Oestrogen receptors in human malignant melanoma. *Lancet* 1976; 2: 337–339.
20. Rumke P, Kleeberg UR, MacKie RM, et al. Tamoxifen as a single agent for advanced melanoma in postmenopausal women. A phase II study of the EORTC malignant melanoma cooperative group. *Melanoma Res* 1992; 2: 153–155.
21. Meyskens FL Jr, Voakes JB. Tamoxifen in metastatic malignant melanoma. *Cancer Treat Rep* 1980; 64: 171–173.

22. Creagan ET, Ingle JN, Green SJ, et al. Phase II study of tamoxifen in patients with disseminated malignant melanoma. *Cancer Treat Rep* 1980; 64: 199–201.
23. Reimer RR, Costanzi J, Fabian C. Southwest Oncology Group experience with tamoxifen in metastatic melanoma. *Cancer Treat Rep* 1982; 66: 1680–1681.
24. Masiel A, Buttrick P, Bitran J. Tamoxifen in the treatment of malignant melanoma. *Cancer Treat Rep* 1981; 65: 531–532.
25. Cocconi G, Bella M, Calabresi F, et al. Treatment of metastatic malignant melanoma with dacarbazine plus tamoxifen. *N Engl J Med* 1992; 327: 516–523.
26. Rusthoven JJ, Quirt IC, Iscoe NA, et al. Randomized, double-blind, placebo-controlled trial comparing the response rates of carmustine, dacarbazine, and cisplatin with and without tamoxifen in patients with metastatic melanoma. *J Clin Oncol* 1996; 14: 2083–2090.
27. Falkson CI, Ibrahim J, Kirkwood JM, et al. Phase III trial of dacarbazine versus dacarbazine with interferon α-2b versus dacarbazine with tamoxifen versus dacarbazine with interferon α-2b and tamoxifen in patients with metastatic malignant melanoma: an Eastern Cooperative Oncology Group study. *J Clin Oncol* 1998; 16: 1743–1751.
28. Kirkwood JM, Ernstoff MS. *Cutaneous Melanoma in Biologic Therapy of Cancer*. DeVita VT, Helman S, Rosenberg SA, eds. J.B. Lippincott, Philadelphia, 1991.
29. Legha SS. The role of interferon alfa in the treatment of metastatic melanoma. *Semin Oncol* 1997; 24(Suppl 4): S4-24–S4-31.
30. Mastrangelo MJ, Bellet RE, Kane MJ, et al. *Chemotherapy of Melanoma in the Chemotherapy Source Book*. Perry MC, ed. Williams and Wilkins, Baltimore, 1992.
31. Bajetta E, Di Leo A, Zampino MG, et al. Multicenter randomized trial of decarbazine alone or in combination with two different doses and schedules of interferon alfa-2a in the treatment of advanced melanoma. *J Clin Oncol* 1994; 12: 806–811.
32. Thomson DB, Adena M, McLeod GR, et al. Interferon-alpha 2a does not improve response or survival when combined with dacarbazine in metastatic malignant melanoma: results of a multi-institutional Australian randomized trial. *Melanoma Res* 1993; 3; 133–138.
33. Kirkwood JM, Ernstoff MS, Giuliano A, et al. Interferon alpha-2a and decarbazine in melanoma. *J Natl Cancer Inst* 1990; 82: 1062–1063.
34. Falkson CI, Falkson G, Falkson HC. Improved results with the addition of interferon alfa-2b to dacarbazine in the treatment of patients with metastatic malignant melanoma. *J Clin Oncol* 1991; 9: 1403–1408.
35. Kirkwood JM, Strawderman MH, Ernstoff MS, et al. Interferon alfa-2b adjuvant therapy of high-risk resected cutaneous melanoma: the Eastern Cooperative Oncology Group trial EST 1684. *J Clin Oncol* 1996; 14: 7–17.
36. Margolin KA, Liu PY, Unger JM, et al. Phase II trial of biochemotherapy with interferon alfa, dacarbazine, cisplatin and tamoxifen in metastatic melanoma: a Southwest Oncology Group trial. *J Cancer Res Clin Oncol* 1999; 125: 292–296.
37. Atkins MB, Lotze MT, Dutcher JP, et al. High-dose recombinant interleukin 2 therapy for patients with metastatic melanoma: analysis of 270 patients treated between 1985 and 1993. *J Clin Oncol* 1999; 17: 2105–2116.
38. West WH, Taver KW, Yannelli JR, et al. Constant infusion recombinant interleukin-2 in adoptive immunotherapy of adoptive cancer. *N Engl J Med* 1987; 316: 898–905.
39. Ehrke MJ, Mihich E, Berd D, et al. Effects of anticancer drugs on the immune system in humans. *Semin Oncol* 1989; 16: 230–253.
40. Mitchell MS. Combining chemotherapy with biological response modifiers in treatment of cancer. *J Natl Cancer Inst* 1988; 8: 1445–1450.
41. Maguire HC Jr, Ettore VL. Enhancement of dinitrochlorobenzene (DNCB) contact sensitization by cyclophosphamide in the guinea pig. *J Invest Dermatol* 1967; 48: 39–43.
42. Berd D, Mastrangelo MJ, Engstrom PF, et al. Augmentation of the human immune response by cyclophosphamide. *Cancer Res* 1982; 42: 4862–4866.

43. Rosenberg B. Possible mechanisms for the antitumor activity of platinum coordination complexes. *Cancer Chemother Rep* 1975; 59: 589–598.
44. Watanabe M, Kawano Y, Kubota T, et al. Mechanism of synergistic antitumor effects of mitomycin-C, 5-fluorouracil and interleukin-2 against human colon cancer. *Proc Am Assoc Cancer Res* 1995; 36: 299.
45. Allavena P, Pirovano P, Bonazzi, et al. In vitro and in vivo effects of cisplatin on the generation of lymphokine-activated killer cells. *J Natl Cancer Inst* 1990; 82: 139.
46. Taylor CW, Gore BH. Effect of cytotoxic chemotherapy drugs on lymphokine activated killer (LAK) cell generation and activity. *Proc Am Assoc Cancer Res* 1990; 31: 268.
47. Sodhi A, Pai K, Singh RK, et al. Activation of human NK cells and monocytes with cisplatin in vitro. *Int J Immunopharmacol* 1990; 12: 893–898.
48. Lichtenstein AK, Pende D. Enhancement of natural killer cytotoxicity by cis-diamminedichloroplatinum (II) in vivo an d in vitro. *Cancer Res* 1986; 46: 639–644.
49. Tsuda H, Kitahashi S, Umesaki N, et al. Abrogation of suppressor cells activity by cis-diamminedichloroplatinum (CDDP) treatment using therapeutic doses in ovarian cancer patients. *Gynecol Oncol* 1994; 52: 218–221.
50. Kleinerman ES, Zwelling LA, Muchmore AV. Enhancement of naturally occurring human spontaneous monocyte-mediated cytotoxicity by cis-diamminedichloroplatinum (II). *Cancer Res* 1980; 40: 3099–3102.
51. Sodhi A, Geetha B. Effect of cisplatin, lipopolysaccharide, muramyl dipeptide, and recombinant interferon-gamma on murine macrophages in vitro. I. *Nat Immun Cell Growth Regul* 1989; 8: 108–116.
52. Kleinerman ES, Zwelling LA, Howser D, et al. Defective monocyte killing in patients with malignancies and restoration of function during chemotherapy. *Lancet* 1980; 2: 1102–1105.
53. Lower EE, Baughman RP. The effect of cancer and chemotherapy on monocyte function. *J Clin Lab Immunol* 1990; 31: 121–125.
54. Samlowski WE, Tom C, McGregor JR, et al. Natural killer and lymphokine activated killer cell sensitivity of multidrug resistant human tumor cell lines. Meeting abstract, sponsored by the National Cancer Institute. In: *Combining Biologic Response Modifiers with Cytotoxics in the Treatment of Cancer: Developing a Rational Approach to a New Therapy*. March 5–7, 1990, Baltimore, MD.
55. Passerini CG, Rivoltini L, Radrizzani M, et al. Susceptibility of human and murine drug-resistant tumor cells to the lytic activity of r-IL-2 activated lymphocytes (LAK). *Cancer Metastasis Rev* 1988; 7: 335–346.
56. Ohtsu A, Sasaki Y, Tamura T, et al. Inhibition of colony formation of drug-resistant human tumor cell lines by combinations of interleukin-2 activated killer cells and antitumor drugs. *Jpn J Cancer Res* 1989; 8: 265–270.
57. Braunschweiger P, Cameron D, Sharp L, et al. Cisplatin and nitric oxide have cynergistic cytotoxicity in cP resistant human melanoma cells. *Proc Annu Meet Am Assoc Cancer Res* 1996; 37: 404.
58. Thomsen LL, Baguley BC, Rustin GJ, et al. Flavone acetic acid (FAA) with recombinant interleukin-2 (IL-2) in advanced malignant melanoma. II. Induction of nitric oxide production. *Br J Cancer* 1992; 66: 723–727.
59. Rhinehart JJ, Triozzi PL, Lee MH, et al. The effect of intensive chemotherapy and recombinant human IL-2 (rhIL-2) in a murine tumor model. *Proc Am Assoc Cancer Res* 1990; 31: 277.
60. Papa MZ, Yang JC, Vetto JT. Combined effect of chemotherapy and interleukin-2 in the therapy of mice with advanced pulmonary tumors. *Cancer Res* 1988; 48: 122–129.
61. Gauny S, Zimmerman RJ, Winkelhake JL. Combination therapies using interleukin-2 and chemotherapeutics in murine tumors. *Proc Am Assoc Cancer Res* 1989; 30: 372.
62. Winkelhade JL, Gauny S, Zimmerman R. Strategies for combining drugs and BRM's using animal tumor models. Meeting abstract, sponsored by the National Cancer Institute. In: *Com-*

bining Biologic Response Modifiers with Cytotoxics in the Treatment of Cancer: Developing a Rational Approach to a New Therapy. March 5–7, 1990, Baltimore, MD.

63. Bernsen MR, Van Barlingen HJ, Van der Velden AW, et al. Dualistic effects of cisdiammine-dichloro-platinum on the anti-tumor efficacy of subsequently applied recombinant interleukin-2 therapy: a tumor-dependent phenomenon. *Int J Cancer* 1993; 54: 513–517.
64. Flaherty LE, Redmen BG, Chabot GG, et al. A phase I-II study of dacarbazine in combination with outpatient interleukin-2 in metastatic malignant melanoma. *Cancer* 1990; 65: 2471–2477.
65. Chabot GG, Flaherty LE, Valdiviesco M, et al. Alteration of dacarbazine (DTIC) pharmacokinetics after interleukin-2 (rIL-2) administration in melanoma patients. *Chemother Pharmacol* 1990; 27: 157–160.
66. Stoter G, Shiloni E, Gundersen S, et al. Alternating recombinant interleukin-2 and dacarbazine in advanced melanoma. A multicenter phase II study. *Cancer Treat Rev* 1989; 16(Suppl A): 59–63.
67. Dillman RO, Oladham RK, Barth NM, et al. Recombinant interleukin-2 and adoptive immunotherapy alternated with dacarbazine therapy in melanoma: a National Biotherapy Study Group trial. *J Natl Cancer Inst* 1990; 82: 1345–1349.
68. Papadopoulos NEJ, Howard JG, Murray JL, et al. Phase II DTIC and interleukin-2 (IL-2) trial for metastatic malignant melanoma. *Proc Am Soc Clin Oncol* 1990; 9: 277.
69. Demchak PA, Mier JW, Robert NJ, et al. A phase II pilot trial of interleukin-2 and high dose cisplatin in patients with metastatic melanoma. *J Clin Oncol* 1991; 9: 1821–1830.
70. Richards JM, Gilewski TA, Ramming K, et al. Effective chemotherapy for melanoma after treatment with interleukin-2. *Cancer* 1992; 69: 427–429.
71. Richards JM, Mehta N, Ramming K, et al. Sequential chemoimmunotherapy in the treatment of metastatic melanoma. *J Clin Oncol* 1992; 10: 1338–1343.
72. Antoine EC, Benhammouda A, Bernard A, et al. Salpetriere hospital experience with biochemotherapy in metastatic melanoma. *Cancer J Sci Am* 1997; 3: S16–S21.
73. Keilholz U, Scheibenbogen C, Tilgen W. Interferon-α and interleukin-2 in the treatment of metastatic melanoma. *Cancer* 1993; 72: 607–614.
74. Keilholz U, Goey SH, Punt CJ, et al. Interferon alfa-2a and interleukin-2 with or without cisplatin in metastatic melanoma: a randomized trial of the European Organization for Research and Treatment of Cancer Melanoma Cooperative Group. *J Clin Oncol* 1997; 15: 2579–2588.
75. O'Day SJ, Gammon G, Boasberg PD, et al. Advantages of concurrent biochemotherapy modified by decrescendo interleukin-2, granulocyte colony-stimulating factor, and tamoxifen for patients with metastatic melanoma. *J Clin Oncol* 1999; 17: 2752–2761.
76. Keilholz U, Conradt C, Legha S, et al. Results of interleukin-2 based treatment in advanced melanoma: a case record-based analysis in 631 patients. *J Clin Oncol* 1998; 16: 2921–2929.
77. Allen IE, Kupelnick B, Kumashiro M. Efficacy of interleukin-2 in the treatment of metastatic melanoma—systemic review and metastasis-analysis. *Cancer Therapeutics* 1998; 1: 168–173.
78. Legha SS, Ring S, Eton O, et al. Development and results of biochemotherapy in metastatic melanoma: the University of Texas M.D. Anderson Cancer Center Experience. *Cancer J Sci Am* 1997; 3: S9–S15.
79. Legha SS, Ring S, Eton O, et al. Development of a biochemotherapy regimen with concurrent administration of cisplatin, vinblastine, dacarbazine, interferon alfa, and interleukin-2 for patients with metastatic melanoma. *J Clin Oncol* 1998; 16: 1752–1759.
80. McDermott DF, Mier JW, Lawrence DP, et al. A phase II pilot trial of concurrent biochemotherapy with cisplatin, vinblastine, dacarbazine (CVD), interleukin-2 (RIL-2) and interferon alpha-2B (IFN) in patients with metastatic melanoma. *Proc Am Soc Clin Oncol* 1998; 17: 507a.

81. Flaherty LE, Robinson W, Redman BG, et al. A phase II study of dacarbazine and cisplatin in combination with outpatient administered interleukin-2 in metastatic malignant melanoma. *Cancer* 1993; 71: 3520–3525.
82. Redman BG, Flaherty L, Chou T, et al. Sequential dacarbazine/cisplatin and IL-2 in metastatic melanoma. *Immunother* 1991; 10: 147–151.
83. Thompson JA, Gold PJ, Markowitz DR, et al. Updated analysis of an outpatient chemo-immunotherapy regimen for treating metastatic melanoma. *Cancer J Sci Am* 1997; 3: S29–S34.
84. Flaherty LE, Atkins M, Sosman J, et al. Randomized phase II trial of chemotherapy and outpatient biotherapy with interleukin-2 (IL-2) and interferon alpha (IFN) in metastatic malignant melanoma (MMM). *Proc Am Soc Clin Oncol* 1999; 18: 536a.
85. Rosenberg SA, Yang JC, Schwartzentruber DJ, et al. Prospective randomized trial of the treatment of patients with metastatic melanoma using chemotherapy with cisplatin, dacarbazine, and tamoxifen alone or in combination with interleukin-2 and interferon alfa-2b. *J Clin Oncol* 1999; 17: 968–975.
86. Keilholz U, Cornelius JA, Punt CJA, et al. Dacarbazine, cisplatin and interferon alpha with or without interleukin-2 in advanced melanoma: interim analysis of EORTC trial 18951. *Proc Am Soc Clin Oncol* 1999; 18: 530a.
87. Eton O, Legha S, Bedikian A, et al. Phase III randomized trial of cisplatin, vinblastine and dacarbazine (CDV) plus interleukin-2 (IL2) and interferon-alpha-2b (INF) versus CVD in patients (Pts) with metastatic melanoma. *Proc Am Soc Clin Oncol* 2000; 19: 552a.
88. Buzaid AC, Bedikian A, Eton O, et al. Importance of major histologic response in melanoma patients (pts) with local regional metastases (LRM) receiving neoadjuvant biochemotherapy. *Proc Am Soc Clin Oncol* 1997; 16: 503a.
89. Atzpodien J, Lopez Hanninen E, Kirchner H, et al. Chemoimmunotherapy of advanced malignant melanoma: sequential administration of subcutaneous interleukin-2 and interferon-alpha after intravenous dacarbazine and carboplatin or intravenous dacarbazine, cisplatin, carmustine and tamoxifen. *Eur J Cancer* 1995; 31A: 876–881.
90. Bernengo MG, Doveil GC, Bertero M, et al. Low-dose integrated chemoimmuno-hormono-therapy with cisplatin, subcutaneous interleukin-2, alpha-interferon and tamoxifen for advanced metastatic melanoma—a pilot study. *Melanoma Res* 1996; 6: 257–265.
91. Guida M, Latorre A, Mastria A, et al. Subcutaneous recombinant interleukin-2 plus chemotherapy with cisplatin and dacarbazine in metastatic melanoma. *Eur J Cancer* 1996; 32A: 730–733.
92. Kamanabrou, P, Straub C, Heinsch M, et al. Sequential Biochemotherapy of INF-a/IL-2, cisplatin (CDDP), dacarbazine (DTIC) and carmustine (BCNU), results of a monocenter phase II study in 109 patients with advanced metastatic malignant melanoma (MMM). *Proc Am Soc Clin Oncol* 1999; 18: 530a.
93. Dillman R, Soori G, Schulof R, et al. Cancer Biotherapy research Group (CBRG) trial 94-11: outpatient subcutaneous interleukin-2 (proleukin) and interferon α 2b (intron A) with combination chemotherapy plus tamoxifen in the treatment of metastatic melanoma. *Proc Am Soc Clin Oncol* 1999; 18: 530a.

11 Signal Transduction Abnormalities as Therapeutic Targets

Ruth Halaban, PhD
and
Maria C. von Willebrand, MD, PhD

Contents

1. INTRODUCTION

The transformation of normal melanocytes to melanoma cells is associated with accumulation of genetic alterations that impact directly and/or indirectly on cell cycle regulators. As a result, melanoma cells acquire the ability to proliferate and resist apoptosis regardless of environmental cues that control normal melanocytes. Although the full scope of the mutations acquired by melanocytes in their malignant progression has not yet been elucidated, the few that have been identified are in regulatory proteins that control cell cycle progression. The transition to self-sufficiency is a step-wise process, initiated as melanocytic lesions advance from benign to dysplastic nevi, to primary superficial spreading melanomas, and further on to invasive, nodular and metastatic lesions *(1,2)*. This aberrant self-proliferating loop is likely to play a role in fixation and propagation of oncogenic mutations *(3)*. Any mechanism-based approach for melanoma therapy requires the detailed knowledge of the critical players in maintaining autonomous cell proliferation. For example, up-regulated activity of receptor kinases has been implicated in the progression of numerous tumors *(4)*. Prominent

From: *Current Clinical Oncology, Melanoma: Biologically Targeted Therapeutics*
Edited by: E. C. Borden

in this category are receptors from the epidermal growth factor receptor (EGFR) family, such as Erb-2 (also called HER or Neu), a tyrosine kinase receptor, which is overexpressed in 20 to 30% of human breast and ovarian tumors *(5–7)*. Erb-2 is the target for current and future therapeutic strategies *(8)*, such as the use of neutralizing antibodies or specific kinase inhibitors *(4,9,10)*. Another example is *bcr-abl* fusion gene, a hallmark of chronic myelogenous leukemia (CML), which encodes the constitutively active abl-kinase fused to Bcr. A competitive inhibitor of the Bcr-Abl kinase, STI571 (CGP57148), is currently one of the most promising treatments of CML *(11–15)*. The discovery of the kinase inhibitor CGP57148, as an effective tumor suppressor specifically for CML, serves as an example for a successful logical mechanistic approach and provides the impetus for searching specific signal transduction targets in other cancers, including melanomas. In fact, as will be described here, investigators and pharmaceutical companies have already developed several inhibitors that target various intermediates in growth factor-mediated signaling, and some of these compounds are already in clinical trials *(4,16,17)*.

To identify candidate signal transduction molecules as targets for intervention in melanomas, the underlying mechanism, which converts growth factor-dependent melanocytes to the self propagating melanoma cells, has to be elucidated, and the relative importance of receptor–ligand systems in this process has to be assessed. Cell proliferation can be restrained at multiple steps; the aim is to find the one that is unique to melanomas that spares the host tissues. Here, we will describe the growth factor–receptor systems critical for normal melanocyte proliferation, the function of signal transduction intermediates, the molecular basis for melanoma cell autonomy, and the various approaches that have been used to validate molecular targets for tumor intervention.

2. CELL CYCLE CONTROLS IN NORMAL MELANOCYTES

The general scheme of stimulation by external factors of normal cells is shared by most cell types (Figs. 1–3). Growth factors activate cell surface receptors, which then trigger intracellular cascades, that impact on nuclear transcription factors and the expression of genes whose protein products promote cell proliferation. The specificity in response is driven by the nature of the receptors expressed at the cell surface and the abundance of the cognate ligands in the environment. Each growth factor–receptor system activate common intermediates, but may retain specificity through interaction with unique set of signal transducers. In general, the immediate biochemical modification stimulated by growth factors involves activation of the receptor intracellular domain, which serves to recruit a complex of proteins near the cell surface (Figs. 1 and 2). This leads to triggering the activation of the Ras-Raf-MAPK intracellular cascade, mediating the extracellular message to the nucleus, and eliciting a biological response.

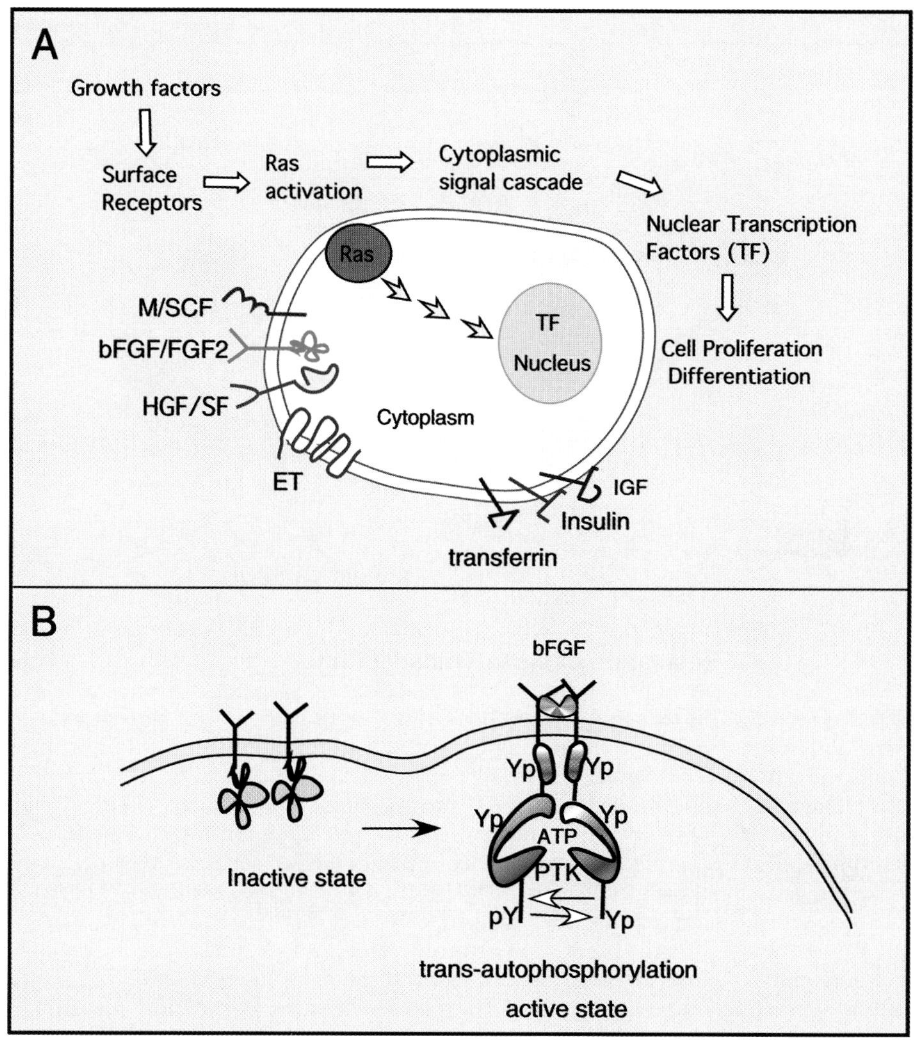

Fig. 1. Schematic representation of normal state of proliferation–differentiation limited by the availability of growth factors in the external domain **(A)** and initial ligand-mediated receptor dimerization and activation **(B)**. **(A)** Normal melanocytes express the "housekeeping" receptors to insulin, insulin-like growth factor, and transferrin, and the receptors to the specific growth factors, bFGF/FGF2, HGF/SF, ET, and Kit. The ligand-binding extracellular portion of each receptor confers specificity to growth factors. The catalytic–regulatory domain in the intracellular portion transmits signals via intracellular intermediates, such as Ras, to the nucleus. **(B)** Binding of growth factors to their receptors causes receptor dimerization, induces conformational changes in their intracellular domain with concomitant activation of the tyrosine kinase domain (ATP) and transphosphorylation of receptor critical tyrosine residues (Yp).

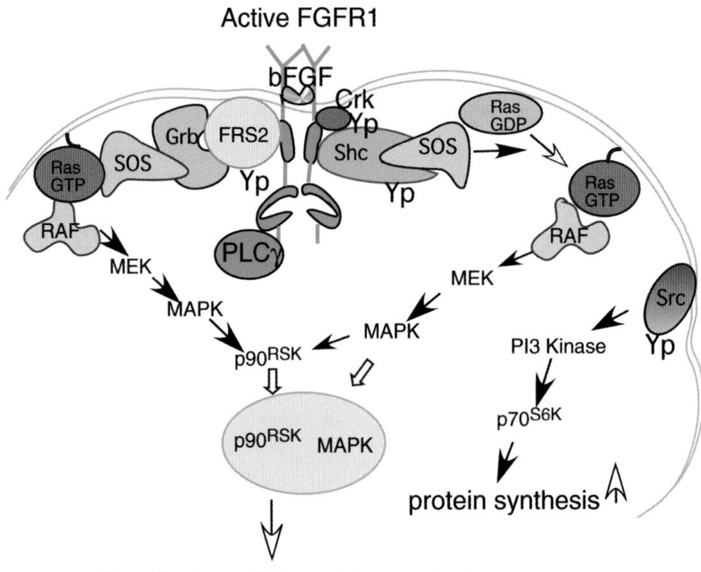

Fig. 2. The critical intermediates in FGFR1 signal transduction. The phosphorylated tyrosine residues on the activated receptor create docking sites to several preformed complexes of proteins (Shc and SOS, or FRS2, Grb, and SOS). SOS activates Ras, by exchanging guanine diphosphate (GDP) with guanine triphosphate (GTP). Ras, in turn, activates a series of tyrosine and serine–threonine kinases known as the MAPK and the PI3K cascades. The message emanating from the cell surface is then delivered to the transcriptional machinery in the nucleus by the translocation of phosphorylated forms of several intermediates, including MAPK and $p90^{RSK}$ to the nucleus. Consequently, growth regulatory, as well as differentiation factors, are induced. Constitutive activation of some members in this pathway, such as the production of growth factors that constantly activate their receptor, overexpression and/or mutational activation of a receptor, activation of Ras (by mutations or by receptor activation) can lead to perpetual mode of proliferation and cellular transformation.

2.1. Melanocyte Growth Factors–Receptors

The proliferation of normal human melanocytes in culture is stringently dependent not only on the presence of serum factors (such as insulin and transferrin, termed “housekeeping”, required by most mammalian cells), but also on synergistically acting ligands, termed “specific” factors, which include fibroblast growth factors (FGFs), mast/stem cell growth factor (M/SCF) (also known as KIT ligand or Steel factor), hepatocyte growth factor/scatter factor (HGF/SF), endothelins (such as ET-1, ET-2, ET-3) and, to some extent, melanotropin (melanocyte stimulating hormone; MSH), see review *(18)* and references within. In chemically-defined medium, in the presence of housekeeping factors, each one of the specific factors by itself is insufficient to elicit proliferation, and individually, only ET maintains viability over several days *(19)*.

The specific growth factors are most likely the natural melanocyte mitogens in vivo. They are produced in the skin by keratinocytes and/or fibroblasts, and their levels are further increased by ultraviolet B (UVB) irradiation, with consequent increase in melanocyte numbers *(20–27)*. These factors can also increase pigmentation of adult skin when injected subcutaneously, as shown for mast/stem cell factor (M/SCF) *(28,29)*, or when taken orally, as shown for MSH *(30–32)*.

The factors listed play a role also in melanocytic stem cells or melanoblast proliferation. Studies with murine and avian neural crest-derived cells demonstrated that bFGF, M/SCF, ET-3 and HGF/SF have profound effect on melanoblast viability, proliferation, and further differentiation into melanocytes *(33–40)*. In the absence of these factors, the melanocyte progenitors undergo apoptosis, as demonstrated by blocking the Kit receptor kinase activity through elimination of M/SCF, or the addition of ACK2, an interfering monoclonal anti-c-Kit antibody *(40)*.

Genetic disorders that disable a specific ligand or receptor activity, further identified critical melanocyte growth factors–receptors during development. The most well known example is piebaldism, a condition characterized by white patches devoid of melanocytes due to inactivation mutation in the KIT receptor *(41–43)*. Likewise, inactivating mutations in the endothelin-B receptor (EDNRB), ET-3, or RET, a receptor tyrosine kinase for glial-cell-line-derived neurotrophic factor, have been identified in patients with Hirschsprung disease (HSCR) and Waardenburg syndrome (WS), which are disorders affecting neural crest-derived cells associated with hypopigmentation *(44–50)*. Inactivation mutations affecting melanocyte viability, division, and possibly migration during embryogenesis, of receptors or ligands such as KIT and MGF/SCF *(41,43)*, as well as the endothelin B receptor or ET-3 *(51,52)* have been also identified, or experimentally induced in the mouse, lending further support to the importance of specific growth factors during development.

2.2. Intracellular Signal Transduction

The melanocyte cell surface receptors listed above belong to the families of transmembrane receptor tyrosine kinases (RTK) and G protein-coupled receptors (GPCRs) containing seven putative transmembrane domains (also referred to as serpentine receptors) (Figs. 1 and 2). The RTKs includes FGFR1, the bFGF/FGF2 receptor, KIT, the M/SCF receptor, and Met, the HGF/SF receptor, whereas the serpentine-type receptors include the ET receptors EDNRA and EDNRB, and the MSH receptor melanocortin. Receptor activation and mitogenic signaling has been elucidated in various cell types *(53–56)*, and full description is beyond the scope of this chapter. Several key aspects will be highlighted here, with bFGF/FGFR1 as the paradigm, because unregulated expression of bFGF/FGF2 and chronic stimulation of this receptor kinase are common features to most melanoma cells *(57–60)*.

Basic FGF/FGF2 mediates cellular functions by binding to specific sites in the extracellular domain of FGFR1, a process requiring heparan sulfate glycosaminoglycans *(61)*. Heparin-derived oligosaccharides induce the dimerization of bFGF/FGF2, augmenting affinity to the receptor *(62,63)*. Initial events following ligand binding include receptor dimerization, a change in intracellular receptor conformation, induction of receptor kinase autocatalytic activity, with concomitant receptor autophosphorylation, and phosphorylation of specific tyrosine residues within the intracellular (domain reviewed in refs. *54,55,64,65*), and schematically presented in Fig. 1B and Fig. 2.

Subsequently, within seconds, the activated intracellular domains serve as docking sites for accessory proteins *(66,67)*. The assembled complex, which includes the adaptor proteins FRS2 or Shc, recruits the guanine nucleotide exchange factor SOS via the associated protein Grb2. SOS activates Ras by exchanging GDP with GTP *(65,68–71)*. GTP-bound Ras is a central player in activating multiple effector pathways *(72)*. Ras activates the mitogen-activated protein kinase (MAPK) cascade via binding to Raf, affecting cell cycle progression as well as apoptosis. The components of the MAPK cascade include several intracellular protein kinases, which transmit signaling by phosphorylation of tyrosine and/or serine–threonine residues. Alternatively, Ras activates the phosphatidylinositol (PI) 3-kinase (PI3K) cascade, up-regulating protein synthesis, and the Mekk cascade, affecting transcription factors of the *c*-Jun *N*-terminal kinase (JNK) family. Other intermediates alter the cytoskeleton, cell–cell junctions and Golgi trafficking *(72–74)*.

In melanocytes, each of the growth factors described above can activate to various degrees the MAPK and PI3K pathways *(19,75,76)*. However, to elicit proliferation, the "cascades" must be sustained at high levels and prolonged duration, an effect accomplished only by the presence of multiple synergistic growth factors in the extracellular milieu *(19)*. Interestingly, as melanocytes become senescent and stop proliferating, they also lose their ability to activate the MAPK cascade *(76)*, in agreement with the pivotal role of this pathway in cell division.

The phosphorylation of some of the intermediates, such as MAPK and $p90^{RSK}$, serves to transport them to the nucleus, where they phosphorylate nuclear factors and change their transcriptional activity via the recruitment of critical elements such as cyclic AMP responsive element binding protein (CREB), CREB binding protein (CBP) *(77–80)*. In normal melanocytes, the phosphorylation state and presumably activity of two transcription factors, microphthalmia transcription factor (MITF) *(81–84)*, and CREB *(19)*, are altered in response to growth factors. MITF is an important regulator of melanocyte-specific gene expression *(84)*.

2.3. Inactivation of pRb Family of Tumor Suppressor Proteins (Pocket Proteins)

The growth factor activated MAPK pathway mediates transit of quiescent cells into DNA synthesis (G_1 to S phase of the cell cycle), in large part, by activating a group of cyclin-dependent kinases (CDKs) responsible for phosphorylating the pRb family of tumor suppressor proteins (pRb, p107, and p130), termed pocket proteins (Fig. 3) *(85–88)*, a process demonstrated also in human melanocytes *(89,90)*. Under normal conditions, pocket proteins undergo cell cycle-dependent phosphorylation and dephosphorylation, which serve to inactivate and activate, respectively, their function as inhibitors of cell cycle progression *(91–94)*. The activity of CDKs, namely CDK4, CDK6, and CDK2 is coordinated by association with the positive partners cyclins, and the negative regulators CDK inhibitors (CKI), as well as by site-specific phosphorylation or dephosphorylation carried out by the cyclin activating kinase (CAK) and Cdc25 phosphatase, respectively *(95,96)*. The pocket proteins are regarded as master regulators of the cell cycle governing the restriction (R) point, i.e., the point of commitment from quiescence (G_0/G_1) to DNA synthesis (S) *(97–100)*. Pocket proteins repress gene transcription by recruiting Rb binding protein (RBP) to pRb, p107, and p130. RBP, in turn, serves as a bridging molecule to recruit histone deacetylase (HDAC) *(101–103)*, and, in addition, provides a second HDAC-independent repression function *(101)*. HDAC in turn, down-regulates gene expression by changing histone conformation through deacetylation *(104)*.

Hyperphosphorylation of pocket proteins releases their suppressive-association with transcription factors from the E2F family (E2F1–E2F5), leading to the accumulation of E2F transcriptional activity and activation of genes responsible for cell cycle progression (cyclin A, cyclin D1, cyclin E, cdc2, p107, and $p21^{CIP}$), DNA synthesis (dihydrofolate reductase and DNA polymerase), and transcription factors c-MYC, c-MYB, B-MYB, as well as E2F1 and E2F2, that participate in induction of early and late response genes *(100,105–109)*. The most abundant transcriptionally active E2F family members in mitogen-stimulated normal melanocytes are E2F2 and E2F4, which accumulate as unbound "free" species; in contrast, in mitogen-deprived normal melanocytes, free E2Fs are present at extremely low levels, below the threshold needed to stimulate cell cycle progression, and complexes containing E2F4, in association with p130 accumulate, possibly serving as transcriptional suppressors, exerting cell cycle arrest *(90)*.

3. MELANOMAS: *ACQUIRED AUTONOMOUS CELL PROLIFERATION*

In vivo malignant progression is expressed in vitro as release from the stringent dependency on exogenously added growth factors, which is char-

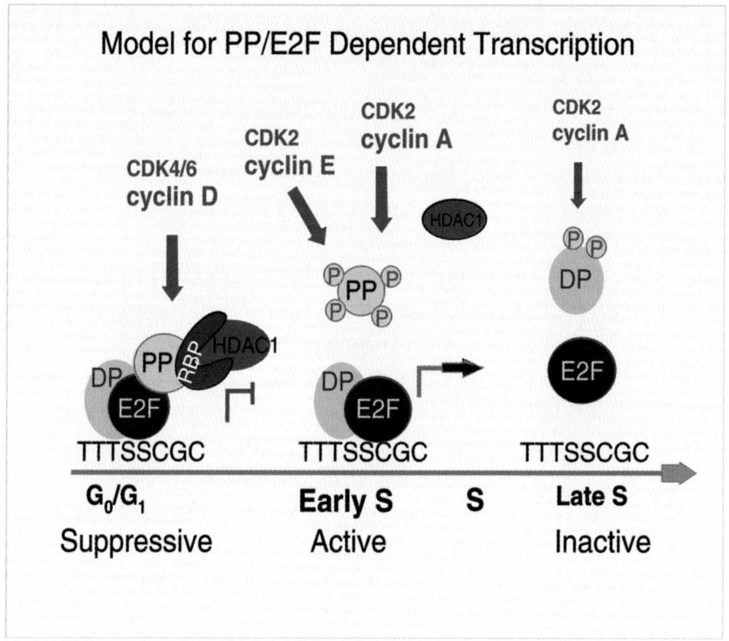

Fig. 3. Control of cell cycle progression by pocket proteins (PP)-regulated E2F transcription factors. The model depicts the accepted notion by which PP from the retinoblastoma tumor suppressor family (pRb, p107, and p130) regulate the transition of cells from quiescence (G_0/G_1 phase) to DNA synthesis (S phase). In their un- or hypophosphorylated forms, PP suppress the expression of genes required for cell cycle progression by tethering to E2F promoter sites through binding to E2F transcription factors. Transcriptional suppression is mediated, at least in part, by recruitment of HDAC1 through association of p130 and pRb with RBP (pocket-binding protein), which in turn induces transcriptionally-unfavorable chromosomal conformation *(101,291)*. It should be noted that HDAC-dependent and -independent repression activities are associated with the RB "pocket". Sequential phosphorylation of pocket proteins by CDK4, CDK6, and CDK2, releases their repressive association with E2F and HDAC1, and allows transcription of gene products required for cell cycle progression. DP is E2F dimerization partner that facilitates E2F/DNA binding. CDK2/cyclin A also phosphorylates DP during the S phase, inducing its dissociation from E2F, detachment from promoter sites and termination of E2F-dependent transcriptional activation. P denotes phosphorylated sites. Not shown are the negative regulators of CDK from the INK and KIP/CIP family discussed in the text.

acteristic of normal human melanocytes (*see* Fig. 1). The transition from growth factor dependency to growth factor self-sufficiency is accomplished in at least three steps:

1. Melanocytes from early primary thin melanomas (up to Breslow depth approx 1 mm) are similar to normal melanocytes in that they require the presence of the full spectrum of specific growth factors, i.e., HGF/SF, bFGF/FGF2,

and ETs, as well as the housekeeping factors, such as insulin and transferrin, in the medium to grow in vitro.

2. Melanocytes from slightly more advanced primaries (Breslow depth approx 2 mm) still require housekeeping, as well as at least one specific growth factor to the external medium, such as ET1, to proliferate in vitro.
3. Only melanocytes from invasive primaries (nodular melanomas) or metastases do not require the addition of specific external growth factors to proliferate well in vitro. Furthermore, some even display independence of, or increased responsiveness to insulin or insulin-like growth factor I (IGF-I) and transferrin *(110,111)*.

The molecular alterations that drive the malignant progression of normal melanocytes are only beginning to be sorted out. Like other tumors, malignant transformation is associated with the acquisition of new functions, which confer growth advantage, and the loss of restraining functions, which exert cell arrest and apoptosis. As discussed below, treatments can be developed to suppress the gain of function capabilities or up-regulate the cell cycle suppressors. In addition, therapy can capitalize on the "abundance" or overactive molecules in cancer cells to deliver or express drugs specifically in the tumor, sparing the normal host tissues. However, as indicated before and demonstrated in other cancers, the mechanism-based drug therapy requires a clear knowledge of the major molecular players in the pathophysiology of melanomas *(4,17)*.

3.1. Autocrine Loops in Melanomas: Growth Factors–Receptors

To this day, constitutive activation of a receptor tyrosine kinase due to activating mutations has not yet been identified in melanomas. Instead, one of the hallmarks of melanomas is ectopic expression of growth factors and/or receptors that are not produced by normal human melanocytes *(112–121)* or up-regulation of a receptor kinase, such as the IGF-1 receptor (IGF-1R) *(122)*. This abnormal expression probably contributes not only to autonomous growth, but also to changes in expression of melanocytic functions *(123,124)*. Some of these growth factors, such as FGF2/bFGF and melanoma growth stimulating activity (MGSA), generate an autocrine loop because ligand and cognate receptor are expressed *(125–128)*, while others act in a paracrine fashion due to melanoma cell increased responsiveness to the ligand in the environment, such as IGF-1 or transferrin *(110)*. In addition, the aberrant production of growth factors such as platelet derived growth factor (PDGF), epidermal growth factor (EGF), or vascular endothelial cell growth factor (VEGF) and bFGF/FGF2 promote melanoma tumor growth by stimulating stroma cells and vascular endothelial cells, up-regulating angiogenesis, and creating a compatible microenvironment *(129–137)*. This concerted activity is likely to contribute to melanoma cell autonomy and unchecked proliferation. It should be noted that other potent receptor kinases, known to induce melanoma when ectopically expressed in their activated form in mouse melanocytes, such as RET *(138–140)* or MET (the HGF/SF receptor) *(141,142)*, are not constitutively active in human melanomas *(143–145)*. The proto-oncogene Kit, on the other hand, can be regarded as an "anti-oncogene," since it is commonly down-regulated in melanomas *(146–148)*, and M/SCF inhibits the growth of Kit-expressing melanoma cells in culture *(147)* and suppressed melanoma tumor growth in vivo *(149)*.

The multiple growth factors abnormalities sustained by melanoma cells may, at first glance, suggest that interference with one pathway is unlikely to be effective in growth suppression due to redundancy in function. However, results from several studies have shown that melanoma cell growth in vitro and in vivo can be impeded by blocking FGF2/FGFR1 or IGF/IGFR activity. It is thus possible that each receptor–kinase is operative to different degrees in different melanomas or that the concerted activity of several systems is required for optimal proliferation, as shown for normal human melanocytes. Since suppression of a single pathway can retard, but does not completely arrest tumor growth, it is possible that targeting more then one receptor–kinase system can produce a synergistic growth arrest.

3.2. Targeting Extracellular Receptor Kinases

3.2.1. Disruption in bFGF/FGFR1 Signal Transduction

The common expression of bFGF in melanoma cells and the persistent presence of its cognate receptor, FGFR1, attracted several investigators to design methods that interrupt ligand–receptor function as a mean for intervention in tumor growth. Furthermore, bFGF plays a role in angiogenesis, and thus, its suppression provides the additional benefit of reduced angiogenesis and blood supply to the tumor. Disruption of FGFR activity in adults may not cause great damage to host tissues because FGF and FGFR are important during development and regenerative events, but are down-regulated in normal adult tissues *(150–152)*.

The first report demonstrating abnormal expression of bFGF in melanoma cells also showed that bFGF antagonistic peptides or intracellular administration of bFGF neutralizing antibodies (but not extracellular) suppressed melanoma cell growth in vitro *(57)*. These results provided the first "proof of principle" regarding FGFR/bFGF role in melanomas, which was subsequently followed by other approaches.

The FGFR has been used to suppress melanoma cell growth in experimental systems as a target for inhibition, or as a vector for drug delivery to receptor-positive malignant cells. FGFR1 activity has been successfully suppressed by intervening with ligand binding, receptor or ligand expression, or tyrosine kinase activity.

3.2.1.1. Interfering with Heparan Sulfate Proteoglycans-Mediated Ligand–Receptor Interaction. As mentioned before, binding of FGFs to the high-affinity FGFR is mediated by complex formation with heparan sulfate proteoglycans (HSPG) *(153)*. FGF failed to bind and activate FGF receptors in Chinese hamster ovary (CHO) mutant cells deficient in endogenous heparan sulfate *(154–156)*. The diminished bFGF receptor binding due to reduced heparin sulfate in mutant cells was associated with reduced mitogenesis, plasminogen activator induction, and in vitro angiogenesis, and was corrected by addition of exogenous heparin *(61,157)*. HSPG mediate FGF sequestration, stabilization, and high-affinity receptor binding and signaling by interacting with the FGFR as well as with FGF *(153,156)*.

These observations motivated targeting HSPG as the mean for inhibiting growth in tumor cells in general and in melanoma cells in particular. Yayon and his collaborators validated the concept by demonstrating that down-regulation of perlecan, a secreted HSPG abundant in proliferating cells, by ectopic expression of antisense cDNA reduced melanoma cell responsiveness to bFGF in vitro *(158)*. Drugs that mimic heparin-like cellular binding sites might be a more effective way of interfering with HSPG-mediated growth factor–receptor recognition in tumor cells in vivo. Examples are RG-13577, a nonsulfated polyanionic aromatic compound *(153,159)*, and synthetic sulfonic acid polymers *(160)* used to suppress endothelial cells. However, these compounds effectiveness in arresting melanoma cells has not been tested, and their toxic side effects in animal models is not known.

3.2.1.2. Dominant Interfering FGFR. A molecular approach for impeding the autocrine loop created by endogenous FGFs is ectopic expression of mutant FGFR that form inactive heterodimers with endogenous FGFRs and prevent receptor autophosphorylation (Fig. 1B). The two main versions are constructs that express a truncated form of FGFR, which lacks most of the intracellular tyrosine kinase, but retains the transmembrane (Tm) anchoring domain, known as dominant-negative FGFR (dnFGFR-Tm) *(161,162)*, or constructs that lack the kinase and transmembrane domain and thus are secreted out of the cell (secreted soluble Dominant-Negative Receptor or sol-DNR) *(163)*. Ectopic expression of mouse dnFGFR-Tm in human metastatic melanoma cells dramatically reduced the basal as well as bFGF-induced growth of these cells in vitro and suppressed their tumorigenic potential in nude mice *(164)*. The mechanism by which interfering with the FGFR1 activity in melanoma cells inhibited growth is not clear, but is likely due to a block in membrane signaling to a critical downstream intermediate. One such intermediate was shown to be a Src-like kinase *(164)*.

However, growth inhibition by dnFGFR-Tm required effective competition for ligand binding with native receptors at the cell surface, attained only by high levels expression of transgene in selected clones *(164)*. A more effective dominant-interfering molecule is the sol-DNR constructed by Merlino and his collaborators, termed dnFGFR-HFc *(163)*. dnFGFR-HFc is a chimeric protein comprising the extracellular ligand-binding domain of the mouse FGFR2b cDNA (that can bind to aFGF, FGF3, FGF7, and FGF10, but not bFGF/FGF2) and the transmembrane domain of mouse Ig heavy chain hinge and Fc domains. The protein was secreted as a disulfide-linked dimer, and its expression in transgenic mice caused severe abnormalities in several organs and limbs *(163)*. A similar construct comprising of FGFR1 capable of binding bFGF might be more effective then dnFGFR1 in suppressing bFGF-dependent melanoma cell growth and tumorigenesis.

3.2.1.3. FGFR1/bFGF Expression and Intracellular Activity. Antisense technology directed against bFGF or FGFR1 provided further support to the notion that this autocrine loop is required for melanoma cell proliferation. Antisense oligonucleotides targeting FGF2 or FGFR1 in human melanomas blocked melanoma cell growth in vitro *(165–167)*. More recently, Becker and Wang have shown that injection of episomal vectors containing antisense-oriented bFGF or FGFR-1 cDNAs into human melanomas grown as subcutaneous tumors in nude mice arrested tumor growth. Some tumors regressed as a result of blocked intratumoral angiogenesis and subsequent necrosis *(168)*.

3.2.1.4. Specific Receptor Protein Kinase Inhibitors. The driving force in receptor-mediated signal transduction is the protein tyrosine kinase activity of the intracellular domain (Figs. 1B and 2). The protein tyrosine kinase catalyzes the transfer of phosphate of adenosine triphosphate (ATP) to tyrosine residues on adjacent receptor dimer and other protein substrates, leading to activation of the signal transduction cascade. The central role of phosphorylation events in cell proliferation and cancer biology inspired a new approach to cancer chemotherapy, i.e., the development of drugs that specifically inhibit kinase activity of cell surface receptors as well as intracellular kinases *(169–171)*. For example, specific, irreversible inhibitors of the ATP-binding cleft of the EGFR have been synthesized that are exceptionally efficient at inhibiting the EGF family of receptors at low concentrations. These inhibitors are already in clinical trials for the treatment of epithelial cancers, such as breast cancer *(8,169,171–173)*.

Likewise, two new families of synthetic compounds capable of inhibiting the FGFR have been developed. One, designated PD 173074, belongs to the pyrido[2,3-d]pyrimidine class and the other, designated SU5402, is of the oxindole type (indolinones). Both are ATP competitive tyrosine kinase inhibitors. PD 173074 selectively inhibits the tyrosine kinase activities of the FGF and VEGF receptors at low concentrations *(174,175)*. The selectivity to the FGFR is due to specific binding to the ATP domain, inducing a conformational change in the nucleotide-binding loop, as determined by crystal structures of the tyrosine kinase domain of FGFR1 in complex with each of the two compounds *(176,177)*. Systemic administration of PD 173074 in mice effectively blocked angiogenesis induced by either FGF or VEGF with no apparent toxicity *(177)*. PD 173074, in combination with photodynamic therapy, displayed potent anti-angiogenic and antimurine mammary tumor activity in vivo *(178)*. The cytotoxicity of these compounds are currently evaluated in phase I trials. So far there are no reports on the effect of these compounds on melanoma cell growth in vivo or in vitro.

3.2.1.5. FGFR as a Vehicle for Drug Delivery. Baird and collaborators were the first to attempt specific bFGF-based delivery of cytotoxic compounds to FGFR expressing tumor cells. The full-length sequence of FGF2 conjugated to saporin, the ribosome-inactivating protein, inhibited human and mouse B16 melanoma cell proliferation in vitro, and B16 melanoma tumor growth in vivo *(179–182)*. However, the usefulness of these compounds against human melanomas in vitro is in question, since no reports have been published over the past 5 yr.

Targeted gene transfer via the FGFR is also an emerging field. Several groups have attempted to modify adenovirus-based gene therapy by targeting specific cell surface receptors including heparan-containing cellular receptors *(183–185)*.

3.2.2. Disruption of IGF-R/IGF-I

Basic FGF-induced autocrine growth in melanoma cells is likely to be complemented by the increased responsiveness to, and/or production of, other growth factors. Herlyn and collaborators have shown a dramatic increase in responsiveness to insulin, IGF-I, and transferrin as melanoma cells advance from primary to metastatic lesions *(110,186)*. The IGF-IR plays a critical role in normal and abnormal growth and is particularly important in anchorage-independent proliferation *(187)*, a characteristic of metastatic melanoma cells *(110,188)*. Increased responsiveness to IGF-I might be a consequence of increased expression of IGF-IR protein as cells progress from benign nevi to metastatic melanoma *(122)*.

Functional IGF-IR is required for cell cycle progression and malignant transformation, since cells lacking this receptor cannot be transformed by a number of oncogenes, including simian virus 40 (SV40) large T antigen and Ras *(189)*. Thus, inhibition of IGF-IR signaling has been assessed as a potential target for anticancer drug development by three different approaches: (*i*) the use of IGF-IR specific antibody (IR-3); (*ii*) ectopic expression of antisense RNA directed to the IGF-IR; and (*iii*) inhibition of the IGF-IR tyrosine kinase with pharmacological inhibitors (tyrphostins AG1024 or AG1034).

3.2.2.1. IGF-IR Specific Antibody. The antibody IR-3 blocks the binding of IGF-I to IGF-IR thus interfering with receptor activation by paracrine loops. The antibody inhibited the in vitro IGF-I- and insulin-mediated growth stimulation of a metastatic melanoma cell line *(110)*, but was not effective toward other cell lines that did not respond to IGF-I stimulation *(111)*. Furthermore, the same pattern of response to the antibody was observed in melanoma xenotransplants into nude mice; i.e., IR-3 inhibited tumor growth of IGF-I responsive melanoma cells, but was not effective toward the other lines. These results demonstrated that IGF-I can be targeted in vivo only in IGF-dependent melanoma cells.

3.2.2.2. Antisense IGF-R RNA. Results of experiments with antisense RNA also validate the usefulness of targeting the IGF-IR. Ectopic expression of IGF-IR antisense oligonucleotides reduced the number of IGF-IR at the cell surface and inhibited the growth of human melanoma cells in vivo *(190)*. The development of tumors in some mice after a long delay was associated with the loss antisense expression and reappearance of normal levels of IGF-IR. Consistent with IGF-I activity, in vitro the antisense RNA did not affect monolayers growth, but reduced the efficiency of colony formation in soft agar.

3.2.2.3. Tyrphostins. The IGF-IR is also inhibited by tyrphostins (AG1024 and AG1034), which act by inhibiting receptor kinase activity *(191)*. Although these compounds effectively inhibited IGF-stimulated NIH-3T3 cell proliferation *(191)*, they have not yet been tested on melanoma cells, and their effectiveness and cytotoxicity in vivo have not been reported. These tyrphostins are promising agents which have to be further evaluated, since they may have undesired effects on other kinases with deleterious effects on normal host tissues.

3.3. Targeting Intracellular Signal Transduction Pathways

3.3.1. Inactivation of Ras Family of Proteins

3.3.1.1. The Role of Activated Ras in Melanomas. Ras proteins are critical regulators of multiple signaling pathways controlling cell growth, differentiation, and apoptosis *(72,192)*, as schematically presented in Figs. 1 and 2. The *ras* gene was one of the first oncogenes to be discovered, and mutations in *ras* are found in a multitude of human cancers. The original reports downplayed the role of activating *ras* mutations in melanoma genesis *(193–195)*. However, more recent results indicate that of the three *ras* genes, H-ras, K-ras, and N-ras, N-ras is mostly involved in melanomas. Although activating mutation in codon 61 of *N-ras* was detected in only approximately 7–15% of human melanomas in general, they are present at higher levels, such as approximately 30%, in sun-exposed head and neck melanomas and nodular melanomas *(196–198)*. The increase in N-ras protein levels as lesions progress from benign, to dysplastic, to metastatic stages may also be an indication for increased Ras participation in tumor growth *(199)*. Aberrant Ras activity may be even more prevalent than that reflected by activating mutations, because ectopic expression of growth factors with the consequent receptor activation, can lead to persistent Ras activity.

Results from experimental mouse models confirmed the high potency of mutant Ras in inducing melanomas. Forced expression of activated mutant Ha-Ras transformed immortalized mouse melanocytes in the absence of any additional oncogenes *(123)*, and melanocytes of transgenic mice expressing Ha-RasV12G developed melanocytic hyperplasia *(200)*, which progressed into melanomas when treated with the carcinogen 7,12-dimethylbenz(a)anthracene (DMBA) *(201)*. Furthermore, in hybrid progeny produced by crossing

Ha-RasV12G transgenic with p16^{INK4A} knock-out mice, the melanocytic hyperplasia advanced to melanomas in a Ras-dependent manner *(202–204)*.

3.3.1.2. Ribozyme-Mediated Ras Inactivation. The few reports on Ras inactivation in melanomas validate Ras as a potential target for tumor suppression. In one set of experiments, H-ras ribozyme designed to cleave activated H-ras RNA, suppressed H-ras expression, melanoma cell proliferation, and the efficiency to form colonies in soft agar *(205,206)*. Furthermore, H-ras ribozyme expression specifically in melanoma cells via the tyrosinase promoter produced similar inhibition, suggesting a way to prevent general Ras inactivation in normal tissues *(207)*. However, the utility of this construct against melanoma cell lines that possess N-ras, but not H- or K-ras mutation, was not tested. Furthermore, the efficiency of this gene-expression approach has not yet been reported to yield results in vivo.

3.3.1.3. Synthetic Antagonists. The universal role of activated *ras* mutations in human tumors inspired efforts to design synthetic Ras antagonists as potential anticancer drugs *(4,17,208)*. Ras activity is dependent on its membrane localization, which is, in turn, mediated by a farnesyl group at the C terminus of the protein. The synthetic antagonists dislodge Ras from its membrane anchor or inhibit the process of farnesylation, preventing its attachment; in both cases, Ras degradation is also accelerated decreasing its expression, and blocking the propagation of Ras signaling to downstream effectors. Jansen and collaborators showed that the disrupting antagonist S-trans-trans-farnesylthiosalicylic acid (FTS) inhibited the growth of two human melanoma cell lines expressing wild-type or activated N-ras in vitro and in vivo in severe combined immunodeficiency (SCID) mice *(209)*.

The farnesyl-protein transferase inhibitors (FTIs) and the geranylgeranyltransferases peptidomimetic inhibitors (GGTIs) *(210,211)* inhibit farnesylation and/or geranylgeranylation of multiple G-proteins, which include Ras, Rho, and Rac, prevent their membrane attachment and cause cell cycle arrest of various cell types *(212–216)*. In vivo studies with human glioma cells demonstrated that farnesyltransferase inhibition was more effective in diminishing growth compared with geranylgeranyltransferases inhibition *(217)*. However, FTIs were apparently disappointing as effective therapy in phase I trials and are currently undergoing clinical evaluation in combination with other therapy *(17)*.

In our experiments, the farnesyltransferase inhibitor FTI 277 and the geranylgeranyltransferase inhibitor GGTI 298 inhibited DNA synthesis of two melanoma cell lines in micromolar amounts (Fig. 4), supporting the notion that inactivation of Ras and/or other small G-proteins could be effective targets in attempts to inhibit melanoma growth.

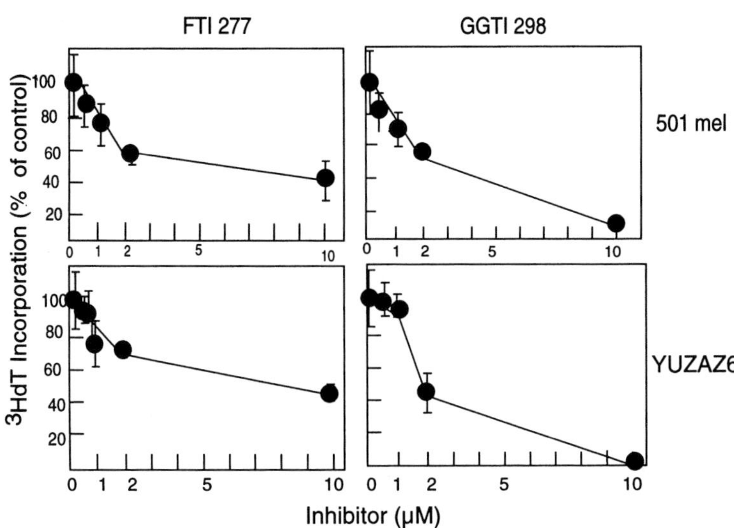

Fig. 4. In vitro growth inhibition of metastatic melanomas 501 mel and YUZAZ6 by the farnesylprotein transferase inhibitor (FTI 277), and the geranylgeranyltransferases inhibitors (GGTI 298). Melanoma cells were seeded in 24-well plates at subconfluent density in serum supplemented Ham's F10 medium. FTI 277 and GGTI 298 were added the following day at the indicated concentrations, and the rate of DNA synthesis was measured at the end of a 24-h incubation with the ^{3}H-thymidine incorporation assay. Each data value is an average of triplicate wells, and express ^{3}H-thymidine incorporation given as percent of control, nontreated cells, ± standard deviation. The FTase-specific peptidomimetic FTI-277 and the GGTase-I-specific GGTI-298 were a gift from Dr. Sebti, S. M. H. Lee Moffitt Cancer Center and Research Institute, Department of Biochemistry and Molecular Biology at the University of South Florida, Tampa, Florida.

3.3.2. Inhibiting Src Family Kinases

Like Ras, the Src family of kinases are signal transducers of several growth factor receptors, e.g. PDGF-R, colony-stimulating factor (CSF)-1 receptor and EGFR *(53,218–222)*. Src itself can phosphorylate unique tyrosine residues on growth factor receptors creating docking sites for downstream signal transducers. Studies with dnFGFR1 indicated that a Src-like kinase is a downstream mediator of the FGFR signal transduction pathway in melanoma cells *(164)*. The importance of Src-signaling in tumorigenesis rendered them an attractive target for the design of potent and selective inhibitors *(223)*. Some of the analogues of the ATP competitive pyrido[2,3-d]pyrimidine tyrosine kinase inhibitors, described in Subheading 3.2.1.4. *(173,177)*, are selective Src kinase inhibitors. They display antiproliferative and antimitotic effect on several tumor cell lines *(174,224,225)*, and are currently being used in advanced clinical trials for the treatment of breast and brain cancers *(173)*. As indicated above, the CML experience with the specific Abl-kinase inhibitor is very promising *(11,12)*, with an important caveat to keep in mind; drug resistance can develop from the selection of clones with *BCL* amplification *(226)* or *BCR/ABL*-negative progenitors *(227)*. Nevertheless, it is very likely that melanoma patients can also benefit from this type of approach.

3.3.3. The MAP Kinase and PI3 Kinase Cascades

Activated Ras binds to the serine–threonine kinase Raf. This results in translocation of Raf to the membrane where it is activated. Raf phosphorylates the dual specificity kinase Mek, which in turn phosphorylates and activates the MAP kinase. Inhibiting any of these protein kinases suppresses growth, since this pathway mediates activation of genes required for cell proliferation. For this reason, several pharmaceutical companies devised compounds that target Raf or the downstream kinases for cancer chemotherapy, and some of these agents are already in phase I trials *(4,17,228)*. For example, phosphorothioate antisense oligonucleotide directed to the 3' untranslated region of the c-Raf-1 mRNA, depletes c-Raf and inhibits the growth of human tumor cell lines in vitro and in vivo in *(228)*. In a phase I trial, intravenous (i.v.) infusion of the antisense oligonucleotide decreased Raf mRNA levels in 4 patients with ovarian, renal, pancreatic, and colon cancer, who remained disease-stable for up to 10 mo *(4,17,229)*. Two pharmacological agents, named PD-98059 and PD-184352, inhibit the protein kinase Mek and the growth of several human tumor cell lines *(230)*.

Another Ras downstream effector is the lipid kinase phosphatidylinositol 3-kinase (PI3 kinase). PI3 kinase is involved in multiple cellular functions, including cell proliferation and transformation, and inhibition of apoptosis. PI3 kinase mediates its anti-apoptotic effect by activating the protein kinase Akt, which is a suppressor of apoptosis. Akt is likely to be activated in melanomas that suffer from mutation in PTEN, the phosphatase that down-regulates Akt activity *(231–233)*. A potent pharmacological inhibitor of PI3 kinase, LY294002, induced apoptosis in Ras-transformed cells when administered in combination with an FTI *(234)*. These cells did not respond to FTI treatment alone, indicating that activation of PI3 kinase and Akt interfered with the pro-apoptotic effect of the FTI. These findings suggest that a PI3 kinase inhibitor and an FTI could be used as combination therapy for the best anticancer effect.

Melanoma cell proliferation was also inhibited in vitro by the PI3-kinase and Mek inhibitors (LY294002 and PD-98059 receptively) (Fig. 5). Our results show that the two suppressed the activated states of intracellular signal intermediates impinging on the expression of cyclins and the pRb family of tumor suppressors (*see* Subheading 3.4.1.). Our results suggesting that inhibition of either pathway might have an effect on melanoma growth and encourage further attempts to use

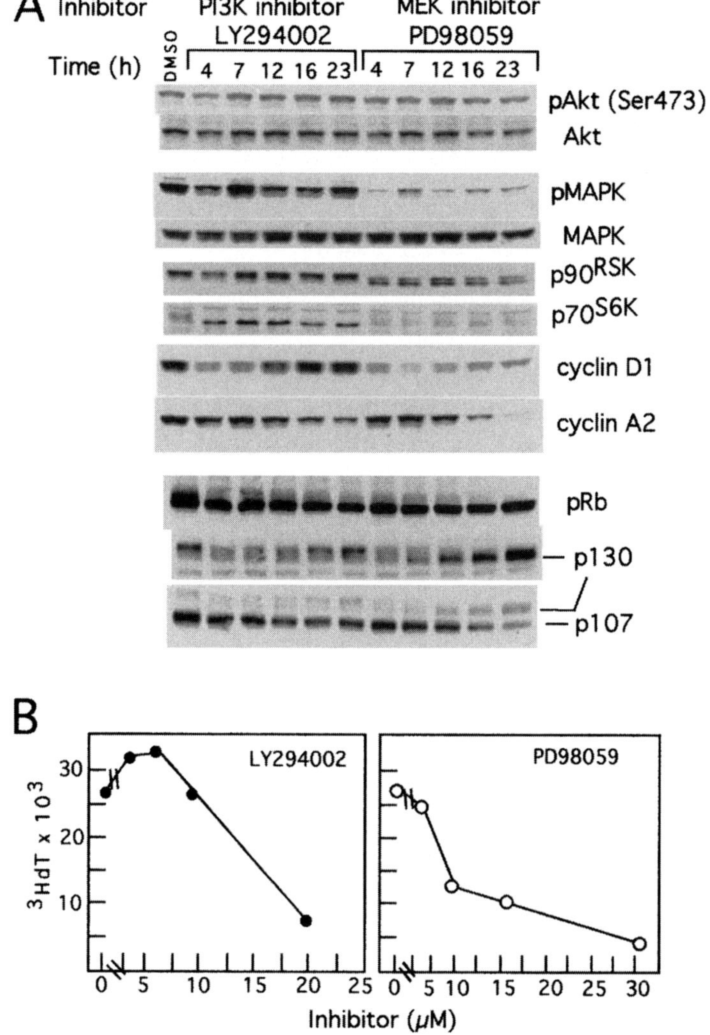

Fig. 5. Inhibition of PI3 kinase or Mek pathways inhibit metastatic melanoma cell proliferation. The PI3K inhibitor LY294002 and MEK inhibitor PD98059 induced changes in cell cycle intermediates **(A),** and arrest metastatic melanoma cell growth in vitro **(B)**. Metastatic melanoma cells 501 mel were incubated with 20 μ*M* LY294002 or 30 μ*M* of PD98059 and harvested at different intervals thereafter as indicated **(A)**. Cell extracts were subjected to Western blotting with antibodies that recognize activated and phosphorylated Akt (pAkt) or the Akt protein (Akt), activates MAPK (pMAPK) or MAPK (MAPK), the $p90^{RSK}$, $p70^{S6K}$, cyclin D1, cyclin A2, and the 3 PPs pRb, p130, and p107. Equal loading was verified by blotting with actin (data not shown). The results show that inhibition of PI3K or MAPK pathways in these cells did not affect the phosphorylation level of Akt, suggesting that Akt is controlled by a an upstream signal. On the other hand, inhibition of PI3 kinase, as expected, reduced the phosphorylation levels of the downstream target $p70^{S6K}$ as observed by the downward mobility shift of the protein (compare lane marked with dimethyl sulfoxide [DMSO] to the 4-h time point with

such inhibitors in combination with another drug that inhibits a different step of the signaling pathway.

3.4. Targeting the Rb/E2F Pathway

3.4.1. pRb/E2F Activity in Melanomas

Sustained inactivation of pocket proteins and elevated free E2F transcriptional activity in melanomas is one of the underlying mechanism for autonomous growth.

Mutations in the pRb "pocket" region (that block binding to E2F) are rare in melanoma tumors *(235,236)*, although retinoblastoma patients and their relatives display an increased risk to develop melanomas, as well as other tumors *(237,238)*. However, the tumor suppression function of pRb and other family members, p107 and p130 in human melanoma tumors and cell lines is commonly inactivated by hyperphosphorylation *(89,90,236)*. Reduced suppressor activity of pocket proteins might be further compounded by diminished expression of an RBBP2 homologue *(239)*, together ensuring that the HDAC-dependent and independent mode of gene suppression are eliminated. Pocket protein inactivation is associated with 5- to 10-fold higher levels of growth promoting free E2F activity in melanoma cells and tumors compared to proliferating melanocytes. The E2F-DNA binding activity contained E2F1, E2F2, E2F3, E2F4, and occasionally E2F5, while the growth suppressive complexes E2F4/p130 seen in deprived normal melanocytes were absent. Western blot analyses showed that the increase in transcriptionally active E2F in melanoma cells compared to normal melanocytes could be accounted for, in large part, by an increase in the protein levels of the dimerization partner DP1 (absolutely required for DNA binding activity) and E2F1 *(90)*. Up-regulated E2F transcriptional activity and elimination of E2F4/p130 transcriptional repression are likely to facilitate the self-sustaining mode of growth of melanoma cells by inducing the expression of specific genes required for cell proliferation.

(figure caption continued from previous page) LY294002 of p70^{S6K} blot). LY294002 had only a temporal effect on cyclin D1 expression, but reduced cyclin A2 levels. On the other hand, inhibiting the MEK caused a marked reduction in the phosphorylation and, thus, the activation state of MAPK (see blot marked pMAPK) and p90^{RSK}. (The latter is shown by downward mobility shift of the protein compared to control DMSO, as well as down-regulation of the two cyclins (D1 and A2). The impact on PPs is more pronounced with PD98059, compared to LY294002, but in both cases, there is reduction in the hyperphosphorylated species (as indicated by the differences in the migration pattern) and reduction in the levels of p107. **(B)** Growth arrest in response to increasing concentration of PI3K and MEK inhibitors LY294002 and PD98059, respectively. The metastatic melanoma cells (501 mel) were exposed to different concentrations of the inhibitors for 24 h, and DNA synthesis was measured by the ^{3}H-thymidine assay as described in the legend to Fig. 4. Data are averages of triplicate wells expressed as total counts per minute (CPM)/well/h.

Constitutively active CDKs, mainly CDK2 and CDK4, are responsible for persistent pocket protein phosphorylation in melanomas *(90)*. The cause for constitutively active CDK is in large part due to persistent high levels of the positive subunits cyclins (Cyclin A, D, and E). CDK activity is strictly dependent upon the presence of these positive regulators, whose expression is normally stringently controlled by extracellular mitogenic stimuli *(93,95,240)*. Sustained expression of cyclins is likely due to aberrant production of autocrine-acting growth factors and the activation of their cognate receptors (*see* Fig. 5). Gene amplification was demonstrated only in the case of cyclin D1 (previously known as PRAD1/BCL1) and also only in one out of 10 melanoma cell lines *(241,242)*.

To some degree, elimination of the negative regulators $p16^{INK4A}$ and $p27^{KIP}$ is also associated with the melanoma phenotype *(89,90,236,243)*. Decreased $p16^{INK4A}$ activity results from gene deletion, transcriptional inactivation, or mutation *(236,244–246)*. In addition, functional ablation of $p16^{INK4A}$ in 2 out of 23 melanoma cell lines and in two independent melanoma-prone pedigrees is mediated indirectly by a single amino acid substitution in CDK4 (arginine 24 to cysteine), which disrupts binding to and, thus, inhibition by $p16^{INK4A}$ *(236,247)*.

3.4.2. Targeting the pRb/E2F Pathway

Two main approaches can be applied to impact the pRb/E2F pathway as a mean for tumor suppression: (*i*) suppression of excess E2F activity; and (*ii*) harnessing the robust tumor cell E2F transcriptional activity for delivery of toxic molecules.

3.4.2.1. Suppression of Excess E2F Activity. CDK activity directly impacts pocket protein activation–inactivation status that control E2F activity. Therefore, various methods are being developed that target this group of enzymes, and some of the CDK inhibitors are already in clinical development *(248)*. A series of potent CDK inhibitors, which act by competing with ATP for binding at the catalytic site, have been recently identified *(249,250)*. Among this group is flavopiridol, an inhibitor of CDK 1, 2, 4, and 7, which blocks cell cycle progression and induces apoptosis in several cancer cell types *(251–256)*. Likewise, in vitro exposure of several melanoma cell strains to 200 n*M* flavopiridol-induced growth arrest, progressive loss of phosphorylated forms of all three pocket proteins, pRb, p107, and p130, as well as reduction in pRb and p107 protein levels, and a sharp decrease in free E2F binding activity, reminiscent of growth factor-deprived normal melanocytes *(90)*. These results suggest that melanoma patients can benefit from flavopiridol therapy, which is undergoing phase I clinical trials *(248,254)*.

The persistently "free" E2F can be directly targeted with novel therapeutic approaches involving application of DNA technology. Double-stranded DNA with high affinity for E2F can serve as a decoy to bind endogenous E2F, sequester it from host promoter sites, and block the activation of genes mediating cell cycle progression *(257)*. Such a decoy inhibited human mesangial cell proliferation *(258)*, and this approach is currently being tested against intimal hyperplasia after vascular injury in human bypass vein grafts with encouraging results *(259)*.

3.4.2.2. E2F Transcriptional Activity for Gene Therapy. The abundant E2F can be exploited to express cytotoxic molecules at high levels, specifically in tumor cells using the gene under the E2F responsive promoter. For example, the high E2F promoter activity in C6 glioma cells was used to express the herpes thymidine kinase (TK) gene at extremely high levels specifically in the cancer cells. Under in vitro conditions, the adenovirus-infected TK gene under the E2F promoter (Ad.E2F1-tk) was expressed at higher levels and was more cytotoxic compared with adenovirus-infected TK gene under the cytomegalovirus (CMV) promoter (Ad.CMV-tk) *(260)*. Furthermore, rats with 6-d-old intracerebral tumors survived longer when treated by stereotactic injections of Ad.E2F1-tk as compared to control galactosidase-expressing vector, in combination with systemic ganciclovir administration *(260)*. Although the Ad.E2F1-tk and Ad.CMV-tk had comparable effect on suppressing tumor growth, the Ad.E2F1-tk expression eradicated established gliomas with significantly less toxicity to normal tissue compared to the Ad.CMV-tk vector *(260)*. We expect the E2F promoter-dependent gene therapy to be more efficient in expressing cytotoxic molecules in melanomas than the tyrosinase-promoter *(261,262)*. The main reason is that all melanomas (cell lines and freshly dissected tumors) so far tested express extremely high levels of free E2F/DNA binding activity, which drive their autonomous growth. On the other hand, some melanomas, especially of the undifferentiated (and most aggressive) kind, lose the capacity to direct expression of genes under the tyrosinase promoter *(263)*. Gene delivery based on the tyrosinase promoter is likely to mediate expression in melanocytic cells, but would eventually select for aggressive cells that no longer express melanocyte-specific genes. The E2F promoter-dependent expression of cytotoxic molecules *(260)* should not be confused with E2F1-mediated growth arrest in human melanomas *(264)*, as overexpression of E2F1 by itself can cause growth arrest and apoptosis in a variety of cell types *(265–272)*, including normal cells, and does not carry the specificity to spare normal adjacent tissues.

3.5. Induction of Apoptosis and Cell Arrest

3.5.1. Inhibition of Anti-Apoptotic Molecules

Melanoma cells overexpress several molecules that confer growth advantage by suppressing apoptosis, such as Bcl-2 *(273–276)* and survivin *(277)*, and attempts are in progress to interfere with the expression or function of these molecules as a possible modality for melanoma therapy. For example, antisense Bcl-2 therapy of melanoma patients is currently under phase I trials. Likewise, interfering with survivin may have a therapeutic effect as expression of the surviving dominant negative mutant (Cys85Ala) triggered apoptosis in a melanoma cell line in the absence of other genotoxic stimuli *(277)*.

3.5.2. Activation of Growth Arrest Genes

As mentioned before, part of the malignant phenotype is the down-regulation of molecules that suppress cell growth, such as inhibitors of CDK activity ($p16^{INK4a}$ and p27) or proteins that can induce differentiation and growth arrest, such as mda-7 *(278)* or AP-2 *(279,280)*. In some cases, down-regulation of growth arrest genes is due to methylation by cytosine DNA methyltransferase (MeTase), which is an enzyme that is hyperactive in cancer cells. Inhibition of DNA MeTase by antagonist or antisense oligonucleotides induced the cell cycle suppressors $p16^{INK4a}$, $p27^{KIP}$, and $p21^{WAF/CIP1}$ and caused growth arrest *(281–284)*. The mechanism of gene reactivation, however, was not always through demethylation, as rapid increase in $p21^{WAF/CIP1}$ protein was not associated with promoter demethylation *(282)*.

3.5.3. Activation of Cell Surface-Mediated Growth Arrest and Apoptosis

It has been known for quite a while that, in some cases, ligands that promote the proliferation of normal melanocytes can arrest the proliferation of melanoma cells. Some examples are the phorbol ester TPA, which is known to stimulate protein kinase C*(285)*, and the Kit-dependent growth arrest by S/MGF, which was discussed previously *(149)*. The molecular basis for this dual effect has not yet been elucidated. A fascinating possibility is differential activation of an inducible switch that modulates proliferative signals. It is possible that stimulation of an already activated cell lead to super-activation of E2F1, which in turn, cause growth arrest via activation of apoptotic signals, such as p53. On the other hand, other molecules might be involved, such as the suppressor of cytokine signaling (SOCS) family of proteins. Socs1 is a downstream component of the Kit receptor signaling pathway in bone marrow-derived mast cells, and overexpression of Socs1 suppressed the mitogenic potential of Kit while maintaining S/MGF-dependent cell survival signals *(286)*. Elucidating the mechanism of differential growth response in normal versus malignant melanocytes might illuminate new ways to keep in check malignant cell proliferation.

3.6. Combined Patient-Tailored Therapy

Melanomas are known to acquire drug resistance, and current therapies utilize, in most cases, a combination of several drugs and/or biological modifiers (such as IL-2 and interferon). Likewise, successful mechanism-based therapies are likely to rely on drugs and/or treatments that intervene at multiple sites of the proliferative pathways to produce a synergistic suppressive effect. For example, the in vitro antiproliferative effect of the tyrosine kinase inhibitor AG957 on CML progenitors was dramatically increased when given in combination with anti-Fas receptor antibody *(227)*. Optimal treatments should exploit the sensitivity of melanomas to a kinase inhibitor, such as flavopiridol, in combination with pro-apoptotic agents, such MeTase antisense oligonucleotides, or a gene transfer vector expressing tumor suppressor protein. Several classes of tyrosine kinase inhibitors are under design by several investigators and pharmaceutical companies (such as Parke Davis and SUGEN). Screening for effectiveness against melanomas is likely to unravel a specific inhibitor that target the "Achilles heel", i.e., the key tyrosine kinase(s) that drives the proliferative machinery of this tumor.

Melanoma is a clinically heterogeneous disease displaying a variety of phenotypes with different capacities to spread to distant sites on the skin, adjacent lymph nodes, visceral organs, to induce host angiogenic response, and to resist specific drugs and/or immunemodulators. This clinical heterogeneity is likely to reflect molecular heterogeneity, which determines patients' response to current therapy and survival. Thus, the common molecular markers shared by melanomas subtypes can be used to predict the course of the disease and help design individual therapeutic modalities. Large-scale gene expression profiles of cell populations can be accomplished with the help of emerging new technologies, such as serial analysis of gene expression (SAGE), DNA microarrays, and proteomics. The gene expression approach has already been applied to breast cancer *(287–289)* and B cell lymphoma *(290)*. In breast cancer, unique pattern of expression of clusters of genes was associated with estrogen receptor status, with clinical tumor stage, or with tumor size *(288)*. Likewise, classification of melanomas on the basis of gene expression accompanied with the profile of protein modification that predicts their activity is likely to contribute toward our understanding the various phenotypes of melanoma tumors and to custom-design treatment to melanoma patients.

ACKNOWLEDGMENTS

This work was supported by a National Institutes of Health (NIH) grant no. 2R01-CA44542 to R.H. and the Finnish Medical Society, for the post-doctoral research award to M.vW. for studies abroad. We thank Dr. Sebti, S.M.H. Lee Moffitt Cancer Center and Research Institute, Department of Biochemistry and Molecular Biology at the University of South Florida, Tampa, FL for the gift of FTI 277 and GGTI 298.

REFERENCES

1. Elder DE, Jucovy PM, Tuthill RJ, Clark WH Jr. The classification of malignant melanoma. *Am J Dermatopathol* 1980; 2: 315–320.
2. Clark WH Jr, Elder DE, Guerry D, Epstein MN, Greene MH, Van Horn M. A study of tumor progression: the precursor lesions of superficial spreading and nodular melanoma. *Hum Pathol* 1984; 15: 1147–1165.

3. Eccles SA, Modjtahedi H, Box G, Court W, Sandle J, Dean CJ. Significance of the c-erbB family of receptor tyrosine kinases in metastatic cancer and their potential as targets for immunotherapy. *Invasion Metastasis* 1994; 14: 337–348.
4. Gibbs JB. Anticancer drug targets: growth factors and growth factor signaling. *J Clin Invest* 2000; 105: 9–13.
5. Slamon DJ, Godolphin W, Jones LA, et al. Studies of the HER-2/*neu* proto-oncogene in human breast and ovarian cancer. *Science* 1989; 244: 707–712.
6. Hynes NE, Stern DF. The biology of erbB-2/neu/HER-2 and its role in cancer. *Biochim Biophys Acta* 1994; 1198: 165–184.
7. Fan QB, Bian ML, Huang SZ, et al. Amplification of the C-erbB-2(HER-2/neu) proto-oncogene in ovarian carcinomas. *Chin Med J (Engl)* 1994; 107: 589–593.
8. Kirschbaum MH, Yarden Y. The ErbB/HER family of receptor tyrosine kinases: a potential target for chemoprevention of epithelial neoplasms. *J Cell Biochem* 2000; 77: 52–60.
9. Dougall WC, Greene MI. Biological studies and potential therapeutic applications of monoclonal antibodies and small molecules reactive with the neu/c-erbB-2 protein. *Cell Biophys* 1994; 25: 209–218.
10. Hurwitz E, Stancovski I, Sela M, Yarden Y. Suppression and promotion of tumor growth by monoclonal antibodies to ErbB-2 differentially correlate with cellular uptake. *Proc Natl Acad Sci USA* 1995; 92: 3353–3357.
11. Sawyers CL, Druker B. Tyrosine kinase inhibitors in chronic myeloid leukemia. *Cancer J Sci Am* 1999; 5: 63–69.
12. Druker BJ, Lydon NB. Lessons learned from the development of an abl tyrosine kinase inhibitor for chronic myelogenous leukemia. *J Clin Invest* 2000; 105: 3–7.
13. Stephenson J. Researchers buoyed by promise of targeted leukemia therapy. *JAMA* 2000; 283: 317, 21.
14. Sausville EA. A Bcr/Abl kinase antagonist for chronic myelogenous leukemia: a promising path for progress emerges. *J Natl Cancer Inst* 1999; 91: 102–103.
15. le Coutre P, Mologni L, Cleris L, et al. In vivo eradication of human BCR/ABL-positive leukemia cells with an ABL kinase inhibitor. *J Natl Cancer Inst* 1999; 91: 163–168.
16. Courtneidge SA, Plowman GD. The discovery and validation of new drug targets in cancer. *Curr Opin Biotechnol* 1998; 9: 632–636.
17. Gibbs JB. Mechanism-based target identification and drug discovery in cancer research. *Science* 2000; 287: 1969–1973.
18. Halaban R. The regulation of normal melanocyte proliferation. *Pigment Cell Res* 2000; 13: 4–14.
19. Böhm M, Moellmann G, Cheng E, et al. Identification of $p90^{RSK}$ as the probable CREB-Ser^{133} kinase in human melanocytes. *Cell Growth Differ* 1995; 6: 291–302.
20. Bull HA, Bunker CB, Terenghi G, et al. Endothelin-1 in human skin: immunolocalization, receptor binding, mRNA expression, and effects on cutaneous microvascular endothelial cells. *J Invest Dermatol* 1991; 97: 618–623.
21. Hara M, Yaar M, Gilchrest BA. Endothelin-1 of keratinocyte origin is a mediator of melanocyte dendricity. *J Invest Dermatol* 1995; 105: 744–748.
22. Halaban R, Tyrrell L, Longley J, Yarden Y, Rubin J. Pigmentation and proliferation of human melanocytes and the effects of melanocyte-stimulating hormone and ultraviolet B light. *Ann NY Acad Sci* 1993; 680: 290–301.
23. Tada A, Suzuki I, Im S, et al. Endothelin-1 is a paracrine growth factor that modulates melanogenesis of human melanocytes and participates in their responses to ultraviolet radiation. *Cell Growth Differ* 1998; 9: 575–584.
24. Pawelek JM, Chakraborty AK, Osber MP, et al. Molecular cascades in UV-induced melanogenesis: a central role for melanotropins? *Pigment Cell Res* 1992; 5: 348–356.

25. Bhardwaj RS, Luger TA. Proopiomelanocortin production by epidermal cells: evidence for an immune neuroendocrine network in the epidermis. *Arch Dermatol Res* 1994; 287: 85–90.
26. Luger TA, Scholzen T, Brzoska T, Becher E, Slominski A, Paus R. Cutaneous immunomodulation and coordination of skin stress responses by alpha-melanocyte-stimulating hormone. *Ann NY Acad Sci* 1998; 840: 381–394.
27. Luger TA. Immunomodulation by UV light: role of neuropeptides. *Eur J Dermatol* 1998; 8: 198–199.
28. Costa JJ, Demetri GD, Harrist TJ, et al. Recombinant human stem cell factor (kit ligand) promotes human mast cell and melanocyte hyperplasia and functional activation in vivo. *J Exp Med* 1996; 183: 2681–2686.
29. Grichnik JM, Burch JA, Burchette J, Shea CR. The SCF/KIT pathway plays a critical role in the control of normal human melanocyte homeostasis. *J Invest Dermatol* 1998; 111: 233–238.
30. Lerner AB, McGuire J. Effect of a- and b-melanocyte-stimulating hormones on the skin colour of man. *Nature* 1961; 189: 176–179.
31. Hadley ME, Sharma SD, Hruby VJ, Levine N, Dorr RT. Melanotropic peptides for therapeutic and cosmetic tanning of the skin. *Ann NY Acad Sci* 1993; 680: 424–439.
32. Hadley ME, Hruby VJ, Blanchard J, et al. Discovery and development of novel melanogenic drugs. Melanotan-I and -II. *Pharm Biotechnol* 1998; 11: 575–595.
33. Stocker KM, Sherman L, Rees S, Ciment G. Basic FGF and TGF-b1 influence commitment to melanogenesis in neural crest-derived cells of avian embryos. *Development* 1991; 111: 635–641.
34. Sherman L, Stocker KM, Morrison R, Ciment G. Basic fibroblast growth factor (bFGF) acts intracellularly to cause the transdifferentiation of avian neural crest-derived Schwann cell precursors into melanocytes. *Development* 1993; 118: 1313–1326.
35. Reid K, Nishikawa S, Bartlett PF, Murphy M. Steel factor directs melanocyte development in vitro through selective regulation of the number of c-kit+ progenitors. *Dev Biol* 1995; 169: 568–579.
36. Guo CS, Wehrle-Haller B, Rossi J, Ciment G. Autocrine regulation of neural crest cell development by steel factor. *Dev Biol* 1997; 184: 61–69.
37. Lahav R, Dupin E, Lecoin L, et al. Endothelin 3 selectively promotes survival and proliferation of neural crest-derived glial and melanocytic precursors in vitro. *Proc Natl Acad Sci USA* 1998; 95: 14214–14219.
38. Lahav R, Ziller C, Dupin E, LeDouarin NM. Endothelin 3 promotes neural crest cell proliferation and mediates a vast increase in melanocyte number in culture. *Proc Natl Acad Sci USA* 1996; 93: 3892–3897.
39. Kos L, Aronzon A, Takayama H, et al. Hepatocyte growth factor/scatter factor-MET signaling in neural crest-derived melanocyte development. *Pigment Cell Res* 1999; 12: 13–21.
40. Ito M, Kawa Y, Ono H, et al. Removal of stem cell factor or addition of monoclonal anti-c-KIT antibody induces apoptosis in murine melanocyte precursors. *J Invest Dermatol* 1999; 112: 796–801.
41. Halaban R, Moellmann G. White mutants in mice shedding light on humans. *J Invest Dermatol* 1993; 100(Suppl): 176s–85s.
42. Spritz RA. Molecular basis of human piebaldism. *J Invest Dermatol* 1994; 103: 137S–140S.
43. Fleischman RA. From white spots to stem cells: the role of the Kit receptor in mammalian development. *Trends Genet* 1993; 9: 285–290.
44. Puffenberger EG, Hosoda K, Washington SS, et al. A missense mutation of the endothelin-B receptor gene in multigenic Hirschsprung's disease. *Cell* 1994; 79: 1257–1266.
45. Attie T, Till M, Pelet A, et al. Mutation of the endothelin-receptor B gene in Waardenburg-Hirschsprung disease. *Hum Mol Genet* 1995; 4: 2407–2409.

46. Edery P, Attie T, Amiel J, et al. Mutation of the endothelin-3 gene in the Waardenburg-Hirschsprung disease (Shah-Waardenburg syndrome). *Nat Genet* 1996; 12: 442–444.
47. Amiel J, Attie T, Jan D, et al. Heterozygous endothelin receptor B (EDNRB) mutations in isolated Hirschsprung disease. *Hum Mol Genet* 1996; 5: 355–357.
48. Seri M, Yin L, Barone V, et al. Frequency of RET mutations in long- and short-segment Hirschsprung disease. *Hum Mutat* 1997; 9: 243–249.
49. Hofstra RM, Osinga J, Tan-Sindhunata G, et al. A homozygous mutation in the endothelin-3 gene associated with a combined Waardenburg type 2 and Hirschsprung phenotype (Shah-Waardenburg syndrome). *Nat Genet* 1996; 12: 445–447.
50. Edery P, Eng C, Munnich A, Lyonnet S. RET in human development and oncogenesis. *Bioessays* 1997; 19: 389–395.
51. Baynash AG, Hosoda K, Giaid A, et al. Interaction of endothelin-3 with endothelin-B receptor is essential for development of epidermal melanocytes and enteric neurons. *Cell* 1994; 79: 1277–1285.
52. Hosoda K, Hammer RE, Richardson JA, et al. Targeted and natural (piebald-lethal) mutations of endothelin-B receptor gene produce megacolon associated with spotted coat color in mice. *Cell* 1994; 79: 1267–1276.
53. Hubbard SR, Mohammadi M, Schlessinger J. Autoregulatory mechanisms in protein-tyrosine kinases. *J Biol Chem* 1998; 273: 11987–11990.
54. Lemmon MA, Schlessinger J. Transmembrane signaling by receptor oligomerization. *Methods Mol Biol* 1998; 84: 49–71.
55. Weiss A, Schlessinger J. Switching signals on or off by receptor dimerization. *Cell* 1998; 94: 277–280.
56. Stoffel RH 3rd, Pitcher JA, Lefkowitz RJ. Targeting G protein-coupled receptor kinases to their receptor substrates. *J Membr Biol* 1997; 157: 1–8.
57. Halaban R, Kwon BS, Ghosh S, Delli Bovi P, Baird A. bFGF as an autocrine growth factor for human melanomas. *Oncogene Res* 1988; 3: 177–186.
58. Rodeck U, Menssen HD, Herlyn M. Growth factors in the pathogenesis of malignant diseases. *Dtsch Med Wochenschr* 1988; 113: 904–906.
59. Albino AP, Shea CR, McNutt NS. Oncogenes in melanomas. *J Dermatol* 1992; 19: 853–867.
60. Meier F, Nesbit M, Hsu MY, et al. Human melanoma progression in skin reconstructs: biological significance of bFGF. *Am J Pathol* 2000; 156: 193–200.
61. Aviezer D, Hecht D, Safran M, Eisinger M, David G, Yayon A. Perlecan, basal lamina proteoglycan, promotes basic fibroblast growth factor-receptor binding, mitogenesis, and angiogenesis. *Cell* 1995; 79: 1005–1013.
62. Safran M, Eisenstein M, Aviezer D, Yayon A. Oligomerization reduces heparin affinity but enhances receptor binding of fibroblast growth factor 2. *Biochem J* 2000; 1: 107–113.
63. DiGabriele AD, Lax I, Chen DI, et al. Structure of a heparin-linked biologically active dimer of fibroblast growth factor. *Nature* 1998; 393: 812–817.
64. Plotnikov AN, Schlessinger J, Hubbard SR, Mohammadi M. Structural basis for FGF receptor dimerization and activation. *Cell* 1999; 98: 641–650.
65. Klint P, Claesson-Welsh L. Signal transduction by fibroblast growth factor receptors. *Front Biosci* 1999; 15: D165–D177.
66. Hadari YR, Kouhara H, Lax I, Schlessinger J. Binding of Shp2 tyrosine phosphatase to FRS2 is essential for fibroblast growth factor-induced PC12 cell differentiation. *Mol Cell Biol* 1998; 18: 3966–3973.
67. Ong SH, Guy GR, Hadari YR, et al. FRS2 proteins recruit intracellular signaling pathways by binding to diverse targets on fibroblast growth factor and nerve growth factor receptors. *Mol Cell Biol* 2000; 20: 979–989.
68. Landgren E, Blumejensen P, Courtneidge SA, Claessonwelsh L. Fibroblast growth factor receptor-1 regulation of Src family kinases. *Oncogene* 1995; 10: 2027–2035.

69. Larsson H, Klint P, Landgren E, Claesson-Welsh L. Fibroblast growth factor receptor-1-mediated endothelial cell proliferation is dependent on the Src homology (SH) 2/SH3 domain-containing adaptor protein Crk. *J Biol Chem* 1999; 274: 25726–25734.
70. Klint P, Kanda S, Kloog Y, Claesson-Welsh L. Contribution of Src and Ras pathways in FGF-2 induced endothelial cell differentiation. *Oncogene* 1999; 18: 3354–3364.
71. Malumbres M, Pellicer A. RAS pathways to cell cycle control and cell transformation. *Front Biosci* 1998; 6: d887–d912.
72. Vojtek AB, Der CJ. Increasing complexity of the Ras signaling pathway. *J Biol Chem* 1998; 273: 19925–19928.
73. Cobb MH. MAP kinase pathways. *Prog Biophys Mol Biol* 1999; 71: 479–500.
74. Lewis TS, Shapiro PS, Ahn NG. Signal transduction through MAP kinase cascades. *Adv Cancer Res* 1998; 74: 49–139.
75. Imokawa G, Yada Y, Kimura M. Signalling mechanisms of endothelin-induced mitogenesis and melanogenesis in human melanocytes. *Biochem J* 1996; 314: 305–312.
76. Medrano EE, Yang F, Boissy R, et al. Terminal differentiation and senescence in the human melanocyte: repression of tyrosine-phosphorylation of the extracellular signal-regulated kinase 2 selectively defines the two phenotypes. *Mol Biol Cell* 1994; 5: 497–509.
77. Montminy M. Transcriptional regulation by cyclic AMP. *Annu Rev Biochem* 1997; 66: 807–822.
78. Eckner R. p300 and CBP as transcriptional regulators and targets of oncogenic events. *Biol Chem* 1996; 377: 685–688.
79. Goldman PS, Tran VK, Goodman RH. The multifunctional role of the co-activator CBP in transcriptional regulation. *Recent Prog Horm Res* 1997; 52: 103–119.
80. De Cesare D, Fimia GM, Sassone-Corsi P. Signaling routes to CREM and CREB: plasticity in transcriptional activation. *Trends Biochem Sci* 1999; 24: 281–285.
81. Bertolotto C, Abbe P, Hemesath TJ, et al. Microphthalmia gene product as a signal transducer in cAMP-induced differentiation of melanocytes. *J Cell Biol* 1998; 142: 827–835.
82. Hemesath TJ, Price ER, Takemoto C, Badalian T, Fisher DE. MAPK links the transcription factor Microphthalmia to c-Kit signaling in melanocytes. *Nature* 1998; 391: 298–301.
83. Sato S, Roberts K, Gambino G, Cook A, Kouzarides T, Goding CR. CBP/p300 as a co-factor for the Microphthalmia transcription factor. *Oncogene* 1997; 14: 3083–3092.
84. Goding CR, Fisher DE. Regulation of melanocyte differentiation and growth. *Cell Growth Differ* 1997; 8: 935–940.
85. Adams PD, Kaelin WG Jr. Transcriptional control by E2F. *Semin Cancer Biol* 1995; 6: 99–108.
86. Adams PD, Kaelin WG Jr. The cellular effects of E2F overexpression. *Curr Top Microbiol Immunol* 1996; 208: 79–93.
87. Sherr CJ. Growth factor-regulated G1 cyclins. *Stem Cells* 1994; 1: 47–55.
88. Sherr CJ. G1 phase progression: cycling on cue. *Cell* 1994; 79: 551–555.
89. Halaban R, Miglarese MR, Smicun Y, Puig S. Melanomas, from the cell cycle point of view. *Int J Mol Med* 1998; 1: 419–425.
90. Halaban R, Cheng C, Smicun Y, Germino J. Deregulated E2F transcriptional activity in autonomously growing melanoma cells. *J Exp Med* 2000; 191: 1005–1016.
91. Weinberg RA. The retinoblastoma protein and cell cycle control. *Cell* 1995; 81: 323–330.
92. Kaelin WG Jr. Recent insights into the functions of the retinoblastoma susceptibility gene product. *Cancer Invest* 1997; 15: 243–254.
93. Sherr CJ. Cancer cell cycles. *Science* 1996; 274: 1672–1677.
94. Zarkowska T, Mittnacht S. Differential phosphorylation of the retinoblastoma protein by G1/S cyclin-dependent kinases. *J Biol Chem* 1997; 272: 12738–12746.
95. Weinberg RA. The molecular basis of carcinogenesis—understanding the cell cycle clock. *Cytokines Mol Ther* 1996; 2: 105–110.

96. Taya Y. Rb kinases and Rb-binding proteins: new points of view. *Trends Biochem Sci* 1997; 22: 14–17.
97. Pardee A. G1 events and regulation of cell proliferation. *Science* 1989; 246: 603–608.
98. Bartek J, Bartkova J, Lukas J. The retinoblastoma protein pathway and the restriction point. *Curr Opin Cell Biol* 1996; 8: 805–814.
99. Planas-Silva MD, Weinberg RA. The restriction point and control of cell proliferation. *Curr Opin Cell Biol* 1997; 9: 768–772.
100. Nevins JR. Toward an understanding of the functional complexity of the E2F and retinoblastoma families. *Cell Growth Differ* 1998; 9: 585–593.
101. Lai A, Lee JM, Yang WM, et al. RBP1 recruits both histone deacetylase-dependent and -independent repression activities to retinoblastoma family proteins. *Mol Cell Biol* 1999; 19: 6632–6641.
102. Magnaghi-Jaulin L, Groisman R, Naguibneva I, et al. Retinoblastoma protein represses transcription by recruiting a histone deacetylase. *Nature* 1998; 391: 601–605.
103. Ferreira R, Magnaghi-Jaulin L, Robin P, Harel-Bellan A, Trouche D. The three members of the pocket proteins family share the ability to repress E2F activity through recruitment of a histone deacetylase. *Proc Natl Acad Sci USA* 1998; 95: 10493–10498.
104. Brehm A, Miska EA, McCance DJ, Reid JL, Bannister AJ, Kouzarides T. Retinoblastoma protein recruits histone deacetylase to repress transcription. *Nature* 1998; 391: 597–601.
105. Jacks T, Weinberg RA. Cell-cycle control and its watchman. *Nature* 1996; 381: 643–644.
106. Weinberg RA. How cancer arises. *Sci Am* 1996; 275: 62–70.
107. Grana X, Garriga J, Mayol X. Role of the retinoblastoma protein family, pRB, p107 and p130 in the negative control of cell growth. *Oncogene* 1998; 17: 3365–3383.
108. Johnson DG, Schneider-Broussard R. Role of E2F in cell cycle control and cancer. *Front Biosci* 1998; 27: d447–d448.
109. Hiyama H, Iavarone A, Reeves SA. Regulation of the CDK inhibitor p21 gene during cell cycle progression is under the control of the transcription factor E2F. *Oncogene* 1998; 16: 1513–1523.
110. Rodeck U, Herlyn M, Menssen HD, Furlanetto RW, Koprowsk H. Metastatic but not primary melanoma cell lines grow in vitro independently of exogenous growth factors. *Int J Cancer* 1987; 40: 687–690.
111. Furlanetto RW, Harwell SE, Baggs RB. Effects of insulin-like growth factor receptor inhibition on human melanomas in culture and in athymic mice. *Cancer Res* 1993; 53: 2522–2526.
112. Halaban R. Receptor tyrosine protein kinases in normal and malignant melanocytes. In: Okhawara A, McGuire J, eds. *The Biology of the Epidermis*. Elsevier, New York, 1992, pp. 133–140.
113. Easty DJ, Ganz SE, Farr CJ, Lai C, Herlyn M, Bennett DC. Novel and known protein tyrosine kinases and their abnormal expression in human melanomas. *J lnvest Dermatol* 1993; 101: 679–684.
114. Scott G, Stoler M, Sarkar S, Halaban R. Localization of basic fibroblast growth factor mRNA in melanocytic lesions by *in situ* hybridization. *J Invest Dermatol* 1991; 96: 318–322.
115. Ueda M, Funasaka Y, Ichihashi M, Mishima Y. Stable and strong expression of basic fibroblast growth factor in naevus cell naevus contrasts with aberrant expression in melanoma. *Br J Dermatol* 1994; 130: 320–324.
116. al-Alousi S, Carlson JA, Blessing K, Cook M, Karaoli T, Barnhill RL. Expression of basic fibroblast growth factor in desmoplastic melanoma. *J Cutan. Pathol* 1996; 23: 118–125.
117. Reed JA, McNutt NS, Albino AP. Differential expression of basic fibroblast growth factor (bFGF) in melanocytic lesions demonstrated by in situ hybridization. Implications for tumor progression. *Am J Pathol* 1994; 144: 329–336.

118. Halaban R. Growth factors and melanomas. *Semin Oncol* 1996; 23: 673–681.
119. Rodeck R, Melber K, Kath R, et al. Constitutive expression of multiple growth factor genes by melanoma cells but not normal melanocytes. *J Invest Dermatol* 1991; 97: 20–26.
120. Rodeck U, Becker D, Herlyn M. Basic fibroblast growth factor in human melanoma. *Cancer Cells* 1991; 3: 308–311.
121. Albino AP. The role of oncogenes and growth factors in progressive melanoma-genesis. *Pigment Cell Res* 1992; 2: 199–218.
122. Kanter-Lewensohn L, Dricu A, Girnita L, Wejde J, Larsson O. Expression of insulin-like growth factor-1 receptor (IGF-1R) and p27Kip1 in melanocytic tumors: a potential regulatory role of IGF-1 pathway in distribution of p27Kip1 between different cyclins. *Growth Factors* 2000; 17: 193–202.
123. Dotto GP, Moellmann G, Ghosh S, Edwards M, Halaban R. Transformation of murine melanocytes by basic fibroblast growth factor cDNA and oncogenes and selective suppression of the transformed phenotype in a reconstituted cutaneous environment. *J Cell Biol* 1989; 109: 3115–3128.
124. Balentien E, Mufson BE, Shattuck RL, Derynck R, Richmond A. Effects of MGSA/GRO alpha on melanocyte transformation. *Oncogene* 1991; 6: 1115–1124.
125. Richmond A. The pathogenic role of growth factors in melanoma. *Semin Dermatol* 1991; 10: 246–255.
126. Tettelbach W, Nanney L, Ellis D, King L, Richmond A. Localization of MGSA/GRO protein in cutaneous lesions. *J Cutan Pathol* 1993; 20: 259–266.
127. Rodeck U, Herlyn M. Growth factors in melanoma. *Cancer Metastasis Rev* 1991; 10: 89–101.
128. Easty DJ, Herlyn M, Bennett DC. Abnormal protein tyrosine kinase gene expression during melanoma progression and metastasis. *Int J Cancer* 1995; 60: 129–136.
129. Ellis DL, Kafka SP, Chow JC, et al. Melanoma, growth factors, acanthosis nigricans, the sign of Leser-Trelat, and multiple acrocordons: a possible role for alpha-transforming growth factor in cutaneous paraneoplastic syndromes. *N Engl J Med* 1987; 317: 1582–1587.
130. Forsberg K, Valyi-Nagy I, Heldin C-H, Herlyn M, Westermark B. Platelet-derived growth factor (PDGF) in oncogenesis: development of a vascular connective tissue stroma in xenotransplanted human melanoma producing PDGF-BB. *Proc Natl Acad Sci USA* 1993; 90: 393–397.
131. Danielsen T, Rofstad EK. The constitutive level of vascular endothelial growth factor (VEGF) is more important than hypoxia-induced VEGF up-regulation in the angiogenesis of human melanoma xenografts. *Br J Cancer* 2000; 82: 1528–1534.
132. Weber F, Sepp N, Fritsch P. Vascular endothelial growth factor and basic fibroblast growth factor in melanoma. *Br J Dermatol* 2000; 142: 392–393.
133. Herold-Mende C, Steiner HH, Andl T, et al. Expression and functional significance of vascular endothelial growth factor receptors in human tumor cells. *Lab Invest* 1999; 79: 1573–1582.
134. Birck A, Kirkin AF, Zeuthen J, Hou-Jensen K. Expression of basic fibroblast growth factor and vascular endothelial growth factor in primary and metastatic melanoma from the same patients. *Melanoma Res* 1999; 9: 375–381.
135. Bayer-Garner IB, Hough AJ Jr, Smoller BR. Vascular endothelial growth factor expression in malignant melanoma: prognostic versus diagnostic usefulness. *Mod Pathol* 1999; 12: 770–774.
136. Rofstad EK, Danielsen T. Hypoxia-induced metastasis of human melanoma cells: involvement of vascular endothelial growth factor-mediated angiogenesis. *Br J Cancer* 1999; 80: 1697–1707.
137. Graeven U, Fiedler W, Karpinski S, et al. Melanoma-associated expression of vascular endothelial growth factor and its receptors FLT-1 and KDR. *J Cancer Res Clin Oncol* 1999; 125: 621–629.

138. Iwamoto T, Takahashi M, Ito M, et al. Aberrant melanogenesis and melanocytic tumour development in transgenic mice that carry a metallothionein/*ret* fusion gene. *EMBO J* 1991; 10: 3167–3175.
139. Kato M, Takahashi M, Akhand AA, et al. Transgenic mouse model for skin malignant melanoma. *Oncogene* 1998; 17: 1885–1888.
140. Kato M, Liu W, Akhand AA, et al. Linkage between melanocytic tumor development and early burst of Ret protein expression for tolerance induction in metallothionein-I/ret transgenic mouse lines. *Oncogene* 1999; 18: 837–842.
141. Takayama H, LaRochelle WJ, Sharp R, et al. Diverse tumorigenesis associated with aberrant development in mice overexpressing hepatocyte growth factor/scatter factor. *Proc Natl Acad Sci USA* 1997; 94: 701–706.
142. Otsuka T, Takayama H, Sharp R, et al. c-Met autocrine activation induces development of malignant melanoma and acquisition of the metastatic phenotype. *Cancer Res* 1998; 58: 5157–5167.
143. Halaban R, Rubin JS, Funasaka Y, et al. Met and hepatocyte growth factor/scatter factor signal transduction in normal melanocytes and melanoma cells. *Oncogene* 1992; 7: 2195–2206.
144. Halaban R. Molecular correlates in the progression of normal melanocytes to melanomas. *Sem Cancer Biol* 1993; 4: 171–181.
145. Halaban R, Rubin W, White W. Met and HGF/SF in normal melanocytes and melanoma cells. In: Goldberg ID, ed. *Hepatocyte Growth Factor-Scatter Factor and the C-Met Receptor*. Birkhäuser Verlag, Basel, Switzerland, 1993, pp. 329–339.
146. Natali PG, Nicotra MR, Sures I, Santoro E, Bigotti A, Ullrich A. Expression of c-kit receptor in normal and transformed human nonlymphoid tissues. *Cancer Res* 1992; 52: 6139–6143.
147. Zakut R, Perlis R, Eliyahu S, et al. KIT ligand (mast cell growth factor) inhibits the growth of KIT-expressing melanoma cells. *Oncogene* 1993; 8: 2221–2229.
148. Lassam N, Bickford S. Loss of c-kit expression in cultured melanoma cells. *Oncogene* 1992; 7: 51–56.
149. Huang SY, Luca M, Gutman M, et al. Enforced C-Kit expression renders highly metastatic human melanoma cells susceptible to stem cell factor-induced apoptosis and inhibits their tumorigenic and metastatic potential. *Oncogene* 1996; 13: 2339–2347.
150. Segev O, Chumakov I, Nevo Z, et al. Restrained chondrocyte proliferation and maturation with abnormal growth plate vascularization and ossification in human FGFR-3(G380R) transgenic mice. *Hum Mol Genet* 2000; 9: 249–258.
151. Monsonego-Ornan E, Adar R, Feferman T, Segev O, Yayon A. The transmembrane mutation G380R in fibroblast growth factor receptor 3 uncouples ligand-mediated receptor activation from down-regulation. *Mol Cell Biol* 2000; 20: 516–522.
152. Garofalo S, Kliger-Spatz M, Cooke JL, et al. Skeletal dysplasia and defective chondrocyte differentiation by targeted overexpression of fibroblast growth factor 9 in transgenic mice. *J Bone Miner Res* 1999; 14: 1909–1915.
153. Vlodavsky I, Miao HQ, Medalion B, Danagher P, Ron D. Involvement of heparan sulfate and related molecules in sequestration and growth promoting activity of fibroblast growth factor. *Cancer Metastasis Rev* 1996; 15: 177–186.
154. Yayon A, Klagsbrun M, Esko JD, Leder P, Ornitz DM. Cell surface, heparin-like molecules are required for binding of basic fibroblast growth factor to its high affinity receptor. *Cell* 1991; 64: 841–848.
155. Ornitz DM, Yayon A, Flanagan JG, Svahn CM, Levi E, Leder P. Heparin is required for cell-free binding of basic fibroblast growth factor to a soluble receptor and for mitogenesis in whole cells. *Mol Cell Biol* 1992; 12: 240–247.

156. Kan M, Wang F, Xu J, Crabb JW, Hou J, McKeehan WL. An essential heparin-binding domain in the fibroblast growth factor receptor kinase. *Science* 1993; 259: 1918–1921.
157. Li LY, Safran M, Aviezer D, Bohlen P, Seddon AP, Yayon A. Diminished heparin binding of a basic fibroblast growth factor mutant is associated with reduced receptor binding, mitogenesis, plasminogen activator induction, and in vitro angiogenesis. *Biochemistry* 1994; 33: 10999–11007.
158. Aviezer D, Iozzo RV, Noonan DM, Yayon A. Suppression of autocrine and paracrine functions of basic fibroblast growth factor by stable expression of perlecan antisense cDNA. *Mol Cell Biol* 1997; 17: 1938–1946.
159. Miao HQ, Ornitz DM, Aingorn E, Ben-Sasson SA, Vlodavsky I. Modulation of fibroblast growth factor-2 receptor binding, dimerization, signaling, and angiogenic activity by a synthetic heparin-mimicking polyanionic compound. *J Clin Invest* 1997; 99: 1565–1575.
160. Liekens S, Leali D, Neyts J, et al. Modulation of fibroblast growth factor-2 receptor binding, signaling, and mitogenic activity by heparin-mimicking polysulfonated compounds. *Mol Pharmacol* 1999; 56: 204–213.
161. Werner S, Weinberg W, Liao X, et al. Targeted expression of a dominant-negative FGF receptor mutant in the epidermis of transgenic mice reveals a role of FGF in keratinocyte organization and differentiation. *EMBO J* 1993; 12: 2635–2643.
162. Peters K, Werner S, Liao X, Wert S, Whitsett J, Williams L. Targeted expression of a dominant negative FGF receptor blocks branching morphogenesis and epithelial differentiation of the mouse lung. *EMBO J* 1994; 13: 3296–3301.
163. Celli G, LaRochelle WJ, Mackem S, Sharp R, Merlino G. Soluble dominant-negative receptor uncovers essential roles for fibroblast growth factors in multi-organ induction and patterning. *EMBO J* 1998; 17: 1642–1655.
164. Yayon A, Ma YS, Safran M, Klagsbrun M, Halaban R. Suppression of autocrine cell proliferation and tumorigenesis of human melanoma cells and fibroblast growth factor transformed fibroblasts by a kinase-deficient FGF receptor 1: evidence for the involvement of Src-family kinases. *Oncogene* 1997; 14: 2999–3009.
165. Becker D, Meier CB, Becker. Proliferation of human malignant melanomas is inhibited by antisense oligodeoxynucleotides targeted against basic fibroblast growth factor. *EMBO J* 1989; 8: 3685–3691.
166. Becker D, Lee PL, Rodeck U, Herlyn M. Inhibition of the fibroblast growth factor receptor 1 (FGFR-1) gene in human melanocytes and malignant melanomas leads to inhibition of proliferation and signs indicative of differentiation. *Oncogene* 1992; 7: 2303–2313.
167. Kato J, Wanebo H, Calabresi P, Clark JW. Basic fibroblast growth factor production and growth factor receptors as potential targets for melanoma therapy. *Melanoma Res* 1992; 2: 13–23.
168. Wang Y, Becker D. Antisense targeting of basic fibroblast growth factor and fibroblast growth factor receptor-1 in human melanomas blocks intratumoral angiogenesis and tumor growth. *Nature Med* 1997; 3: 887–893.
169. Traxler P, Furet P. Strategies toward the design of novel and selective protein tyrosine kinase inhibitors. *Pharmacol Ther* 1999; 82: 195–206.
170. al-Obeidi FA, Wu JJ, Lam KS. Protein tyrosine kinases: structure, substrate specificity, and drug discovery. *Biopolymers* 1998; 47: 197–223.
171. Fry DW. Inhibition of the epidermal growth factor receptor family of tyrosine kinases as an approach to cancer chemotherapy: progression from reversible to irreversible inhibitors. *Pharmacol Ther* 1999; 82: 207–218.
172. Klapper LN, Kirschbaum MH, Sela M, Yarden Y. Biochemical and clinical implications of the ErbB/HER signaling network of growth factor receptors. *Adv Cancer Res* 2000; 77: 25–79.
173. Klohs WD, Fry DW, Kraker AJ. Inhibitors of tyrosine kinase. *Curr Opin Oncol* 1997; 9: 562–568.

174. Hamby JM, Connolly CJ, Schroeder MC, et al. Structure-activity relationships for a novel series of pyrido[2,3- d]pyrimidine tyrosine kinase inhibitors. *J Med Chem* 1997; 40: 2296–2303.
175. Showalter HD, Kraker AJ. Small molecule inhibitors of the platelet-derived growth factor receptor, the fibroblast growth factor receptor, and Src family tyrosine kinases. *Pharmacol Ther* 1997; 76: 55–71.
176. Mohammadi M, McMahon G, Sun L, et al. Structures of the tyrosine kinase domain of fibroblast growth factor receptor in complex with inhibitors. *Science* 1997; 276: 955–960.
177. Mohammadi M, Froum S, Hamby JM, et al. Crystal structure of an angiogenesis inhibitor bound to the FGF receptor tyrosine kinase domain. *EMBO J* 1998; 17: 5896–5904.
178. Dimitroff CJ, Klohs W, Sharma A, et al. Anti-angiogenic activity of selected receptor tyrosine kinase inhibitors, PD166285 and PD173074: implications for combination treatment with photodynamic therapy. *Invest New Drugs* 1999; 17: 121–135.
179. Lappi DA, Ying W, Barthelemy I, et al. Expression and activities of a recombinant basic fibroblast growth factor-saporin fusion protein. *J Biol Chem* 1994; 269: 12552–12558.
180. Beitz JG, Davol P, Clark JW, et al. Antitumor activity of basic fibroblast growth factor-saporin mitotoxin in vitro and in vivo. *Cancer Res* 1992; 52: 227–230.
181. Ying WB, Martineau D, Beitz J, Lappi DA, Baird A. Anti-B16-B10 melanoma activity of a basic fibroblast growth factor-saporin mitotoxin. *Cancer* 1994; 74: 848–853.
182. Lappi DA. Tumor targeting through fibroblast growth factor receptors. *Semin Cancer Biol* 1995; 6: 279–288.
183. Michael SI, Curiel DT. Strategies to achieve targeted gene delivery via the receptor-mediated endocytosis pathway. *Gene Ther* 1994; 1: 223–232.
184. Wickham TJ, Roelvink PW, Brough DE, Kovesdi I. Adenovirus targeted to heparan-containing receptors increases its gene delivery efficiency to multiple cell types. *Nat Biotechnol* 1996; 14: 1570–1573.
185. Kochanek S. High-capacity adenoviral vectors for gene transfer and somatic gene therapy. *Hum Gene Ther* 1999; 10: 2451–2459.
186. Rodeck U, Herlyn M. Characteristics of cultured human melanocytes from different stages of tumor progression. *Cancer Treat Res* 1988; 43: 3–16.
187. Baserga R. The IGF-I receptor in cancer research. *Exp Cell Res* 1999; 253: 1–6.
188. Herlyn M, Balaban G, Bennicelli J, et al. Primary melanoma cells of the vertical growth phase: similarities to metastatic cells. *J Natl Cancer Inst* 1985; 74: 283–289.
189. Baserga R. The insulin-like growth factor I receptor: a key to tumor growth? *Cancer Res* 1995; 55: 249–252.
190. Resnicoff M, Coppola D, Sell C, Rubin R, Ferrone S, Baserga R. Growth inhibition of human melanoma cells in nude mice by antisense strategies to the type 1 insulin-like growth factor receptor. *Cancer Res* 1994; 54: 4848–4850.
191. Parrizas M, Gazit A, Levitzki A, Wertheimer E, LeRoith D. Specific inhibition of insulin-like growth factor-1 and insulin receptor tyrosine kinase activity and biological function by tyrphostins. *Endocrinology* 1997; 138: 1427–1433.
192. Khosravifar R, White MA, Westwick JK, et al. Oncogenic ras activation of raf/mitogen-activated protein kinase-independent pathways is sufficient to cause tumorigenic transformation. *Mol Cell Biol* 1996; 16: 3923–3933.
193. Albino AP, Nanus DM, Mentle IR, et al. Analysis of ras oncogenes in malignant melanoma and precursor lesions: correlation of point mutations with differentiation phenotype. *Oncogene* 1989; 4: 1363–1374.
194. Albino AP, Nanus DM, Davis ML, McNutt NS. Lack of evidence of Ki-ras codon 12 mutations in melanocytic lesions. *J Cutan Pathol* 1991; 18: 273–278.
195. O'Mara SM, Todd AV, Russell PJ. Analysis of expressed N-ras mutations in human melanoma short-term cell lines with allele specific restriction analysis induced by the polymerase chain reaction. *Eur J Cancer* 1992; 28: 9–11.

196. Jiveskog S, Ragnarsson-Olding B, Platz A, Ringborg U. N-ras mutations are common in melanomas from sun-exposed skin of humans but rare in mucosal membranes or unexposed skin. *J Invest Dermatol* 1998; 111: 757–761.
197. Carr J, Mackie RM. Point mutations in the N-ras oncogene in malignant melanoma and congenital naevi. *Br J Dermatol* 1994; 131: 72–77.
198. van Elsas A, Zerp SF, van der Flier S, et al. Relevance of ultraviolet-induced N-ras oncogene point mutations in development of primary human cutaneous melanoma. *Am J Pathol* 1996; 149: 883–893.
199. Platz A, Ringborg U, Grafstrom E, Hoog A, Lagerlof B. Immunohistochemical analysis of the N-ras p21 and the p53 proteins in naevi, primary tumours and metastases of human cutaneous malignant melanoma—increased immunopositivity in hereditary melanoma. *Melanoma Res* 1995; 5: 101–106.
200. Powell MB, Hyman P, Bell OD, et al. Hyperpigmentation and melanocytic hyperplasia in transgenic mice expressing the human T24 Ha-ras gene regulated by a mouse tyrosinase promoter. *Mol Carcinog* 1995; 12: 82–90.
201. Powell MB, Gause PR, Hyman P, et al. Induction of melanoma in TPras transgenic mice. *Carcinogenesis* 1999; 20: 1747–1753.
202. Chin L, Tam A, Pomerantz J, et al. Essential role for oncogenic Ras in tumour maintenance. *Nature* 1999; 400: 468–472.
203. Chin L, Pomerantz J, Polsky D, et al. Cooperative effects of *INK4a* and *ras* in melanoma susceptibility in vivo. *Genes Dev* 1997; 11: 2822–2834.
204. Chin L, Merlino G, DePinho RA. Malignant melanoma: modern black plague and genetic black box. *Genes Dev* 1998; 12: 3467–3481.
205. Ohta Y, Tone T, Shitara T, et al. H-ras ribozyme-mediated alteration of the human melanoma phenotype. *Ann NY Acad Sci* 1994; 716: 242–253.
206. Kashani-Sabet M, Funato T, Florenes VA, Fodstad O, Scanlon KJ. Suppression of the neoplastic phenotype in vivo by an anti-ras ribozyme. *Cancer Res* 1994; 54: 900–902.
207. Ohta Y, Kijima H, Ohkawa T, Kashani-sabet M, Scanlon KJ. Tissue-specific expression of an anti-ras ribozyme inhibits proliferation of human malignant melanoma cells. *Nucleic Acids Res* 1996; 24: 938–942.
208. Prendergast GC. Farnesyltransferase inhibitors: antineoplastic mechanism and clinical prospects. *Curr Opin Cell Biol* 2000; 12: 166–173.
209. Jansen B, Schlagbauer-Wadl H, Kahr H, et al. Novel Ras antagonist blocks human melanoma growth. *Proc Natl Acad Sci USA* 1999; 96: 14019–14024.
210. Gibbs BS, Zahn TJ, Mu Y, Sebolt-Leopold JS, Gibbs RA. Novel farnesol and geranylgeraniol analogues: a potential new class of anticancer agents directed against protein prenylation. *J Med Chem* 1999; 42: 3800–3808.
211. Gelb MH, Scholten JD, Sebolt-Leopold JS. Protein prenylation: from discovery to prospects for cancer treatment. *Curr Opin Chem Biol* 1998; 2: 40–48.
212. Vogt A, Qian Y, McGuire TF, Hamilton AD, Sebti SM. Protein geranylgeranylation, not farnesylation, is required for the G1 to S phase transition in mouse fibroblasts. *Oncogene* 1996; 13: 1991–1999.
213. Vogt A, Sun J, Qian Y, Hamilton AD, Sebti SM. The geranylgeranyltransferase-I inhibitor GGTI-298 arrests human tumor cells in G0/G1 and induces p21(WAF1/CIP1/SDI1) in a p53-independent manner. *J Biol Chem* 1997; 272: 27224–27229.
214. Lerner EC, Zhang TT, Knowles DB, Qian Y, Hamilton AD, Sebti SM. Inhibition of the prenylation of K-Ras, but not H- or N-Ras, is highly resistant to CAAX peptidomimetics and requires both a farnesyltransferase and a geranylgeranyltransferase I inhibitor in human tumor cell lines. *Oncogene* 1997; 15: 1283–1288.
215. Miquel K, Pradines A, Sun J, et al. GGTI-298 induces G0-G1 block and apoptosis whereas FTI-277 causes G2-M enrichment in A549 cells. *Cancer Res* 1997; 57: 1846–1850.

216. Sun J, Qian Y, Chen Z, Marfurt J, Hamilton AD, Sebti SM. The geranylgeranyltransferase I inhibitor GGTI-298 induces hypophosphorylation of retinoblastoma and partner switching of cyclin-dependent kinase inhibitors. A potential mechanism for GGTI-298 antitumor activity. *J Biol Chem* 1999; 274: 6930–6934.
217. Pollack IF, Bredel M, Erff M, Hamilton AD, Sebti SM. Inhibition of Ras and related guanosine triphosphate-dependent proteins as a therapeutic strategy for blocking malignant glioma growth: II—preclinical studies in a nude mouse model. *Neurosurgery* 1999; 45: 1208–1214.
218. Liu X, Brodeur SR, Gish G, et al. Regulation of c-Src tyrosine kinase activity by the Src SH2 domain. *Oncogene* 1993; 8: 1119–1126.
219. Pawson T, Schlessinger J. SH2 and SH3 domains. *Curr Biol* 1993; 3: 434–442.
220. Schlessinger J. New roles for Src kinases in control of cell survival and angiogenesis. *Cell* 2000; 100: 293–296.
221. Pawson T. Protein modules and signalling networks. *Nature* 1995; 373: 573–580.
222. Pawson T, Hunter T. Signal transduction and growth control in normal and cancer cells. *Curr Opin Genet Dev* 1994; 4: 1–4.
223. Lawrence DS, Niu J. Protein kinase inhibitors: the tyrosine-specific protein kinases. *Pharmacol Ther* 1998; 77: 81–114.
224. Moasser MM, Srethapakdi M, Sachar KS, Kraker AJ, Rosen N. Inhibition of Src kinases by a selective tyrosine kinase inhibitor causes mitotic arrest. *Cancer Res* 1999; 59: 6145–6152.
225. Roginskaya V, Zuo S, Caudell E, Nambudiri G, Kraker AJ, Corey SJ. Therapeutic targeting of Src-kinase Lyn in myeloid leukemic cell growth. *Leukemia* 1999; 13: 855–861.
226. le Coutre P, Tassi E, Varella-Garcia M, et al. Induction of resistance to the Abelson inhibitor STI571 in human leukemic cells through gene amplification. *Blood* 2000; 95: 1758–1766.
227. Carlo-Stella C, Regazzi E, Sammarelli G, et al. Effects of the tyrosine kinase inhibitor AG957 and an Anti-Fas receptor antibody on CD34(+) chronic myelogenous leukemia progenitor cells. *Blood* 1999; 93: 3973–3982.
228. O'Dwyer PJ, Stevenson JP, Gallagher M, et al. c-raf-1 depletion and tumor responses in patients treated with the c-raf-1 antisense oligodeoxynucleotide ISIS 5132 (CGP 69846A). *Clin Cancer Res* 1999; 5: 3977–3982.
229. Cunningham CC, Holmlund JT, Schiller JH, et al. A phase I trial of c-Raf kinase antisense oligonucleotide ISIS 5132 administered as a continuous intravenous infusion in patients with advanced cancer. *Clin Cancer Res* 2000; 6: 1626–1631.
230. Sebolt-Leopold JS, Dudley DT, Herrera R, et al. Blockade of the MAP kinase pathway suppresses growth of colon tumors in vivo. *Nat Med* 1999; 5: 810–816.
231. Guldberg P, thor Straten P, Birck A, Ahrenkiel V, Kirkin AF, Zeuthen J. Disruption of the MMAC1/PTEN gene by deletion or mutation is a frequent event in malignant melanoma. *Cancer Res* 1997; 57: 3660–3663.
232. Robertson GP, Furnari FB, Miele ME, et al. In vitro loss of heterozygosity targets the PTEN/MMAC1 gene in melanoma. *Proc Natl Acad Sci USA* 1998; 95: 9418–9423.
233. Tsao H, Zhang X, Benoit E, Haluska FG. Identification of PTEN/MMAC1 alterations in uncultured melanomas and melanoma cell lines. *Oncogene* 1998; 16: 3397–3402.
234. Du W, Liu A, Prendergast GC. Activation of the PI3'K-AKT pathway masks the proapoptotic effects of farnesyltransferase inhibitors. *Cancer Res* 1999; 59: 4208–4212.
235. Horowitz JM, Park S-H, Bogenman E, et al. Frequent inactivation of the retinoblastoma anti-oncogene is restricted to a subset of human tumor cells. *Proc Natl Acad Sci USA* 1990; 87: 2772–2779.
236. Bartkova J, Lukas J, Guldberg P, et al. The p16-cyclin D/Cdk4-pRb pathway as a functional unit frequently altered in melanoma pathogenesis. *Cancer Res* 1996; 56: 5475–5483.

237. Bataille V, Hiles R, Bishop JA. Retinoblastoma, melanoma and the atypical mole syndrome. *Br J Dermatol* 1995; 132: 134–138.
238. Moll AC, Imhof SM, Bouter LM, Tan KE. Second primary tumors in patients with retinoblastoma. A review of the literature. *Ophthalmic Genet* 1997; 18: 27–34.
239. Vogt T, Kroiss M, McClelland M, et al. Deficiency of a novel retinoblastoma binding protein 2-homolog is a consistent feature of sporadic human melanoma skin cancer. *Lab Invest* 1999; 79: 1615–1627.
240. Sherr CJ. Mammalian G1 cyclins and cell cycle progression. *Proc Assoc Am Physicians* 1995; 107: 181–186.
241. Halaban R, Funasaka Y, Lee P, Rubin J, Ron D, Birnbaum D. Fibroblast growth factors in normal and malignant melanocytes. *Ann NY Acad Sci* 1991; 638: 232–243.
242. Gaudray P, Szepetowski P, Escot C, Birnbaum D, Theillet C. DNA amplification at 11q13 in human cancer: from complexity to perplexity. *Mutat Res* 1992; 276: 317–328.
243. Halaban R. Melanoma cell autonomous growth: the Rb/E2F pathway. *Cancer Metastasis Rev* 1999; 8: 333–343.
244. Nobori T, Miura K, Wu DJ, Lois A, Takabayashi K, Carson DA. Deletions of the cyclin-dependent kinase-4 inhibitor gene in multiple human cancers. *Nature* 1994; 368: 753–756.
245. Kamb A, Gruis NA, Weaver-Feldhaus J, et al. A cell cycle regulator potentially involved in genesis of many tumor types. *Science* 1994; 264: 436–440.
246. Kamb A, Shattuck-Eidens D, Eeles R, et al. Analysis of the p16 gene (CDKN2) as a candidate for the chromosome 9p melanoma susceptibility locus. *Nat Genet* 1994; 8: 23–26.
247. Wolfel T, Hauer M, Schneider J, et al. A $p16^{INK4a}$-insensitive CDK4 mutant targeted by cytolytic T lymphocytes in a human melanoma. *Science* 1995; 269: 1281–1284.
248. Senderowicz AM, Sausville EA. Preclinical and clinical development of cyclin-dependent kinase modulators. *J Natl Cancer Inst* 2000; 92: 376–387.
249. Gray N, Detivaud L, Doerig C, Meijer L. ATP-site directed inhibitors of cyclin-dependent kinases. *Curr Med Chem* 1999; 6: 859–875.
250. Hajduch M, Havlieek L, Vesely J, Novotny R, Mihal V, Strnad M. Synthetic cyclin dependent kinase inhibitors. New generation of potent anti-cancer drugs. *Adv Exp Med Biol* 1999; 457: 341–353.
251. Carlson BA, Dubay MM, Sausville EA, Brizuela L, Worland PJ. Flavopiridol induces G1 arrest with inhibition of cyclin-dependent kinase (CDK) 2 and CDK4 in human breast carcinoma cells. *Cancer Res* 1996; 56: 2973–2978.
252. Patel V, Senderowicz AM, Pinto D Jr, et al. Flavopiridol, a novel cyclin-dependent kinase inhibitor, suppresses the growth of head and neck squamous cell carcinomas by inducing apoptosis. *J Clin Invest* 1998; 102: 1674–1681.
253. Schrump DS, Matthews W, Chen GA, Mixon A, Altorki NK. Flavopiridol mediates cell cycle arrest and apoptosis in esophageal cancer cells. *Clin Cancer Res* 1998; 4: 2885–2890.
254. Senderowicz AM. Flavopiridol: the first cyclin-dependent kinase inhibitor in human clinical trials. *Invest New Drugs* 1999; 17: 313–320.
255. Li Y, Bhuiyan M, Alhasan S, Senderowicz AM, Sarkar FH. Induction of apoptosis and inhibition of c-erbB-2 in breast cancer cells by flavopiridol. *Clin Cancer Res* 2000; 6: 223–229.
256. Carlson B, Lahusen T, Singh S, et al. Down-regulation of cyclin D1 by transcriptional repression in MCF-7 human breast carcinoma cells induced by flavopiridol. *Cancer Res* 1999; 59: 4634–4641.
257. Morishita R, Gibbons GH, Horiuchi M, et al. A gene therapy strategy using a transcription factor decoy of the E2F binding site inhibits smooth muscle proliferation in vivo. *Proc Natl Acad Sci USA* 1995; 92: 5855–5859.
258. Maeshima Y, Kashihara N, Yasuda T, et al. Inhibition of mesangial cell proliferation by E2F decoy oligodeoxynucleotide in vitro and in vivo. *J Clin Invest* 1998; 101: 2589–2597.

259. Mann MJ, Whittemore AD, Donaldson MC, et al. Ex-vivo gene therapy of human vascular bypass grafts with E2F decoy: the PREVENT single-centre, randomised, controlled trial. *Lancet* 1999; 354: 1493–1498.
260. Parr MJ, Manome Y, Tanaka T, et al. Tumor-selective transgene expression in vivo mediated by an E2F-responsive adenoviral vector. *Nat Med* 1997; 3: 1145–1149.
261. Park BJ, Brown CK, Hu Y, et al. Augmentation of melanoma-specific gene expression using a tandem melanocyte-specific enhancer results in increased cytotoxicity of the purine nucleoside phosphorylase gene in melanoma. *Hum Gene Ther* 1999; 10: 889–898.
262. Siders WM, Halloran PJ, Fenton RG. Melanoma-specific cytotoxicity induced by a tyrosinase promoter-enhancer/herpes simplex virus thymidine kinase adenovirus. *Cancer Gene Ther* 1998; 5: 281–291.
263. Eberle J, Garbe C, Wang NP, Orfanos CE. Incomplete expression of the tyrosinase gene family (tyrosinase, TRP-1, and TRP-2) in human malignant melanoma cells in vitro. *Pigment Cell Res* 1995; 8: 307–313.
264. Dong YB, Yang HL, Jane M, et al. Adenovirus-mediated E2F-1 gene transfer efficiently induces apoptosis in melanoma cells. *Cancer* 1999; 86: 2021–2033.
265. Kowalik TF, DeGregori J, Schwarz JK, Nevins JR. E2F1 overexpression in quiescent fibroblasts leads to induction of cellular DNA synthesis and apoptosis. *J Virol* 1995; 69: 2491–2500.
266. Phillips AC, Bates S, Ryan KM, Helin K, Vousden KH. Induction of DNA synthesis and apoptosis are separable functions of E2F-1. *Genes Dev* 1997; 11: 1853–1863.
267. Holmberg C, Helin K, Sehested M, Karlstrom O. E2F-1-induced p53-independent apoptosis in transgenic mice. *Oncogene* 1998; 17: 143–155.
268. DeGregori J, Leone G, Miron A, Jakoi L, Nevins JR. Distinct roles for E2F proteins in cell growth control and apoptosis. *Proc Natl Acad Sci USA* 1997; 94: 7245–7250.
269. Shan B, Farmer AA, Lee WH. The molecular basis of E2F-1/DP-1-induced S-phase entry and apoptosis. *Cell Growth Differ* 1996; 7: 689–697.
270. Trimarchi JM, Fairchild B, Verona R, Moberg K, Andon N, Lees JA. E2F-6, a member of the E2F family that can behave as a transcriptional repressor. *Proc Natl Acad Sci USA* 1998; 95: 2850–2855.
271. Cartwright P, Muller H, Wagener C, Holm K, Helin K. E2F-6: a novel member of the E2F family is an inhibitor of E2F-dependent transcription. *Oncogene* 1998; 17: 611–623.
272. Gaubatz S, Wood JG, Livingston DM. Unusual proliferation arrest and transcriptional control properties of a newly discovered E2F family member, E2F-6. *Proc Natl Acad Sci USA* 1998; 95: 9190–9195.
273. Kanitakis J, Montazeri A, Ghohestani R, Faure M, Claudy A. Bcl-2 oncoprotein expression in benign nevi and malignant melanomas of the skin. *Eur J Dermatol* 1995; 5: 501–507.
274. Rutberg SE, Goldstein IM, Yang YM, Stackpole CW, Ronai Z. Expression and transcriptional activity of AP-1, CRE, and URE binding proteins in B16 mouse melanoma subclones. *Mol Carcinog* 1994; 10: 82–87.
275. Saenz-Santamaria MC, Reed JA, McNutt NS, Shea CR. Immunohistochemical expression of BCL-2 in melanomas and intradermal nevi. *J Cutan Pathol* 1994; 21: 393–397.
276. Borner C, Schlagbauer Wadl H, Fellay I, Selzer E, Polterauer P, Jansen B. Mutated N-ras upregulates Bcl-2 in human melanoma in vitro and in SCID mice. *Melanoma Res* 1999; 9: 347–350.
277. Grossman D, McNiff JM, Li F, Altieri DC. Expression and targeting of the apoptosis inhibitor, survivin, in human melanoma. *J Invest Dermatol* 1999; 113: 1076–1081.
278. Madireddi MT, Dent P, Fisher PB. Regulation of mda-7 gene expression during human melanoma differentiation. *Oncogene* 2000; 19: 1362–1368.
279. Bar-Eli M. Role of AP-2 in tumor growth and metastasis of human melanoma. *Cancer Metastasis Rev* 1999; 18: 377–385.

280. Huang S, Jean D, Luca M, Tainsky MA, Bar-Eli M. Loss of AP-2 results in downregulation of c-KIT and enhancement of melanoma tumorigenicity and metastasis. *EMBO J* 1998; 17: 4358–4369.
281. Fournel M, Sapieha P, Beaulieu N, Besterman JM, MacLeod AR. Down-regulation of human DNA-(cytosine-5) methyltransferase induces cell cycle regulators p16(ink4A) and p21(WAF/Cip1) by distinct mechanisms. *J Biol Chem* 1999; 274: 24250–24256.
282. Milutinovic S, Knox JD, Szyf M. DNA methyltransferase inhibition induces the transcription of the tumor suppressor p21(WAF1/CIP1/sdi1). *J Biol Chem* 2000; 275: 6353–6359.
283. Ramchandani S, MacLeod AR, Pinard M, von Hofe E, Szyf M. Inhibition of tumorigenesis by a cytosine-DNA, methyltransferase, antisense oligodeoxynucleotide. *Proc Natl Acad Sci USA* 1997; 94: 684–689.
284. Slack A, Cervoni N, Pinard M, Szyf M. DNA methyltransferase is a downstream effector of cellular transformation triggered by simian virus 40 large T antigen. *J Biol Chem* 1999; 274: 10105–10112.
285. Halaban R, Ghosh S, Duray P, Kirkwood JM, Lerner AB. Human melanocytes cultured from nevi and melanomas. *J Invest Dermatol* 1986; 87: 95–101.
286. De Sepulveda P, Okkenhaug K, Rose JL, Hawley RG, Dubreuil P, Rottapel R. Socs1 binds to multiple signalling proteins and suppresses steel factor-dependent proliferation. *EMBO J* 1999; 18: 904–915.
287. Martin KJ, Kritzman BM, Price LM, et al. Linking gene expression patterns to therapeutic groups in breast cancer. *Cancer Res* 2000; 60: 2232–2238.
288. Perou CM, Jeffrey SS, van de Rijn M, et al. Distinctive gene expression patterns in human mammary epithelial cells and breast cancers. *Proc Natl Acad Sci USA* 1999; 96: 9212–9217.
289. Nacht M, Ferguson AT, Zhang W, et al. Combining serial analysis of gene expression and array technologies to identify genes differentially expressed in breast cancer. *Cancer Res* 1999; 59: 5464–5470.
290. Alizadeh AA, Eisen MB, Davis RE, et al. Distinct types of diffuse large B-cell lymphoma identified by gene expression profiling. *Nature* 2000; 403: 503–511.
291. Lai A, Marcellus RC, Corbeil HB, Branton PE. RBP1 induces growth arrest by repression of E2F-dependent transcription. *Oncogene* 1999; 18: 2091–2100.

12 Tumor Angiogenesis

Bela Anand-Apte, MBBS, PhD
and
Paul L. Fox, PhD

Contents

1. INTRODUCTION

As early as the 1960s, the observation of hyperemia and increased vascularity of tumors was considered to be due to a dilation of pre-existing host vessels stimulated by necrotic tumor products *(1,2)*. Despite early reports, that suggested this phenomenon could result from induction of new vessels rather than vasodilation *(3,4)*, a debate persisted about whether tumors were supplied by existing vessels or by neovascularization. Subsequent experiments, in which a transparent chamber was implanted into a rabbit ear, permitted the observation of angiogenesis in vivo *(5)*. Critical experiments which marked a turning point in the field were initiated in 1963 by Folkman and his collaborators *(6,7)*. They showed that tumors, implanted into isolated perfused organs, were restricted in their growth to spheroids of about 1 mm^3 or less. This limited growth was accompanied by a

From: *Current Clinical Oncology, Melanoma: Biologically Targeted Therapeutics*
Edited by: E. C. Borden

complete absence of angiogenesis, due to a degeneration of capillary endothelium following prolonged perfusion. However, when the tumor spheroid was transplanted to the mouse strain from which it originated, the tumors became vascularized and grew rapidly beyond the 1 mm^3 limit and killed their hosts.

The term angiogenesis was first used to describe the formation of new blood vessels in the placenta. It is defined as the sprouting of new capillary blood vessels in any tissue from preexisting capillaries and post-capillary venules. The establishment and maintenance of a patent vascular network appears to be a critical requirement for the growth of neoplastic tissues. It is now widely recognized that for a tumor to grow beyond a critical size, it must recruit endothelial cells from the surrounding stroma to form a network of blood vessels to feed itself and meet its increased metabolic requirements. With this idea in mind, much current research is aimed towards understanding the basic biology of neovascularization, as well as towards designing antiangiogenic therapies that may have potential usefulness as anticancer agents.

2. TUMORS ARE ANGIOGENESIS-DEPENDENT

2.1. The Hypothesis

"Once tumor take has occurred, every increase in tumor cell population must be preceded by an increase in new capillaries that converge upon the tumor" *(8)*.

2.2. The Evidence

Following the observations of restricted tumor growth in isolated perfused organs, a large body of evidence, both indirect and direct, has been amassed to test the hypothesis. These have been reviewed previously *(9,10)* and are summarized here:

1. Vascularization induced exponential growth of tumors in two experimental models, subcutaneous transparent chambers and avascular rabbit cornea *(4,11)*.
2. Tumors inoculated into the aqueous fluid of the anterior chamber of the eye were unable to grow beyond 1 mm^3, but were capable of inducing vascularization of the iris. Subsequent implantation of the tumor spheroid contiguous to the iris vessels resulted in an induction of tumor neovascularization and rapid growth *(12)*. Similarly, the vitreous of the rabbit eye permitted only slow tumor growth due to the lack of a vascular network. However, once the tumor reached the retinal surface, it became neovascularized and grew very rapidly *(13)*. In addition, in the avascular cornea, the rate of proliferation of tumor cells, as measured by the [^{3}H]thymidine labeling index, was seen as a gradient. The highest labeling index was observed in cells closest to an open capillary, and a decreased rate of proliferation was seen in cells further away from the capillary *(11)*.
4. Tumors implanted on the chick chorioallantoic membrane (CAM) were restricted in growth during the early avascular phase, but underwent rapid growth following vascularization *(14)*. In addition, tumors implanted on the CAMs of older embryos grew at slower rates corresponding to the alteration of endothelial turnover with age *(14)*.

5. Increased growth and metastasis of human melanoma was associated with the appearance of new blood vessels at the base of the tumor *(15)*.
6. In transgenic mice engineered to develop spontaneous carcinomas of the pancreatic islets, tumors arose from the subset of preneoplastic hyperplastic islets that had become vascularized *(16–18)*.
7. Subcutaneous injection of neoplastic cells in mice resulted in tumors that became vascularized at approximately 0.4 mm^3. As vascularization increased, the tumor size increased in parallel *(19)*.
8. In nude mice, growth of colon carcinoma lacking basic fibroblast growth factor (FGF) receptors increased following systemic injection of basic FGF. This stimulated an increase in the density and branching of blood vessels in the tumor. Neutralizing antibodies to basic FGF retarded the increase in tumor growth. This was the first direct evidence that changes in growth rate of tumor blood vessels directly regulated tumor growth *(20–22)*.
9. Fibroblasts, transfected with a cDNA encoding basic FGF, secreted the growth factor in vitro and stimulated angiogenesis and tumor formation when implanted into mice *(23)*. Neutralizing antibody to basic FGF resulted in decreased tumor neovascularization and tumor volume *(23)*.
10. Neutralizing antibody to vascular endothelial growth factor (VEGF) decreased the growth of several tumors that secreted VEGF *(24)*.
11. Introduction of a dominant-negative mutant of the VEGF receptor (Flk-1) into endothelial cells by retrovirus resulted in an inhibition of angiogenesis and growth of brain tumors in nude mice *(25,26)*.
12. Several angiogenesis inhibitors have been described, which inhibit tumor growth in vivo but not in vitro *(27–29)*.

The experiments described above presented strong experimental evidence that the expansion of a tumor cell population is dependent on the onset of angiogenesis. As a corollary, the absence of angiogenesis in the early preneovascular phase prevents the expansion and growth of the tumor irrespective of the proliferative capacity of the tumor cells.

3. ANGIOGENESIS AND TUMOR METASTASIS

Metastasis is a highly selective and sequential process involving tumor cell proliferation, invasion of basement membranes, evasion of host defenses, loss of adhesion, cell motility, embolization, adhesion and arrest, extravasation, and proliferation at the secondary site (*see* Fig. 1 for schematic). Besides its role in tumor expansion, it is now becoming increasingly clear that angiogenesis is a critical component of metastasis, and highly vascular tumors have the potential to produce metastases at a higher rate than less angiogenic tumors *(30)*. This idea is based on two principles. First, the number of circulating tumor cells shed from the primary tumor correlates directly with the cellular mass of the primary tumor *(31,32)*. Thus, if angiogenesis inhibition can reduce the growth of the primary

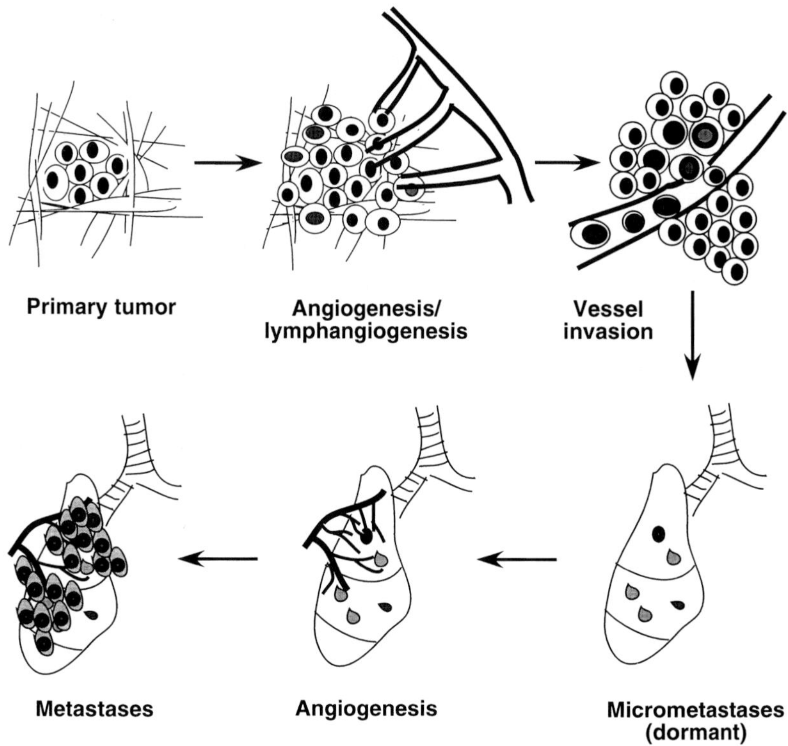

Fig. 1. Angiogenesis and tumor metastases.

tumor, then it, in turn, has the potential to inhibit the capacity of the tumor to form clinically relevant metastases. Secondly, increased vascularization provides the tumor with a larger surface area over which tumor cells and blood vessels interact, allowing a greater probability of the shedding of tumor cells into the blood stream. In addition, tumor angiogenesis induces vessels that are immature, highly permeable, and containing fewer intercellular junctional complexes, all of which facilitates the entry of tumor cells into the circulation.

The experimental evidence supporting a role for tumor angiogenesis in metastasis can be summarized as follows:

1. In animal models of cancer, treatment of the primary tumor with well-characterized angiogenesis inhibitors results in decreased vascularity of the tumors and a subsequent decrease in the formation of metastatic colonies *(33–45)*.
2. Metastases in liver and peritoneum rarely grow beyond a diameter of a few millimeters until after vascularization *(46)*.
3. Dormant micrometastases have increased rates of apoptosis secondary to decreased angiogenesis *(47)*.

4. Implantation of melanoma cells transfected with VEGF increases the number of lung metastases compared to controls *(48)*. Similarly, antibodies to VEGF can decrease metastases in experimental models. However, a recent study reports that the expression of VEGF in ciliochoroidal melanomas correlates with the presence of necrosis, but not with the occurrence of systemic metastases or tumor angiogenesis *(49)*.
5. Many studies in patients with a variety of cancers have shown a correlation between vascular density and increased metastases and decreased survival *(50–57)*.

It has been proposed that angiogenesis, primary tumor growth, and metastases are regulated by an imbalance of positive and negative effectors *(17,58)*. Given the heterogeneity of tumors, it is highly likely that the regulation of tumor angiogenesis is dependent on multiple organ- and tumor type-specific factors.

Endothelial cells and pericytes line newly-formed capillaries and have the potential to generate complete capillary networks. Formation of a primitive vascular plexus during development occurs following differentiation of angioblasts from mesoderm. Mesoderm-inducing factors of the fibroblast growth factor family *(59,60)*, as well as VEGF appear to be critical in this process. There is evidence for the existence of a bipotential hemangioblast (precursor for hematopoietic cells and angioblasts), but the factors that determine its commitment to the angioblastic or hematopoietic lineage have yet to be identified. Mouse embryos lacking the gene for VEGF-R2 exhibit a defect in both the hematopoietic as well as angioblast lineages, suggesting that this receptor and its ligands may play a critical role in this process *(61–65)*.

3.1. Sprouting and Nonsprouting Angiogenesis

Following the formation of the primary capillary plexus, new capillaries can be generated by sprouting or by splitting from their vessel of origin *(59)*. Sprouting angiogenesis is the process by which new capillaries are formed from preexisting blood vessels (Fig. 2A). It is a multistep process, requiring the degradation of the basement membrane, endothelial cell migration, capillary tube formation, and endothelial cell proliferation *(66,67)*. The process is usually initiated by a localized breakdown of the basement membrane of the parent vessel. A precise spatial and temporal regulation of extracellular proteolytic activity appears to be critical in this initial process of endothelial cell invasion into the extracellular matrix (ECM). Endothelial cells then migrate into the surrounding ECM within which they form a capillary sprout. Elongation of the sprout occurs by further migration and by endothelial cell proliferation behind the migrating front, resulting in the formation of a lumen. Anastomoses of contiguous tubular sprouts forms a functional capillary loop, which is followed by reconstitution of the basement membrane and vessel maturation.

Nonsprouting angiogenesis occurs by proliferation of endothelial cells inside a vessel, producing a wide lumen that can be split by transcapillary pillars of

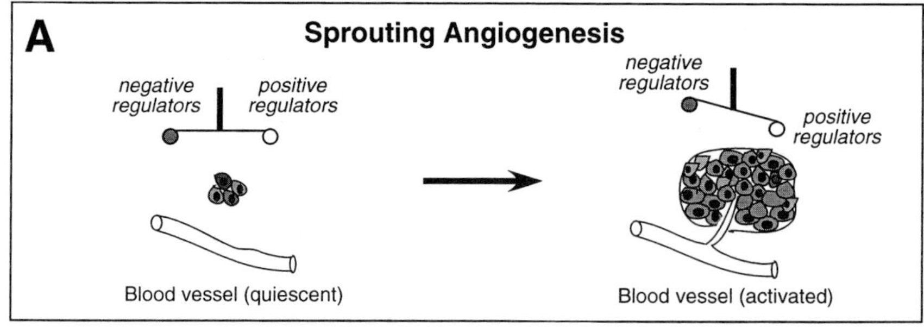
A
Sprouting Angiogenesis
negative regulators
positive regulators
Blood vessel (quiescent)
negative regulators
positive regulators
Blood vessel (activated)

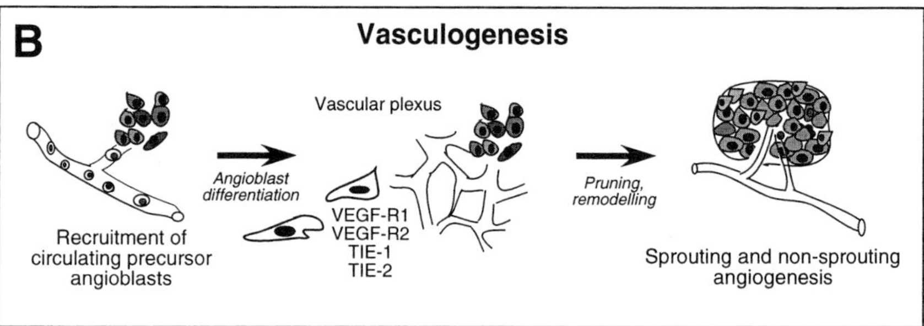
B
Vasculogenesis
Recruitment of circulating precursor angioblasts
Angioblast differentiation
Vascular plexus
VEGF-R1
VEGF-R2
TIE-1
TIE-2
Pruning, remodelling
Sprouting and non-sprouting angiogenesis

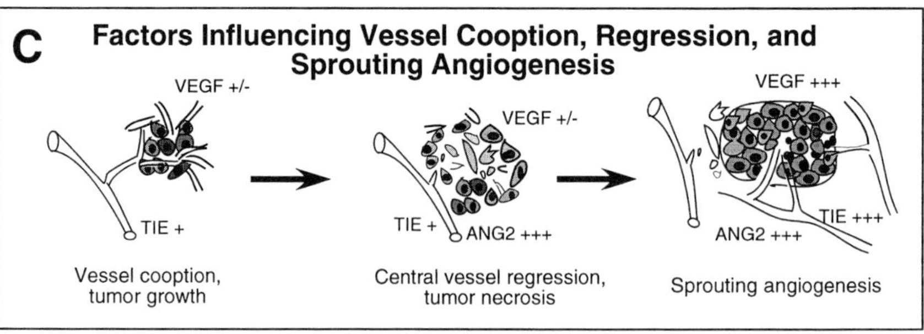
C
Factors Influencing Vessel Cooption, Regression, and Sprouting Angiogenesis
VEGF +/-
TIE +
Vessel cooption, tumor growth
VEGF +/-
TIE +
ANG2 +++
Central vessel regression, tumor necrosis
VEGF +++
TIE +++
ANG2 +++
Sprouting angiogenesis

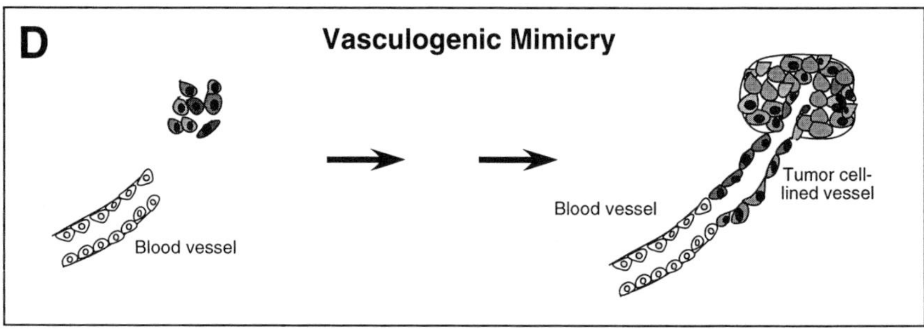
D
Vasculogenic Mimicry
Blood vessel
Blood vessel
Tumor cell-lined vessel

Fig. 2. Potential mechanisms of tumor angiogenesis.

extracellular matrix *(68)*. It is possible that both forms of angiogenesis occur concurrently in vivo. The presence of endogenous precursors, in addition to high vascularity, may predispose an organ to the nonsprouting form of angiogenesis, while the absence of angioblasts in an organ may stimulate sprouting angiogenesis under the appropriate conditions *(69)*. Targeted mutations of VEGF receptors and the Tie (tyrosine kinase that contains immunoglobulin-like loops and epidermal growth factor similar domains) ligands suggest that these factors may play an important role in both these processes *(70–73)*.

3.2. Pruning and Remodeling

Once the initial vascular plexus is formed, it is rapidly remodeled to generate a mature network of vessels (Fig. 2B). Excess endothelial cells generated by vasculogenesis are lost prior to the onset of circulation. The pruning of vessels may be due to a decrease in endothelial cell survival factors such as VEGF, first described in embryonic retina *(74)*. It is possible that pruned endothelial cells undergo apoptosis (although this has been difficult to demonstrate), or they may migrate to reassemble into other vessels, or they may simply dedifferentiate *(59)*. Factors regulating the pruning of the vascular network have yet to be determined. In addition, it is unclear whether this pruning is random or whether the spacing between invading sprouts is predetermined and tightly controlled.

3.3. Vessel Maturation

The mechanisms by which a newly forming vasculature becomes a stable mature vessel bed is unknown. This process of maturation includes, investment of vessels with mural cells (pericytes or smooth muscle cells), production of basement membrane, and induction of vessel bed specializations. Some have suggested that the process is initiated by circulating factors such as VEGF, transforming growth factor-β, tissue factor, and platelet-derived growth factor. Cell–cell interactions, as well as cell–matrix interactions, affecting the adhesion of endothelial cells may regulate maturation. Other signals, such as shear stress and hypoxia may also have important roles *(75)*. The physical association between a nascent vascular tube and mural cells, such as pericytes, may signal vessel stabilization by inhibiting endothelial cell proliferation *(76–78)* or growth factor dependence *(79)*. Angiopoietin (Ang)-1 and -2 are also believed to play a critical, albeit undefined, role in the stabilization process. The relationship between the maturation or regression of vessels and the tissue or organ they supply is complex and not well-understood. A number of questions have not yet been answered. For example: is the maturation process regulated in a tissue-specific manner? Are all vascular beds similar, or are there tissue-specific differences? What is the specific role of pericytes in the regulation of blood vessel maturation? What is the role of growth factors, specifically VEGF, and the basement membrane in this process? The mechanisms involved in the development of quiescent organ-specific and mature endothelium of the adult needs to be investigated in further detail.

While it is well-accepted that tumors acquire new blood vessels by the process of sprouting angiogenesis, some variations in this paradigm have been proposed recently. The incorporation of endothelial progenitors or angioblasts from circulating blood into sites of ischemia-driven angiogenesis suggests the possible utilization of these precursor cells in tumor angiogenesis *(80,81)*. A process of vessel co-option has been suggested in which tumors initially co-opt the existing vasculature, which then regresses causing necrosis, and the tumor is subsequently revascularized at the periphery by sprouting angiogenesis *(82,83)* (Fig. 2C). The possibility that cancer cells may themselves participate in the formation of blood vessels in tumors had been proposed as early as 1948 *(84)*. Subsequently, investigators using histological and ultrastructural techniques confirmed the contribution of cancer cells to wall formation of tumor vessels *(85–87)*. More recently the term "vasculogenic mimicry" has been ascribed to the process by which uveal melanomas generate nonendothelial lined channels delimited by ECM and surrounded by tumor cells *(88)* (Fig. 2D). Although this finding has created a controversy regarding methodologies and interpretations *(89,90)*, because of its potential significance, the presence and pathophysiological significance of tumor cells within tumor blood vessels merits further investigation.

Although tumor angiogenesis structurally resembles embryonic angiogenesis, it is likely that distinguishing factors are present. Whether physiological angiogenesis (ovarian cycle) and pathological angiogenesis (tumors) are regulated by similar mechanisms is still unclear. Also, it has not been shown definitively that the induced vessels are similar or identical. Clearly, additional processes are likely to be critical for the induction of neovascularization in tumors, for example cell cycle progression, induction of proteolysis, changes in cell adhesions and junctions, and imbalance of inducers and inhibitors of angiogenesis.

4. MICROVASCULATURE OF TUMORS

Tumor vessels differ from normal vessels both structurally as well as histologically. Most tumor vessels have an abnormal branching pattern and irregular diameter with thin walls that are not usually coated by mural cells *(91–97)*. Some tumor vessels exhibit an incomplete basement membrane and may show increased binding and uptake of cationic liposomes and abnormal expression of integrins and growth factors and their receptors when compared with normal vessels *(59,83,97)*. Tumor vessels have been shown to be unusually leaky *(94,98)*, which may enhance extravasation of plasma proteins and erythrocytes and even provide a permissive exit route for tumor cells to enter the blood stream and form metastases *(99)*. Increased expression of VEGF, structural transendothelial holes, vesiculo-vacuolar organelles, intercellular gaps, and fenestrae have been reported in the endothelium of tumor vessels and may all contribute to the leakiness observed *(100)*. Tumor vessels have been described with a defective cellular lining composed of disorganized branched, loosely connected, and overlapping endothelial cells *(101)*. This abnormal endothelial structure may contribute significantly to tumor vessel leakiness. The possible participation of tumor cells in formation of the blood vessel wall *(88)* may also contribute significantly to alterations in vessel wall properties.

5. REGULATION OF ANGIOGENESIS

In healthy adults, endothelial cell turnover is generally extremely slow except during the response to tissue injury and in the female reproductive organs. Endothelial cells are thought to be maintained in a quiescent state by a balance of endogenous pro-angiogenic and antiangiogenic factors. Multiple in vitro and in vivo bioassays have been developed to screen for potential angiogenesis inducers (and inhibitors). These assays were designed to apparently mimic the complex process of angiogenesis *(102)*. Measurement of in vitro endothelial cell proliferation and migration have been widely used to screen for potential angiogenesis regulatory molecules *(103)*. Because of their inherent limitations, these assays are usually complemented by in vivo assays, such as implantation into chick CAM or into the avascular cornea of rabbits or rodents (corneal micropocket assay). Factors that regulate angiogenesis are often derived from tumor cells, stroma, and infiltrating cells such as macrophages and fibroblasts (*see* Fig. 3 for schematic). Multiple factors have been identified that have angiogenesis-inducing properties in experimental settings (Table 1). However, in most cases, their role in physiological and pathological regulation of neovascularization in an intact organism has not been proven.

5.1. Vascular Endothelial Growth Factor

VEGF is the most potent direct-acting angiogenic protein and appears to fulfill most of the criteria of being an endogenous physiological positive regulator of angiogenesis *(61,62,65,104)*. It is a diffusible endothelial cell-specific growth factor, which acts by stimulating a family of primarily endothelial cell-specific receptor tyrosine kinases including Flk-1/KDR/VEGFR-2, Flt-1/VEGFR-1, and Flt-4/VEGFR-3 *(105)*. More recently, it has been reported that VEGF splice variants differentially bind to a novel VEGF receptor, neuropilin-1, which is highly expressed by tumor cells *(106)*. Analysis of genetically engineered mice lacking VEGF, or its receptors Flt-1 or KDR, confirms the critical role of these molecules in blood vessel development. VEGF and its receptor, KDR/Flk-1, are required for the initial stages of endothelial differentiation and vascular development in the embryo. Melanoma cell lines have been shown to express

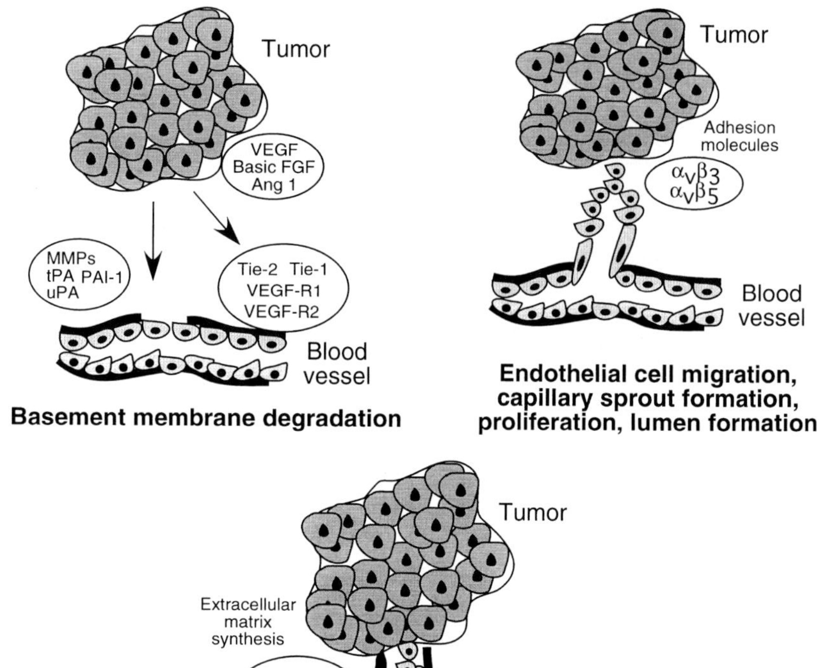

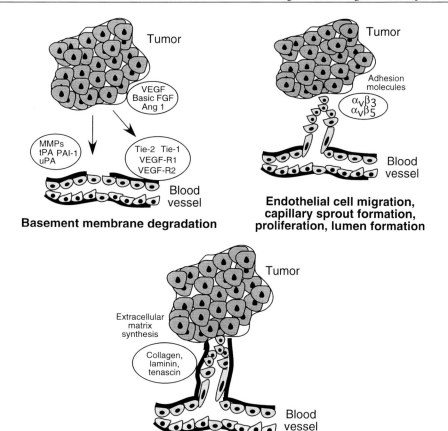

Fig. 3. Morphogenetic events and factors involved in tumor-induced angiogenesis.

the VEGF receptor, KDR, and respond to exogenously added VEGF, suggesting that VEGF may play a role in autocrine as well as paracrine stimulation of melanoma growth *(107)*, particularly in response to hypoxia *(108)*. VEGF expression is up-regulated by oxygen deprivation *(109–111)* and mediated in some cases by adenosine *(112,113)* via up-regulation of the KDR receptor *(114)*. VEGF is also induced by cytokines such as interleukin (IL)-1β *(115)* and IL-6 *(116)*, altered tumor suppressor genes *(117,118)*, oncogenes such as v-Raf and v-Src *(119,120)*, growth factors such as transforming growth factor-β *(121)* and insulin-like growth factor *(122)*, and hormones such as progestins and estrogen *(123,124)*. Four additional VEGF-related molecules, VEGF-B, VEGF-C, VEGF-D, and placenta growth factor (PlGF) have been identified *(125)*. There appears to be a heterogenous expression of VEGF and VEGF-related molecules in human

Table 1
Positive Regulators of Angiogenesis

Angiogenic factor	*MW (daltons)*	*In vivo angiogenesis assay*	*EC migration*	*EC mitogen*	*References*
Angiogenin	14,100	Rabbit cornea	↑	–	*255*
		Chick CAM			
Angiopoietin-1	55,000			–	
Fibroblast growth factor, basic acidic	18,000	Rabbit cornea	↑	+	*256,257*
	16,400	Chick CAM	↑	+	
Granulocyte colony-stimulating factor	17,000	Rabbit cornea	↑	+	*258,259*
Hepatocyte growth factor	92,000	Rat cornea	↑	+	*260–262*
Interleukin-8	40,000	Rat cornea	↑	+	*263*
Placental growth factor	25,000	Rabbit cornea	↑	±	*264*
		Chick CAM			
Platelet-derived endothelial growth factor	45,000	Rat cornea	↑	+	*265*
		Chick CAM			
Proliferin	35,000	Rat cornea	↑	+	*266,267*
Transforming growth factor-α	5,500	Hamster cheek pouch	↑	+	*268*
Transforming growth factor-β	25,000	Newborn mouse skin	No	±	*269*
		Chick CAM			
Tumor necrosis factor-α	17,000	Rat cornea	↑	–	*270–272*
		Chick CAM			
Vascular endothelial growth factor	45,000	Rat cornea	↑	+	*273–275*
		Chick CAM			
		Transgenic mice			

Effect of angiogenic factors on EC migration, proliferation, and in vivo argiogenesis. EC, endothelial cell; CAM, check chorioallantoic membrane; ↑, induction of EC migration; +, induction of EC proliferation; –, no induction of EC proliferation.

neoplasms *(126)*. VEGF-C and VEGF-D may play a role in lymphangiogenesis and lymph node metastasis.

Tumors in their initial state of avascular growth may be hypoxic due to insufficient vascularization. This hypoxia up-regulates the production of VEGF, which then contributes to the initiation of tumor-associated angiogenesis *(127)*. Human melanoma cell lines (SKMEL-2), which express minimal constitutive and hypoxia-inducible VEGF, produce small poorly vascularized tumors in immunodeficient mice *(48)*. Overexpression of VEGF in these cells results in the ability to form large vascularized tumors with hyperpermeable blood vessels and minimal necrosis along with increased tumor colonization in the lung *(48)*. Cellular expression of VEGF and its receptors appears to correlate directly with tumor aggressiveness and metastatic capability. Consistent with this hypothesis, several approaches using anti-VEGF therapies have been used to slow the growth of tumors *(24,25,128–130)*. Recently, VEGF has been shown to have an important role in promoting the survival of new vessels induced by tumors that have not been stabilized by interactions with ECM and supporting cells *(79,131)*. Thus, the anti-VEGF therapies currently under study may be useful, not only for suppressing angiogenesis, but also for their potential to cause regression of tumor vessels that are immature and tenuous in nature.

5.2. Angiopoietins

Ang-1 and -2 are recently identified ligands for the Tie2 receptor *(72,73, 132,133)*. Ang-mediated responses appear to be endothelium-specific due to the restricted expression of Tie2 receptors to the endothelium. Genetically engineered mice, which lack the Tie2 receptor, die later than those that lack VEGF or VEGF receptors, suggesting that the Tie2 receptor and its ligands exert their effects during the later stages of embryonic blood vessel development. Some evidence suggests that Tie2 regulates the ability of endothelial cells to recruit stromal cells and pericytes surrounding the endothelial tubes in order to stabilize vascular integrity *(70,134)*. Transgenic mice, which overexpress Ang-1, show a marked increase in vascularization, which may result from vascular remodeling and inhibition of vascular pruning *(135)*. Ang-1 may also have a role in the stabilization of blood vessels by promoting the survival of differentiated endothelial cells *(136,137)*. Ang-2 is a naturally occurring antagonist of the Ang-1/Tie2 receptor interaction *(132)*. Expression patterns of Ang-1 and Ang-2 in vivo have led to the proposal that Ang-2 plays a facilitative role at sites of vascular remodeling by blocking the constitutive stabilizing action of Ang-1. The destabilizing activity of Ang-2 in the presence of high levels of VEGF may prime the vessels to mount an angiogenic response. In contrast, destabilization of the vessels by Ang-2 in the absence of VEGF leads to vessel regression.

Recent studies of the role of angiopoietins in tumor angiogenesis suggest that the prevailing view, that most tumors originate as avascular masses and sub-

Table 2
Negative Regulators of Angiogenesis

Factor	*Inhibits endothelial cell migration*	*Presence in the circulation*	*Presence in the ECM*	*References*
Angiostatin	Yes	Yes	nt	*147*
Endostatin	Yes	Yes	nt	*42,150*
Angiopoietin-2	Yes	nt	nt	*276*
Interferon-α	Yes	Yes	nt	*153,277,278*
Placental proliferin-related protein	Yes	Yes	nt	*266*
Platelet factor 4	Yes	Yes	No	*279,280*
Prolactin (16-kDa fragment)	Yes	nt	nt	*281,282*
Thrombospondin 1	Yes	Yes	Yes	*283–286*
Tissue inhibitors of metalloproteinases:				
TIMP-1	No	Yes	No	*239,240*
TIMP-2	No	Yes	No	*287*
TIMP-3	Yes	nt	Yes	*159*

nt, not tested

sequently induce angiogenic support, may require modification *(82,83,138)*. These studies have led to an alternate hypothesis in which there is rapid co-opting of host vessels by an establishing tumor to form an initially well-vascularized tumor mass. This process is followed by a widespread regression of co-opted vessels by an apoptotic mechanism, which may involve a disruption of interactions of endothelial cells with the surrounding ECM and stromal cells, leading to avascular necrosis of the tumor. The tumor then mounts an angiogenic response at its rim, leading to secondary growth of the tumor. It should be noted, however, that newly formed tumor vessels are tenuous, poorly differentiated, and unstable. It is possible that continued expression of Ang-2 by newly formed vessels leads to a persistent blocking of Tie2 signaling, which prevents vessel maturation and stabilization.

Endogenous inhibitors of angiogenesis have been identified that counterbalance the effects of positive regulators of angiogenesis (Table 2). These have been reviewed previously *(139)* and are discussed in Subheadings 5.3.–5.6. briefly and in more detail in Chapter 13.

5.3. Thrombospondin

Thrombospondin (TSP1) is an extracellular matrix glycoprotein, which is a potent inhibitor of angiogenesis in both in vitro (endothelial cell proliferation

[140], migration *[140]*, and morphogenesis *[141]*) and in vivo assays *(142)*. The antiangiogenic activity of TSP1 correlates with the expression of a tumor suppressor gene *(143)*. In human bladder cancers, the expression of TSP1 has been shown to be inversely related to p53 expression and angiogenesis *(144)*. The antiangiogenic region of TSP1 maps to the type 1 (properdin) repeats. Based on sequence homology with these regions, two proteins METH-1 and METH-2 (containing metalloproteinase and disintegrin sequences) have been identified and shown to have antiangiogenic properties *(145)*.

5.4. Angiostatin and Endostatin

Angiostatin, a 38-kDa fragment of the clotting cascade protease precursor plasminogen, was the first tumor-derived angiogenesis inhibitor to be isolated *(146)*. After systemic administration, purified angiostatin results in apoptosis in metastases *(47)* and can sustain the dormancy of several human tumors implanted subcutaneously into nude mice *(147)*. Macrophage-derived metalloelastase is responsible for the generation of angiostatin in Lewis lung carcinoma *(148)*. The angiogenesis inhibitor endostatin is a 20-kDa C-terminal fragment of collagen XVIII, a proteoglycan–collagen found in vessel walls and basement membranes *(149,150)*. The generation of endostatin or endostatin-like collagen XVIII fragments is catalyzed by proteolytic enzymes, including cathepsin L *(151)* and metalloelastase *(152)*, which cleave peptide bonds within the protease-sensitive hinge region of the C-terminal domain. In experimental settings, endostatin is a potent inhibitor of tumor growth and metastasis *(42)*.

5.5. Interferon

Interferons have antiangiogenic activity in vivo *(153)*. Hemangioma growth is inhibited by interferon *(154,155)*, and this effect may be mediated by its ability to block the production or activity of angiogenic factors produced by tumor cells *(156)*.

5.6. Metalloproteinase Inhibitors

Matrix metalloproteinases (MMPs) may be important regulators of angiogenesis as well as tumor metastasis *(157,158)*. Naturally occurring MMP inhibitors, known as tissue inhibitor of metalloproteinases (TIMPs) are potent inhibitors of angiogenesis and tumor growth *(157–160)*. A protein with TIMP-like domains and potent antiangiogenic activity has been isolated from cartilage *(161)*. These enzymes are also involved in the processing of angiogenic regulators such as FGF receptor-1, tumor necrosis factor (TNF)-α, and TNF-α receptor ectodomain, as well as the angiogenesis inhibitors, angiostatin, and endostatin *(158)*.

The vasculature in the normal adult mammal is usually quiescent except during the process of ovulation, menstruation, implantation, and pregnancy in the female reproductive cycle. A tightly regulated balance between positive and negative endogenous regulators of angiogenesis has been hypothesized to keep the endothelial cells quiescent (Fig. 2A). Thus, the switch to the angiogenic state may involve either the loss or inactivation of a negative regulator, the induction of a positive regulator, or both.

6. ANGIOGENIC SWITCH IN TUMORS

The dependence of tumor growth and metastases on the establishment and maintenance of a vascular supply raises a question on the temporal nature of these events, specifically, when is angiogenesis activated during the development of a tumor? Using transgenic mouse models of cancer, as well as human tumors, the patterns and mechanisms of the angiogenic switch that occurs during tumorigenesis are beginning to be elucidated *(17)*. It is now evident that the angiogenic switch often occurs during the early preneoplastic stages in the development of the tumor and may be a rate-limiting step in the progression of the cancer. These studies were done in transgenic mice with modeled multistage tumorigenesis, such as insulinomas in RIP-Tag transgenic mice *(16)*, dermal fibrosarcoma *(162)*, and squamous carcinoma *(163–165)*. In addition, human cancers such as breast cancers *(166–168)*, cervical carcinoma *(163,169)*, and cutaneous melanomas *(170)* showed a similar stage-specific angiogenic switch during their development. The balance between angiogenic inducers and inhibitors is thought to play a major role in the development of the angiogenic switch. Under normal physiological settings endogenous angiostatic molecules may counteract and balance the constitutive expression of endogenous angiogenic factors to keep the growth of new capillaries in check. Tumor suppressor genes such as p53 and oncogenes can play a role in maintaining this balance, enabling them to interfere with or induce the tumor phenotype of which angiogenesis is a major component *(171,172)*. Another mechanism of inducing the angiogenic switch may be the release of sequestered inducers and/or inhibitors. Several angiogenic factors, for example VEGF and basic FGF, are sequestered in the ECM and are, therefore, unavailable for stimulation of angiogenesis. Matrix breakdown by proteases may release these factors, which in turn activate endothelial cells. It is becoming evident that a subset of angiogenesis inhibitors are cryptic fragments of larger molecules, which by themselves do not possess angiostatic properties. Release of these fragments from the parent molecule by proteases or sequestration in the parent protein may contribute to the delicate balance that regulates angiogenesis. Thus, integrity of matrix, as well as proteins that house angiostatic fragments, may be critical targets utilized by both host defenses, as well as tumors during tumorigenesis. Finally, keeping in mind the possibility that the tumor cells themselves may form the vessels that supply blood to the tumor, the angiogenic switch may also include a change in the aggressive tumor cells, which allows them to metamorphose into vessels that could provide microcirculation to itself *(173)*.

Whether the angiogenic switch results from increased inducers or decreased inhibitors of angiogenesis (or both) is unclear. Multiple strategies for increasing activator levels or reducing inhibitor levels may be utilized by different tissues and tumor types. It is possible that tissues, which are well-demarcated from the vasculature by basement membrane and stroma, such as epidermis, may favor increases in positive regulators to induce angiogenesis. Endocrine organs such as pancreatic islets, which are in close proximity to blood vessels at all times, may utilize angiogenic inhibitors to maintain a quiescent state. Thus, a decrease in inhibitor activity may contribute to tumor growth in this milieu.

Inadequate vascularization of tumors has been classically believed to induce necrotic cell death. However, apoptotic cell death of tumor cells has also been shown to occur in the presence of angiogenesis inhibitors. Some angiogenesis inhibitors can induce endothelial cell apoptosis, and this may contribute to loss of neovascularization. With this evidence in hand, it is important to consider the design of therapeutic strategies targeting the angiogenic switch in cancers, which have been detected early, as well as those aimed at ongoing neovascularization in well-established tumors.

7. QUANTITATION OF ANGIOGENESIS

Measurement of blood vessel density in a tumor is a direct measurement of its vascular status. Immunohistochemistry of the tumor microvasculature using endothelial cell-specific antibodies such as Factor VIII-related antigen (von Willebrand Factor; vWF), CD31, and CD34 permits the quantitation of vessels within a specified area of the tumor *(174)*. The quantitation can be done by several methods, including image analysis to count vessels in a high-powered field *(175)* or by calculating the number of instances that a grid overlies a vessel *(176)*.

The potential role of vessel counts in prognosis was shown by Weidner and his collaborators in 1991 *(50)*. Subsequently, several tumor types have been studied to assess the potential of tumor microvessel density (MVD) as a prognostic marker in progressive cancers. Quantitation of microvessels has been shown to have some value in predicting the behaviors of malignant melanoma *(15,177)*, gastric carcinoma *(55)*, prostatic carcinoma *(54)*, head and neck tumors *(57)*, and node-negative non-small cell carcinoma of the lung *(178)*. Many studies have subsequently examined the prognostic value of microvessel density in breast cancer and the findings to date have been conflicting. Several reports show a strong association between microvessel density and survival *(168,179–183)*. However, there are reports that do not find this association *(184–189)*. This discrepancy may be due to the variability in the methodology utilized to assess angiogenesis, as well as the heterogeneity of cancers. There is not a consensus on the preferred endothelial antigen for immunohistochemical detection. In addition, methods of tissue fixation and antigen retrieval may modify reactivity. A major factor contributing to methodological discrepancies may be the quantification of microvessels. Although guidelines *(174)* have been set and apparently followed, variability occurs between analyses performed by different people on the same region of similar tumors *(185)*. One of the requirements for assessment of MVD is that the section be scanned at low magnification to select neovascular "hot spots" prior to analyses, which introduces an element of unavoidable subjectivity to the measurements. A recent study, however, does provide evidence that the Chalkely score, when applied in series from different centers, showed a good agreement among pathologists and had prognostic value *(190)*.

Quantitation of MVD gives an indication of a tissue vascularization, but does not necessarily reflect angiogenic activity. Few studies have quantitated angiogenic activity by assessing the percentage of proliferating endothelial cells *(191,192)* and the recruitment of pericytes *(193)* in human tumors. In general, considerable heterogeneity was observed in the degree of active angiogenesis within each tumor, as well as between different tumor types. Surprisingly, even in the most angiogenic tumors, angiogenesis was far less intense than the physiologic angiogenesis observed in granulation tissue and the growing ovarian corpus rubrum. Furthermore, intratumoral endothelial cell proliferation index in prostatic carcinoma and breast carcinoma did not correlate with intratumoral MVD *(194,195)*.

The use of specific marker molecules, which quantitate active angiogenesis during MVD measurements, may provide better specificity in determining the angiogenic index of a tumor. New methods for detection of angiogenic activity in tumors have been developed and are being currently evaluated. The measurement of angiogenic factors as tumor markers has been under investigation *(196–199)*. VEGF protein is expressed in human breast cancer *(126,200,201)*, and correlations have been made between VEGF expression and angiogenesis *(202,203)*. Serum VEGF is elevated in patients with aggressive breast cancers *(204,205)* and colorectal cancer *(206)*. Serum levels of basic FGF are also increased in patients with a wide variety of cancers *(206–213)*. These retrospective studies suggest that angiogenic factors play an important role in the progression of various solid tumors. More recent studies have assessed in tumors the expression of specific integrins *(214)*, microvascular permeability utilizing contrast-enhanced magnetic resonance imaging *(215)*, and angiogenic peptides in the cytosol by immunoassay *(216)*.

Microvascular patterns are good prognostic indicators for uveal melanomas *(217–220)*. Recent studies suggest that interactions between microvascular patterns, cell-type, and tumor location may modify their relative prognostic ability. Microvascular patterns have predicted poor outcome of choroidal melanomas, but have had no prognostic power for tumors of the ciliary body *(221,222)*. It is, thus, critical that additional prospective studies be done on a large number of patients to assess the clinical utility of using angiogenic index as a prognostic marker for various tumors *(223)*. Novel imaging techniques in combination with improved MVD analysis will be necessary to consistently identify the angiogenic index of individual tumor patients.

It is likely that the value of assessing angiogenic activity will be dependent on the tumor type being investigated. Vessel count is a stronger prognostic factor than nodal status in a number of studies *(179,224)*. Besides being prognostic indicators, the ability to assess angiogenic activity may be useful as a guide to therapy. If patients with highly angiogenic tumors are more likely to develop distant metastases, then this group of patients will most likely require adjuvant therapy, which include the use of antiangiogenic agents.

8. THERAPEUTIC TARGETING OF TUMOR ANGIOGENESIS

The inhibition of angiogenesis in tumors is an attractive therapeutic strategy currently in clinical trials. Conceptually, this approach has multiple advantages. Since physiological angiogenesis occurs only rarely in a healthy adult (wound healing and menstrual cycle), therapies targeting pathological angiogenesis may be highly specific and have minimal adverse side effects. In addition, since the development of neovascularization is a physiological host response, pharmacological inhibition of this process may not be susceptible to developed resistance *(225)*. This contrasts with therapies targeting tumor cell determinants, which change according to selection pressures *(226)*. Based on the described molecular mechanisms and morphogenetic events involved in angiogenesis, approaches using endogenous as well as synthetic molecules have been undertaken to inhibit tumor-induced neovascularization *(227)* (Table 3).

8.1. Inhibition of VEGF and VEGF Receptor Signaling

Inhibitors of angiogenic cytokines, e.g., neutralizing antibodies to VEGF and specific inhibitors of VEGF receptors and their downstream targets, are attractive candidates as antiangiogenic agents. Several additional strategies have been utilized for the same purpose, including the use of soluble VEGF receptors, antisense VEGF, dominant-negative truncated form of VEGF receptor-2, and a VEGF-toxin conjugate *(228,229)*.

8.2. Inhibition of Endothelial Cell Function

TNP-470 is a synthetic derivative of fumagillin, which is an angiostatic product of the fungus *Aspergillus fumigatus fresenius* and inhibits the proliferation of endothelial cells. Phase II studies with this agent are ongoing for several solid tumor types. α_v/β_3 integrin is a receptor for vitronectin and is important in endothelial cell adhesion to ECM. Vitaxin, a humanized monoclonal antibody (LM609) against α_v/β_3 integrin, inhibits tumor neovascularization and subsequent growth in preclinical studies *(214,230)*.

Table 3
Antiangiogenic Therapeutic Strategies in Clinical Trials *(288)*

Agent	*Source/function/trial status*
Endogenous inhibitors	
Angiostatin	Plasminogen fragment.
Endostatin	Collagen XVIII fragment/phase I solid tumors.
Interleukin-12	Induces interferon-gamma-inducible protein-10/ phase I/II Kaposis sarcoma.
Angiopoietin 2	Inhibits angiopoietin-1 and blood vessel maturation.
Interferon-α	Inhibition of VEGF and basic FGF production/ phase III infant hemangiomas.
Platelet Factor 4	Inhibits endothelial cell proliferation.
Biological antagonists	
VEGF Inhibitors	Humanized neutralizing antibody/ phase I refractory solid tumors, phase II metastatic renal cancer antisense oligonucleotides.
VEGF Receptor Blockers	Receptor tyrosine kinase antagonists, SU5416/phase II prostate cancer, colorectal cancer, metastatic melanoma, multiple myeloma, malignant mesothelioma/ phase III metastatic colorectal cancer. SU 6668/phase I advanced tumors.
Soluble Receptors	Angiogenesis inhibition with soluble VEGF or Tie2 receptors.
α_v/β_3 Integrin Antagonists	Induction of apoptosis by monoclonal antibodies LM609 and 9G2.1.3.
Synthetic inhibitors	
Metalloproteinase Inhibitors	Marimastat/phase III non-small cell lung carcinoma, small cell lung carcinoma, breast cancers. AG3340/phase III non-small cell lung carcinoma, hormone refractory prostate cancer. COL-3/phase I/II brain tumors. Neovastat/phase III renal cell cancer, non-small cell lung carcinoma. BMS-275291/phase I.
Thalidomide	Phase I/II advanced melanoma. Phase II head and neck cancer ovarian, metastatic prostate and Kaposis sarcoma, gynecologic sarcomas, liver cancer/phase III non-small cell lung carcinoma, renal cancer, refractory multiple myeloma.
Squalamine	Inhibits sodium-hydrogen exchanger, NHE3/phase II non-small cell lung cancer, ovarian cancer.

(continued)

Table 3 *(continued)*

Agent	*Source/function/trial status*
Synthetic inhibitors	
Combretastatin A-4 Prodrug	Induction of apoptosis in proliferating endothelial cells/ phase I solid tumors.
TNP-470	Inhibits endothelial cell migration and proliferation/phase III breast carcinoma, Kaposis sarcoma, cervical carcinoma.
CAI (carboxyamidotriazole)	Calcium channel blocker/ phase III non-small cell lung cancer, phase II ovarian cancer, advanced renal cancer.

8.3. Matrix Metalloproteinase Inhibitors

Endothelial cell invasion of the ECM is an initiating step during angiogenesis. The importance of matrix protease activity in angiogenic responses is supported by several lines of evidence: (*i*) angiogenic factors induce the synthesis of matrix proteases by endothelial cells *(231–236)*; (*ii*) antiangiogenic activity of interferon and glucocorticoids correlate with their ability to inhibit the induction of matrix protease genes *(237)*; (*iii*) antiprotease antibodies and protease inhibitors, such as phenanthroline, block angiogenesis *(234,238)*; and (*iv*) endogenous tissue inhibitors of MMPs TIMP-1, TIMP-2, and TIMP-3 inhibit angiogenic responses in vitro and in vivo *(159,161,238–240)*. Synthetic MMP inhibitors, alone or in combination with other angiogenesis inhibitors, are being assessed in clinical trials. These approaches are directed against the development of newly formed blood vessels rather than established vessels and, thus, may be more beneficial as adjuvant therapies perhaps to prevent the growth of dormant micrometastases.

8.4. Endogenous Inhibitors of Angiogenesis

More recently, two endogenous angiogenesis inhibitors derived from tumors, angiostatin and endostatin, have been shown to be potent inducers of tumor regression *(42,146)*. Repeated cycles of antiangiogenic therapy with endostatin has been shown to result in prolonged tumor dormancy without further treatment *(225)*. Endostatin has recently entered phase I clinical trials. Interferon-α2a has already been shown to be efficacious in inducing early resolution of juvenile hemangiomas, and this effect may be mediated by its antiangiogenic activity *(241,242)*.

8.5. Vascular Targeting

Another approach being tested is that of vasculature-targeted chemotherapy. This involves the destruction of tumor blood vessels with cytotoxic agents by utilizing specific molecular determinants of newly formed vessels. Endothelial cells involved in pathological angiogenesis appear to be quite distinct from their counterparts in mature blood vessels, and these differences may be exploited for drug delivery *(227)*. Additionally, this approach may minimize the problems of poor tissue penetration and drug resistance seen with conventional tumor targeting *(243)*. Phage display has identified proteins containing the Arg-Gly-Asp (RGD) (α_v integrin-binding) and Asn-Gly-Arg (NGR) motifs as specific for tumor-induced endothelial cells, and, thus, as potential vehicles for drug delivery *(244,245)*. RGD peptides target the α_v/β_3 integrin dimer expressed on endothelial cells only during angiogenesis. Preliminary studies coupling the anticancer drug doxorubicin to RGD or NGR peptides enhanced the efficacy of the drug against human breast cancer xenografts in nude mice and also reduced its toxicity *(246)*. Aminopeptidase N is a receptor for NGR tumor-homing peptide and can serve as a target for delivering drugs into tumors and inhibiting angiogenesis *(247)*. These results indicate that it may be possible to develop targeted chemotherapy strategies based on selective expression of receptors in tumor vasculature.

It has been established that growth of most tumors is angiogenesis-dependent; however, recent studies suggest that some tumors may grow without neovascularization if a suitable vascular bed is available. Investigations of the pattern of vascularization in a series of 500 primary stage I, non-small cell lung carcinomas determined that at least 16% (80/500) of the tumors grew in an alveolar-like way, along preexisting blood vessels, and were characterized by a lack of parenchymal destruction and absence of both tumor-associated stroma and new vessels *(248)*. It has thus been proposed that both angiogenesis-dependent and angiogenesis-independent growth may be present in the same tumor. This can explain discrepancies in intratumoral MVD counting studies. High intratumoral MVD counts may reflect active angiogenesis and poor prognosis, but on the other hand low MVD counts may not necessarily indicate a better prognosis. This may be an important consideration in designing strategies aimed to inhibit tumor growth by vascular targeting or by inhibition of angiogenesis.

Since most antiangiogenic therapies target active angiogenesis rather than established vessels, it seems unlikely that they will replace conventional cytotoxic therapy. Surprisingly, a number of research groups have demonstrated that a variety of conventional chemotherapeutic drugs exhibit significant antiangiogenic or antivascular effects, which can be potentiated by continuous low-dose therapy now termed "antiangiogenic scheduling" *(249)*. Improvement in therapeutic efficacy has been seen by combination of antiangiogenic drugs with conventional chemotherapy *(250)*. More recently, continuous low-dose therapy with vinblastine and VEGF receptor-2 antibody has been found to induce sustained tumor regression without any increase in toxicity *(251)*. These results suggest the need to optimize and evaluate combinatorial therapies with particular emphasis on antivascular dosing and scheduling characteristics, and their effects on different tumors.

Determination of the most effective method of delivery of anticancer drugs will be a critical issue in the future *(252)*. Specific and more effective delivery methods of the antiangiogenic recombinant proteins, synthetic molecules, or even genes themselves, targeted to the vascular bed of a tumor may provide improved therapeutic efficacy. Gene delivery systems such as adenovirus-mediated gene transfer *(253)*, direct DNA injection, and liposome-mediated gene transfer are all currently being tested *(254)*.

9. CONCLUSIONS

There is much variability in the mechanisms and regulation of tumor angiogenesis at different stages in the natural history of cancer. Thus, the therapeutic approaches will probably need to be different depending on the stage of cancer at the time of diagnosis. At this point, multimodality therapy, in which antiangiogenic strategies are combined with more conventional chemotherapy and/or radiotherapy, might prove to be most beneficial to the patient. A deeper understanding of the angiogenesis-dependent and -independent regulation of tumor growth and metastasis is likely to lead to the development of more efficient therapies.

ACKNOWLEDGMENT

This work was supported by National Institutes of Health grant no. R01 HL/CA54519 and National Aeronautics and Space Administration grant no. 96-HEDS-04 (to P.L.F.) and by National Institutes of Health grant no. R29 EY12109-03 (to B.A.-A.).

REFERENCES

1. Coman D, Sheldon W. The significance of hyperemia around tumor implants. *Am J Pathol* 1946; 22: 821–831.
2. Warren B, Greenblatt M, Kommineni V. Tumour angiogenesis: ultrastructure of endothelial cells in mitosis. *Br J Exp Pathol* 1972; 53: 216–224.
3. Ide A, Baker N, Warren SL. Vascularization of the Brown-Pearce rabbit epithelioma transplant as seen in the transparent ear chamber. *Am J Roentgenol* 1939; 42: 891–899.
4. Algire G, Chalkely H, Legallais F, et al. Vascular reactions of normal and malignant tumors in vivo. I. Vascular reactions of mice to wounds and to normal and neoplastic transplants. *J Natl Cancer Inst* 1945; 6: 73–85.
5. Clark E, Clark E. Microscopic observations on the growth of blood capillaries in the living mammal. *Am J Anat* 1939; 64: 251–301.
6. Folkman J. Tumor angiogenesis: therapeutic implications. *N Engl J Med* 1971; 285: 1182–1186.
7. Folkman J, Cole P, Zimmerman S. Tumor behaviour in isolated perfused organs: in vitro growth and metastasis of biopsy material in rabbit thyroid and canine intestinal segment. *Ann Surg* 1966; 164: 491–502.
8. Folkman J. *Biology of Endothelial Cells*. In: Jaffe E, ed. Martinus Nijhoff, Boston, 1984, pp. 412–428.

9. Folkman J. What is the evidence that tumors are angiogenesis dependent? *J Natl Cancer Inst* 1990; 82: 4–6.
10. Folkman J. Tumor angiogenesis. In: Mendelsohn J, Howley PM, Israel MA, Liotta LA, eds. *The Molecular Basis for Cancer*. W.B. Saunders, Philadelphia, 1995, pp. 206–232.
11. Gimbrone MJ, Cotran R, Leapman S, Folkman J. Tumor growth and neovascularization: an experimental model using the rabbit cornea. *J Natl Cancer Inst* 1974; 52: 413–427.
12. Gimbrone MJ, Leapman S, Cotran R, Folkman J. Tumor dormancy in vivo by prevention of neovascularization. *J Exp Med* 1972; 136: 261–276.
13. Brem S, Brem H, Folkman J, Finkelstein D, Patz A. Prolonged tumor dormancy by prevention of neovascularization in the vitreous. *Cancer Res* 1976; 36: 2807–2812.
14. Knighton D, Ausprunk D, Tapper D, Folkman J. Avascular and vascular phases of tumour growth in the chick embryo. *Br J Cancer* 1977; 35: 347–356.
15. Srivastava A, Laidler P, Davies RP, Horgan K, Hughes LE. The prognostic significance of tumor vascularity in intermediate-thickness (0.76–4.0 mm thick) skin melanoma. A quantitative histologic study. *Am J Pathol* 1988; 133: 419–423.
16. Folkman J, Watson K, Ingber D, Hanahan D. Induction of angiogenesis during the transition from hyperplasia to neoplasia. *Nature* 1989; 339: 58–61.
17. Hanahan D, Folkman J. Patterns and emerging mechanisms of the angiogenic switch during tumorigenesis. *Cell* 1996; 86: 353–364.
18. Hanahan D, Christofori G, Naik P, Arbeit J. Transgenic mouse models of tumour angiogenesis: the angiogenic switch, its molecular controls, and prospects for preclinical therapeutic models. *Eur J Cancer* 1996; 32A: 2386–2393.
19. Thompson WD, Shiach KJ, Fraser RA, McIntosh LC, Simpson JG. Tumours acquire their vasculature by vessel incorporation, not vessel ingrowth. *J Pathol* 1987; 151: 323–332.
20. Gross JL, Herblin WF, Dusak BA, Czerniak P, Diamond M, Dexter DL. Modulation of solid tumor growth in vivo by bFGF. *Proc Am Assoc Cancer Res* 1990; 31: 79.
21. Gross JL, Herblin WF, Eidsvoog K, Horlick R, Brem SS. Tumor growth regulation by modulation of basic fibroblast growth factor. *EXS* 1992; 61: 421–427.
22. Gross JL, Herblin WF, Dusak BA, et al. Effects of modulation of basic fibroblast growth factor on tumor growth in vivo. *J Natl Cancer Inst* 1993; 85: 121–131.
23. Hori A, Sasada R, Matsutani E, et al. Suppression of solid tumor growth by immunoneutralizing monoclonal antibody against human basic fibroblast growth factor. *Cancer Res* 1991; 51: 6180–6184.
24. Kim KJ, Li B, Winer J, et al. Inhibition of vascular endothelial growth factor-induced angiogenesis suppresses tumour growth in vivo. *Nature* 1993; 362: 841–844.
25. Millauer B, Shawver LK, Plate KH, Risau W, Ullrich A. Glioblastoma growth inhibited in vivo by a dominant-negative Flk-1 mutant. *Nature* 1994; 367: 576–579.
26. Millauer B, Longhi MP, Plate KH, et al. Dominant-negative inhibition of Flk-1 suppresses the growth of many tumor types in vivo. *Cancer Res* 1996; 56: 1615–1620.
27. Folkman J. New perspectives in clinical oncology from angiogenesis research. *Eur J Cancer* 1996; 32A: 2534–2539.
28. Folkman J. Angiogenesis research: from laboratory to clinic. *Forum (Genova)* 1999; 9: 59–62.
29. Folkman J. Angiogenesis in cancer, vascular, rheumatoid and other disease. *Nat Med* 1995; 1: 27–31.
30. Zetter B. Angiogenesis and tumor metastasis. *Annu Rev Med* 1998; 49: 407–424.
31. Fidler IJ. Metastasis: quantitative analysis of distribution and fate of tumor embolilabeled with 125 I-5-iodo-2'-deoxyuridine. *J Natl Cancer Inst* 1970; 45: 773–782.
32. Liotta LA, Kleinerman J, Saidel GM. Quantitative relationships of intravascular tumor cells, tumor vessels, and pulmonary metastases following tumor implantation. *Cancer Res* 1974; 34: 997–1004.

33. Taylor S, Folkman J. Protamine is an inhibitor of angiogenesis. *Nature* 1982; 297: 307–312.
34. Crum R, Szabo S, Folkman J. A new class of steroids inhibits angiogenesis in the presence of heparin or a heparin fragment. *Science* 1985; 230: 1375–1378.
35. D'Amato RJ, Loughnan MS, Flynn E, Folkman J. Thalidomide is an inhibitor of angiogenesis. *Proc Natl Acad Sci USA* 1994; 91: 4082–4085.
36. Ingber D, Fujita T, Kishimoto S, et al. Synthetic analogues of fumagillin that inhibit angiogenesis and suppress tumour growth. *Nature* 1990; 348: 555–557.
37. Konno H, Tanaka T, Matsuda I, et al. Comparison of the inhibitory effect of the angiogenesis inhibitor, TNP-470, and mitomycin C on the growth and liver metastasis of human colon cancer. *Int J Cancer* 1995; 61: 268–271.
38. Mori S, Ueda T, Kuratsu S, Hosono N, Izawa K, Uchida A. Suppression of pulmonary metastasis by angiogenesis inhibitor TNP-470 in murine osteosarcoma. *Int J Cancer* 1995; 61: 148–152.
39. Weinstat-Saslow DL, Zabrenetzky VS, VanHoutte K, Frazier WA, Roberts DD, Steeg PS. Transfection of thrombospondin 1 complementary DNA into a human breast carcinoma cell line reduces primary tumor growth, metastatic potential, and angiogenesis. *Cancer Res* 1994; 54: 6504–6511.
40. Weinstat-Saslow D, Steeg PS. Angiogenesis and colonization in the tumor metastatic process: basic and applied advances. *FASEB J* 1994; 8: 401–407.
41. O'Reilly MS, Holmgren L, Shing Y, et al. Angiostatin: a novel angiogenesis inhibitor that mediates the suppression of metastases by a Lewis lung carcinoma. *Cell* 1994; 79: 315–328.
42. O'Reilly MS, Boehm T, Shing Y, et al. Endostatin: an endogenous inhibitor of angiogenesis and tumor growth. *Cell* 1997; 88: 277–285.
43. Kolber DL, Knisely TL, Maione TE. Inhibition of development of murine melanoma lung metastases by systemic administration of recombinant platelet factor 4. *J Natl Cancer Inst* 1995; 87: 304–309.
44. Watson SA, Morris TM, Robinson G, Crimmin MJ, Brown PD, Hardcastle JD. Inhibition of organ invasion by the matrix metalloproteinase inhibitor batimastat (BB-94) in two human colon carcinoma metastasis models. *Cancer Res* 1995; 55: 3629–3633.
45. Watson SA, Morris TM, Parsons SL, Steele RJ, Brown PD. Therapeutic effect of the matrix metalloproteinase inhibitor, batimastat, in a human colorectal cancer ascites model. *Br J Cancer* 1996; 74: 1354–1358.
46. Lien WM, Ackerman NB. The blood supply of experimental liver metastases. II. A microcirculatory study of the normal and tumor vessels of the liver with the use of perfused silicone rubber. *Surgery* 1970; 68: 334–340.
47. Holmgren L, O'Reilly MS, Folkman J. Dormancy of micrometastases: balanced proliferation and apoptosis in the presence of angiogenesis suppression. *Nat Med* 1995; 1: 149–153.
48. Claffey KP, Brown LF, del Aguila LF, et al. Expression of vascular permeability factor/vascular endothelial growth factor by melanoma cells increases tumor growth, angiogenesis, and experimental metastasis. *Cancer Res* 1996; 56: 172–181.
49. Sheidow TG, Hooper PL, Crukley C, Young J, Heathcote JG. Expression of vascular endothelial growth factor in uveal melanoma and its correlation with metastasis. *Br J Ophthalmol* 2000; 84: 750–756.
50. Weidner N, Semple JP, Welch WR, Folkman J. Tumor angiogenesis and metastasis—correlation in invasive breast carcinoma. *N Engl J Med* 1991; 324: 1–8.
51. Gasparini G, Harris A. Clinical importance of the determination of tumor angiogenesis in breast carcinoma: much more than a new prognostic tool. *J Clin Oncol* 1995; 13: 765–782.
52. Gasparini G, Bevilacqua P, Bonoldi E, et al. Predictive and prognostic markers in a series of patients with head and neck squamous cell invasive carcinoma treated with concurrent chemoradiation therapy. *Clin Cancer Res* 1995; 1: 1375–1383.

53. Ellis LM, Takahashi Y, Fenoglio CJ, Cleary KR, Bucana CD, Evans DB. Vessel counts and vascular endothelial growth factor expression in pancreatic adenocarcinoma. *Eur J Cancer* 1998; 34: 337–340.
54. Weidner N, Carroll PR, Flax J, Blumenfeld W, Folkman J. Tumor angiogenesis correlates with metastasis in invasive prostate carcinoma. *Am J Pathol* 1993; 143: 401–409.
55. Maeda K, Chung YS, Takatsuka S, et al. Tumor angiogenesis as a predictor of recurrence in gastric carcinoma. *J Clin Oncol* 1995; 13: 477–481.
56. Wiggins D, Granai C, Steinhoff M, Calabresi P. Tumor angiogenesis as a prognostic factor in cervical carcinoma. *Gynecol Oncol* 1995; 56: 353–356.
57. Gasparini G, Weidner N, Maluta S, et al. Intratumoral microvessel density and p53 protein: correlation with metastasis in head-and-neck squamous-cell carcinoma. *Int J Cancer* 1993; 55: 739–744.
58. Liotta LA, Steeg PS, Stetler-Stevenson WG. Cancer metastasis and angiogenesis: an imbalance of positive and negative regulation. *Cell* 1991; 64: 327–336.
59. Risau W. Mechanisms of angiogenesis. *Nature* 1997; 386: 671–674.
60. Risau W. Development and differentiation of endothelium. *Kidney Int Suppl* 1998; 67: S3–S6.
61. Fong GH, Rossant J, Gertsenstein M, Breitman ML. Role of the Flt-1 receptor tyrosine kinase in regulating the assembly of vascular endothelium. *Nature* 1995; 376: 66–70.
62. Carmeliet P, Ferreira V, Breier G, et al. Abnormal blood vessel development and lethality in embryos lacking a single VEGF allele. *Nature* 1996; 380: 435–439.
63. Ferrara N, Carver-Moore K, Chen H, et al. Heterozygous embryonic lethality induced by targeted inactivation of the VEGF gene. *Nature* 1996; 380: 439–442.
64. Breier G, Damert A, Plate KH, Risau W. Angiogenesis in embryos and ischemic diseases. *Thromb Haemost* 1997; 78: 678–683.
65. Shalaby F, Rossant J, Yamaguchi TP, et al. Failure of blood-island formation and vasculogenesis in Flk-1-deficient mice. *Nature* 1995; 376: 62–66.
66. Ausprunk DH, Folkman J. Migration and proliferation of endothelial cells in preformed and newly formed blood vessels during tumor angiogenesis. *Microvasc Res* 1977; 14: 53–65.
67. Pepper MS. Manipulating angiogenesis. From basic science to the bedside. *Arterioscler Thromb Vasc Biol* 1997; 17: 605–619.
68. Patan S, Haenni B, Burri PH. Implementation of intussusceptive microvascular growth in the chicken chorioallantoic membrane (CAM): 1. pillar formation by folding of the capillary wall. *Microvasc Res* 1996; 51: 80–98.
69. Pardanaud L, Yassine F, Dieterlen-Lievre F. Relationship between vasculogenesis, angiogenesis and haemopoiesis during avian ontogeny. *Development* 1989; 105: 473–485.
70. Sato TN, Tozawa Y, Deutsch U, et al. Distinct roles of the receptor tyrosine kinases Tie-1 and Tie-2 in blood vessel formation. *Nature* 1995; 376: 70–74.
71. Davis S, Aldrich TH, Jones PF, et al. Isolation of angiopoietin-1, a ligand for the TIE2 receptor, by secretion-trap expression cloning. *Cell* 1996; 87: 1161–1169.
72. Davis S, Yancopoulos GD. The angiopoietins: Yin and Yang in angiogenesis. *Curr Top Microbiol Immunol* 1999; 237: 173–185.
73. Suri C, Jones PF, Patan S, et al. Requisite role of angiopoietin-1, a ligand for the TIE2 receptor, during embryonic angiogenesis. *Cell* 1996; 87: 1171–1180.
74. Alon T, Hemo I, Itin A, Pe'er J, Stone J, Keshet E. Vascular endothelial growth factor acts as a survival factor for newly formed retinal vessels and has implications for retinopathy of prematurity. *Nat Med* 1995; 1: 1024–1028.
75. Franke RP, Grafe M, Dauer U, Schnittler H, Mittermayer C. Stress fibres (SF) in human endothelial cells (HEC) under shear stress. *Klin Wochenschr* 1986; 64: 989–992.
76. Crocker DJ, Murad TM, Geer JC. Role of the pericyte in wound healing. An ultrastructural study. *Exp Mol Pathol* 1970; 13: 51–65.

77. Hirschi KK, Rohovsky SA, Beck LH, Smith SR, D'Amore PA. Endothelial cells modulate the proliferation of mural cell precursors via platelet-derived growth factor-BB and heterotypic cell contact. *Circ Res* 1999; 84: 298–305.
78. Hirschi KK, D'Amore PA. Control of angiogenesis by the pericyte: molecular mechanisms and significance. *EXS* 1997; 79: 419–428.
79. Benjamin LE, Golijanin D, Itin A, Pode D, Keshet E. Selective ablation of immature blood vessels in established human tumors follows vascular endothelial growth factor withdrawal. *J Clin Invest* 1999; 103: 159–165.
80. Asahara T, Murohara T, Sullivan A, et al. Isolation of putative progenitor endothelial cells for angiogenesis. *Science* 1997; 275: 964–967.
81. Asahara T, Masuda H, Takahashi T, et al. Bone marrow origin of endothelial progenitor cells responsible for postnatal vasculogenesis in physiological and pathological neovascularization. *Circ Res* 1999; 85: 221–228.
82. Holash J, Wiegand SJ, Yancopoulos GD. New model of tumor angiogenesis: dynamic balance between vessel regression and growth mediated by angiopoietins and VEGF. *Oncogene* 1999; 18: 5356–5362.
83. Holash J, Maisonpierre PC, Compton D, et al. Vessel cooption, regression, and growth in tumors mediated by angiopoietins and VEGF. *Science* 1999; 284: 1994–1998.
84. Willis RA. *Pathology of Tumors*. Butterworths, London, 1948, p. 136.
85. Konerding MA, Steinberg F, Streffer C. The vasculature of xenotransplanted human melanomas and sarcomas on nude mice. II. Scanning and transmission electron microscopic studies. *Acta Anat (Basel)* 1989; 136: 27–33.
86. Warren BA. The vascular morphology of tumors. In: Peterson HI, ed. *Tumor Blood Circulation: Angiogenesis, Vascular Morphology and Blood Flow of Experimental and Human Tumors*. CRC Press, Boca Raton, 1979, pp. 1–48.
87. Francois J, Neetens A. Physico-anatomical studies of spontaneous and experimental ocular new growths: vascular supply. *Bibl Anat* 1967; 9: 403–411.
88. Maniotis AJ, Folberg R, Hess A, et al. Vascular channel formation by human melanoma cells in vivo and in vitro: vasculogenic mimicry. *Am J Pathol* 1999; 155: 739–752.
89. Folberg R, Hendrix M, Maniotis A. Vasculogenic mimicry and tumor angiogenesis. *Am J Pathol* 2000; 156: 361–381.
90. McDonald DM, Munn L, Jain RK. Vasculogenic mimicry: how convincing, how novel, and how significant? *Am J Pathol* 2000; 156: 383–388.
91. Konerding MA, Miodonski AJ, Lametschwandtner A. Microvascular corrosion casting in the study of tumor vascularity: a review. *Scanning Microsc* 1995; 9: 1233–1243.
92. Konerding MA, Malkusch W, Klapthor B, et al. Evidence for characteristic vascular patterns in solid tumours: quantitative studies using corrosion casts. *Br J Cancer* 1999; 80: 724–732.
93. Papadimitrou JM, Woods AE. Structural and functional characteristics of the microcirculation in neoplasms. *J Pathol* 1975; 116: 65–72.
94. Peterson HI, Appelgren L. Tumour vessel permeability and transcapillary exchange of large molecules of different size. *Bibl Anat* 1977; 262–265.
95. Peterson HI. Tumor angiogenesis inhibition by prostaglandin synthetase inhibitors. *Anticancer Res* 1986; 6: 251–253.
96. Dvorak HF, Detmar M, Claffey KP, Nagy JA, van de Water L, Senger DR. Vascular permeability factor/vascular endothelial growth factor: an important mediator of angiogenesis in malignancy and inflammation. *Int Arch Allergy Immunol* 1995; 107: 233–235.
97. Dvorak HF, Nagy JA, Feng D, Brown LF, Dvorak AM. Vascular permeability factor/vascular endothelial growth factor and the significance of microvascular hyperpermeability in angiogenesis. *Curr Top Microbiol Immunol* 1999; 237: 97–132.
98. Peterson HI. Modification of tumour blood flow—a review. *Int J Radiat Biol* 1991; 60: 201–210.

99. Liotta LA. Cancer cell invasion and metastasis. *Sci Am* 1992; 266: 54–63.
100. Dvorak HF, Nagy JA, Dvorak JT, Dvorak AM. Identification and characterization of the blood vessels of solid tumors that are leaky to circulating macromolecules. *Am J Pathol* 1988; 133: 95–109.
101. Hashizume H, Baluk P, Morikawa S, et al. Openings between defective endothelial cells explain tumor vessel leakiness. *Am J Pathol* 2000; 156: 1363–1380.
102. Cockerill GW, Gamble JR, Vadas MA. Angiogenesis: models and modulators. *Int Rev Cytol* 1995; 159: 113–160.
103. Anand-Apte B, Zetter B. Biological principles of angiogenesis. In: D'Amore P, Voest E, eds. *Tumor Angiogenesis and Microcirculation*. Marcel Dekker, New York, 2000.
104. Ferrara N, Bunting S. Vascular endothelial growth factor, a specific regulator of angiogenesis. *Curr Opin Nephrol Hypertens* 1996; 5: 35–44.
105. Mustonen T, Alitalo K. Endothelial receptor tyrosine kinases involved in angiogenesis. *J Cell Biol* 1995; 129: 895–898.
106. Soker S, Takashima S, Miao HQ, Neufeld G, Klagsbrun M. Neuropilin-1 is expressed by endothelial and tumor cells as an isoform-specific receptor for vascular endothelial growth factor. *Cell* 1998; 92: 735–745.
107. Liu B, Earl HM, Baban D, et al. Melanoma cell lines express VEGF receptor KDR and respond to exogenously added VEGF. *Biochem Biophys Res Commun* 1995; 217: 721–727.
108. Namiki A, Brogi E, Kearney M, et al. Hypoxia induces vascular endothelial growth factor in cultured human endothelial cells. *J Biol Chem* 1995; 270: 31189–31195.
109. Minchenko A, Bauer T, Salceda S, Caro J. Hypoxic stimulation of vascular endothelial growth factor expression in vitro and in vivo. *Lab Invest* 1994; 71: 374–379.
110. Levy AP, Levy NS, Wegner S, Goldberg MA. Transcriptional regulation of the rat vascular endothelial growth factor gene by hypoxia. *J Biol Chem* 1995; 270: 13333–13340.
111. Levy AP, Levy NS, Goldberg MA. Hypoxia-inducible protein binding to vascular endothelial growth factor mRNA and its modulation by the von Hippel-Lindau protein. *J Biol Chem* 1996; 271: 25492–25497.
112. Takagi H, King GL, Robinson GS, Ferrara N, Aiello LP. Adenosine mediates hypoxic induction of vascular endothelial growth factor in retinal pericytes and endothelial cells. *Invest Ophthalmol Vis Sci* 1996; 37: 2165–2176.
113. Hashimoto E, Kage K, Ogita T, Nakaoka T, Matsuoka R, Kira Y. Adenosine as an endogenous mediator of hypoxia for induction of vascular endothelial growth factor mRNA in U-937 cells. *Biochem Biophys Res Commun* 1994; 204: 318–324.
114. Brogi E, Schatteman G, Wu T, et al. Hypoxia-induced paracrine regulation of vascular endothelial growth factor receptor expression. *J Clin Invest* 1996; 97: 469–476.
115. Li J, Perrella MA, Tsai JC, et al. Induction of vascular endothelial growth factor gene expression by interleukin-1 beta in rat aortic smooth muscle cells. *J Biol Chem* 1995; 270: 308–312.
116. Cohen T, Nahari D, Cerem LW, Neufeld G, Levi BZ. Interleukin 6 induces the expression of vascular endothelial growth factor. *J Biol Chem* 1996; 271: 736–741.
117. Mukhopadhyay D, Tsiokas L, Sukhatme VP. Wild-type p53 and v-Src exert opposing influences on human vascular endothelial growth factor gene expression. *Cancer Res* 1995; 55: 6161–6165.
118. Mukhopadhyay D, Tsiokas L, Sukhatme VP. High cell density induces vascular endothelial growth factor expression via protein tyrosine phosphorylation. *Gene Expr* 1998; 7: 53–60.
119. Grugel S, Finkenzeller G, Weindel K, Barleon B, Marme D. Both v-Ha-Ras and v-Raf stimulate expression of the vascular endothelial growth factor in NIH 3T3 cells. *J Biol Chem* 1995; 270: 25915–25919.
120. Rak J, Filmus J, Finkenzeller G, Grugel S, Marme D, Kerbel RS. Oncogenes as inducers of tumor angiogenesis. *Cancer Metastasis Rev* 1995; 14: 263–277.

121. Pertovaara L, Kaipainen A, Mustonen T, et al. Vascular endothelial growth factor is induced in response to transforming growth factor-beta in fibroblastic and epithelial cells. *J Biol Chem* 1994; 269: 6271–6274.
122. Warren RS, Yuan H, Matli MR, Ferrara N, Donner DB. Induction of vascular endothelial growth factor by insulin-like growth factor 1 in colorectal carcinoma. *J Biol Chem* 1996; 271: 29483–29488.
123. Hyder SM, Stancel GM. Regulation of angiogenic growth factors in the female reproductive tract by estrogens and progestins. *Mol Endocrinol* 1999; 13: 806–811.
124. Hyder SM, Stancel GM. Regulation of VEGF in the reproductive tract by sex-steroid hormones. *Histol Histopathol* 2000; 15: 325–334.
125. Nicosia RF. What is the role of vascular endothelial growth factor-related molecules in tumor angiogenesis? *Am J Pathol* 1998; 153: 11–16.
126. Salven P, Lymboussaki A, Heikkila P, et al. Vascular endothelial growth factors VEGF-B and VEGF-C are expressed in human tumors. *Am J Pathol* 1998; 153: 103–108.
127. Shweiki D, Neeman M, Itin A, Keshet E. Induction of vascular endothelial growth factor expression by hypoxia and by glucose deficiency in multicell spheroids: implications for tumor angiogenesis. *Proc Natl Acad Sci USA* 1995; 92: 768–772.
128. Asano M, Yukita A, Matsumoto T, Kondo S, Suzuki H. Inhibition of tumor growth and metastasis by an immunoneutralizing monoclonal antibody to human vascular endothelial growth factor/vascular permeability factor121. *Cancer Res* 1995; 55: 5296–5301.
129. Goldman CK, Kendall RL, Cabrera G, et al. Paracrine expression of a native soluble vascular endothelial growth factor receptor inhibits tumor growth, metastasis, and mortality rate. *Proc Natl Acad Sci USA* 1998; 95: 8795–8800.
130. Warren RS, Yuan H, Matli MR, Gillett NA, Ferrara N. Regulation by vascular endothelial growth factor of human colon cancer tumorigenesis in a mouse model of experimental liver metastasis. *J Clin Invest* 1995; 95: 1789–1797.
131. Benjamin LE, Keshet E. Conditional switching of vascular endothelial growth factor (VEGF) expression in tumors: induction of endothelial cell shedding and regression of hemangioblastoma-like vessels by VEGF withdrawal. *Proc Natl Acad Sci USA* 1997; 94: 8761–8766.
132. Maisonpierre PC, Suri C, Jones PF, et al. Angiopoietin-2, a natural antagonist for Tie2 that disrupts in vivo angiogenesis. *Science* 1997; 277: 55–60.
133. Davis GE, Camarillo CW. Regulation of endothelial cell morphogenesis by integrins, mechanical forces, and matrix guidance pathways. *Exp Cell Res* 1995; 216: 113–123.
134. Vikkula M, Boon LM, Carraway KL 3rd, et al. Vascular dysmorphogenesis caused by an activating mutation in the receptor tyrosine kinase TIE2. *Cell* 1996; 87: 1181–1190.
135. Suri C, McClain J, Thurston G, et al. Increased vascularization in mice overexpressing angiopoietin-1. *Science* 1998; 282: 468–471.
136. Papapetropoulos A, Garcia-Cardena G, Dengler TJ, Maisonpierre PC, Yancopoulos GD, Sessa WC. Direct actions of angiopoietin-1 on human endothelium: evidence for network stabilization, cell survival, and interaction with other angiogenic growth factors. *Lab Invest* 1999; 79: 213–223.
137. Papapetropoulos A, Fulton D, Mahboubi K, et al. Angiopoietin-1 inhibits endothelial cell apoptosis via the Akt/survivin pathway. *J Biol Chem* 2000; 275: 9102–9105.
138. Zagzag D, Hooper A, Friedlander DR, et al. In situ expression of angiopoietins in astrocytomas identifies angiopoietin-2 as an early marker of tumor angiogenesis. *Exp Neurol* 1999; 159: 391–400.
139. Auerbach W, Auerbach R. Angiogenesis inhibition: a review. *Pharmacol Ther* 1994; 63: 265–311.
140. Vogel T, Guo NH, Krutzsch HC, et al. Modulation of endothelial cell proliferation, adhesion, and motility by recombinant heparin-binding domain and synthetic peptides from the type I repeats of thrombospondin. *J Cell Biochem* 1993; 53: 74–84.

141. Iruela-Arispe ML, Bornstein P, Sage H. Thrombospondin exerts an antiangiogenic effect on cord formation by endothelial cells in vitro. *Proc Natl Acad Sci USA* 1991; 88: 5026–5030.
142. Tolsma SS, Volpert OV, Good DJ, Frazier WA, Polverini PJ, Bouck N. Peptides derived from two separate domains of the matrix protein thrombospondin-1 have anti-angiogenic activity. *J Cell Biol* 1993; 122: 497–511.
143. Bouck N. P53 and angiogenesis. *Biochim Biophys Acta* 1996; 1287: 63–66.
144. Grossfeld GD, Ginsberg DA, Stein JP, et al. Thrombospondin-1 expression in bladder cancer: association with p53 alterations, tumor angiogenesis, and tumor progression. *J Natl Cancer Inst* 1997; 89: 219–227.
145. Iruela-Arispe ML, Vazquez F, Ortega MA. Antiangiogenic domains shared by thrombospondins and metallospondins, a new family of angiogenic inhibitors. *Ann NY Acad Sci* 1999; 886: 58–66.
146. O'Reilly MS. Angiostatin: an endogenous inhibitor of angiogenesis and of tumor growth. *EXS* 1997; 79: 273–294.
147. O'Reilly MS, Holmgren L, Chen C, Folkman J. Angiostatin induces and sustains dormancy of human primary tumors in mice. *Nat Med* 1996; 2: 689–692.
148. Dong Z, Kumar R, Yang X, Fidler IJ. Macrophage-derived metalloelastase is responsible for the generation of angiostatin in Lewis lung carcinoma. *Cell* 1997; 88: 801–810.
149. Zatterstrom UK, Felbor U, Fukai N, Olsen BR. Collagen XVIII/endostatin structure and functional role in angiogenesis. *Cell Struct Funct* 2000; 25: 97–101.
150. Yamaguchi N, Anand-Apte B, Lee M, et al. Endostatin inhibits VEGF-induced endothelial cell migration and tumor growth independently of zinc binding. *EMBO J* 1999; 18: 4414–4423.
151. Felbor U, Dreier L, Bryant RA, Ploegh HL, Olsen BR, Mothes W. Secreted cathepsin L generates endostatin from collagen XVIII. *EMBO J* 2000; 19: 1187–1194.
152. Wen W, Moses MA, Wiederschain D, Arbiser JL, Folkman J. The generation of endostatin is mediated by elastase. *Cancer Res* 1999; 59: 6052–6056.
153. Sidky YA, Borden EC. Inhibition of angiogenesis by interferons: effects on tumor- and lymphocyte-induced vascular responses. *Cancer Res* 1987; 47: 5155–5161.
154. Chang E, Boyd A, Nelson CC, et al. Successful treatment of infantile hemangiomas with interferon-alpha-2b. *J Pediatr Hematol Oncol* 1997; 19: 237–244.
155. Ezekowitz RA, Mulliken JB, Folkman J. Interferon alfa-2a therapy for life-threatening hemangiomas of infancy. *N Engl J Med* 1992; 326: 1456–1463.
156. Singh RK, Gutman M, Bucana CD, Sanchez R, Llansa N, Fidler IJ. Interferons alpha and beta down-regulate the expression of basic fibroblast growth factor in human carcinomas. *Proc Natl Acad Sci USA* 1995; 92: 4562–4566.
157. Powell WC, Matrisian LM. Complex roles of matrix metalloproteinases in tumor progression. *Curr Top Microbiol Immunol* 1996; 213: 1–21.
158. Moses MA. The regulation of neovascularization of matrix metalloproteinases and their inhibitors. *Stem Cells* 1997; 15: 180–189.
159. Anand-Apte B, Pepper MS, Voest E, et al. Inhibition of angiogenesis by tissue inhibitor of metalloproteinase-3. *Invest Ophthal Vis Sci* 1997; 38: 817–823.
160. Anand-Apte B, Bao L, Smith R, et al. A review of tissue inhibitor of metalloproteinases-3 (TIMP-3) and experimental analysis of its effect on primary tumor growth. *Biochem Cell Biol* 1996; 74: 853–862.
161. Moses MA, Sudhalter J, Langer R. Identification of an inhibitor of neovascularization from cartilage. *Science* 1990; 248: 1408–1410.
162. Kandel J, Bossy-Wetzel E, Radvanyi F, Klagsbrun M, Folkman J, Hanahan D. Neovascularization is associated with a switch to the export of bFGF in the multistep development of fibrosarcoma. *Cell* 1991; 66: 1095–1104.

163. Smith-McCune KK, Weidner N. Demonstration and characterization of the angiogenic properties of cervical dysplasia. *Cancer Res* 1994; 54: 800–804.
164. Smith-McCune K, Zhu YH, Hanahan D, Arbeit J. Cross-species comparison of angiogenesis during the premalignant stages of squamous carcinogenesis in the human cervix and K14-HPV16 transgenic mice. *Cancer Res* 1997; 57: 1294–1300.
165. Smith-McCune K. Angiogenesis in squamous cell carcinoma in situ and microinvasive carcinoma of the uterine cervix. *Obstet Gynecol* 1997; 89: 482–483.
166. Brown LF, Berse B, Jackman RW, et al. Expression of vascular permeability factor (vascular endothelial growth factor) and its receptors in breast cancer. *Hum Pathol* 1995; 26: 86–91.
167. Guidi AJ, Fischer L, Harris JR, Schnitt SJ. Microvessel density and distribution in ductal carcinoma in situ of the breast. *J Natl Cancer Inst* 1994; 86: 614–619.
168. Weidner N, Folkman J, Pozza F, et al. Tumor angiogenesis: a new significant and independent prognostic indicator in early-stage breast carcinoma. *J Natl Cancer Inst* 1992; 84: 1875–1887.
169. Guidi AJ, Abu-Jawdeh G, Berse B, et al. Vascular permeability factor (vascular endothelial growth factor) expression and angiogenesis in cervical neoplasia. *J Natl Cancer Inst* 1995; 87: 1237–1245.
170. Rak JW, St Croix BD, Kerbel RS. Consequences of angiogenesis for tumor progression, metastasis and cancer therapy. *Anticancer Drugs* 1995; 6: 3–18.
171. Dameron KM, Volpert OV, Tainsky MA, Bouck N. The p53 tumor suppressor gene inhibits angiogenesis by stimulating the production of thrombospondin. *Cold Spring Harb Symp Quant Biol* 1994; 59: 483–489.
172. Volpert OV, Stellmach V, Bouck N. The modulation of thrombospondin and other naturally occurring inhibitors of angiogenesis during tumor progression. *Breast Cancer Res Treat* 1995; 36: 119–126.
173. Bissell MJ. Tumor plasticity allows vasculogenic mimicry, a novel form of angiogenic switch. A rose by any other name? *Am J Pathol* 1999; 155: 675–679.
174. Vermeulen PB, Gasparini G, Fox SB, et al. Quantification of angiogenesis in solid human tumours: an international consensus on the methodology and criteria of evaluation. *Eur J Cancer* 1996; 32A: 2474–2484.
175. Barbareschi M, Gasparini G, Morelli L, Forti S, Dalla Palma P. Novel methods for the determination of the angiogenic activity of human tumors. *Breast Cancer Res Treat* 1995; 36: 181–192.
176. Fox SB, Leek RD, Weekes MP, Whitehouse RM, Gatter KC, Harris AL. Quantitation and prognostic value of breast cancer angiogenesis: comparison of microvessel density, Chalkley count, and computer image analysis. *J Pathol* 1995; 177: 275–283.
177. Srivastava A, Laidler P, Hughes LE, Woodcock J, Shedden EJ. Neovascularization in human cutaneous melanoma: a quantitative morphological and Doppler ultrasound study. *Eur J Cancer Clin Oncol* 1986; 22: 1205–1209.
178. Macchiarini P, Fontanini G, Hardin MJ, Squartini F, Angeletti CA. Relation of neovascularisation to metastasis of non-small-cell lung cancer. *Lancet* 1992; 340: 145–146.
179. Toi M, Kashitani J, Tominaga T. Tumor angiogenesis is an independent prognostic indicator in primary breast carcinoma. *Int J Cancer* 1993; 55: 371–374.
180. Heimann R, Ferguson D, Powers C, Recant WM, Weichselbaum RR, Hellman S. Angiogenesis as a predictor of long-term survival for patients with node-negative breast cancer. *J Natl Cancer Inst* 1996; 88: 1764–1769.
181. Gasparini G, Weidner N, Bevilacqua P, et al. Tumor microvessel density, p53 expression, tumor size, and peritumoral lymphatic vessel invasion are relevant prognostic markers in node-negative breast carcinoma. *J Clin Oncol* 1994; 12: 454–466.
182. Fox SB, Leek RD, Smith K, Hollyer J, Greenall M, Harris AL. Tumor angiogenesis in node-negative breast carcinomas—relationship with epidermal growth factor receptor, estrogen receptor, and survival. *Breast Cancer Res Treat* 1994; 29: 109–116.

183. Bosari S, Lee AK, DeLellis RA, Wiley BD, Heatley GJ, Silverman ML. Microvessel quantitation and prognosis in invasive breast carcinoma. *Hum Pathol* 1992; 23: 755–761.
184. Hall NR, Fish DE, Hunt N, Goldin RD, Guillou PJ, Monson JR. Is the relationship between angiogenesis and metastasis in breast cancer real? *Surg Oncol* 1992; 1: 223–229.
185. Axelsson K, Ljung BM, Moore DH 2nd, et al. Tumor angiogenesis as a prognostic assay for invasive ductal breast carcinoma. *J Natl Cancer Inst* 1995; 87: 997–1008.
186. Costello P, McCann A, Carney DN, Dervan PA. Prognostic significance of microvessel density in lymph node negative breast carcinoma. *Hum Pathol* 1995; 26: 1181–1184.
187. Goulding H, Abdul Rashid NF, Robertson JF, et al. Assessment of angiogenesis in breast carcinoma: an important factor in prognosis? *Hum Pathol* 1995; 26: 1196–1200.
188. Morphopoulos G, Pearson M, Ryder W, Howell A, Harris M. Tumour angiogenesis as a prognostic marker in infiltrating lobular carcinoma of the breast. *J Pathol* 1996; 180: 44–49.
189. Van Hoef ME, Knox WF, Dhesi SS, Howell A, Schor AM. Assessment of tumour vascularity as a prognostic factor in lymph node negative invasive breast cancer. *Eur J Cancer* 1993; 29A: 1141–1145.
190. Gasparini G, Fox SB, Verderio P, et al. Determination of angiogenesis adds information to estrogen receptor status in predicting the efficacy of adjuvant tamoxifen in node-positive breast cancer patients. *Clin Cancer Res* 1996; 2: 1191–1198.
191. Hirst DG, Denekamp J, Hobson B. Proliferation kinetics of endothelial and tumour cells in three mouse mammary carcinomas. *Cell Tissue Kinet* 1982; 15: 251–261.
192. Hobson B, Denekamp J. Endothelial proliferation in tumours and normal tissues: continuous labelling studies. *Br J Cancer* 1984; 49: 405–413.
193. Eberhard A, Kahlert S, Goede V, Hemmerlein B, Plate KH, Augustin HG. Heterogeneity of angiogenesis and blood vessel maturation in human tumors: implications for antiangiogenic tumor therapies. *Cancer Res* 2000; 60: 1388–1393.
194. Fox SB, Gatter KC, Bicknell R, et al. Relationship of endothelial cell proliferation to tumor vascularity in human breast cancer. *Cancer Res* 1993; 53: 4161–4163.
195. Vartanian RK, Weidner N. Endothelial cell proliferation in prostatic carcinoma and prostatic hyperplasia: correlation with Gleason's score, microvessel density, and epithelial cell proliferation. *Lab Invest* 1995; 73: 844–850.
196. Mattern J, Koomagi R, Volm M. Association of vascular endothelial growth factor expression with intratumoral microvessel density and tumour cell proliferation in human epidermoid lung carcinoma. *Br J Cancer* 1996; 73: 931–934.
197. Toi M, Inada K, Hoshina S, Suzuki H, Kondo S, Tominaga T. Vascular endothelial growth factor and platelet-derived endothelial cell growth factor are frequently coexpressed in highly vascularized human breast cancer. *Clin Cancer Res* 1995; 1: 961–964.
198. Takahashi Y, Cleary KR, Mai M, Kitadai Y, Bucana CD, Ellis LM. Significance of vessel count and vascular endothelial growth factor and its receptor (KDR) in intestinal-type gastric cancer. *Clin Cancer Res* 1996; 2: 1679–1684.
199. Takahashi Y, Bucana CD, Cleary KR, Ellis LM. p53, vessel count, and vascular endothelial growth factor expression in human colon cancer. *Int J Cancer* 1998; 79: 34–38.
200. Salven P, Ruotsalainen T, Mattson K, Joensuu H. High pre-treatment serum level of vascular endothelial growth factor (VEGF) is associated with poor outcome in small-cell lung cancer. *Int J Cancer* 1998; 79: 144–146.
201. Salven P, Perhoniemi V, Tykka H, Maenpaa H, Joensuu H. Serum VEGF levels in women with a benign breast tumor or breast cancer. *Breast Cancer Res Treat* 1999; 53: 161–166.
202. Guidi AJ, Berry DA, Broadwater G, et al. Association of angiogenesis in lymph node metastases with outcome of breast cancer. *J Natl Cancer Inst* 2000; 92: 486–492.
203. Guidi AJ, Schnitt SJ, Fischer L, et al. Vascular permeability factor (vascular endothelial growth factor) expression and angiogenesis in patients with ductal carcinoma in situ of the breast. *Cancer* 1997; 80: 1945–1953.

204. Yamamoto Y, Toi M, Kondo S, et al. Concentrations of vascular endothelial growth factor in the sera of normal controls and cancer patients. *Clin Cancer Res* 1996; 2: 821–826.
205. Gasparini G. Prognostic value of vascular endothelial growth factor in breast cancer. *Oncologist* 2000; 5: 37–44.
206. Dirix LY, Vermeulen PB, Pawinski A, et al. Elevated levels of the angiogenic cytokines basic fibroblast growth factor and vascular endothelial growth factor in sera of cancer patients. *Br J Cancer* 1997; 76: 238–243.
207. Fujimoto K, Ichimori Y, Kakizoe T, et al. Increased serum levels of basic fibroblast growth factor in patients with renal cell carcinoma. *Biochem Biophys Res Commun* 1991; 180: 386–392.
208. Fujimoto K, Ichimori Y, Yamaguchi H, et al. Basic fibroblast growth factor as a candidate tumor marker for renal cell carcinoma. *Jpn J Cancer Res* 1995; 86: 182–186.
209. Duensing S, Grosse J, Atzpodien J. Increased serum levels of basic fibroblast growth factor (bFGF) are associated with progressive lung metastases in advanced renal cell carcinoma patients. *Anticancer Res* 1995; 15: 2331–2333.
210. Sliutz G, Tempfer C, Obermair A, Dadak C, Kainz C. Serum evaluation of basic FGF in breast cancer patients. *Anticancer Res* 1995; 15: 2675–2677.
211. Sliutz G, Tempfer C, Obermair A, Reinthaller A, Gitsch G, Kainz C. Serum evaluation of basic fibroblast growth factor in cervical cancer patients. *Cancer Lett* 1995; 94: 227–231.
212. Meyer GE, Yu E, Siegal JA, Petteway JC, Blumenstein BA, Brawer MK. Serum basic fibroblast growth factor in men with and without prostate carcinoma. *Cancer* 1995; 76: 2304–2311.
213. Nguyen M, Watanabe H, Budson AE, Richie JP, Folkman J. Elevated levels of the angiogenic peptide basic fibroblast growth factor in urine of bladder cancer patients. *J Natl Cancer Inst* 1993; 85: 241–242.
214. Brooks P, Stromblad S, Klemke R, Visscher D, Sarkar F, Cheresh D. Antiintegrin alpha v beta 3 blocks human breast cancer growth and angiogenesis in human skin. *J Clin Invest* 1995; 96: 1815–1822.
215. Degani H, Gusis V, Weinstein D, Fields S, Strano S. Mapping pathophysiological features of breast tumors by MRI at high spatial resolution. *Nat Med* 1997; 3: 780–782.
216. Mori K, Hasegawa M, Nishida M, et al. Expression levels of thymidine phosphorylase and dihydropyrimidine dehydrogenase in various human tumor tissues. *Int J Oncol* 2000; 17: 33–38.
217. Folberg R, Mehaffey M, Gardner LM, Meyer M, Rummelt V, Pe'er J. The microcirculation of choroidal and ciliary body melanomas. *Eye* 1997; 11: 227–238.
218. Mehaffey MG, Gardner LM, Folberg R. Distribution of prognostically important vascular patterns across multiple levels in ciliary body and choroidal melanomas. *Am J Ophthalmol* 1998; 126: 373–378.
219. Mueller AJ, Folberg R, Freeman WR, et al. Evaluation of the human choroidal melanoma rabbit model for studying microcirculation patterns with confocal ICG and histology. *Exp Eye Res* 1999; 68: 671–678.
220. Rummelt V, Mehaffey MG, Campbell RJ, et al. Microcirculation architecture of metastases from primary ciliary body and choroidal melanomas. *Am J Ophthalmol* 1998; 126: 303–305.
221. Makitie T, Summanen P, Tarkkanen A, Kivela T. Microvascular density in predicting survival of patients with choroidal and ciliary body melanoma. *Invest Ophthalmol Vis Sci* 1999; 40: 2471–2480.
222. Makitie T, Summanen P, Tarkkanen A, Kivela T. Microvascular loops and networks as prognostic indicators in choroidal and ciliary body melanomas. *J Natl Cancer Inst* 1999; 91: 359–367.
223. Ellis LM, Walker RA, Gasparini G. Is determination of angiogenic activity in human tumours clinically useful? *Eur J Cancer* 1998; 34: 609–618.

224. Horak ER, Leek R, Klenk N, et al. Angiogenesis, assessed by platelet/endothelial cell adhesion molecule antibodies, as indicator of node metastases and survival in breast cancer. *Lancet* 1992; 340: 1120–1124.
225. Boehm T, Folkman J, Browder T, O'Reilly MS. Antiangiogenic therapy of experimental cancer does not induce acquired drug resistance. *Nature* 1997; 390: 404–407.
226. Yoshiji H, Harris SR, Thorgeirsson UP. Vascular endothelial growth factor is essential for initial but not continued in vivo growth of human breast carcinoma cells. *Cancer Res* 1997; 57: 3924–3928.
227. Eatock MM, Schatzlein A, Kaye SB. Tumour vasculature as a target for anticancer therapy. *Cancer Treat Rev* 2000; 26: 191–204.
228. Saleh M, Stacker SA, Wilks AF. Inhibition of growth of C6 glioma cells in vivo by expression of antisense vascular endothelial growth factor sequence. *Cancer Res* 1996; 56: 393–401.
229. Ramakrishnan S, Olson TA, Bautch VL, Mohanraj D. Vascular endothelial growth factor-toxin conjugate specifically inhibits KDR/flk-1-positive endothelial cell proliferation in vitro and angiogenesis in vivo. *Cancer Res* 1996; 56: 1324–1330.
230. Mitjans F, Sander D, Adan J, et al. An anti-alpha v-integrin antibody that blocks integrin function inhibits the development of a human melanoma in nude mice. *J Cell Sci* 1995; 108: 2825–2838.
231. Gross JL, Moscatelli D, Jaffe EA, Rifkin DB. Plasminogen activator and collagenase production by cultured capillary endothelial cells. *J Cell Biol* 1982; 95: 974–981.
232. Moscatelli D, Jaffe E, Rifkin DB. Tetradecanoyl phorbol acetate stimulates latent collagenase production by cultured human endothelial cells. *Cell* 1980; 20: 343–351.
233. Moscatelli DA, Rifkin DB, Jaffe EA. Production of latent collagenase by human umbilical vein endothelial cells in response to angiogenic preparations. *Exp Cell Res* 1985; 156: 379–390.
234. Montesano R, Orci L. Tumor-promoting phorbol esters induce angiogenesis in vitro. *Cell* 1985; 42: 469–477.
235. Zucker S, Conner C, Di Massmo BI, et al. Thrombin induces the activation of progelatinase A in vascular endothelial cells. Physiologic regulation of angiogenesis. *J Biol Chem* 1995; 270: 23730–23738.
236. Cornelius LA, Nehring LC, Roby JD, Parks WC, Welgus HG. Human dermal microvascular endothelial cells produce matrix metalloproteinases in response to angiogenic factors and migration. *J Invest Dermatol* 1995; 105: 170–176.
237. Shapiro SD, Campbell EJ, Kobayashi DK, Welgus HG. Immune modulation of metalloproteinase production in human macrophages. Selective pretranslational suppression of interstitial collagenase and stromelysin biosynthesis by interferon-gamma. *J Clin Invest* 1990; 86: 1204–1210.
238. Mignatti P, Tsuboi R, Robbins E, Rifkin DB. In vitro angiogenesis on the human amniotic membrane: requirement for basic fibroblast growth factor-induced proteinases. *J Cell Biol* 1989; 108: 671–682.
239. Johnson MD, Kim HR, Chesler L, Tsao-Wu G, Bouck N, Polverini PJ. Inhibition of angiogenesis by tissue inhibitor of metalloproteinase. *J Cell Physiol* 1994; 160: 194–202.
240. Takigawa M, Nishida Y, Suzuki F, Kishi J, Yamashita K, Hayakawa T. Induction of angiogenesis in chick yolk-sac membrane by polyamines and its inhibition by tissue inhibitors of metalloproteinases (TIMP and TIMP-2). *Biochem Biophys Res Commun* 1990; 171: 1264–1271.
241. White CW, Sondheimer HM, Crouch EC, Wilson H, Fan LL. Treatment of pulmonary hemangiomatosis with recombinant interferon alfa-2a. *N Engl J Med* 1989; 320: 1197–1200.
242. White CW, Wolf SJ, Korones DN, Sondheimer HM, Tosi MF, Yu A. Treatment of childhood angiomatous diseases with recombinant interferon alfa-2a. *J Pediatr* 1991; 118: 59–66.

243. Arap W, Pasqualini R, Ruoslahti E. Chemotherapy targeted to tumor vasculature. *Curr Opin Oncol* 1998; 10: 560–565.
244. Pasqualini R, Koivunen E, Ruoslahti E. Alpha v integrins as receptors for tumor targeting by circulating ligands. *Nat Biotechnol* 1997; 15: 542–546.
245. Pasqualini R. Vascular targeting with phage peptide libraries. *Q J Nucl Med* 1999; 43: 159–162.
246. Arap W, Pasqualini R, Ruoslahti E. Cancer treatment by targeted drug delivery to tumor vasculature in a mouse model. *Science* 1998; 279: 377–380.
247. Pasqualini R, Koivunen E, Kain R, et al. Aminopeptidase N is a receptor for tumor-homing peptides and a target for inhibiting angiogenesis. *Cancer Res* 2000; 60: 722–727.
248. Pezzella F, Pastorino U, Tagliabue E, et al. Non-small-cell lung carcinoma tumor growth without morphological evidence of neo-angiogenesis. *Am J Pathol* 1997; 151: 1417–1423.
249. Browder T, Butterfield CE, Kraling BM, et al. Antiangiogenic scheduling of chemotherapy improves efficacy against experimental drug-resistant cancer. *Cancer Res* 2000; 60: 1878–1886.
250. Kakeji Y, Teicher BA. Preclinical studies of the combination of angiogenic inhibitors with cytotoxic agents. *Invest New Drugs* 1997; 15: 39–48.
251. Klement G, Baruchel S, Rak J, et al. Continuous low-dose therapy with vinblastine and VEGF receptor-2 antibody induces sustained tumor regression without overt toxicity. *J Clin Invest* 2000; 105: R15–R24.
252. Sato TN. A new approach to fighting cancer? *Proc Natl Acad Sci USA* 1998; 95: 5843–5844.
253. Griscelli F, Li H, Bennaceur-Griscelli A, et al. Angiostatin gene transfer: inhibition of tumor growth in vivo by blockage of endothelial cell proliferation associated with a mitosis arrest. *Proc Natl Acad Sci USA* 1998; 95: 6367–6372.
254. Liu Y, Thor A, Shtivelman E, et al. Systemic gene delivery expands the repertoire of effective antiangiogenic agents. *J Biol Chem* 1999; 274: 13338–13344.
255. Hu G, Riordan JF, Vallee BL. Angiogenin promotes invasiveness of cultured endothelial cells by stimulation of cell-associated proteolytic activities. *Proc Natl Acad Sci USA* 1994; 91: 12096–12100.
256. Herbert JM, Laplace MC, Maffrand JP. Effect of heparin on the angiogenic potency of basic and acidic fibroblast growth factors in the rabbit cornea assay. *Int J Tissue React* 1988; 10: 133–139.
257. Esch F, Baird A, Ling N, et al. Primary structure of bovine pituitary basic fibroblast growth factor (FGF) and comparison with the amino-terminal sequence of bovine brain acidic FGF. *Proc Natl Acad Sci USA* 1985; 82: 6507–6511.
258. Bussolino F, Ziche M, Wang JM, et al. In vitro and in vivo activation of endothelial cells by colony-stimulating factors. *J Clin Invest* 1991; 87: 986–995.
259. Bussolino F, Colotta F, Bocchietto E, Guglielmetti A, Mantovani A. Recent developments in the cell biology of granulocyte-macrophage colony-stimulating factor and granulocyte colony-stimulating factor: activities on endothelial cells. *Int J Clin Lab Res* 1993; 23: 8–12.
260. Bussolino F, Di Renzo MF, Ziche M, et al. Hepatocyte growth factor is a potent angiogenic factor which stimulates endothelial cell motility and growth. *J Cell Biol* 1992; 119: 629–641.
261. Grant DS, Kleinman HK, Goldberg ID, et al. Scatter factor induces blood vessel formation in vivo. *Proc Natl Acad Sci USA* 1993; 90: 1937–1941.
262. Polverini PJ, Nickoloff BJ. The role of scatter factor and the c-met proto-oncogene in angiogenic responses. *EXS* 1995; 74: 51–67.
263. Koch AE, Polverini PJ, Kunkel SL, et al. Interleukin-8 as a macrophage-derived mediator of angiogenesis. *Science* 1992; 258: 1798–1801.
264. Ziche M, Maglione D, Ribatti D, et al. Placenta growth factor-1 is chemotactic, mitogenic, and angiogenic. *Lab Invest* 1997; 76: 517–531.

265. Ishikawa F, Miyazono K, Hellman U, et al. Identification of angiogenic activity and the cloning and expression of platelet-derived endothelial cell growth factor. *Nature* 1989; 338: 557–562.
266. Jackson D, Volpert OV, Bouck N, Linzer DI. Stimulation and inhibition of angiogenesis by placental proliferin and proliferin-related protein. *Science* 1994; 266: 1581–1584.
267. Groskopf JC, Syu LJ, Saltiel AR, Linzer DI. Proliferin induces endothelial cell chemotaxis through a G protein-coupled, mitogen-activated protein kinase-dependent pathway. *Endocrinology* 1997; 138: 2835–2840.
268. Grotendorst GR, Soma Y, Takehara K, Charette M. EGF and TGF-alpha are potent chemoattractants for endothelial cells and EGF-like peptides are present at sites of tissue regeneration. *J Cell Physiol* 1989; 139: 617–623.
269. Yang EY, Moses HL. Transforming growth factor beta 1-induced changes in cell migration, proliferation, and angiogenesis in the chicken chorioallantoic membrane. *J Cell Biol* 1990; 111: 731–741.
270. Leibovich SJ, Polverini PJ, Shepard HM, Wiseman DM, Shively V, Nuseir N. Macrophage-induced angiogenesis is mediated by tumour necrosis factor-alpha. *Nature* 1987; 329: 630–632.
271. Frater-Schroder M, Risau W, Hallmann R, Gautschi P, Bohlen P. Tumor necrosis factor type alpha, a potent inhibitor of endothelial cell growth in vitro, is angiogenic in vivo. *Proc Natl Acad Sci USA* 1987; 84: 5277–5281.
272. Olivo M, Bhardwaj R, Schulze-Osthoff K, Sorg C, Jacob HJ, Flamme I. A comparative study on the effects of tumor necrosis factor-alpha (TNF-alpha), human angiogenic factor (h-AF) and basic fibroblast growth factor (bFGF) on the chorioallantoic membrane of the chick embryo. *Anat Rec* 1992; 234: 105–115.
273. Koch AE, Harlow LA, Haines GK, et al. Vascular endothelial growth factor. A cytokine modulating endothelial function in rheumatoid arthritis. *J Immunol* 1994; 152: 4149–4156.
274. Wilting J, Christ B, Bokeloh M, Weich HA. In vivo effects of vascular endothelial growth factor on the chicken chorioallantoic membrane. *Cell Tissue Res* 1993; 274: 163–172.
275. Yoshida A, Anand-Apte B, Zetter BR. Differential endothelial migration and proliferation to basic fibroblast growth factor and vascular endothelial growth factor. *Growth Factors* 1996; 13: 57–64.
276. Witzenbichler B, Maisonpierre PC, Jones P, Yancopoulos GD, Isner JM. Chemotactic properties of angiopoietin-1 and -2, ligands for the endothelial-specific receptor tyrosine kinase Tie2. *J Biol Chem* 1998; 273: 18514–18521.
277. Brouty-Boye D, Zetter BR. Inhibition of cell motility by interferon. *Science* 1980; 208: 516–518.
278. Dvorak HF, Gresser I. Microvascular injury in pathogenesis of interferon-induced necrosis of subcutaneous tumors in mice. *J Natl Cancer Inst* 1989; 81: 497–502.
279. Maione TE, Gray GS, Petro J, et al. Inhibition of angiogenesis by recombinant human platelet factor-4 and related peptides. *Science* 1990; 247: 77–79.
280. Gengrinovitch S, Greenberg SM, Cohen T, et al. Platelet factor-4 inhibits the mitogenic activity of VEGF121 and VEGF165 using several concurrent mechanisms. *J Biol Chem* 1995; 270: 15059–15065.
281. D'Angelo G, Struman I, Martial J, Weiner RI. Activation of mitogen-activated protein kinases by vascular endothelial growth factor and basic fibroblast growth factor in capillary endothelial cells is inhibited by the antiangiogenic factor 16-kDa N-terminal fragment of prolactin. *Proc Natl Acad Sci USA* 1995; 92: 6374–6378.
282. Clapp C, Martial JA, Guzman RC, Rentier-Delure F, Weiner RI. The 16-kilodalton N-terminal fragment of human prolactin is a potent inhibitor of angiogenesis. *Endocrinology* 1993; 133: 1292–1299.

283. Dameron KM, Volpert OV, Tainsky MA, Bouck N. Control of angiogenesis in fibroblasts by p53 regulation of thrombospondin-1. *Science* 1994; 265: 1582–1584.
284. Good DJ, Polverini PJ, Rastinejad F, et al. A tumor suppressor-dependent inhibitor of angiogenesis is immunologically and functionally indistinguishable from a fragment of thrombospondin. *Proc Natl Acad Sci USA* 1990; 87: 6624–6628.
285. Rastinejad F, Polverini PJ, Bouck NP. Regulation of the activity of a new inhibitor of angiogenesis by a cancer suppressor gene. *Cell* 1989; 56: 345–355.
286. Taraboletti G, Roberts D, Liotta LA, Giavazzi R. Platelet thrombospondin modulates endothelial cell adhesion, motility, and growth: a potential angiogenesis regulatory factor. *J Cell Biol* 1990; 111: 765–772.
287. Murphy AN, Unsworth EJ, Stetler-Stevenson WG. Tissue inhibitor of metalloproteinases-2 inhibits bFGF-induced human microvascular endothelial cell proliferation. *J Cell Physiol* 1993; 157: 351–358.
288. Angiogenesis inhibitors in clinical trials. (http://cancertrials.nci.nih.gov/news/angio/table.html), 2000.

13 Antiangiogenic Therapy for Melanoma

Vann P. Parker, PhD

Contents

1. INTRODUCTION

The field of antiangiogenesis for the treatment of cancer can be traced back to a seminal paper from Judah Folkman thirty years ago. In it, he described an ecosystem between tumor cells and the surrounding endothelial cells. The proliferation of each of these cell populations is dependent upon the other for continued expansion. The concept of "antiangiogenesis" was introduced, and speculation was made that this may be an area worthy of "serious exploration" *(1)*. More recently, studies have examined specific angiogenic growth factors elaborated in the melanoma tumor microenvironment *(2–7)*. A correlation of angiogenesis with melanoma disease stage and prognosis has been made for patients *(8–15)*. Similar correlations have been made for most other solid tumors *(16–23)* and for some of the hematopoietic cancers *(24)*.

The endothelial cells that make up the new blood architecture surrounding tumors are normal cells that have been stimulated to proliferate and differentiate in response to specific factors produced by the tumor cells. Angiogenesis does not occur in adults, other than transiently as part of wound healing or in the

From: *Current Clinical Oncology, Melanoma: The New Biotherapeutics for Solid Tumors*
Edited by: E. C. Borden © Humana Press Inc., Totowa, NJ

female reproductive cycle *(25,26)*. To the extent that the process for stimulating angiogenesis is common to different tumor types, it may be possible to block the growth of any tumor with an antiangiogenic approach. An understanding of the steps involved in angiogenesis has suggested several avenues of approach for inhibition. Preclinical models have led to the discovery of many different molecules that have entered into development. Currently, more than 30 inhibitors are undergoing clinical testing in a variety of tumor types. The National Cancer Institute (NCI) maintains a portion of their web site devoted specifically to this field (http://cancertrials.nci.nih.gov/news/angio/table.html), as does the private Angiogenesis Foundation (http://www.angio.org/). The clinical potential for antiangiogenic therapy should be realized as results from many of these trials become available in the next few years.

2. APPROACHES TO INHIBITING ANGIOGENESIS

In the past few years, there has been a dramatic increase in the number of biologic agents with antiangiogenic properties under development for the therapy of cancer. These have been directed at all stages of the formation and maintenance of new blood vessels.

Matrix metalloproteinases (MMPs) are enzymes involved in the degradation of the extracellular matrix that surrounds tissues. This class of enzymes may be an attractive target for therapeutic intervention, as MMPs are involved in events leading to the remodeling of the blood vasculature. Participation of MMPs has been postulated for both early stages of extravasation of cells from a primary tumor and in remodeling associated with maturation of new blood vessels *(27)*. Thus, blocking the activity of MMPs may affect both metastatic and primary tumor growth. The MMP inhibitors are orally available small molecule drugs *(28)*. Of the agents in testing as antiangiogenics, this class has been in clinical trials for the longest period of time. Phase II/III or phase III clinical trials have been initiated for marimastat *(27)*, prinomastat, BAY 12-9566, and BMS-275291.

Vascular endothelial growth factor (VEGF) is an endothelial-specific growth factor produced by tumors that has been shown to be important for the proliferation, differentiation, and survival of endothelial cells (*see* Chapter 12). VEGF binds to two high-affinity cell surface tyrosine kinase receptors *(29,30)*, designated VEGFR-1 and VEGFR-2 (also known as Flt-1 and KDR). Several different classes of agents are being developed to interrupt this pathway (*see* Table 1). Monoclonal antibodies targeting VEGF are under clinical development at Genentech *(31,32)* and Protein Design Labs. A monoclonal antibody directed against VEGFR-2 recently began phase I testing *(33)*. A ribozyme directed against the VEGFR-1 mRNA has been designated ANGIOZYME and is entering expanded phase II clinical trials *(34)*. The compound SU5416 is a parenterally delivered small molecule that blocks the signal transduction of VEGFR-2 by

Table 1
Angiogenesis Inhibitors in Clinical Trials

Drug	*Sponsor*	*Phase*	*Mechanism of action*
Anti-VEGF MAb	Genentech	III	Monoclonal antibody to VEGF.
Interferon-α	Commercial	III	Inhibits release of endothelial growth factors.
Marimastat	British Biotech	III	Broad spectrum MMP inhibitor.
Neovastat	Aeterna/NCI	III	Shark cartilage-based MMP inhibitor.
TNP-470	TAP Pharma	III	Fumigillin analog that blocks MetAP-2 activity.
BMS-275291	Bristol-Meyers Squibb	II/III	Synthetic MMP inhibitor.
SU5416	SUGEN	II/III	VEGFR-2 tyrosine kinase inhibitor.
Prinomastat (AG3340)	Agouron	II	MMP inhibitor.
Squalamine	Magainin	II	Synthetic version of shark-derived inhibitor.
Thalidomide	Celgene	II	Unknown mechanism.
Vitaxin	Ixsys/MedImmune	II	MAb to α_v/β_3 integrin.
CAI	NCI	I/II	Nonspecific inhibitor of cell invasion and motility.
ANGIOZYME	Ribozyme Pharmaceuticals, Inc./Chiron	II	Ribozyme targeting VEGFR-1 mRNA.
BB-3644	British Biotech	I	Next generation MMP inhibitor.
Col-3 (Metastat)	Collagenex/NCI	I	Tetracycline analog (nonantimicrobial) that inhibits MMP-2.
Combretastatin A-4	Oxigene/BMS	I	African bark extract, binds to tubulin; targets tumor vasculature.
EMD-121974	Merck KGaA	I	Cyclic α_v/β_5 integrin antagonist.
Endostatin	EntreMed/NCI	I	Naturally occurring collagen fragment, inhibits angiogenesis.
IMC-lC11	ImClone	I	MAb to VEGFR-2.
2ME2 (2-Methoxy-estradiol)	EntreMed	I	Unknown mechanism of action.
MMI270	Novartis	I	Synthetic MMP inhibitor.
PTK787/ZK22584	Novartis	I	Blocks VEGF receptor signaling.
SU6668	SUGEN	I	Small molecule inhibitor of PDGF, bFGF, and VEGFR-2 tyrosine kinase activities.
Angiostatin	Entremed	I	Blocks endothelial cell growth.
VEGF MAb	Protein Design Labs/ Toagosei	I	Humanized monoclonal to VEGF.

PDGF, platelet-derived growth factor; MAb, monoclonal antibody.

interfering with intracellular protein phosphorylation *(35)*. Phase III trials in colorectal cancer are underway using SU5416.

Other agents targeting endothelial cell growth and function are also under development. This group includes angiostatin *(36)*, endostatin *(37)*, interferon *(38)*, carboxyamidotriazole (CAI) *(39)*, combretastatin A-4 *(40)*, thalidomide *(41)*, interleukin (IL)-10 *(42)*, and IL-12.

Not included in this review are other agents targeting farnesyltransferase inhibitors, growth factors such as epidermal growth factor (EGF), and other cytostatic and cytotoxic agents exerting their effect through more indirect antiangiogenic mechanisms. Recent reviews of these agents are available *(43,44)*.

3. PRECLINICAL EVIDENCE FOR ANTIANGIOGENICS IN CANCER THERAPY

Experimental models of melanoma include syngeneic mouse tumors, established human melanoma xenografts, and explants of primary human tumors to mice or rats. These systems can be exploited to attempt to dissect the important elements for tumor growth and progression. The participation of angiogenesis has been unequivocally demonstrated in such model systems. Modulation of angiogenesis using the human cell line SK-MEL-2 was accomplished by transfection of a murine sense or antisense mRNA. When these cell lines were introduced into rats, there was a significant difference in the growth of tumors that expressed exogenous VEGF relative to control and antisense constructs. Likewise, the cells expressing lower levels of VEGF as a result of transfection with an antisense VEGF grew less vigorously than the untransfected line. The pattern of tumor growth was correlated with vascularization of the tumors, blood volume, blood flow, and vascular permeability *(45)*. A similar series of experiments was undertaken using mice as the recipient of transfected SK-MEL-2 cells. In addition to effects on primary tumor growth, an inhibition of metastatic potential was seen. SK-MEL-2 cells overexpressing VEGF, which were injected intravenously, had a fiftyfold increase in lung tumor colonization compared to the parental SK-MEL-2 cell line or the antisense expressing line *(46)*.

The contribution of specific factors to angiogenesis is complex and includes positive and negative regulators. Malignant progression involves the activation of oncogenes and inactivation of tumor suppressor genes, many of the same factors that control angiogenesis. These factors can act in an autocrine or paracrine manner. The elaboration of regulatory molecules varies as cells progress from normal melanocytes to melanoma *(47,48)*. Confounding the analysis of antiangiogenic therapies for melanoma is the widespread expression of receptors for angiogenic factors on melanoma cells. It has been well documented that melanoma cells express receptors for fibroblast growth factor (bFGF) *(49)*, VEGF

(50), and IL-8 *(51)*. Inhibitors of these factors have the potential to directly inhibit tumor cells in addition to endothelial cells.

Animal models have been used by many groups to identify specific factors associated with tumor angiogenesis. The pivotal role of VEGF has been demonstrated through the manipulation of tumor cells as described above, by inhibition using monoclonal antibodies directed either toward VEGF or its receptor VEGFR-2 *(33,52)*, by ribozymes targeting VEGFR-1 or VEGFR-2 *(34)*, and by molecules designed to interrupt the signal transduction pathway of VEGF *(35)*. Other studies have shown inhibition of tumor growth through the inhibition of tyrosine kinase that contains immunoglobulin-like loops and EGF-like domains (Tie-2) *(4)*, perlican *(53)*, IL-8 *(54)*, or bFGF *(55)*. The macrophage-derived cytokines tumor necrosis factor (TNF)-α and IL-1 can lead to the expression of angiogenic factors from adjacent tumor cells. The use of antibodies to either TNF-α or IL-1 blocks the expression of VEGF and IL-8, thereby inhibiting angiogenesis and tumor growth *(56)*.

Naturally occurring negative regulators of angiogenesis also exist. Members of this class of molecules include the interferons *(38,57,58)*, angiostatin *(36)*, endostatin *(37)*, interferon-gamma-inducible protein 10 (IP)-10 *(59)*, IL-12 *(60)*, and thrombospondin *(61)*. Addition of these agents was shown to block tumor progression in animal models. Several subsequent studies have shown that the combination of one of these naturally occurring antiangiogenic molecules with other antiangiogenic moieties leads to additive or synergistic effects *(62–64)*. The interferons are pleiotropic cytokines that have been shown to block angiogenesis as well as having effects on the immune system. An important element in translating these observations to the clinic is developing an understanding of the importance of dose and schedule for their use. Low-dose continuous exposure to interferon has been more effective than high-dose treatment in murine models *(65)*. This observation may be secondary to induction of signal transduction inhibitory proteins at higher doses in mice *(66–68)*. However, how this relates to human doses remains unclear.

Angiostatin and endostatin were discovered by a systematic search for naturally occurring antiangiogenic molecules. It was reasoned that metastatic growth of tumors is a product of the balance of positive and negative regulators. Pathologic examination of tissue often reveals the presence of micrometastatic lesions. The clinical observation that removal of a primary tumor can lead to the rapid growth at metastatic sites led to the hypothesis that the tumor itself was making a factor or factors capable of inhibiting angiogenesis and, thus, growth at the distant site. Biochemical purification led to the discovery of angiostatin and endostatin *(36,37)*. Cloning and expression of these molecules has facilitated their testing in preclinical and clinical trials. An important series of experiments showed that endostatin is able to cause tumor regression in animal models, including the B16F10 melanoma cell line. Following treatment with endostatin, the tumor shrank to minimal size. When treatment was discontinued, the tumor regrew. Retreatment was again capable of causing the tumor to regress. Remarkably, after several rounds of tumor growth and regression, the tumors failed to grow back and stayed in remission for the duration of the animal's life. The authors showed that this was due to a local effect on the tumor, by demonstrating that implantation of tumor cells elsewhere on the animal led to robust tumor growth and that a small dormant tumor could be seen at the original site *(69)*.

The therapeutic potential of blocking a single molecular pathway is controversial. For example, both bFGF and VEGF are capable of inducing an angiogenic response when given exogenously *(70,71)*. Furthermore, overexpression of any of a number of oncogenes is sufficient to induce tumor growth *(72)*. Thus, blocking of a single pathway may block growth of a given tumor, but not be generally applicable. There is not a master switch that is uniformly involved in all cancers. Another potential problem is that modulation of one pathway by a specific inhibitor may lead to compensatory activation of another. Studies that have looked at multiple factors and their involvement in progression of tumors in animal models suggest that blockade at multiple points may be required *(3,5)*. An alternative hypothesis has recently been proposed, specifically, that angiogenesis is a tightly coordinated process relying on an intricate balance of different factors. Consequently, interruption at any one of a number of different points may be sufficient to disrupt the balance and block angiogenesis *(73)*. Support for this comes from a series of experiments using human-derived melanoma cell lines. Monoclonal antibodies to VEGF, IL-8, platelet-derived endothelial cell growth factor (PD-ECGF), and bFGF were used to probe the contributions of different angiogenic molecules to the growth of tumors introduced into mice. Different cell lines were shown to have distinct expression patterns for these molecules. In cell lines expressing multiple factors, monoclonal antibody treatment directed against a single factor blocked angiogenesis and was not compensated for by the other pro-angiogenic factors *(74)*.

Several lines of evidence suggest that at least part of the activity of standard chemotherapeutic agents is through their effect on endothelial cells. The cycling time of tumor endothelium is approximately 5 d. This is similar to the turnover rate of tumor cells, gastrointestinal (GI), and bone marrow. By contrast, the turnover time for mature vessels is about 1500 d. The therapeutic index of chemotherapeutic drugs is defined by the ability to impact cancer cells without excess toxicity to normal cellular compartments. Tumor endothelium, because of its rapid proliferation, is also a viable candidate to be impacted by chemotherapy *(75)*. Low doses of chemotherapy, given on a more frequent schedule, is being tried as a means of targeting tumor endothelium *(44)*. Recent studies have shown that combining low-dose frequent administration of cyclophosphamide in combination with the antiangiogenic agent TNP-470 leads to a synergistic effect on antiangiogenic and antitumor activity. The combination appears to lead to an increase in apoptosis of endothelial cells *(76)*. Low-dose vinblastine was added to therapy with a monoclonal antibody targeting VEGFR-2. Both therapies were shown to be antiangiogenic, although response to single agents was transient. The combination led to a lasting regression of established tumors *(77)*. Low-dose doxorubicin was not observed to be antiangiogenic in several breast cancer models, but did produce a significant difference when added to a VEGF monoclonal antibody *(78)*. Perhaps in similar fashion, the combination of standard chemotherapy has been shown to augment the antitumor effects of antiangiogenic agents *(79,80)*.

4. CLINICAL CORRELATES IN MELANOMA

Several studies have looked at the clinical correlation of angiogenesis and melanoma growth. The notion of an angiogenic switch in the course of melanoma development is supported by the observation that transition from horizontal to vertical growth phase is accompanied by an increase in angiogenesis *(10)*. The increased vascular density was further correlated with an increase in the production of VEGF protein *(15)*. Positive staining for VEGF was seen in 90% of malignant melanomas, but in only 32% of primary cutaneous melanomas *(13)*. However, in this study, they did not see a correlation between VEGF expression and thickness of the primary melanoma lesion, overall survival, or size of metastases. Studies in larger patient cohorts have seen prognostic correlates of angiogenesis and outcome. In a study of 102 patients with vertical growth phase melanomas, increased microvessel density was correlated with tumor diameter, ulceration, and decreased patient survival *(12)*. Another study examining the role of VEGF in 70 patients with metastatic disease found survival to be significantly shorter in patients with high blood vessel counts in their tumors. They also found that the degree of VEGF expression was significantly correlated with blood vessel density *(14)*. A study looking at the number of microvessels in primary melanomas in a matched set of patients with or without metastases showed a significantly higher level of microvessels in the metastatic set. Furthermore, patients with distant metastases had higher microvessel counts than patients who only had lymph node metastases *(11)*. A study looking at the level of angiogenic factors in the serum of melanoma patients found that increased levels of VEGF, bFGF, and IL-8 were strongly correlated with time to disease progression and overall survival *(7)*.

5. CLINICAL TRIALS OF ANTIANGIOGENIC MOLECULES

The promise of antiangiogenic molecules for the treatment of cancer remains great, but clinical validation is still needed. The mechanism of action of antiangiogenic agents suggests that they should be cytostatic rather than cytotoxic. Specifically, if a compound was capable of halting the growth of new blood vessels, an existing tumor should be able to continue to be nourished by the existing blood supply, but be incapable of continued growth or metastasis. This notion has led to a different paradigm for drug development *(81)*. Classically, phase II trials have used tumor shrinkage (response rate) as a clinical surrogate for activity. This was based on the assumption that patient survival, the common phase III endpoint, would likely be increased in patients whose tumors responded to therapy. Since antiangiogenic agents were assumed not to lead to tumor shrinkage, other indicators of activity needed to be used to advance a clinical candidate to pivotal trials. Recent evidence showing tumor responses to agents targeting VEGF (see below), as well as the preclinical experience with endostatin *(69)*, are challenging the notion that antiangiogenic agents will only have cytostatic properties. It should be noted that the effects of VEGF inhibition may lead to regression of recently formed vessels through an apoptotic mechanism *(82–84)*. This could lead to tumor regression by cutting off some of the existing blood supply for tumors.

Further clouding the issue of response to antiangiogenic agents is the choice of patients for phase I/II studies. Since this phase of development is primarily concerned with safety of a new agent, patients tend to be those who have later stage disease for whom other therapeutic options are limited. However, the ideal patient for an antiangiogenic agent may, in fact, be a patient with minimal disease. This makes the likelihood of seeing a clinical effect in early studies more remote. The development of a good surrogate marker of activity may aid in the decision to proceed. However, these have not been uniformly available or validated. Decisions to move forward have thus been based on solid preclinical evidence and perhaps anecdotal responses in early trials. Rather than study response rate in phase II, a more appropriate endpoint for activity could be time to progression (TTP). For many late-stage cancers, the median TTP does not differ greatly from the median survival. To reach a meaningful conclusion for TTP, the size and length of the trial approaches what would be required of a traditional phase III study. Faced with this dilemma, several biotechnology and pharmaceutical companies have chosen to embark on pivotal trials with early stopping rules.

5.1. MMP Inhibitors

Marimastat is an orally available MMP inhibitor with nanomolar inhibitory concentration of 50% (IC_{50}) inhibition of MMP-1, -2, 3, -7, -9, and -12. Multiple phase III trials were undertaken beginning in 1996. During phase II, changes in the rate of increase of serum tumor markers were used as a surrogate of activity *(85)*. Adverse events attributable to drug included myalgias and arthralgias consistent with inhibition of MMPs. The primary endpoint for each of the phase III trials is median survival of the patients. It has been proposed that one of the shortcomings of these trials may be the use of late-stage patients who may not be able to benefit from inhibition of MMPs. Other ongoing trials include patients at an earlier stage of progression, including trials in small cell lung cancer (SCLC) and ovarian cancer. Results from a recent trial in gastric cancer fell just shy of achieving significance *(86)*. In this trial, patients were given marimastat or placebo and followed until 85% of the patients in one arm had died. At that time, 86% of the patients assigned to placebo had died, and 77% of the patients taking marimastat had died ($p = 0.084$). The secondary endpoint of progression-free survival did achieve significance. However, with continued follow-up, a significant difference in survival was eventually seen *(86)*. Controlled trials in melanoma have not been performed using marimastat.

The compound BAY12-9566 is an inhibitor of MMP-2 and -9. Pivotal studies were designed for non-small cell lung cancer (NSCLC), SCLC, and pancreatic cancer. Results from the pancreatic cancer trial were disappointing as patients taking BAY12-9566 at a dose of 800 mg 2×/d (BID) did significantly worse than patients taking gemcitabine. Median overall survival was 3.2 mo for patients taking BAY12-9566 and 6.4 mo for gemcitabine ($p = 0.0001$) *(87)*. In September, 1999, Bayer stopped all clinical trials of the compound following the recommendation of a Data Safety Monitoring Board for the SCLC trial. They reported that patients on the drug were performing worse than those on placebo.

Prinomastat (formerly AG3340) is an inhibitor of MMP-2, -9, -13, and -14. Prinomastat entered into phase II/III trials for NSCLC and hormone refractory prostate cancer in 1998. A Data Safety Monitoring Board halted the trials in August, 2000 due to lack of efficacy. Phase II studies exploring other indications and endpoints are continuing.

BMS-275291 entered a phase II/III trial in first-line NSCLC in combination with carboplatin and paclitaxel in September, 2000. The trial is being run in Canada, France, and Germany. Data from prior trials have not been released.

Neovastat is a synthetic version of a compound discovered in shark cartilage. It has inhibitory effects on MMP-2, -9, and -12. NCI-sponsored trials of this orally active compound in renal and NSCLC patients are underway.

5.2. VEGF Inhibitors

A humanized monoclonal antibody to VEGF is under development by Genentech. Preliminary results from phase II studies in breast, colorectal, and NSCLS have been reported *(88–90)*. In breast cancer, patients with refractory disease were treated with the antibody as a monotherapy. In addition to disease stabilization, several partial responses and one complete response were seen *(88)*. The lung and colon cancer studies were done in combination with standard chemotherapy. For lung cancer, a statistically significant increase in TTP was seen for the high-dose group relative to the control arm. There was also a trend to improved response and survival *(90)*. The colorectal trial showed a significant improvement in TTP and response rate for the low-dose group, with a trend toward improved survival. Paradoxically, the high-dose group did not show the same level of improvement *(89)*. However, these therapies were associated with an increased chance of bleeding. In the lung cancer study, 6 of the 86 patients treated with the anti-VEGF antibody experienced sudden and life threatening hemoptysis. Four of them died. In all trials, episodes of epistaxis were reported in up to 50% of patients. The company has announced plans to take this molecule into phase III studies in colorectal cancer, breast cancer, and NSCLC.

A humanized monoclonal antibody targeting VEGFR-2 has recently begun phase I clinical testing. This molecule was shown to have a synergistic effect in preclinical models when given with an altered schedule of low-dose frequent chemotherapy *(77)*.

SU5416 is a small molecule inhibitor of VEGFR-2 signaling. Preliminary phase II results of an uncontrolled trial in combination with 5-FU and leucovorin for chemotherapy naïve metastatic colorectal cancer patients have been reported. Of 28 patients treated, there was 1 complete response, 10 partial responses, 3 mixed responses, and 10 patients with stable disease. Median survival was more than 50% longer than expected for the population enrolled *(91)*. A phase III trial in this setting is underway.

ANGIOZYME is a ribozyme targeting the VEGFR-1 mRNA. Phase II testing will include a trial in melanoma. Ribozymes bind to a target sequence through base pairing. By manipulation of the length of the binding arms, ribozymes can be designed to recognize a unique sequence in the human mRNA population. After binding to a target sequence, ribozymes effect a catalytic cleavage of the target RNA backbone. This disruption of the mRNA sequence results in a non-functional message and down-modulation of the corresponding protein. Base pairing of a ribozyme to the cleaved product is thermodynamically less stable than to the original target sequence. This results in dissociation of the cleavage products from the ribozyme, allowing binding to another intact target RNA and repeat of the cycle *(92)*. In contrast, antisense molecules can only work in stoiciometric fashion. Lack of toxicity, due to the exquisite specificity of ANGIOZYME predicted from its structure and preclinical activity, has been borne out in early clinical trials *(93,94)*.

5.3. Other Molecules in Development

The teratogenic effects of thalidomide seen with its use in the 1950s are now thought to be a result of inhibition of angiogenesis in the developing limb buds of the fetus. Thalidomide was recently approved for the treatment of moderate to severe cutaneous manifestations of *mycobacterium leprae* infections and is again commercially available, although under very strict regulations. Its use in treating cancer patients has increased dramatically in the last few years. The NCI maintains a registry of patients taking thalidomide and is sponsoring controlled clinical trials to determine whether thalidomide is effective in treating cancer. A Swedish study showed that thalidomide is effective against multiple myeloma *(95)*. Preliminary results in solid tumors have not been as encouraging. A study in late stage melanoma patients failed to show any benefit *(41,96)*. Studies using other patients, different dosing regimens, and in combination with chemotherapeutic agents are all underway.

Interferon at low doses has been shown to inhibit angiogenesis *(65)*. This may be through the regulation of bFGF, particularly in skin *(57)*. Establishment of appropriate dose and schedule for treatment may be a balance between indirect effects through two independent mechanisms. Controlled clinical trials sponsored by the NCI are being run to determine if and how interferons should be used in cancer therapy.

6. FUTURE PROSPECTS

A better understanding of the molecular events involved in tumor growth has led to the current targeted approaches to cancer therapy. Further refinements to our knowledge base can be anticipated as a result of new technologies and information spawned from efforts to sequence the human genome. Already, microarray technology has been used to characterize the expression pattern of various tumor types. Using an array of 8150 cDNAs, 31 melanoma samples were tested for their pattern of expression. A distinct cluster of 19 of the samples could be identified using several different analyses *(97)*. In this study, no clinical correlates were seen between expression patterns and patient status or outcome. By characterizing the pattern of genes expressed, it may be possible to define which patients may benefit from a specific therapy, including antiangiogenic approaches, and which may not. Furthermore, it may be possible to follow response to treatment of an individual patient. An examination of the circulating levels of angiogenic factors following treatment with chemotherapeutic agents (dacarbazine, cisplatin, temozolomide, vincristine) or interferon-α revealed different patterns of change. Treatment with chemotherapy led to an increase in angiogenin, bFGF, and IL-8. Treatment with interferon led to an increase of only IL-8. The circulating levels of VEGF were not impacted by either treatment modality *(7)*. Using gene array profiles, it may be possible to define with greater precision response to therapy, aiding both the drug development process and management of individual patients.

The general applicability of antiangiogenic agents, coupled with an anticipated lower incidence of side effects, has generated tremendous enthusiasm for their use in the treatment of cancer. As yet, no agent has been shown to possess clinical efficacy in controlled clinical trials. Results expected in the next few years are eagerly anticipated by clinicians and patients alike.

REFERENCES

1. Folkman J. Tumor angiogenesis: therapeutic implications. *N Engl J Med* 1971; 285: 1182–1186.
2. al-Alousi S, Barnhill R, Blessing K, Barksdale S. The prognostic significance of basic fibroblast growth factor in cutaneous malignant melanoma. *J Cutan Pathol* 1996; 23: 506–510.
3. Danielsen T, Rofstad EK. VEGF, bFGF and EGF in the angiogenesis of human melanoma xenografts. *Int J Cancer* 1998; 76: 836–841.
4. Siemeister G, Schirner M, Weindel K, et al. Two independent mechanisms essential for tumor angiogenesis: inhibition of human melanoma xenograft growth by interfering with either the vascular endothelial growth factor receptor pathway or the Tie-2 pathway. *Cancer Res* 1999; 59: 3185–3191.
5. Westphal JR, Van't Hullenaar R, Peek R, et al. Angiogenic balance in human melanoma: expression of VEGF, bFGF, IL-8, PDGF and angiostatin in relation to vascular density of xenografts in vivo. *Int J Cancer* 2000; 86: 768–776.
6. Pötgens AJG, Lubsen NH, van Altena MC, Schoenmakers JGG, Ruiter DJ, de Waal RM. Vascular permeability factor expression influences tumor angiogenesis in human melanoma lines xenografted to nude mice. *Am J Pathol* 1995; 146: 197–209.
7. Ugurel S, Rappl G, Tilgen W, Reinhold U. Increased serum concentration of angiogenic factors in malignant melanoma patients correlates with tumor progression and survival. *J Clin Oncol* 2001; 19: 577–583.
8. Denijn M, Ruiter DJ. The possible role of angiogenesis in the metastatic potential of human melanoma. Clinicopathological aspects. *Melanoma Res* 1993; 3: 5–14.
9. Graham CH, Rivers J, Kerbel RS, Stankiewicz KS, White WL. Extent of vascularization as a prognostic indicator in thin (< 0.76 mm) malignant melanomas. *Am J Pathol* 1994; 145: 510–514.
10. Marcoval J, Moreno A, Graells J, et al. Angiogenesis and malignant melanoma. Angiogenesis is related to the development of vertical (tumorigenic) growth phase. *J Cutan Pathol* 1997; 24: 212–218.
11. Neitzel LT, Neitzel CD, Magee KL, Malafa MP. Angiogenesis correlates with metastasis in melanoma. *Ann Surg Oncol* 1999; 6: 70–74.
12. Straume O, Salvesen HB, Akslen LA. Angiogenesis is prognostically important in vertical growth phase melanomas. *Int J Oncol* 1999; 15: 595–599.
13. Salven P, Heikkilä P, Joensuu H. Enhanced expression of vascular endothelial growth factor in metastatic melanoma. *Br J Cancer* 1997; 76: 930–934.
14. Vlaykova T, Laurila P, Muhonen T, et al. Prognostic value of tumour vascularity in metastatic melanoma and association of blood vessel density with vascular endothelial growth factor expression. *Melanoma Res* 1999; 9: 59–68.
15. Erhard H, Rietveld FJ, van Altena MC, Bröcker EB, Ruiter DJ, de Waal RM. Transition of horizontal to vertical growth phase melanoma is accompanied by induction of vascular endothelial growth factor expression and angiogenesis. *Melanoma Res* 1997; 7(Suppl 2): S19–S26.
16. Weidner N, Semple JP, Welch WR, Folkman J. Tumor angiogenesis and metastasis—correlation in invasive breast carcinoma. *N Engl J Med* 1991; 324: 1–8.
17. Macchiarini P, Fontanini G, Hardin MJ, Squartini F, Angeletti CA. Relation of neovascularisation to metastasis of non-small-cell lung cancer. *Lancet* 1992; 340: 145–146.
18. Takahashi Y, Kitadai Y, Bucana CD, Cleary KR, Ellis LM. Expression of vascular endothelial growth factor and its receptor, KDR, correlates with vascularity, metastasis, and proliferation of human colon cancer. *Cancer Res* 1995; 55: 3964–3968.
19. Weidner N, Carroll PR, Flax J, Blumenfeld W, Folkman J. Tumor angiogenesis correlates with metastasis in invasive prostate carcinoma. *Am J Pathol* 1993; 143: 401–409.

20. Yoshino S, Kato M, Okada K. Prognostic significance of microvessel count in low stage renal cell carcinoma. *Int J Urol* 1995; 2: 156–160.
21. Salven P, Ruotsalainen T, Mattson K, Joensuu H. High pre-treatment serum level of vascular endothelial growth factor (VEGF) is associated with poor outcome in small-cell lung cancer. *Int J Cancer* 1998; 79: 144–146.
22. Hollingsworth HC, Kohn EC, Steinberg SM, Rothenberg ML, Merino MJ. Tumor angiogenesis in advanced stage ovarian carcinoma. *Am J Pathol* 1995; 147: 33–41.
23. Ikeda N, Adachi M, Taki T, et al. Prognostic significance of angiogenesis in human pancreatic cancer. *Br J Cancer* 1999; 79: 1553–1563.
24. Bellamy WT, Richter L, Frutiger Y, Grogan TM. Expression of vascular endothelial growth factor and its receptors in hematopoietic malignancies. *Cancer Res* 1999; 59: 728–733.
25. Torry RJ, Rongish BJ. Angiogenesis in the uterus: potential regulation and relation to tumor angiogenesis. *Am J Reprod Immunol* 1992; 27: 171–179.
26. Ruiter DJ, Schlingemann RO, Westphal JR, Denijn M, Rietveld FJ, De Waal RM. Angiogenesis in wound healing and tumor metastasis. *Behring Inst Mitt* 1993: 258–272.
27. Brown PD, Giavazzi R. Matrix metalloproteinase inhibition: a review of anti-tumour activity. *Ann Oncol* 1995; 6: 967–974.
28. Wojtowicz-Praga S. Clinical potential of matrix metalloprotease inhibitors. *Drugs R D* 1999; 1: 117–129.
29. Kanno S, Oda N, Abe M, et al. Roles of two VEGF receptors, Flt-1 and KDR, in the signal transduction of VEGF effects in human vascular endothelial cells. *Oncogene* 2000; 19: 2138–2146.
30. Neufeld G, Tessler S, Gitay-Goren H, Cohen T, Levi BZ. Vascular endothelial growth factor and its receptors. *Prog Growth Factor Res* 1994; 5: 89–97.
31. Gordon MS, Margolin K, Talpaz M, et al. Phase I safety and pharmacokinetic study of recombinant human anti-vascular endothelial growth factor in patients with advanced cancer. *J Clin Oncol* 2001; 19: 843–850.
32. Margolin K, Gordon MS, Holmgren E, et al. Phase Ib trial of intravenous recombinant humanized monoclonal antibody to vascular endothelial growth factor in combination with chemotherapy in patients with advanced cancer: pharmacologic and long-term safety data. *J Clin Oncol* 2001; 19: 851–856.
33. Prewett M, Huber J, Li Y, et al. Antivascular endothelial growth factor receptor (fetal liver kinase 1) monoclonal antibody inhibits tumor angiogenesis and growth of several mouse and human tumors. *Cancer Res* 1999; 59: 5209–5218.
34. Pavco PA, Bouhana KS, Gallegos AM, et al. Antitumor and antimetastatic activity of ribozymes targeting the messenger RNA of vascular endothelial growth factor receptors. *Clin Cancer Res* 2000; 6: 2094–2103.
35. Fong TA, Shawver LK, Sun L, et al. SU5416 is a potent and selective inhibitor of the vascular endothelial growth factor receptor (Flk-1/KDR) that inhibits tyrosine kinase catalysis, tumor vascularization, and growth of multiple tumor types. *Cancer Res* 1999; 59: 99–106.
36. O'Reilly MS, Holmgren L, Shing Y, et al. Angiostatin: a novel angiogenesis inhibitor that mediates the suppression of metastases by a Lewis lung carcinoma. *Cell* 1994; 79: 315–328.
37. O'Reilly MS, Boehm T, Shing Y, et al. Endostatin: an endogenous inhibitor of angiogenesis and tumor growth. *Cell* 1997; 88: 277–285.
38. Sidky YA, Borden EC. Inhibition of angiogenesis by interferons: effects on tumor- and lymphocyte-induced vascular responses. *Cancer Res* 1987; 47: 5155–5161.
39. Christian MC, Pluda JM, Ho PT, Arbuck SG, Murgo AJ, Sausville EA. Promising new agents under development by the Division of Cancer Treatment, Diagnosis, and Centers of the National Cancer Institute. *Semin Oncol* 1997; 24: 219–240.

40. Dark GG, Hill SA, Prise VE, Tozer GM, Pettit GR, Chaplin DJ. Combretastatin A-4, an agent that displays potent and selective toxicity toward tumor vasculature. *Cancer Res* 1997; 57: 1829–1834.
41. Eisen T, Boshoff C, Mak I, et al. Continuous low dose thalidomide: a phase II study in advanced melanoma, renal cell, ovarian and breast cancer. *Br J Cancer* 2000; 82: 812–817.
42. Huang S, Xie K, Bucana CD, Ullrich SE, Bar-Eli M. Interleukin 10 suppresses tumor growth and metastasis of human melanoma cells: potential inhibition of angiogenesis. *Clin Cancer Res* 1996; 2: 1969–1979.
43. Seymour L. Novel anti-cancer agents in development: exciting prospects and new challenges. *Cancer Treat Rev* 1999; 25: 301–312.
44. Kerbel RS, Viloria-Petit A, Klement G, Rak J. "Accidental" anti-angiogenic drugs. Anti-oncogene directed signal transduction inhibitors and conventional chemotherapeutic agents as examples. *Eur J Cancer* 2000; 36: 1248–1257.
45. Oku T, Tjuvajev JG, Miyagawa T, et al. Tumor growth modulation by sense and antisense vascular endothelial growth factor gene expression: effects on angiogenesis, vascular permeability, blood volume, blood flow, fluorodeoxyglucose uptake, and proliferation of human melanoma intracerebral xenografts. *Cancer Res* 1998; 58: 4185–4192.
46. Claffey KP, Brown LF, del Aguila LF, et al. Expression of vascular permeability factor/vascular endothelial growth factor by melanoma cells increases tumor growth, angiogenesis, and experimental metastasis. *Cancer Res* 1996; 56: 172–181.
47. Lazar-Molnar E, Hegyesi H, Toth S, Falus A. Autocrine and paracrine regulation by cytokines and growth factors in melanoma. *Cytokine* 2000; 12: 547–554.
48. Rak J, Filmus J, Kerbel RS. Reciprocal paracrine interactions between tumour cells and endothelial cells: the "angiogenesis progression" hypothesis. *Eur J Cancer* 1996; 32A: 2438–2450.
49. Halaban R. Growth factors and tyrosine protein kinases in normal and malignant melanocytes. *Cancer Metastasis Rev* 1991; 10: 129–140.
50. Gitay-Goren H, Halaban R, Neufeld G. Human melanoma cells but not normal melanocytes express vascular endothelial growth factor receptors. *Biochem Biophys Res Commun* 1993; 190: 702–708.
51. Norgauer J, Metzner B, Schraufstatter I. Expression and growth-promoting function of the IL-8 receptor beta in human melanoma cells. *J Immunol* 1996; 156: 1132–1137.
52. Yuan F, Chen Y, Dellian M, Safabakhsh N, Ferrara N, Jain RK. Time-dependent vascular regression and permeability changes in established human tumor xenografts induced by an anti-vascular endothelial growth factor/vascular permeability factor antibody. *Proc Natl Acad Sci USA* 1996; 93: 14765–14770.
53. Sharma B, Handler M, Eichstetter I, Whitelock JM, Nugent MA, Iozzo RV. Antisense targeting of perlecan blocks tumor growth and angiogenesis in vivo. *J Clin Invest* 1998; 102: 1599–1608.
54. Bar-Eli M. Role of interleukin-8 in tumor growth and metastasis of human melanoma. *Pathobiology* 1999; 67: 12–18.
55. Wang Y, Becker D. Antisense targeting of basic fibroblast growth factor and fibroblast growth factor receptor-1 in human melanomas blocks intratumoral angiogenesis and tumor growth. *Nat Med* 1997; 3: 887–893.
56. Torisu H, Ono M, Kiryu H, et al. Macrophage infiltration correlates with tumor stage and angiogenesis in human malignant melanoma: possible involvement of TNFalpha and IL-1alpha. *Int J Cancer* 2000; 85: 182–188.
57. Dinney CP, Bielenberg DR, Perrotte P, et al. Inhibition of basic fibroblast growth factor expression, angiogenesis, and growth of human bladder carcinoma in mice by systemic interferon-alpha administration. *Cancer Res* 1998; 58: 808–814.

58. Dong Z, Greene G, Pettaway C, et al. Suppression of angiogenesis, tumorigenicity, and metastasis by human prostate cancer cells engineered to produce interferon-beta. *Cancer Res* 1999; 59: 872–879.
59. Arenberg DA, Kunkel SL, Polverini PJ, et al. Interferon-gamma-inducible protein 10 (IP-10) is an angiostatic factor that inhibits human non-small cell lung cancer (NSCLC) tumorigenesis and spontaneous metastases. *J Exp Med* 1996; 184: 981–992.
60. Voest EE, Kenyon BM, O'Reilly MS, Truitt G, D'Amato RJ, Folkman J. Inhibition of angiogenesis in vivo by interleukin 12. *J Natl Cancer Inst* 1995; 87: 581–586.
61. Good DJ, Polverini PJ, Rastinejad F, et al. A tumor suppressor-dependent inhibitor of angiogenesis is immunologically and functionally indistinguishable from a fragment of thrombospondin. *Proc Natl Acad Sci USA* 1990; 87: 6624–6628.
62. Lindner DJ, Borden EC. Effects of tamoxifen and interferon-beta or the combination on tumor-induced angiogenesis. *Int J Cancer* 1997; 71: 456–461.
63. Lingen MW, Polverini PJ, Bouck NP. Retinoic acid and interferon alpha act synergistically as antiangiogenic and antitumor agents against human head and neck squamous cell carcinoma. *Cancer Res* 1998; 58: 5551–5558.
64. Minischetti M, Vacca A, Ribatti D, et al. TNP-470 and recombinant human interferon-alpha2a inhibit angiogenesis synergistically. *Br J Haematol* 2000; 109: 829–837.
65. Slaton JW, Perrotte P, Inoue K, Dinney CP, Fidler IJ. Interferon-alpha-mediated down-regulation of angiogenesis-related genes and therapy of bladder cancer are dependent on optimization of biological dose and schedule. *Clin Cancer Res* 1999; 5: 2726–2734.
66. Naka T, Narazaki M, Hirata M, et al. Structure and function of a new STAT-induced STAT inhibitor. *Nature* 1997; 387: 924–929.
67. Endo TA, Masuhara M, Yokouchi M, et al. A new protein containing an SH2 domain that inhibits JAK kinases. *Nature* 1997; 387: 921–924.
68. Chung CD, Liao J, Liu B, et al. Specific inhibition of Stat3 signal transduction by PIAS3. *Science* 1997; 278: 1803–1805.
69. Boehm T, Folkman J, Browder T, O'Reilly MS. Antiangiogenic therapy of experimental cancer does not induce acquired drug resistance. *Nature* 1997; 390: 404–407.
70. Wilting J, Weich HA, Christ B. Effects of vascular endothelial growth factor and basic fibroblast growth factor: application with corneal grafts on the chorioallantoic membrane. *Acta Anat (Basel)* 1993; 147: 207–215.
71. Kenyon BM, Voest EE, Chen CC, Flynn E, Folkman J, D'Amato RJ. A model of angiogenesis in the mouse cornea. *Invest Ophthalmol Vis Sci* 1996; 37: 1625–1632.
72. Black RJ, Friedman RM. Cytokines and oncogene activity. *Cancer Surv* 1989; 8: 725–739.
73. Yancopoulos GD, Davis S, Gale NW, Rudge JS, Wiegand SJ, Ho J. Vascular-specific growth factors and blood vessel formation. *Nature* 2000; 407: 242–248.
74. Rofstad EK, Halsor EF. Vascular endothelial growth factor, interleukin 8, platelet-derived endothelial cell growth factor, and basic fibroblast growth factor promote angiogenesis and metastasis in human melanoma xenografts. *Cancer Res* 2000; 60: 4932–4938.
75. Folkman J, Hahnfeldt P, Hlatky L. The logic of anti-angiogenic therapy. In: Friedmann T, ed. *The Development of Human Gene Therapy*, Vol. 36. CSH Laboratory Press, Cold Spring Harbor, NY, 1999, p. 540.
76. Browder T, Butterfield CE, Kraling BM, et al. Antiangiogenic scheduling of chemotherapy improves efficacy against experimental drug-resistant cancer. *Cancer Res* 2000; 60: 1878–1886.
77. Klement G, Baruchel S, Rak J, et al. Continuous low-dose therapy with vinblastine and VEGF receptor-2 antibody induces sustained tumor regression without overt toxicity. *J Clin Invest* 2000; 105: R15–R24.
78. Borgstrom P, Gold DP, Hillan KJ, Ferrara N. Importance of VEGF for breast cancer angiogenesis in vivo: implications from intravital microscopy of combination treatments with an

anti-VEGF neutralizing monoclonal antibody and doxorubicin. *Anticancer Res* 1999; 19: 4203–4214.

79. Teicher BA, Holden SA, Ara G, Korbut T, Menon K. Comparison of several antiangiogenic regimens alone and with cytotoxic therapies in the Lewis lung carcinoma. *Cancer Chemother Pharmacol* 1996; 38: 169–177.
80. Herbst RS, Takeuchi H, Teicher BA. Paclitaxel/carboplatin administration along with antiangiogenic therapy in non-small-cell lung and breast carcinoma models. *Cancer Chemother Pharmacol* 1998; 41: 497–504.
81. Pluda JM. Tumor-associated angiogenesis: mechanisms, clinical implications, and therapeutic strategies. *Semin Oncol* 1997; 24: 203–218.
82. Gupta K, Kshirsagar S, Li W, et al. VEGF prevents apoptosis of human microvascular endothelial cells via opposing effects on MAPK/ERK and SAPK/JNK signaling. *Exp Cell Res* 1999; 247: 495–504.
83. Meeson AP, Argilla M, Ko K, Witte L, Lang RA. VEGF deprivation-induced apoptosis is a component of programmed capillary regression. *Development* 1999; 126: 1407–1415.
84. Watanabe Y, Dvorak HF. Vascular permeability factor/vascular endothelial growth factor inhibits anchorage-disruption-induced apoptosis in microvessel endothelial cells by inducing scaffold formation. *Exp Cell Res* 1997; 233: 340–349.
85. Nemunaitis J, Poole C, Primrose J, et al. Combined analysis of studies of the effects of the matrix metalloproteinase inhibitor marimastat on serum tumor markers in advanced cancer: selection of a biologically active and tolerable dose for longer-term studies. *Clin Cancer Res* 1998; 4: 1101–1109.
86. Fielding J, Scholefield J, Stuart R, et al. A randomized double-blind placebo-controlled study of marimastat in patients with inoperable gastric adenocarcinoma. *Proc Am Soc Clin Oncol* 2000; 19: 240a.
87. Moore MJ, Hamm J, Eisenberg P, et al. A comparison between gemcitabine (GEM) and the matrix metalloproteinase (MMP) inhibitor BAY 12-9566 in patients (Pts) with advanced pancreatic cancer. *Proc Am Soc Clin Oncol* 2000; 19: 240a.
88. Sledge G, Miller K, Novotny W, Gaudreault J, Ash M, Colbleigh M. A phase II trial of single-agent rhuMAb VEGF (recombinant humanized monoclonal antibody to vascular endothelial cell growth factor) in patients with relapsed metastatic breast cancer. *Proc Am Soc Clin Oncol* 2000; 19: 3a.
89. Bergsland E, Hurwitz H, Fehrenbacher L, et al. A randomized Phase II trial comparing rhuMAb VEGF (recombinant humanized monoclonal antibody to vascular endothelial cell growth factor) plus 5-fluorouracil/leucovorin (FU/LV) alone in patients with metastatic colorectal cancer. *Proc Am Soc Clin Oncol* 2000; 19: 242a.
90. DeVore RF, Fehrenbacher L, Herbst RS, et al. A randomized phase II trial comparing Rhumab VEGF (recombinant humanized monoclonal antibody to vascular endothelial growth factor) plus carboplatin/paclitaxel (CP) to CP alone in patients with stage IIIB/IV NSCLC. *Proc Am Soc Clin Oncol* 2000; 19: 485a.
91. Rosen PJ, Amado R, Hecht JR, et al. A phase I/II study of SU5416 in combination with 5-FU/leucovorin in patients with metastatic colorectal cancer. *Proc Am Soc Clin Oncol* 2000; 19: 3a.
92. Usman N, Stinchcomb DT. Design, synthesis, and function of therapeutic hammerhead ribozymes. In: Eckstein R, Lilley DMJ, eds. *Nucleic Acids and Molecular Biology*, Vol. 10. Springer-Verlag, Berlin, 1996, pp. 243–264.
93. Parker VP, Sandberg JA, Smith J, et al. Phase I and pharmacokinetic studies of Angiozyme, a synthetic ribozyme targeting the VEGF receptor Flt-1. *Proc Am Soc Clin Oncol* 2000; 19: 181a.
94. Weng DE, Weiss P, Kellacky C, et al. A phase I/II study of repetitive dose Angiozyme, a ribozyme targeting the Flt-1 receptor for VEGF. *EORTC* 2000.

95. Singhal S, Mehta J, Desikan R, et al. Antitumor activity of thalidomide in refractory multiple myeloma. *N Engl J Med* 1999; 341: 1565–1571.
96. Gutman M, Szold A, Ravid A, Lazauskas T, Merimsky O, Klausner JM. Failure of thalidomide to inhibit tumor growth and angiogenesis in vivo. *Anticancer Res* 1996; 16: 3673–3677.
97. Bittner M, Meltzer P, Chen Y, et al. Molecular classification of cutaneous malignant melanoma by gene expression profiling. *Nature* 2000; 406: 536–540.

Index

From: *Current Clinical Oncology, Melanoma: Biologically Targeted Therapeutics*
Edited by: E. C. Borden © Humana Press Inc., Totowa, NJ

D

E

F

G

H

I

R

S